Intrauterine Growth Restriction

Springer
London
Berlin
Heidelberg
New York
Barcelona
Hong Kong
Milan
Paris
Singapore
Tokyo

John Kingdom and Philip Baker (Eds)

Intrauterine Growth Restriction

Aetiology and Management

Foreword by Martin Whittle

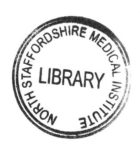

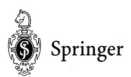

Springer

John Kingdom, MD, FRCS(C), MRCP (UK), MRCOG
Maternal-Fetal Medicine, Mount Sinai Hospital, Suite 775B, University of
Toronto, 600 University Avenue, Toronto, Ontario M5G 1X5, Canada

Philip Baker, BM BS, MRCOG
School of Human Development, City Hospital, Nottingham University,
Hucknall Road, Nottingham. NG5 1PB. UK

ISBN 1-85233-191-7 Springer-Verlag London Berlin Heidelberg

British Library Cataloguing in Publication Data
Intrauterine growth restriction: aetiology and management
  1. Fetal growth retardation – Etiology   2. Fetal growth
  retardation – Treatment
  I. Kingdom, John   II. Baker, Philip
  618.3′62
  ISBN 1852331917

Library of Congress Cataloging-in-Publication Data
Intrauterine growth restriction: aetiology and management/John Kingdom and
  Philip Baker, eds.
      p.   cm.
    Includes bibliographical references and index.
    ISBN 1-85233-191-7
    1. Fetal growth retardation.   2. Fetus–Growth.   3. Pregnancy – Complications.
  I. Kingdom, John, 1959–   .   II. Baker, Philip, 1962–   .
    [DNLM: 1. Fetal Growth Retardation – etiology.   2. Fetal Growth
  Retardation – therapy.   WQ 211 1616 1999]
  RG629.G76154 1999
  618.3′2–dc21
  DNLM/DLC
  for Library of Congress   99–37272

Typeset by EXPO Holdings, Kuala Lumpur, Malaysia
Printed and bound at The Cromwell Press, Trowbridge, Wiltshire, England
28/3830-543210 Printed on acid-free paper SPIN 10636675

Foreword

Intrauterine growth retardation remains a significant clinical problem in modern obstetrics. This book draws together the aetiology of the condition, the underlying mechanisms which may be responsible and the clinical management. In fact the book offers an outstanding insight into the difficulties and challenges which exist in the subject both clinically and scientifically.

The story about intrauterine growth has been a long one and although this book provides a cohesive view of where we are just now, it also makes it obvious that we have some way to go before the final chapter is reached. The configuration of the book reflects the fact that both of the editors are not only obstetricians but also effective clinical scientists. What is particularly exciting is the fact that they have used authors who in general are themselves both young and conversant with the science of molecular and cellular biology.

This exciting mix has produced a book which is relevant for today's practice whilst at the same time offering an useful and intriguing scientific resource. All who have contributed, and especially the authors, are to be congratulated.

Martin Whittle

Preface

This book was conceived at the 4th Tox talks meeting in Mill Valley, California, in June 1996, a multidisciplinary group that focusses on pre-eclampsia. As mild obesity began to set in, we challenged each other to a weight reduction contest for the following SGI meeting in March 1997, and set about creating a book that dealt with the complexities of reduced fetal growth. We were delighted with the enthusiasm shown by the leading investigators that we approached to help with this task. Our aim was to create a text that blends modern clinical practice in maternal-fetal medicine alongside clinical epidemiology and cutting edge basic research.

We would like to thank the efficient and encouraging staff of Springer who have guided us through the project, especially Christopher Greenwell, Nick Mowat and Roger Dobbing.

John Kingdom
Philip Baker

Dedication

To our wives and children who would rather have had us at home.

Contents

Contributors

Dr Ganesh Acharya
Department of Obstetrics and Gynaecology
University College London Medical School
86-96 Chenies Mews
London WC1E 6HX, UK

Professor Asif S. Ahmed
Molecular Reproductive Vascular Biology Unit
Department of Obstetrics & Gynaecology
Birmingham Women's Hospital
Edgbaston, Birmingham B15 2TG, UK

Dr Janet Ashworth
Department of Obstetrics and Gynaecology
Chesterfield and North Derbyshire Royal Hospital
Calow, Chesterfield
Derbyshire S44 5BL, UK

Dr Paul Ayuk
Departments of Child Health and Obs and Gyn
University of Manchester
St Mary's Hospital
Hathersage Road
Manchester M13 9PT, UK

Professor Philip Baker
Professor of Obstetrics & Gynaecology
Academic Department of Obstetrics & Gynaecology
Nottingham City Hospital
Hucknall Road
Nottingham, NG5 1PB, UK

Dr Eve Blair
Western Australian Research Institute for Child Health
Princess Margaret Hospital for Children
P.O. Box D184
Perth, Western Australia 6001, Australia

Dr Jeremy Chipchase
Department of Obstetrics and Gynaecology
University College London Medical School
86-96 Chenies Mews
London WC1E 6HX, UK

Dr James C. Cross
Program in Development and Fetal Health
Samuel Lunenfeld Research Institute
Mount Sinai Hospital
600 University Avenue
Toronto, Ontario M5G 1X5, Canada

Professor Gustaaf Dekker
Department of Obstetrics and Gynaecology
Lyell McEwin Health Service
University of Adelaide
North Terrace
Adelaide 5005, Australia

Dr Caroline Dunk
Postdoctoral Fellow
Program in Development and Fetal Health
Samuel Lunenfeld Research Institute
Mount Sinai Hospital
600 University Avenue
Toronto, Ontario MSG 1X5, Canada

Professor Harold Fox
Department of Pathological Sciences
Stopford Building
University of Manchester
Oxford Road
Manchester M13 9PT, UK

Dr Keith M. Godfrey
MRC Clinical Scientist and Honorary Consultant
MRC Environmental Epidemiology Unit
University of Southampton
Southampton General Hospital
Tremona Road
Southampton SO16 6YD, UK

Professor Mark Hanson
Fetal and Neonatal Physiology Unit
Department of Obstetrics & Gynaecology
University College London Medical School
86-96 Chenies Mews
London WC1E 6HX, UK

Dr Sheena Hodgett
Specialist Registrar
West Midlands Region
Department of Obstetrics and Gynaecology
Royal Shrewsbury Hospital
Mytton Oak Road
Shrewsbury, Shropshire SY3 8XQ, UK

Dr Janet Hornbuckle
Research Fellow in Obstetrics and Gynaecology
Centre for Reproduction Growth and Development
University of Leeds
34 Hyde Terrace
Leeds LS2 9LN, UK

Dr David C. Howe
Specialist Registrar, Lothian Region
Department of Obstretrics and Gynaecology
Royal Infirmary of Edinburgh
Lauriston Place
Edinburgh EH3 9YW, UK

Dr John Hughes
Departments of Child Health and Obs and Gyn
University of Manchester
St Mary's Hospital
Hathersage Road
Manchester M13 9PT, UK

Dr Duncan W. Irons
Consultant Obstetrician and Gynaecologist
Dryburn Hospital
North Road
Durham DH1 5TW, UK

Dr Eric Jauniaux
Reader/Consultant in Fetal Medicine
Department of Obstetrics and Gynaecology
University College London Medical School
86-96 Chenies Mews
London WC1E 6HX, UK

Dr Frank Johnstone
Consultant/Senior Lecturer in Obstetrics & Gynaecology
Reproductive Medicine Service, Ward 35
Royal Infirmary of Edinburgh
Lauriston Place
Edinburgh EH3 9YW, UK

Professor Peter Kaufmann
Department of Anatomy
Klinikum der RWTH
Wendligweg 2
D 52057 Aachen, Germany

Dr Mark Kilby
Reader/Consultant in Maternal/Fetal Medicine
Academic Department of Obstetrics & Gynaecology
University of Birmingham
Birmingham Women's Hospital
Edgbaston, Birmingham B15 2TG, UK

Dr John Kingdom
Associate Professor of Obstretrics and Gynaecology and Pathology
Staff Obstetrician, Maternal Fetal Medicine Division
University of Toronto
Mount Sinai Hospital
600 University Avenue
Toronto, Ontario M5G 1X5, Canada

Professor Torvid Kiserud
Department of Obstetrics and Gynaecology
Bergen University Hospital
N-5021 Bergen, Norway

Dr Gaby Kohnen
Specialist Registrar in Pathology
Department of Pathology
Algernon Firth Building
Leeds General Infirmary
Great George Street
Leeds LS1 3EX, UK

Dr Fiona Lyall
Senior Lecturer
Maternal and Fetal Medicine Section
University of Glasgow
Institute of Medical Genetics
Yorkhill, Glasgow G3 8SJ, UK

Professor Neil Marlow
Professor of Neonatal Medicine
Division of Child Health
Level E, East Block
Queens Medical Centre
Nottingham, NG7 2UH, UK

Dr Karel Maršál
Department of Obstetrics and Gynaecology
University Hospital
SE-221 85 Lund, Sweden

Dr Gurmit S. Pahal
Research Fellow
Department of Obstetrics and Gynaecology
University College London Medical School
86-96 Chenies Mews
London WC1E 6HX, UK

Dr Donald M. Peebles
Senior Lecturer/Consultant
Department of Obstetrics and Gynaecology
University College London Medical School
86-96 Chenies Mews
London WC1E 6HX, UK

Dr Rebecca Reynolds
Wellcome Clinical Research Fellow
MRC Environmental Epidemiology Unit
University of Southampton
Southampton General Hospital
Tremona Road
Southampton SO16 6YD, UK

Professor Steve Robson
Department of Fetal Medicine
Royal Victoria Infirmary
Leazas Wing
Richardson Road
Newcastle upon Tyne NE1 4LP, UK

Professor Colin Sibley
Academic Unit of Child Health
St Mary's Hospital
Hathersage Road
Manchester M13 0JH, UK

Professor Graeme N. Smith
Assistant Professor
Department of Obstetrics and Gynaecology,
    Pharmacology and Toxicology
Queen's University
Kingston General Hospital
76 Stuart Street
Kingston, Ontario, Canada K7L 2V7

Dr Clare Steyn
Postdoctoral Fellow
Department of Obstetrics & Gynaecology
University College London Medical School
86-96 Chenies Mews
London WC1E 6HX, UK

Dr Jim G. Thornton
Reader in Obstetrics and Gynaecology
Centre for Reproduction Growth and Development
University of Leeds
34 Hyde Terrace
Leeds LS2 9LN, UK

Professor James J. Walker
School of Medicine
Worsley Medical and Dental Building
Clarendon Way
Leeds LS2 9NL, UK

Professor Mark Walker
Fellow in Maternal-Fetal Medicine
Department of Obstetrics and Gynaecology
University of Toronto
600 University Avenue
Toronto, Ontario M5G 1X5, Canada

Professor Martin Whittle
Academic Department of Obstetrics and Gynaecology
The University of Birmingham
Birmingham Women's Hospital
Edgbaston, Birmingham B15 2TG, UK

Dr Rory Windrim
Assistant Professor of Obstetrics and Gynaecology
University of Toronto
Staff Obstetrician
Maternal-Fetal Medicine Division
Mount Sinai Hospital
600 University Avenue
Toronto, Ontario M5G 1X5, Canada

Dr John Wolstenholme
Cytogenics Laboratory
Department of Human Genetics
19–20 Clarmont Place
University of Newcastle
Newcastle upon Tyne NE2 4AA, UK

Dr Chris Wright
Department of Pathology
Royal Victoria Infirmary
Queen Victoria Road
Newcastle upon Tyne NE1 4LP, UK

1 Definitions of Intrauterine Growth Restriction

John Kingdom, Philip Baker and Eve Blair

Introduction

Intrauterine growth restriction (IUGR) is a concept signifying that the fetus has not achieved its optimal growth. There are several ways in which fetal growth may be inhibited, and these are discussed in the following chapters. Despite the diversity of causes of IUGR, they all have in common the fact that the IUGR baby would have been bigger were it not for suboptimal genetic and/or environmental factors.

By contrast, the concept of small for gestational age (SGA) is purely statistical. Provided the distribution of birthweight for gestational age is available for an appropriate population and that the gestational age of the pregnancy is accurately known, the position of the infant's birthweight on the distribution of the appropriate population (for example, as a percentile position) can be determined.

IUGR and SGA are thus not synonymous. At least 50 per cent of newborn infants weighing < 10th percentile for sex and gestation will have been normally nourished in utero, and many infants weighing more than the 10th percentile will have failed to reach their optimal growth potential [1].

However, these terms are frequently used in an interchangeable manner because it is not always easy to assess whether or not restriction has occurred, particularly if only retrospective data are available, as is the case in many epidemiological studies.

Approaches to the Recognition and Measurement of IUGR

Birthweight for Gestational Age

Routine pregnancy dating by ultrasound in the developed world has been established for only at most 20 years [2]. Epidemiological studies before this time were subject to pregnancy dating errors, although the concept of impaired fetal growth was becoming recognised [3]. Neonatal dating, using the Dubowitz scoring system, provided a clinically based tool for avoiding dating errors [4], and gestation-specific birthweight percentile charts were developed from pregnancies of women with accurately recalled menstrual dates [5]. Unfortunately the latter data were obtained at high altitude, which in itself is known to limit fetal growth through hypobaric hypoxia. Most investigators now use local percentile growth curves.

A number of non-pathological factors are known to influence birthweight. These include infant gender, the number of previous births, maternal height and weight and ethnicity, where a genetic rather than environment effect on growth can be demonstrated [6,7]. The validity of adjusting the categorisation of SGA for these determinants, in addition to gestational age, is demonstrated by the better discrimination between healthy and sick newborns using adjusted rather than unadjusted SGA categorisation [8,9].

Percentile charts of birthweight for gestational age have an additional flaw. At lower gestational ages at delivery, the birth is more likely to have a pathological cause and this pathological cause may also restrict growth. Therefore a greater proportion of all preterm newborns are likely to be IUGR. If the same proportion of preterm as term infants are categorised SGA (i.e. the same birthweight for gestation percentile is used to define SGA) a greater proportion of preterm IUGR will go unrecognised [10]. The extent to which unavoidable misclassification of infants at birth impinges on the validity of a study depends on the study design. Since SGA (as estimated by customised growth charts, for example) is a statistical concept it gives valid results when applied to population-based epidemiological studies; however, it is less robust at predicting outcomes at the individual level or in small case series selected on the basis of birthweight percentile. (Smith and Kingdom develop the latter point in Ch. 13.)

A different approach to using the dichotomous SGA categorisation is to regard IUGR as a continuous measure and assess degree of smallness. The accuracy of percentiles at the extremes of birthweight distribution is crucial. The percentiles are very sensitive to sample size, data errors and general health of the reference population (e.g. the Denver percentiles at high altitude). The common practice of excluding outliers runs the risk of excluding the extremely IUGR fetus or newborn, as does the exclusion of stillborn individuals. The positions of percentile extremes are therefore sensitive to data quality.

Neonatal Morphology

IUGR does not affect fetal organ size equally. Growth of the fetal abdomen, especially the liver, is disproportionately affected, resulting in an increased head circumference (HC) to abdominal circumference (AC) ratio. This difference has been used to infer IUGR where there is a high percentile position of the ratio of head/abdominal circumference. Since the fetal liver represents a substantial proportion of fetal weight, IUGR has also been inferred from a low ponderal index (PI) (weight/length) of the newborn, because weight is also disproportionately affected in comparison with fetal length. Whilst the concept of PI may be appropriate in the neonatal period for the detection of IUGR secondary to placental insufficiency, no ultrasound parameters to date, such as HC/AC ratio, correlate closely enough with this neonatal measure [11,12]. Length is a critical component, but cannot be measured accurately in the fetus now that static-mode ultrasound equipment has become obsolete [13]. The accurate measurement of fetal organ volumes using techniques such as echo–planar magnetic resonance imaging (MRI) [14] has the potential to contribute to intrauterine fetal assessment.

Serial Ultrasound Estimates of Fetal Weight

Early studies of fetal growth employed measurements of the fetal head since this part was most easily visualised by early equipment. Whilst restricted head growth during postnatal life is an important measure of neurological development [15], restricted head growth in utero is unusual. Of all fetal parameters measured ultrasonically, fetal weight correlates most closely with the fetal abdominal size [16]. AC has been considered the most appropriate single ultrasound parameter for the evaluation of fetal growth velocity but fetal abdominal area may be even more appropriate. In a recent study that used receiver operator characteristic curves to determine the most discriminatory cut-off points for fetal abdominal area velocities, values $\geq$ two standard deviations (s) below the mean predicted a skinfold thickness < 10th percentile at birth with a likelihood ratio of 10.4 (95 per cent confidence interval (CI) 3.9–26), values $\geq 1.55\ s$ below the mean predicted a ponderal index < 25th percentile at birth with a likelihood ratio of 9.5 (95 per cent CI 4.6–19) [17].

A Dynamic Diagnosis of IUGR by Ultrasound

Much of the above discussion on the diagnosis of IUGR during fetal life is viewed with scepticism by obstetricians who perform ultrasound evaluations on a daily basis. With serial ultrasound measurements, expert ultrasonographers can distinguish the SGA from the IUGR fetus with ease, using good equipment, since they obtain information on size and health in a stepwise manner. The typical sequence is:

1. Derive an estimate of fetal weight and plot against gestational age.
2. Check HC/AC ratio, amniotic fluid and placental maturation (Grannum grade).
3. For fetuses < 34 weeks, check umbilical artery Doppler waveforms to search for impaired fetal–placental perfusion.
4. Where the fetus is > 36 weeks, check both uterine artery and middle cerebral artery Doppler and complete examination with a biophysical profile.

Kingdom and Smith expand on this multiparameter approach in Ch. 13. At a one-to-one clinical level, particularly in a referral setting, this is an effective way of distinguishing the healthy SGA fetus from its IUGR counterpart [18]. However, it is expensive in terms of equipment and staff resources. A recently completed comprehensive ultrasound evaluation of a cohort of 1,600 unselected singleton pregnancies by one of the authors (JK) proved an enormous effort, with little association between findings and subsequent perinatal mortality or morbidity [19]. These data fit with evidence from an earlier randomised control trial, albeit using static B-mode scanners lacking Doppler facilities [13]. Thus it is not surprising that the majority of epidemiological research workers in the field of IUGR do not have the luxury of access to comprehensive prenatal ultrasound information. However, where carefully applied to identify homogeneous subgroups of IUGR pregnancies, ultrasound facilitates new insights into the underlying mechanisms of IUGR [20]. This practice is becoming more widespread [21] and it is hoped the journal peer review process will increasingly demand such standards [22].

References

1. Wilcox A. Intrauterine growth retardation: beyond birthweight criteria. Early Hum Dev 1983;8:189–93.
2. Gardosi J, Geirsson RT. Routine ultrasound is the method of choice for dating pregnancy. Br J Obstet Gynaecol 1998;105:933–6.
3. Drillien C. The small-for-date infant:etiology and prognosis. Pediatr Clin North Am 1970;17:9–24.
4. Dubowitz L. Assessment of gestational age in newborn: a practical scoring system. Arch Dis Child 1969;44:782.
5. Lubchenco LO, Hansman C, Dressler M, Boyd E. Intrauterine growth as estimated from liveborn birthweight data at 24 to 42 weeks of gestation. Pediatrics 1963;32:793–800.
6. Gardosi J, Chang A, Kalyan B, Sahota D, Symonds EM. Customised antenatal growth charts. Lancet 1992;339:283–7.
7. Blair E. Why do Aboriginal newborns weight less? Determinants of birthweight for gestation. J Pediatr Child Health: 1996;32:498–503.
8. Mongelli M, Gardosi J. Reduction of false positive diagnosis of fetal growth restriction by application of customised fetal growth standards. Obstet Gynecol 1996;88:844–8.
9. Sciscione AC, Gorman R, Callan NA. Adjustment of birthweight standards for maternal and infant characteristics improves the prediction of outcome in the small-for-gestational-age infant. Am J Obstet Gynecol 1996;175:544–7.
10. Hediger ML, Scholl TO, Schall JI, Miller LW, Fischer RL. Fetal growth and the etiology of preterm delivery. Obstet Gynecol 1995;85:175–82.
11. Colley NV, Tremble JM, Henson GL, Cole TJ. Head circumference/abdominal circumference ratio, ponderal index and fetal malnutrition. Br J Obstet Gynaecol 1991;98:524–7.
12. Cole TJ, Henson GL, Tremble JM, Colley NV. Birthweight for length: ponderal index, body mass index or Benn index? Ann Hum Biol 1997;24:289–98.
13. Neilson JP, Munjanja SP, Whitfield CR. Screening for small for dates fetuses: a controlled trial. BMJ 1984;289:1179–82.
14. Baker PN, Johnson IR, Gowland PA, Hykin J, Adams V, Mansfield P, et al. Measurement of fetal liver, brain and placental volumes with echo-planar magnetic resonance imaging. Br J Obstet Gynaecol 1995;102:35–9.
15. Strauss RS, Dietz WH. Growth and development of term children born with low birth weight: effects of genetic and environmental factors. J Pediatr 1998;133:67–72.
16. Smith GC, Smith MF, McNay MB, Fleming JE. The relation between fetal abdominal circumference and birthweight: findings in 3512 pregnancies. Br J Obstet Gynaecol 1997;104:186–90.
17. Owen P, Khan KS. Fetal growth velocity in the prediction of intrauterine growth retardation in a low risk population. Br J Obstet Gynaecol 1998;105:536–40.
18. Fong et al. 1999; submitted to Radiology.
19. Geary M, Kingdom J, Persaud M, Wilshin J, Hindmarsh P, Rodeck C. Incidence of uterine notching in the third trimester and association with obstetric outcome. J Obstet Gynaecol 1998;18 (Suppl 1):S58.
20. Krebs C, Macara LM, Leiser R, Bowman AW, Greer IA, Kingdom JC. Intrauterine growth restriction with absent end-diastolic flow velocity in the umbilical artery is associated with maldevelopment of the placental terminal villous tree. Am J Obstet Gynecol 1996;175:1534–42.
21. Somerset DA, Li XF, Afford S, Strain AJ, Ahmed A, Sangha RK, et al. Ontogeny of hepatocyte growth factor (HGF) and its receptor (c-met) in human placenta: reduced HGF expression in intrauterine growth restriction. Am J Pathol 1998;153:1139–47.
22. Kingdom J. Adraina and Luisa Castellucci Award Lecture 1997. Placental pathology in obstetrics: adaptation or failure of the villous tree. Placenta 1998;19:347–51.

Section 1
Aetiology and Pathogenesis

2 Genes, Chromosomes and IUGR

John Wolstenholme and Chris Wright

Introduction

The growth potential of the fetus is determined by genetic factors, but fulfilment of this potential is dependent on maternal and environmental factors, as discussed in Ch. 4 [1,2]. Winick [3] proposed the model that envisaged early fetal growth (including the embryonic phase and organogenesis) as predominantly a consequence of cell proliferation (hyperplasia), the latter part of pregnancy (from about 32 weeks) as a period of cell growth (hypertrophy), and an intermediate phase with significant contributions from both hyperplasia and hypertrophy. Agents that damage the fetus during the first trimester phase of cell proliferation may reduce the cell population and permanently impede growth potential, while those acting in late pregnancy reduce cell size, with the likelihood of later catch-up growth [4].

Such a model does not of course take account of the fact that growth and development of different organs vary throughout pregnancy, but despite its apparent simplicity it is broadly consistent with clinical and pathological experience, as demonstrated, for example, by the work of Naeye [5]. Genetic abnormalities, like infection and other agents that directly injure the fetus during the first trimester, can reduce cell number and growth potential, with a roughly uniform reduction in the size of all organs (symmetrical growth restriction) [5,6]. Maternal and/or placental factors causing a reduction in nutrient supply (which typically exert their greatest effect in later pregnancy, since the absolute fetal growth is greatest during the last 6–7 weeks of pregnancy) may result in growth impairment associated with a reduction in cell cytoplasm [7,8]; as a result of redistribution of cardiac output brain growth is relatively spared (asymmetrical or malnutrition type growth restriction). In practice, of course, it is difficult in any particular case to exclude the possibility that both mechanisms are active, since agents such as genetic factors and infection can influence fetal growth both directly and through effects on the placenta.

For the purposes of this review, genetic alterations associated with growth restriction are divided into:

1. Chromosome abnormalities
2. Confined placental mosaicism and uniparental disomy
3. Syndromes.

Chromosome Abnormalities

Chromosome abnormalities make a significant contribution to fetal growth restriction detected antenatally. In a report from cytogenetic laboratories serving one area of France, an abnormal karyotype was detected in 12 (6.7 per cent) of 180 SGA infants who otherwise appeared morphologically normal, and 18 (32 per cent) of 57 where there was associated fetal malformation [9]; analyses were undertaken at a mean gestational age of 30 weeks. Snijders et al. [10], in a study of cases referred to a fetal medicine unit at a mean gestation of 29 weeks, made similar observations. In that study there were abnormal karyotypes in 4 (2 per cent) of 243 small but otherwise normally formed fetuses, and 85 (40 per cent) of 215 that were both small and showed ultrasound evidence of malformation. In another report from a referral centre, Heydanus et al. [11] found 20 abnormal karyotypes (7 per cent) out of a total of 307 SGA fetuses (non-malformed and malformed) examined at a mean gestation of 28 weeks. In these three reports the commonest abnormalities detected were triploidy and trisomies 13, 18 and 21.

Trisomies and Structural Abnormalities

Direct measurement of fetuses aborted between 7 and 20 weeks gestation has demonstrated reduced crown–rump length (CRL) in association with aneuploidy, triploidy and structural abnormalities [12]. Recent first trimester ultrasound studies have reported reduction in CRL in trisomies 18 and 13, but not 21[13–15]. Schemmer et al. [14] noted that growth rate appeared to be a better discriminator between aneuploid and euploid fetuses than CRL. In the second trimester, growth restriction remains a more consistent finding in trisomy 18 and 13 than in trisomy 21 [16]. It has been suggested that shortening detected by ultrasound is only apparent and actually reflects late release of ova related to aneuploidy (leading to incorrect dating) rather than reduced growth, but this would not account for normal first trimester CRL with trisomy 21.

In keeping with the first and second trimester findings, birthweights at term for trisomies 18, 13 and 21 are about 65 per cent, 75 per cent and 85 per cent, respectively, of controls [1,17]. There is some evidence that weights of trisomy 21 fetuses are similar to those of controls until about 30 weeks' gestation [1,18]. Birthweights for translocation trisomy 21 do not differ from those of primary trisomy 21 [19].

Growth restriction is a very frequent observation in association with other trisomies and with structural chromosomal defects resulting in either excess or loss of chromosomal material, including many of the more frequent anomalies such as 4p–, 5p–, trisomy 9, 13q–, 18p– and 18q– [1,20,21].

Individuals with mosaic karyotypes comprising one normal and one abnormal cell line tend to have phenotypes (including birthweights) intermediate between those with normal and those with fully abnormal karyotypes, in keeping with an ameliorating effect of the normal cells. The common trisomies (chromosomes 13, 18 and 21) are seen in their mosaic form alongside a normal cell line in around 15 per cent, 10 per cent and 3 per cent of cases reaching term respectively. Other fetal trisomies are sufficiently lethal that the only time that they are seen in later gestation pregnancies is in their mosaic form; most are also extremely rare.

It cannot always be assumed, however, that the phenotypic abnormalities in mosaic fetuses are solely attributable to the cell line with major abnormalities of chromosome number or structure, since in some cases there may be uniparental disomy in the apparently normal diploid cell line as a consequence of trisomic zygote rescue. Moreover, while growth restriction might reasonably result from intrinsic chromosomal anomalies in the fetus, it should be remembered that the placenta will also in general be karyotypically and possibly functionally abnormal, and that this may contribute to the impairment of growth (see under confined placental mosaicism and uniparental disomy for a more detailed discussion of both these effects).

Triploidy

The complete extra set of chromosomes in triploidy is a consequence of either double fertilisation of the ovum (diandry) or failure of the ovum to extrude the polar body (digyny) [22,23]. Antenatally, fetal growth restriction in triploidy can been detected in the first and second trimesters [10,11,14,24].

Two distinct fetal and placental phenotypes are recognisable in association with a triploid karyotype (Fig. 2.1). In type I, fetal growth is not severely impaired but there is frequently microcephaly and the placenta shows changes of partial hydatidiform mole. Type 2 triploid fetuses are markedly but asymmetrically growth restricted with very thin trunk and limbs and relative head sparing; the placentas are small, and do not show molar change. These two phenotypes show correlation with the origin of the additional set of chromsomes: type 1 is of paternal origin (diandry) and type 2 maternal (digyny) [25]. These two phenotypes provide an example of the effects of genomic imprinting.

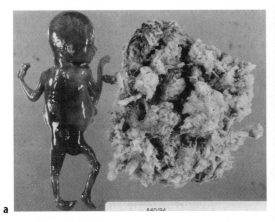
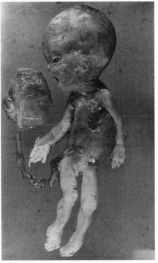

Fig. 2.1 The two phenotypes of human triploidy: **a** Type 1, paternal origin (diandry). Growth-impaired fetus with lumbar myelocoele and a bulky placenta showing changes of hydatidiform mole. **b** Type 2, maternal origin (digyny). Fetus showing very marked asymmetric growth restriction. The placenta is small with no molar change.

Monosomy X (Turner syndrome)

Fetal growth impairment associated with monosomy X has not been detected in first trimester ultrasound studies (although these did include relatively small numbers of cases) [14,15] but is observable during the second trimester [26]. About half of the cases of Turner phenotype have a 45,X karyotype, with the remainder showing a range of abnormalities including 46,X,i(Xq) and various mosaics [27]. The phenotype (including the degree of growth restriction) is consequently variable, with 45,X/46,XX mosaics having a higher birthweight and 45,X/46,X,i(Xq) mosaics a lower birthweight than 45,X individuals, whose weight is about 80–85% of that expected for gestational age [1]. Studies of cases with X chromosome deletions suggests that height is less affected by losses from the long arm than by those from the short arm [27].

Other Abnormalities of Sex Chromosome Number

Review of the small numbers of cases reported suggests that there is evidence for a linear fall in birthweight with increasing number of sex chromsomes, with each extra X chromosome resulting in an approximately 300 g reduction in birthweight [28,29]. The effect of Y chromosome number is unclear, although of lesser importance than the X chromosome [28].

Confined Placental Mosaicism and Uniparental Disomy

Mosaicism

In an important subset of chromosome abnormalities, two or more cell lines with different karyotypes are present, both being derived from the same zygote. Such mosaic karyotypes usually involve coexistence of one normal and one abnormal cell line, although more complex combinations are well described.

The direct growth-retarding effects of fetal mosaicism have been discussed above under trisomies. Prenatally, however, the interaction between mosaicism and IUGR should be considered not just in the context of the fetal karyotype, but in that of the whole fetoplacental unit. Any uneven distribution of abnormal cells adds the complication that growth restriction effects may be attributable to the level of abnormality in the fetus, the level of abnormality in the placenta, or a combination of the two. This would be somewhat an academic point in the clinical situation were it not for an extreme but a suprisingly common form of non-random distribution of abnormal cells – an apparently normal fetus with an abnormal or mosaic abnormal placenta – a combination that may have quite profound effects on growth, development and pregnancy outcome, depending on quite how and when it arises.

Confined Placental Mosaicism and Uniparental Disomy

Karyotypic abnormalities restricted to extraembryonic tissues, subsequently termed confined placental mosaicism (CPM), were known to early cytogeneticists, but were infrequently studied. Their potential effects on fetal development were not appreciated until the report of two such cases among a series of 31 IUGR pregnancies [30]. Although these authors' observations have been confirmed by those of others [31], much of our current understanding of the effects of CPM on fetal growth arises not from direct analysis of term IUGR but from first trimester chorion villus sampling (CVS), which was being developed as an alternative to amniocentesis at the time. Data from CVS demonstrated that discordance between the extraembryonic karyotype and that of the fetus was remarkably common, being present in as many as 2 per cent of pregnancies tested [32–34]. Initially, the main consequence of this phenomenon was considered to be the hazard to accurate prenatal diagnosis using extraembryonic tissues. Fortunately, with greater experience, it soon became apparent which findings could safely be regarded as being unlikely to be representative of the fetal karyotype [32]. This minimised the number of pregnancies requiring additional prenatal testing and made CVS a reliable alternative to amniocentesis. As more cases accumulated, however, it was apparent that larger groups of CPM pregnancies had up to 5–10% more adverse outcomes than would be anticipated by chance [35,36]. Unfortunately in this latter context, the prognostic value of individual first trimester findings was exceptionally poor. We now know that this is because what is seen as CPM is an extremely heterogeneous entity:

- CPM involves a wide range of cytogenetic abnormalities, both numerical (missing or extra chromosomes) and structural (rearranged chromosomes).
- The proportion of abnormal cells varies enormously.
- Abnormal cells may be distributed thoughout the extraembryonic tissues in different ways.
- Apparently identical anomalies may be derived from different types of genetic error with different genetic consequences.

CVS can be usefully thought of as an indirect way of looking at genetic events taking place very early in, and prior to, embryological development.

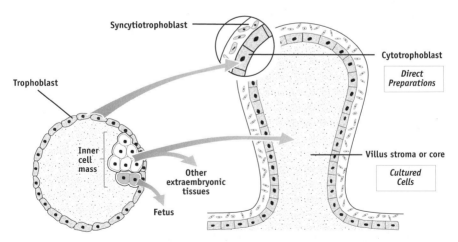

Fig. 2.2 Simplified diagram (not to scale) showing how the first differentiation stage in the pre-implantation embryo produces (i) the trophoblast, which is destined to form the CTB and the syncytiotrophoblast, and (ii) the ICM, which is destined to form other extraembryonic tissues including the villus stroma or core and the fetus itself. The relationship to laboratory methods for analysis of diagnostic CVS is also shown.

Two techniques are commonly used by cytogeneticists to process villus samples (Fig. 2.2):

- direct preparations from the initial biopsy that look at spontaneously dividing cells in the cytotrophoblast (CTB) layer; these cells are derived from the trophoblast cells present in the early blastocyst
- culture of cells from the villus stroma; these cells are derived from the extraembryonic mesoderm (EEM), a lineage derived from the inner cell mass (ICM).

In the majority of cases of CPM, abnormal cells are restricted to only one of these two cell lineages. In around 15 per cent, however, they are present in both. Fig. 2.3, based on the model first developed by Crane and Cheung [37], shows how these observed patterns can be explained by errors producing mosaicism prior to blastocyst formation.

Early models assumed that all CPM was a consequence of errors arising in normal conceptions. Subsequent molecular genetic analysis of trisomic CPMs, the most common and best-studied group of abnormalities involved, shows that this is not the whole picture. Analysis of patterns of inheritance of parental DNA

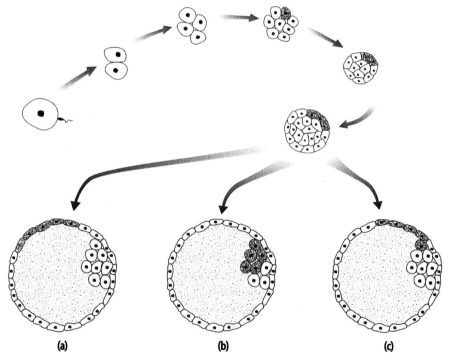

(a)   (b)   (c)

Fig. 2.3 An error in a normal conception, in this case producing one abnormal cell at the eight-cell stage. Blastocysts representing three of the possible resulting abnormal cell distributions are shown: **a** Mosaic abnormality of the trophoblast. **b** Mosaic abnormality of the ICM. **c** Mosaic abnormality of both cell lineages. (For clarity, not all cells are shown beyond the eight-cell stage. Errors occurring earlier in development will have higher proportions of abnormal cells, those occurring later will have lower proportions. Errors may also arise at cell divisions after blastocyst formation; these will, however, result in diminishingly relevant numbers of abnormal cells the later they occur.)

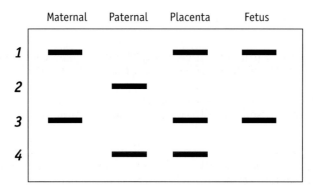

Fig. 2.4 Determination of origin of mosaic trisomy using polymorphic DNA markers. Variations in length of known highly polymorphic repeat sequences throughout the human genome can be used to follow inheritance of chromosomes. In this case, of trisomy 16, alleles 1 and 3 of a known polymorphism, at a locus closely linked to the centromere, identify the maternal chromosomes. Likewise, alleles 2 and 4 identify the paternal chromosomes. The trisomic placenta has one paternal and both maternal alleles indicating an error in maternal meiosis I. The normal cell line in the fetus has been produced by correction involving loss of the paternally derived chromosome.

polymorphisms in normal and abnormal cell lineages in these cases (Fig. 2.4) demonstrates that not one but two primary mechanisms of generation are occurring [38].

- The majority, termed mitotic or somatic errors, arise (as predicted in the early models) from normal conceptions, and appear to result from a non-disjunction event in a mitotic division postfertilisation.
- The remainder, however, arise from trisomic conceptions. These are termed meiotic errors. Here an initial error, which may arise in either meiotic division in either parent, undergoes a correcting mitotic event, loss of one of the offending chromosomes, to produce a normal cell line, a phenomenon known as reduction to disomy or trisomic zygote rescue.

Ignoring any selection mechanisms for or against abnormal cells that might be occurring in early fetal development (see later), two diverging patterns of abnormal cell distribution can then be anticipated, fitting closely with what is seen in late first trimester CVS [39]:

1. For normal conceptions, already shown in Fig. 2.3, at each cell division post-fertilisation the potential contribution of abnormal cells from associated mitotic non-disjunction errors to the developing fetoplacental unit will be progressively less and less as development proceeds. The majority of trisomic CPM is characterised by a corresponding low level of abnormal cells, often restricted to either the CTB or EEM-derived cells, although occasionally it is present in both. In general this type of CPM seems fairly benign and adverse pregnancies are rare. Relatively few low level CPM pregnancies have had their origin investigated, but what evidence there is confirms the primarily mitotic nature of this group.
2. In contrast, for meiotic errors producing abnormal conceptions (Fig. 2.5), any delay in the timing of the correcting event will result in higher and higher proportions of abnormal cells as development proceeds. Experience has shown that

CPM pregnancies with IUGR have much higher proportions of abnormal cells in the CTB or EEM-derived cells, frequently in both, with many cases having 100 per cent of the cells affected. Because of their clinical importance, far more of these cases have had their origins investigated, particularly those with adverse outcomes. Where investigated, adverse outcomes with high levels of trisomic cells in the extraembryonic tissues are usually of meiotic origin.

It should be made quite clear that these patterns of abnormal cell distribution relate to analysis of large series of CPM cases. It it not possible to perform the reverse analysis and extrapolate directly from the cell distribution in individual cases, often only studied at a single biopsy site, to the origin of that abnormality, in anything other than in terms of probability, without supporting molecular genetic studies.

Several mechanisms by which CPM can affect fetal development have been described; three are well established:

- The presence of trisomic cells in the extraembryonic cell lineages may result in reduced placental size, altered placental morphology or, by mechanisms as yet

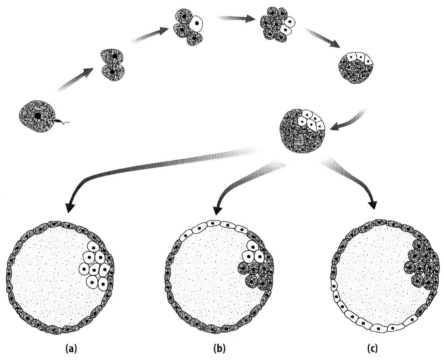

Fig. 2.5 Correction of a trisomic conception, in this case producing one normal cell at the four-cell stage. Blastocysts representing three of the possible abnormal cell distributions are shown: **a** Abnormality of the trophoblast only, in this case 100 per cent abnormality. **b** Mosaic abnormality in both the trophoblast and the the ICM. The fetus may develop from either normal or abnormal cells or a mixture of both. **c** Mosaic trophoblast with a totally abnormal ICM. The fetus will always be abnormal. (For clarity, not all cells are shown beyond the eight-cell stage. In contrast to the mitotic errors in normal conceptions shown in Fig. 2.3, correction of a zygote with an abnormal abnormal karyotype results in higher proportions of abnormal cells if it occurs at later divisions.)

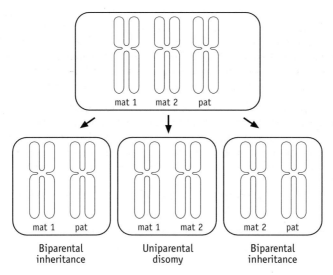

mat 1   mat 2   pat

mat 1 pat	mat 1 mat 2	mat 2 pat
Biparental inheritance	Uniparental disomy	Biparental inheritance

Fig. 2. 6 Correction of trisomy by chromosome loss, showing how uniparental disomy results in one in three cases.

undefined, reduced or aberrant placental function. For some trisomies this may be the main cause of associated IUGR. [In theory, both meiotic and somatic errors may produce such effects, but corrected meiotic errors, with predictably higher levels of abnormal cells, might be considered more prone.]

- Most cases of meiotic origin CPM result from correction of non-disjunction errors that occurred during oogenesis (Fig. 2.6). Reduction to the disomic state by loss of either one of the two maternally derived chromosomes or the paternally derived chromosome will produce a normal-looking karyotype in all cases. Loss of the paternal chromosome, however, produces an unusual genetic state whereby, instead of normal biparental inheritance, both remaining chromosome homologues are maternally derived, termed maternal uniparental disomy (UPDmat), or, if referring to a specific chromosome, upd(x)mat (e.g. upd(16)mat if referring to chromosome 16). The exact opposite combination of events can produce paternal UPD (UPDpat) by comparable correction of the rarer paternal meiotic errors. It is now known that several human chromosomes possess segments where genes are imprinted, with the paternally and maternally derived copies functioning in different manners. This makes it crucial for normal fetal development that one maternal and one paternal gene is present. The presence of UPD in CPM for trisomies of imprinted chromosomes is known to be associated with various problems including IUGR. As the function and development of either or both fetal and extraembryonic cell lineages may be influenced by imprinted genes, the effects of UPD could relate to its presence in the fetus or in the normal placental cells, or a combination of the two. [This applies to corrected meiotic errors only.]

- As a result of normal crossing over between pairs of homologous chromosomes during meiosis I, any cases of UPD produced by the above mechanism will additionally have segments where genetic material has been inherited not just from one parent but from the same original chromosome (Fig. 2.7).

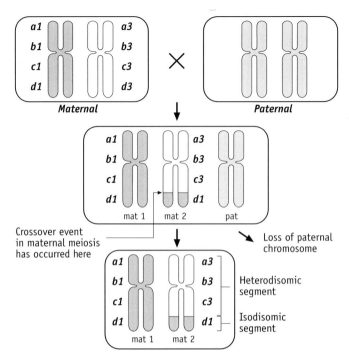

Fig. 2.7 Correction of trisomy by a maternal meiosis error, followed by loss of the paternal homo-logue, to produce a cell line with an apparently normal karyotype with maternal uniparental disomy. Polymorphic repeat sequences at four loci (**a–d**) on the original maternal chromosome pair are used to demonstrate the heterodisomic and isodisomic segments resulting from a crossover in maternal meiosis. For simplicity and to aid comparison with Fig. 2.4, at each locus the allele on the maternal chromosome on the left is shown as allele 1, with the corresponding allele at the locus on the maternal chromosome on the right being allele 3; paternal alleles 2 and 4 have been omitted for clarity.

In the trisomic cells both maternal alleles 1 and 3 are present for loci **a–c** (the centromeric locus **b** is in fact the example used previously in Fig. 2.4). Due to crossing over in maternal meiosis, however, analysis at loci **d** shows inheritance of two copies of allele 1. This means that, if the paternally derived chromosome is lost, any deleterious recessive genes on the isodisomic maternally derived segment, represented by loci **d**, will be expressed.

NB. In practice, analysis is usually rather more complicated. Each set of alleles is unlikely to be fully informative and several crossovers may have taken place.

Homologous segments where both copies from one parent are present are termed heterodisomic; homologous segments where only one original chromosome is represented are termed isodisomic. Isodisomy will unmask any recessive genes present. Several examples have been described. [This applies to corrected meiotic errors only.]

At least two other factors may also be contributing, although in practice these are rather difficult to prove or disprove in individual cases:

● What we see as CPM at the end of the first trimester and at later gestations may not reflect the distribution of abnormal cells during very early embryo-logical development. Trisomic cells present in the fetus proper during the very early first trimester may have been eliminated or outgrown by normal cells but their effects on development may remain [meiotic or somatic].

● Establishment of fetal karyotype abnormality is often restricted to a small number of easily analysed tissues (typically lymphocytes and skin fibroblasts). Although we may see cases as CPM, residual levels of trisomic cells may be present in other fetal tissues [meiotic or somatic].

It is important to appreciate that these mechanisms are not mutually exclusive; placental abnormality, UPD, isodisomy and undetected fetal trisomy may all coexist in the same pregnancy, making the analysis of their relative contributions to IUGR, if present, rather problematical.

Using trisomy CPM as a model one makes the assumption that this group of errors can regarded as a homogeneous entity. However, although some useful conclusions can be drawn, we now know that each trisomy itself needs to be considered separately as several other factors may be superimposed on the general patterns indicated above.

● Analysis of the more common trisomic CPMs shows that each has its own pattern of origin. Maternal meiotic non-disjunction of chromosome 16 is remarkably common; approximately 1.5 per cent of all human pregnancies are trisomy 16 at fertilisation. Correction of trisomy 16 conceptions is a major source of CPM in these pregnancies. In contrast, however, non-disjunction for chromosome 16 in the mitotic divisions postfertilisation in normal conceptions seems to be a comparatively rare event [40]. Exactly the opposite situation prevails for chromosome 7: comparative stability in meiotic division but a high rate of non-disjunction in the early postfertilisation mitotic divisions. Predicted patterns of origin can also be deduced for the other more common trisomic CPMs: 2, 3, 8, 9, 15 and 22 [39].

● Some trisomies (e.g. 4, 6, 17 and 19) are very rarely seen as CPM, which suggests relative stability in both meiotic and early postfertilisation mitotic divisions. However, direct information regarding the incidence of individual trisomies at fertilisation is sparse, particularly for mosaicism. With the exception of trisomy 16, it is not possible to establish a base level of abnormality at conception that can be followed through correction, subsequent fetal development and/or pregnancy wastage. Although when compared with trisomy 16, these rare trisomies are less common at fertilisation, just how much less is unclear. Such mosaic preimplantation embryos may also have poor viability in utero or trisomic cells may be outgrown by their normal counterparts, both of which would also reduce the apparent incidence at later gestations. For rare trisomies, how what we see at later gestations relates to what is present in early development is largely unknown.

● Intuitively, the detailed mechanisms whereby trisomic conceptions are corrected seem unlikely to be random events; they may form part of more general mechanisms that maintain karyotype stability throughout somatic tissues. There is no reason to believe that they function equally well for each trisomy.

● There may be specific mechanisms for directing abnormal cells to some or all of the extraembryonic tissues [39], or equally likely, normal cells to those that will eventually form the fetus itself. Normally-developing, spare in vitro fertilisation (IVF) preimplantation embryos often show a high incidence of cells with abnormal, often bizarre karyotypes that are unlikely to figure in normal

Table 2.1 Cytogenetic abnormalities restricted to the placenta that have been associated with IUGR. A full analysis of their relative contribution is not possible at present, but the number of symbols (•) provides a semiquantitative estimate

CPM abnormality	Incidence in IUGR cases
trisomy 16	••••••
trisomy 22	•••
trisomy 9	•••
trisomy 2	••
trisomy 7	•
trisomy 15	•
trisomy 18 or 21	•?
other trisomies	•
sex chromosome aneuploidies	•
double trisomies	••
structural abnormalities	•
tetraploidy	•

fetal development [41]. Again, there is no reason to presuppose that any such mechanisms will apply equally well to all trisomies.

Athough we can now see how CPM can produce adverse pregnancy outcomes, how it contributes to the overall problem of IUGR in the clinical context is, to say the least, still an emerging picture. In the UK, less than 1 per cent of all pregnancies undergo CVS and considerably fewer have useful diagnostic investigations of the placental karyotype in relation to IUGR. Less than one in ten trisomic CPM pregnancies in published series have any information about their mechanism of generation; the origins of CPM for other (non-trisomic) cytogenetic anomalies are virtually unstudied. Most investigations are still very much in the research environment and published data are heavily biased towards problem outcomes. The relative contributions of CPM for different cytogenetic abnormalities to IUGR are given in Table 2.1. Available information on the long term prognosis for affected individuals is very limited indeed.

Trisomy 16

Trisomy 16 CPM is common, occurring in 1 in 3,000 diagnostic CVS. High levels of abnormal cells are usually present, often throughout the placenta. The majority of these cases, at least 80 per cent and probably more, are corrections of maternal meiosis I errors, reflecting the origins of non-mosaic trisomy 16 [42]. The incidence of UPDmat corresponds closely to the one in three chance of random loss of the paternal chromosome 16 during reduction to disomy, giving an estimated incidence of 1 in 10,000 in the same patient group. This will be higher than the population risk, as CVS patients have a significant maternal age referral bias, which will itself relate to an increased frequency of maternal meiotic errors available to be corrected. Reports linking trisomy 16 CPM to IUGR and late pregnancy losses are numerous. In the order of 50 per cent of pregnancies with trisomy 16 CPM detected in the first trimester are compromised in some way [40]. The primary mechanism generating IUGR is unclear, and likely to remain so until a big enough body of unselected cases accumulates. IUGR is encountered in both the upd(16)mat and biparental inheritance groups, suggesting that it is the presence of abnormal cells in the placenta that is the significant factor [43]. There is some evidence that upd(16)mat cases are more frequently affected and that they are associated with a more severe IUGR (below the 3rd percentile) and earlier delivery [40]; there are certainly more published cases of associated stillbirths and intrauterine deaths. This may, however, simply reflect the level of abnormal cells in these cases, or a reporting bias. Unfortunately, comparable information on the birthweight and UPD status of "normal outcome" trisomy 16 CPM pregnancies is relatively sparse. There is the reasonable assumption that these represent in the main biparental inheritance cases, but this is far from proven. Maternal UPD in association with normal birthweight has been reported [44]. Several reports link trisomy 16 CPM to an atypical alpha fetoprotein/human chorionic gonadotrophin (AFP/hCG) profile, both being elevated during routine maternal serum screening for trisomy 21 in the mid second trimester, which is suggestive of altered placental development or function at this stage [45]. Most publications including cases of trisomy 16 CPM are primarily of a cytogenetic/ molecular genetic nature and associated placental histopathological data are limited. In general, the placenta is small and immature for gestational age; various non-specific degenerative changes have been described [42,46,47]. Placental thickening and sonolucencies have been reported in some cases [42,46].

One feature, reported in a small subset of individuals with upd(16)mat, is anal atresia [48]. The intriguing possibility of a link to the anal atresia in Townes–Brock syndrome, associated in some cases with chromosome rearrangements involving proximal 16q, remains to be elucidated. Cardiac abnormalities, primarily septal defects, are a recognised feature of true fetal mosaicism; this is a plausible explanation of their occasional finding in supposed CPM, but cardiac abnormalities may also be an inconsistent component of a upd(16)mat syndrome. Other abnormalities have also been reported in apparent CPM cases: unilateral renal agenesis in a child with upd(16)mat [49], and polysplenia and hydrocephalus in a fetus with biparental inheritance [50].

Trisomy 7

CPM for trisomy 7 is the most commonly reported placental abnormality in CVS, being detected in 1 in 1,100 diagnostic samples. Most (> 85 per cent) present with low levels of abnormal cells restricted to either CTB or cultured extraembryonic mesoderm-derived cells, occasionally both; follow-up data suggest that at these levels trisomy 7 cells have minimal or no subsequent clinical effects [39]. Molecular genetic analysis indicates that trisomy 7 CPM predominantly arises from postfertilisation somatic errors [51]. A small subset of cases, however, have much higher percentages of abnormal cells, often in both cell lineages, corresponding with anticipated corrected meiotic errors. One such report of CPM for trisomy 7, resulting from correction of a maternal meiosis I error and leading to upd(7)mat and IUGR (1560 g at 36 weeks' gestation), has been published [52]. The child was not dysmorphic and at age 3 years 9 months, although remaining small, was recorded as being developmentally normal. Placental histopathology was unremarkable. Interestingly, around 10 per cent of Silver–Russell syndrome patients (see also under Syndromes) have upd(7)mat [53,54], possibly being derived from correction of trisomic conceptions. Unfortunately, as might be expected in these cases, placental material was not available for analysis. Uniparental disomy, with isodisomy of the whole chromosome or the appropriate segments, has also been detected in several infants with recessive genetic conditions mapping to chromosome 7, notably cystic fibrosis. Those with UPDmat were growth restricted [55]; the one with paternal UPD was not [56]. Again placental material was not available for analysis. There is an unusual case of a growth-restricted infant with isochromosomes of both the long arms and short arms of chromosome 7, resulting in paternal isodisomy for the short arms and maternal isodisomy for the long arms (a condition unlikely to have been associated with a trisomic placenta), which suggests that in CPM for trisomy 7 the primary cause of growth restriction is maternal uniparental disomy for the long arm of chromosome 7, rather than the presence of trisomic cells in placental tissue [57]. This is a logical conclusion, but some caution should always be taken when extrapolating from very small numbers of informative cases. An imprinted candidate gene *PEG1/MEST*, homologous to a gene expressed during embryological development in the mouse, has been mapped to the distal long arm of chromosome 7 in humans [58]; however, screening for mutations and altered methylation patterns in this gene in Silver–Russell patients has proved negative [59].

Trisomy 2

Trisomy 2 CPM is observed in 1 in 1,600 diagnostic CVS. As for trisomy 7 CPM, there is a large group of cases (> 80 per cent) with low levels of trisomic cells, a postfertilisation somatic error origin where tested, and little observable in the way of clinical effect [39,60]. Although of no known relevance to IUGR, in these cases trisomy is almost exclusively found among the ICM-derived cells. Again, adverse outcomes are found among a small heterogeneous subgroup of cases with high levels of abnormal cells, often 100 per cent, in both the CTB and cultured cells. The majority are corrected maternal errors, both meiosis I and II [61–63]; one corrected paternal meiosis I error has been reported [64]. Two cases, with biparental inheritance of chromosomes 2 in the fetus, one correction of a maternal meiosis I error [63], the other that of the corrected paternal meiosis I error [64], both showed IUGR. This indicates that IUGR is a consequence of the placental trisomy rather than UPD.

Oligohydramnios is a common feature of trisomy 2 CPM with or without UPD; raised AFP and hCG levels have been detected during mid second trimester maternal serum screening [36,64,65]. The three well-documented upd(2)mat cases [61,62,65] showed additional inconsistent clinical features: renal failure, vesicoureteric reflux, patent ductus arteriosus, congenital pyloric stenosis, hiatus hernia, hypospadias, undescended testes and hypothyroidism. The smallest, 510 g at 36/52, died soon after birth; the others, 765 g at 31/52 and 1710 g at 36/52, were alive but with continuing clinical problems at age 24 and 31 months. Both remained small. but development was otherwise normal. It is unclear, however, whether these features are part of an ill-defined upd(2)mat syndrome. There is a report [66] of a 36-year-old woman with maternal isodisomy for the whole of chromosome 2 as the result of a rare isochromosome rearrangement, but with a normal phenotype, normal intelligence, and a recorded normal birthweight; its authors claim this as strong evidence for the lack of imprinted genes on chromosome 2, and attribute the phenotypic findings in prenatally detected upd(2)mat cases to undetected trisomic cells in the fetus. Only detailed analysis of further cases will resolve this issue.

Trisomy 15

Mosaicism for trisomy 15 is encountered in about 1 in 5,000 diagnostic CVS. A large collaborative European Study [67] indicates that the same two meiotic and somatic error groups can be predicted, in roughly equal numbers. Meiotic errors appear to be primarily of maternal origin. The primary clinical considerations are Prader–Willi syndrome (PWS) as a consequence of upd(15)mat and/or the presence of trisomic cells in fetal cells. In most published reports, birthweight data is missing, but IUGR has been recorded in PWS outcomes. Approximately 10 per cent of PWS detected postnatally appears to arise from correction of a maternally derived trisomy 15, and it is a reasonable assumption that if placental investigation had been undertaken it would have revealed significant levels of trisomy in most cases. Short stature and low birthweight are part of the overall spectrum of PWS features. The aetiology of IUGR in CPM cases is unknown.

Other Trisomies

Several reports [30,31,68,69] link a minority of cases of placental trisomy 9 and trisomy 22 to IUGR. These trisomies are relatively infrequent causes of CPM, about 1 in 3,500 and 1 in 7,000 diagnostic CVS respectively. Outcome data are too poor to come to any definitive conclusions regarding aetiology, but correction of trisomy has been reported for both these chromosomes and it is likely that problem outcomes will be concentrated in this group. A very thorough report [70] of a growth-restricted infant with placental trisomy 22 and upd(22)mat is complicated by the presence of trisomic cells in fetal tissue; clinical features including a perimembranous VSD, consistent with the fetal trisomy 22 mosaicism, were present. One report of IUGR with apparent CPM for trisomy 22 also described cardiac features [31]. The relative contributions of placental trisomy, UPD and low level residual trisomy in the fetus to IUGR and congenital abnormality remain to be elucidated.

Analysis of trisomy 9 CPM cases is also complicated by the possibility of undetected low levels of trisomic cells in fetal tissue. Demonstrable mosaic trisomy 9 is a rare but recognised syndrome; IUGR is a consistent feature [71]. Most cases do not have associated cytogenetic studies of placental material, making predictive interpretation of prenatally detected extraembryonic abnormality somewhat problematical.

IUGR has been reported in conjunction with rarer CPMs for trisomy 11 [72] and trisomy 14 [73], and also with a minority of cases of trisomy 18 and trisomy 21. The trisomy 11 case died in utero and was an unusual example of a paternal uniparental disomy. As upd(11)pat might intuitively be expected to influence known imprinted genes on the short arm of chromosome 11 producing the overgrowth Beckwith–Wiedemann syndrome, there is a strong argument that the primary aetiology in this case is the presence of trisomic cells in the placenta rather than the UPD. Growth restriction and mental retardation with precocious puberty are features of an emerging upd(14)mat syndrome. Affected individuals with inappropriate inheritance of familial chromosome rearrangements [74] (i.e. unlikely to involve placental trisomy) suggest UPD as the primary cause of reduced stature. The relevance of the small number of trisomy 18 and trisomy 21 cases is unknown; they may possibly be coincidental. Upd(21)mat has been described in early pregnancy loss [75], further confusing the situation.

Other Methods for Correction of Trisomy

Several reports demonstrate correction of trisomy not by loss of the entire chromosome but by some equally poorly understood fragmentation process. This reduces the third chromosome to a small centromeric marker (non-centromeric fragments are lost during cell division) sometimes identifiable as a ring chromosome [76]. Subsequent loss of the marker chromosome, producing an apparently normal cell line, may also occur, giving the potential for three-way trisomy/marker/normal mosaicism. Such correction can again produce IUGR owing to either extraembryonic cytogenetic abnormality or the generation of UPD. A fetus with a proportion of cells having a small marker chromosome might be expected to be more viable than a fetus with a similar proportion of cells with the corresponding intact chromosome. Based on the detection rate of mosaic marker chromosomes in first trimester CVS, correction of trisomy in this way is probably comparatively rare.

A further potential source of UPD is the total exclusion of the third chromosome such that no trisomic cell line remains. As the established method of screening for UPD in IUGR pregnancies relies almost exclusively on first detecting trisomic cells, clearly, unless detected fortuitously, all such cases will have been missed. A recently published example [77] may represent a one-off event or the tip of a completely undiagnosed iceberg.

It should also be appreciated that not all uniparental disomy arises as a consequence of corrected trisomy. Several alternative mechanisms involving gamete complementation (chance fusion of a disomic and a matching nullisomic gamete), chromosome duplication in monosomic conceptions, or inappropriate inheritance of familial rearrangements, have been described [78].

CPM for other Chromosome Abnormalities in Association with IUGR

IUGR has been described in a minority of cases of CPM for sex chromosome abnormalities, structural abnormalities and double (or more) aneuploidies. Why a mosaic karyotype such as 47,XXX/46,XX or 47,XXY/46,XY confined to the placenta should cause problems is unclear. Some interaction with patterns of X inactivation may be involved.

Structurally abnormal chromosomes, particularly those such as deletions and duplications involving only a single chromosome, may also, at least in theory, undergo correction either by loss of the abnormal chromosome and duplication of the normal or by a mitotic interchange event. This would result in uniparental disomy for either all or part of the chromosome concerned. Alternatively, unbalanced chromosome abnormalities, particularly those involving deleted segments, may have a direct effect on placental growth or function.

If CPM for a single trisomy can produce IUGR, rarer cases of CPM where the abnormal cell line has multiple trisomies might be anticipated to be more problematical.

Until formally demonstrated, all these explanations should be regarded as speculative.

Syndromes

Intrauterine fetal growth restriction occurs as part of the phenotype of a large number of syndromic disorders. Some of these show mendelian inheritance, others are sporadic (possibly resulting from dominant mutations or submicroscopic chromosomal deletions). These disorders can be broadly subclassified into two groups:

Conditions due Primarily to Disturbance of Bone Growth

These conditions frequently present with non-uniform (disproportionate) involvement of different parts of the skeletal system. This group includes the osteochondrodysplasias (developmental disorders of chondro-osseus tissue of the whole skeleton, such as thanatophoric dysplasia and osteogenesis imperfecta) and dysostoses (developmental disorders of single bones, such as hemivertebrae and limb reduction defects) [79]. The molecular genetics of a number of the osteochondrodysplasias is now understood [80].

Conditions Associated with a Generalised (Proportionate) Reduction in Body Growth

These syndromes are numerous and include the chromosome breakage syndromes (Fanconi, Bloom, Cockayne), and the de Lange, Donohue, Rubinstein–Taybi, Neu–Laxova, Dubowitz, Seckel, Johanson–Blizzard and Silver–Russell syndromes [81]. Many of these disorders show autosomal recessive inheritance, and for several the gene loci involved have now been identified. For example, the importance of insulin in fetal growth is illustrated by Donohue syndrome (leprechaunism) in which there are mutations in the insulin receptor [82,83]. Silver–Russell syndrome appears to be aetiologically heterogeneous, with some cases probably due to new dominant mutations involving chromosome 17q [84], and others associated with maternal uniparental disomy of chromosome 7 [53,54].

Conclusions

Genetic abnormalities make a significant contribution to intrauterine growth restriction. Fetal growth and development result from the complex coordination of processes including cell proliferation, differentiation and migration. Hypothetically, genetic regulation of these mechanisms can be envisaged as acting at the level of (for example) hormones, growth factors and extracellular matrix proteins, cell surface receptors of these macromolecules, postreceptor signal transduction, cell cycle control proteins and programmed cell death. In addition, placental structure and function will also be influenced by the genetic constitution of the conceptus. Understanding of these normal regulatory mechanisms is expanding rapidly [85,86], providing clues to the aetiology and pathogenetic mechanisms underlying fetal growth restriction. Study of fetal growth impairment is delivering new insight into normal mechanisms of growth control.

Exclusion of an underlying genetic abnormality should be seen as an important part of clinical management in cases of IUGR, although in practice this is, at the moment, very rarely fully undertaken. Prenatally, detailed ultrasound may identify associated congenital abnormality helpful in making a more specific diagnosis. Currently, second or third trimester CVS is probably the most useful initial approach to further invasive testing, particularly if intervention, either termination of pregnancy or early delivery, is being considered. This technique provides sufficient material for both DNA extraction and a rapid karyotype, as appropriate. Unlike amniocentesis or fetal blood sampling (FBS) it will also detect cases where placental cytogenetic abnormality is either the cause of the problem, or an indicator of uniparental disomy or low level mosaicism in the fetus itself. The lack of a technique for rapid screening for UPD is hampering understanding of its contribution to IUGR.

References

1. Polani PE. Chromosomal and other genetic influences on birth weight variation. In: Elliott K, Knight J, editors. Size at birth. Ciba Foundation Symposium 27 (new series). Amsterdam: Elsevier, 1974;127–64.
2. Magnus P. Further evidence for a significant effect of fetal genes on variation in birth weight. Clin Genet 1984;26:289–96.
3. Winick M. Nutrition and fetal development. New York: Wiley, 1974.
4. Singer DB, Sung CJ, Wigglesworth JS. Fetal growth and maturation: with standards for body and organ development. In: Wigglesworth JS, Singer DB, editors. Textbook of fetal and perinatal pathology. Boston: Blackwell, 1991;11–47.
5. Naeye RL. Prenatal organ and cellular growth with various chromosomal disorders. Biol Neonat 1967;11:248–60.
6. Naeye RL, Blanc WA. Pathogenesis of congenital rubella. JAMA 1965;194:1277–83.
7. Naeye RL. Effects of maternal nutrition on the human fetus. Pediatrics 1973;52:494–503.
8. Naeye RL. Malnutrition. Probable cause of fetal growth retardation. Arch Pathol 1965;79:284–91.
9. Eydoux P, Choiset A, Le Porrier N, Thepot F, Szpiro-Tapia S, Alliet J, et al. Chromosomal prenatal diagnosis: study of 936 cases of intrauterine abnormalities after ultrasound assessment. Prenat Diagn 1989;9:255–68.
10. Snijders RJM, Sherrod C, Gosden CM, Nicolaides KH. Fetal growth retardation: associated malformations and chromosomal abnormalities. Am J Obstet Gynecol 1993;168:547–55.
11. Heydanus R, van Splunder IP, Wladimiroff JW. Tertiary centre referral of small-for-gestational age pregnancies: a 10-year retrospective analysis. Prenat Diagn 1994;14:105–8.
12. Wright EV. Chromosomes and human fetal development. In: Roberts DF, Thomson AM, editors. The biology of human fetal growth. London: Taylor & Francis, 1976;237–52.
13. Kuhn P, Brizot M deL, Pandya PP, Snijders RJ, Nicolaides KH. Crown–rump length in chromosomally abnormal fetuses at 10 to 13 weeks' gestation. Am J Obstet Gynecol 1995;172:32–5.
14. Schemmer G, Wapner RJ, Johnson A, Schemmer M, Norton HJ, Anderson WE. First-trimester growth patterns of aneuploid fetuses. Prenat Diagn 1997;17:155–9.
15. Bahado-Singh RO, Lynch L, Deren O, Morroti R, Copel JA, Mahoney MJ, Williams J III. First-trimester restriction and fetal aneuploidy: the effect of type of aneuploidy and gestational age. Am J Obstet Gynecol 1997;176:976–80.
16. Twining P. Ultrasound diagnosis of chromosomal disease. In: Reed GB, Claireaux AE, Cockburn F, editors. Diseases of the fetus and newborn. London: Chapman and Hall, 1996;939–53.
17. Chen ATL, Chan Y-K, Falek A. The effects of chromosome abnormalities on birth weight in man. II. Autosomal defects. Hum Hered 1972;22:209–24.
18. Kucera J, Dolezalova V. Prenatal development of malformed fetuses at 28–42 weeks of gestational age (anencephalus, hydrocephalus, Down's syndrome, cleft lip and palate, and hypospadia). I Weight gains. Biol Neonate 1972;20:253–61.
19. Matsunaga E, Tonomura A. Parental age and birth weight in translocation Down's syndrome. Ann Hum Genet 1972;36:209–19.

20. Roberts DF. The genetics of human fetal growth. In: Falkner F, Tanner JM, editors. Human Growth. A comprehensive treatise: vol 3: Methodology. Ecological, genetic, and nutritional effects on growth, 2nd edn. New York: Plenum Press, 1986;113–43.
21. Gilbert-Barness E. Chromosomal abnormalities. In: Gilbert-Barness E, editors. Potter's pathology of the fetus and infant, Mosby, St Louis: Mosby, 1997;388–432.
22. Niebuhr E. Triploidy in man. Humangenetik 1974;21:103–25.
23. Jacobs PA, Angell RR, Buchanan IM, Hassold TJ, Matsuyama AM, Manuel B. The origin of human triploids. Ann Hum Genet 1978;42:49–57.
24. Jauniaux E, Brown R, Rodeck C, Nicolaides KH. Prenatal diagnosis of triploidy during the second trimester of pregnancy. Obstet Gynecol 1996;88:983–9.
25. McFadden DE, Kwong LC, Yam IYL, Langlois S Parental origin of triploidy in human fetuses: evidence for genomic imprinting. Hum Genet 1993;92:465–9.
26. Fitzsimmons J, Fantel A, Shepard TH. Growth parameters in mid-trimester fetal Turner syndrome. Early Hum Dev 1994;38:121–9.
27. de la Chapelle A. Sex chromosome abnormalities. In: Emery AEH, Rimoin DL, editors. Principle and practice of medical genetics. Edinburgh: Churchill Livingstone, 1990;273–99.
28. Chen ATL, Chan Y-K, Falek A. The effects of chromosome abnormalities on birth weight. I. Sex chromosome disorders. Hum Hered 1971;21:543–56.
29. Barlow PW. The influence of inactive chromosomes on human development. Anomalous sex chromosome complements and the phenotype. Hum Genet 1973;17:105–36.
30. Kalousek DK, Dill FJ. Chromosomal mosaicism confined to the human placenta in human conceptions. Science 1983;221:665–7.
31. Wolstenholme J, Rooney DE, Davison EV. Confined placental mosaicism, IUGR, and adverse pregnancy outcome: a controlled retrospective UK collaborative study. Prenat Diagn 1994;14:345–61.
32. Association of Clinical Cytogeneticists Working Party on chorionic villi in Prenatal Diagnosis (1994) Cytogenetic analysis of chorionic villi for prenatal diagnosis: an ACC collaborative study of UK data. Prenat Diagn 14:363–79.
33. Ledbetter DH, Zachary JM, Simpson JL, Golbus MS, Pergament E, Jackson L, et al. Cytogenetic results from the US collaborative study on CVS. Prenat Diagn 1992;12:317–45.
34. Hahnemann JM, Vejerslev LO. Accuracy of cytogenetic findings on chorionic villus sampling (CVS) – diagnostic consequences of CVS mosaicism and non-mosaic discrepancy in centres contributing to EUROMIC 1986–1992. Prenat Diagn 1997;17:801–20.
35. Johnson A, Wapner RJ., Davis GH, Jackson LG. Mosaicism in chorionic villus sampling: an association with poor perinatal outcome. Obstet Gynecol 1990;75:573–7.
36. Fryburg JS, Dimaio MS, Yang-Feng TL, Mahoney MJ. Follow-up of pregnancies complicated by placental mosaicism diagnosed by chorionic villus sampling. Prenat Diagn 1993;13:481–94.
37. Crane JP, Cheung SW. An embryonic model to explain cytogenetic inconsistencies observed in chorionic villus versus fetal tissue. Prenat Diagn 1988;8:119–29.
38. Simoni G, Sirchia SM. Confined placental mosaicism. Prenat Diagn 1994;14:1185–9.
39. Wolstenholme J. Confined placental mosaicism for trisomies 2, 3, 7, 8, 9, 16 and 22: their incidence, likely origins and mechanisms for cell lineage compartmentalisation. Prenat Diagn 1996;16:511–24.
40. Wolstenholme J. An audit of trisomy 16 in man. Prenat Diagn 1995;15:109–21.
41. Delhanty JDA, Handyside AH. The origin of genetic defects in the human and their detection in the preimplantation embryo. Hum Reprod Update 1995;1:201–15.
42. Kalousek DK, Langlois S, Barrett I, Yam I, Wilson DR, Howard-Peebles PN, et al. Uniparental disomy for chromosome 16 in humans. Am J Hum Genet 1993;52:8–16.
43. Kalousek DK, Barrett I. Genomic imprinting related to prenatal diagnosis. Prenat Diagn 1994;14:1191–201.
44. van Opstal D, van den Berg C, Deelen WH, Brandenburg H, Cohen-Overbeek TE, Halley DJJ, et al. Prospective prenatal investigations on potential uniparental disomy in cases of confined placental trisomy. Prenat Diagn 1998;18:35–44.
45. Groli C, Cerri V, Tarantini M, Bellotti D, Jacobello C, Gianello R, et al. Maternal serum screening and trisomy 16 confined to the placenta. Prenat Diagn 1996;16:685–9.
46. Williams J III, Wang BBT, Rubin CH, Clark RD, Mohandas TK. Apparent non-mosaic trisomy 16 in chorionic villi: diagnostic dilemma or clinically significant finding? Prenat Diagn 1992;12:163–8.
47. Paulyson KJ, Sherer DM, Christian SL, Lewis KM, Ledbetter DH, Salafia CM, et al. Prenatal diagnosis of an infant with mosaic trisomy 16 of paternal origin. Prenat Diagn 1996;16:1021–6.
48. Vaughan JI, Ali Z, Bower S, Bennett P, Chard T, Moore G. Human maternal uniparental disomy for chromosome 16 and fetal development. Prenat Diagn 1994;14:751–6.

49. Woo V, Bridge PJ, Bamforth JS. Maternal uniparental disomy for chromosome 16: case report. Am J Med Genet 1997;70:387–90.

50. Sánchez JM, López de Díaz S, Panal MJ, Moya G, Kenny A, Iglesias D, et al. Severe fetal malformations associated with trisomy 16 confined to the placenta. Prenat Diagn 1997;17:777–9.

51. Kalousek DK, Langlois S, Robinson WP, Telenius A, Bernard L. Barrett IJ, et al. Trisomy 7 CVS mosaicism: pregnancy outcome, placental and DNA analysis in 14 cases. Am J Med Genet 1990;65:348–52.

52. Langlois S, Yong SL, Wilson RD, Kwong LC, Kalousek DK. Prenatal and postnatal growth failure associated with maternal heterodisomy for chromosome 7. J Med Genet 1995;32:871–5.

53. Kotzot D, Schmitt S, Bernasconi F, Robinson WP, Lurie IW, Ilyina H, et al. Uniparental disomy 7 in Silver–Russell syndrome and primordial growth retardation. Hum Mol Genet 1995;4:583–7.

54. Preece MA, Price SM, Davies V, Clough L, Stanier P, Trembath RC et al. Maternal uniparental disomy 7 in Silver-Russell syndrome. J Med Genet 1997;34:6–9.

55. Spence JE, Perciaccante RG, Greig GM, Willad HF, Ledbetter DH, Hejtmancik JF, et al. Uniparental disomy as a mechanism for human genetic disease. Am J Hum Genet 1988;42:217–26.

56. Hoglund P, Holmberg C, de la Chapelle A, Kere J. Paternal isodisomy for chromosome 7 is compatible with normal growth and development in a patient with congenital chloride diarrhoea. Am J Hum Genet 1994;55:747–52.

57. Eggerding FA, Schonberg SA, Chehab FF, Norton ME, Cox VA, Epstein CJ. Uniparental disomy for paternal 7p and maternal 7q in a child with mental retardation. Am J Hum Genet 1994;55:253–65.

58. Kobayashi S, Kohda T, Miyoshi N, Kuroiwa Y, Aisaka K, Tsutsumi O, et al. Human *PEG1/MEST*, an imprinted gene on chromosome 7. Hum Mol Genet 1997;6:781–6.

59. Riesewijk AM, Blagitko N, Schinzel AA, Hu L, Schulz U, Hamel BCJ, et al. Evidence against a major role of *PEG1/MEST* in Silver-Russell syndrome. Eur J Hum Genet 1998;6:114–20.

60. Shaffer LG, Langlois S, McCaskill C, Main DM, Robinson WP, Barrett IJ, et al. Analysis of nine pregnancies with confined placental mosaicism for trisomy 2. Prenat Diagn 1996;16:899–905.

61. Webb AL, Sturgiss S, Warwicker P, Robson SC, Goodship JA, Wolstenholme J. Maternal uniparental disomy for chromosome 2 in association with confined placental mosaicism for trisomy 2 and severe intrauterine growth retardation. Prenat Diagn 1996;16:958–62.

62. Hansen WF, Bernard LE, Langlois S, Rao KW, Chescheir NC, Aylsworth AS, et al. Maternal uniparental disomy of chromosome 2 and confined placental mosaicism for trisomy 2 in a fetus with intrauterine growth restriction, hypospadias, and oligohydramnios. Prenat Diagn 1997;17:443–50.

63. Gibbons B, Cheng HH, Yoong AKH, Brown S. Confined placental mosaicism for trisomy 2 with intrauterine growth retardation and severe oligohydramnios in the absence of uniparental disomy in the fetus. Prenat Diagn 1997;17:689–90.

64. Ariel I, Lerer I, Yagel S, Cohen R, Ben-Neriah Z, Abelovich D. Trisomy 2: confined placental mosaicism in a fetus with intrauterine growth retardation. Prenat Diagn 1997;17:180–3.

65. Harrison K, Eisenger K, Anyane-Yeboa K, Brown S. Maternal uniparental disomy of chromosome 2 in a baby with trisomy 2 mosaicism in amniotic fluid culture. Am J Med Genet 1995;58:147–51.

66. Bernasconi F, Karagüzel A, Celep F, Keser I, Lüleci G, Dutly F, et al. Normal phenotype with m-ternal isodisomy in a female with two isichromosomes: i(2p) and i(2q). Am J Hum Genet 1996;59:1114–18.

67. EUCROMIC The origins of trisomy 15 CPM and the risk of fetal UPD. Prenat Diagn 1999:19:29–35.

68. Appleman Z, Rosensaft J, Chemke J, Caspi B, Ashkenazi M, Mogilner MB. Trisomy 9 confined to the placenta: prenatal diagnosis and neonatal follow-up. Am J Med Genet 1991;40:464–6.

69. Stioui S, De Silvestris M, Molinari A, Stripparo L, Ghisoni L, Simoni G. Trisomic 22 placenta in a case of severe intrauterine growth retardation. Prenat Diagn 1989;9:673–6.

70. de Pater JM, Schuring-Blom GH, van den Bogaard R, van der Sijs-Bos CJM, Christiaens GCML, Stoutenbeek P, et al. Maternal uniparental disomy for chromosome 22 in a child with generalized mosaicism for trisomy 22. Prenat Diagn 1997;17:81–6.

71. Tarina L, Colloridi F, Raguso G, Rizzuti A, Bruni L, Tozzi MC, et al. Trisomy 9 mosaic syndrome. A case report and review of the literature. Ann Génét 1994;37:14–20.

72. Webb A, Beard J, Wright C, Robson S, Wolstenholme J, Goodship J. A case of paternal uniparental disomy for chromosome 11. Prenat Diagn 1995;15:773–7.

73. Artan S, Basaran N, Hassa H, Özalp S, Sener T, Sayli BS, et al. Confined placental mosaicism in term placentae: analysis of 125 cases. Prenat Diagn 1995;15:1135–42.

74. Temple IK, Cockwell A, Hassold T, Pettay D, Jacobs P. Maternal uniparental disomy for chromosome 14. J Med Genet 1991;28:511–14.

75. Henderson JD, Sherman LS, Loughna SC, Bennett PR, Moore EG. Early embryonic failure associated with uniparental disomy for human chromosome 21. Hum Mol Genet 1994;3:1373–6.

76. James RS, Temple IK, Dennis NR, Crolla JA. A search for uniparental disomy in carriers of supernumerary marker chromosomes. Eur J Hum Genet 1995;3:21–6.
77. Los FJ, van Opstal D, van den Berg C, Braat APG, Verhoef S, Wesby-van Swaay E, et al. Uniparental disomy with and without confined placental mosaicism: a model for trisomic zygote rescue. Prenat Diagn 1998;18:659–68.
78. Engel E, DeLozier-Blanchet CD. Uniparental disomy, isodisomy, and imprinting: probable effects in man and strategies for their detection. Am J Med Genet 1991;40:432–9.
79. Yang SS, Gilbert-Barness E. Skeletal system. In: Gilbert-Barness, editor. Potter's pathology of the fetus and infant. St Louis: Mosby, 1997;1423–81.
80. Francomano CA, McIntosh I, Wilkin DJ. Bone dysplasias in man: molecular insights. Curr Opin Genet Dev 1996;6:301–8.
81. Jones KL. Smith's recognisable patterns of human malformation, 5th edn. Philadelphia: WB Saunders, 1997.
82. Psiachou H, Mitton S, Alaghband-Zadeh J, Hone J, Taylor SI, Sinclair L. Leprechaunism and homozygous nonsense mutation in the insulin receptor. Lancet 1993;342:924.
83. Hone J, Accili D, Al-Gazali LI, Lestringant G, Orban T, Taylor SI. Homozygosity for a new mutation (ile119-to-met) in the insulin receptor gene in five sibs with familial insulin resistance. J Med Genet 1994;31:715–16.
84. Midro AT, Debek K, Sawicka A, Marcinkiewicz D, Rogowska M. Second observation of Silver–Russell syndrome in a carrier of a reciprocal translocation with one breakpoint at site 17q25. Clin Genet 1993;44:53–5.
85. Han VKM, Fowden AL. Paracrine regulation of fetal growth. In: Ward RHT, Smith SK, Donnai D (eds) Early fetal growth and development. London: RCOG Press, 1994;275–91.
86. Alsat E, Marcotty C, Gabriel R, Igout A, Frankenne F, Hennen G et al. Molecular approach to intrauterine growth retardation: an overview of recent data. Reprod Fertil Dev 1995;7:1457–64.

3 Perinatal Viral Infections as a Cause of Intrauterine Growth Restriction

Mark Kilby and Sheena Hodgett

Introduction

IUGR is a major cause of perinatal morbidity and mortality; indeed with increasing incidence of detection and "salvage" of the very low birthweight fetus such complications will continue to rise [1].

Classically aetiological factors that affect the fetal genome (and fetal viraemia is one such factor) will tend to present at a relatively early gestational age (prior to 28 weeks). The ultrasound assessment of such affected fetuses often (but not exclusively) reveals a "symmetrical" growth velocity, which in itself carries a worsening outcome, with an associated 50 per cent mortality [2,3]. However, the exact intrauterine presentation will depend very much on the gestational age at which maternal–fetal transmission and fetal viraemia occurs. Both animal models and epidemiological human data indicate that IUGR is most common if infection occurs early in gestation [4]. Fetal Doppler velocimetry may reveal waveforms associated with the presence of abnormal villous development [5] as fetal viral infections may commonly be associated with placental pathology [6]. The presence of associated fetal structural anomalies (i.e. cardiac disease or ventriculomegaly) or ultrasound signs (i.e. hyperechogenic bowel) in the presence of associated IUGR raise the possibility of fetal viral infections, commonly those of congenital rubella or cytomegalovirus infections [7–9].

A reduction in fetal growth velocity, presenting as IUGR, is thought to arise as a result of capillary endothelial damage during organogenesis, causing a decreased number of cells that have a cytoplasmic mass within the normal range and direct cytopathic effects [10].

There is sufficient evidence to support a direct causal relationship between IUGR and congenital infectious disease for only two main viruses: rubella [11] and cytomegalovirus (CMV)[12]. However, a possible relationship also exists for varicella–zoster virus (VZV) [13] and human immunodeficiency virus (HIV) [14].

Although the incidence of maternal infections with various organisms may be as high as 15 per cent, the incidence of congenital infections is estimated at approximately 5 per cent. It is currently estimated that infectious disease accounts for 5–10% of all cases of human IUGR [15].

The prenatal diagnosis of congenital viral infections, along with potential therapeutic interventions, is a poorly established area in the subspecialty of fetal medicine, with much anecdote prevailing. Screening policies (if they exist at all) vary greatly in different parts of the world, reflecting, to a certain extent, epidemiological differences in prevalence and in the perceived importance of such infections.

Properties of Viruses and their Replication

Properties

Viruses are small, obligate parasites that are either eukaryotic or prokaryotic and contain one species of nucleic acid, either DNA or RNA. The generation of viral mRNAs that must compete with host cellular mRNA for the protein synthesising machinery is crucial to the replication of all viruses. The nucleic acid is protected by a capsid (coat) consisting of protein subunits called *capsomeres*. Each capsomere is made of one to three polypeptides. Some viruses have a lipid envelope. The nucleic acid is often in a complex with a protein and the nucleic acid core and capsid together are known as a *nucleocapsid*. The complete viral particle is termed the *viron*. The nucleocapsids of nearly all viruses are built either like helices or like isosahedra. Viruses are classified into families according to the characteristics of their nucleic acid, the number of strands and their polarity.

Mechanisms of Infection

The virus initially adheres to the host cell with a receptor-binding protein complex. The stages of viral infection of cells are then cellular recognition, internalisation, followed by genome transcription to form RNA. Once this occurs, mRNA translation and genome replication occur with release of new virus particles from the cell. The complete cell cycle varies between different families but characteristically takes 6 to 8 hours.

Some RNA-containing viruses are positively stranded and their genome acts directly as messenger RNA. In contrast, negative-stranded RNA viruses possess a virally associated enzyme RNA transcriptase that produces a messenger RNA transcript from the genome RNA. Postive-stranded viruses may translate their mRNA directly. Transcription of DNA viruses is carried out by cellular DNA-dependent RNA polymerases. Viral mRNAs may be spliced, thus allowing several messages to be carried in a single piece of genome. Viruses may "burst" from infected cells in waves or may be released instantaneously by cell lysis.

Many viruses kill the cells in which they replicate and, therefore, have cytopathic effects. These effects occur in the intact host cell as well as in cell cultures. They may include cell lysis, where the parasitic virus encoded protein "shuts down" the synthesis of endogenous macromolecules of the host cell. These viruses cause death of the cell and then lysis, releasing large numbers of viron particles, which may reinfect adjacent cells.

Cell fusion may occur with specific kinds of viruses and the fusion proteins that mediate entry of the viruses through the host plasma membrane may also cause the formation of multinucleated giant cells. This is relatively common in paramyxoviruses. These viruses, therefore, behave in a way that they can pass from cell to cell rather than causing cell death.

Tests

The first class of immunoglobulin to be synthesised by the fetus is IgM. Although endogenous B cells are present in the fetal circulation from the late first trimester and primitive plasma cells secrete IgM by 20 weeks' gestation, only significant amounts of IgM antibody (10 per cent of the adult concentration) are present by the third trimester [16]. This immunological ontogeny means that the assay of a specific IgM prior to 20 weeks is unreliable as a means of excluding a viral infection in the fetus and, even in the third trimester, the sensitivity of such tests may be as low as 28 per cent [17]. At birth, umbilical cord blood IgM concentrations may underestimate the risk of a specific viraemia, as the IgM peak may have occurred much earlier in gestation. Maternal IgG transport across the placenta occurs as early as the late first trimester but is relatively inefficient [18] with low fetal circulating concentrations until late second trimester when endogenous production and transplacental uptake increase. The presence of a specific IgG in fetal blood is thus likely to reflect maternal levels and only persistent levels into childhood correlate with intrauterine infection. Thus maternal (and or fetal) serology may not be high in its sensitivity and specificity in the detection of fetal viraemia. The application of molecular biological techniques such as polymerase chain reaction (PCR) allows the amplification of relatively small amounts of DNA from the infectious agent's genome, making a specific prospective diagnosis more likely. However, false positive diagnosis may be made owing to maternal contamination. Also, false negative diagnoses may be made if there is genetic variability of specific strains of virus, if the replication cycle for the virus is very long or if the virus is not secreted into the body compartment being tested. However, such diagnostic tests allow the prospective evaluation of a growth-restricted fetus, so that aetiology, prognosis and possible therapy can be considered.

Effects on the Fetus

Thus, the virus may cause direct cytopathic damage or induce a host immune response that may lead to secondary damage. In the fetoplacental unit, the timing of the fetal viraemia as well as the degree of cytopathic damage and/or modification of the host cell genome will determine the degree of morphological and cellular damage.

Evidence of infection per se does not imply fetal damage or long term sequelae. It is not unexpected that, given the uncertainties about the true rate of fetal infection for any specific disease, the frequency of congenital abnormalities is even less precisely assessed. However, the association with an identified fetal viraemia and the onset of reduced fetal growth velocity (and perhaps other prospective ultrasound evidence of fetal anomaly) may lead to difficult diagnostic and therapeutic dilemmas. Termination of pregnancy has been offered or requested since prenatal diagnosis has become available. Various treatments may have become accepted in clinical practice without proper randomised controlled trials. However, it would be fair to say that, in general terms, the identification of IUGR and either direct or indirect evidence of maternal/fetal viral infection significantly increase perinatal mortality and morbidity. The specific examples of congenital viral infections of rubella, CMV, varicella zoster and HIV that may cause IUGR will now be discussed in further detail.

Cytomegalovirus

Cytomegalic inclusion disease is due to infection with CMV, a large, enveloped DNA virus. Human CMV is species specific and, therefore, will not infect other animals. Although genetically homologous, there is considerable variation in DNA sequences (variants) and thus molecular methods may be used to trace infection in epidemiological studies. Although the characteristic large cells with prominent intranuclear inclusion bodies seen in the tissues infected with this virus have been recognised since the early 20th century, the virus itself was not isolated until 1956. CMV was initially considered to be a relatively rare problem as only overt clinical disease was noted. However, it is now appreciated that the disease may well be a "silent" one in which there are few clinical manifestations [19]. Indeed, like many herpes-type viruses, after the initial infection there is a long latent period when the host is completely asymptomatic and the severe overt infection becomes apparent only when reactivation of the virus occurs if, for example, the patient becomes relatively immunocompromised. This virus is now recognised as being a common and serious cause of infection in utero. Congenital infection has been reported in up to 2.5 per cent of all babies delivered [20]. It is probable that between 1 and 3 per cent of neonates excrete CMV, but only 5–10 per cent will show clinical symptoms in the newborn period [20]. Approximately 1 per cent of all women are infected with CMV during pregnancy. Primary maternal infection, in pregnancy, poses the greatest risk to the fetus. It is estimated that 5–10% of congenitally affected babies will have neurological [21,22]. Severe symptomatic cytomegalic inclusion disease occurs in approximately 1 in 10,000 neonates and has been estimated by the Communicable Disease Surveillance Centre in the UK (1992–3) as being responsible for 42 of all 1615 (2.6 per cent) CMV infections during this period [23].

In children and adults, CMV infection is almost always asymptomatic. The patient occasionally complains of "influenza-like" symptoms of fever, headache, pharyngitis, cervical lymphadenopathy, myalgia and occasionally an erythroform rash. CMV infection is more severe and prolonged in immuocompromised individuals, which may be a result of either adjunct viral infections such as HIV or pharmacotherapy [24]. CMV may be transmitted by way of secretions and sexual contact. Rarely, individuals are infected by blood transfusion or infected organ transplantation. CMV seropositivity is more common amongst the lower socio-economic groups (Fig. 3.1), but is not particularly associated with those who work with children or the immunosuppressed [25]. In developed countries, up to 50 per cent of the population may escape infection until adulthood [24] and, thus the female population is the group particularly at risk of congenital CMV infection [26].

CMV has developed a remarkably successful form of parasitism in human populations. It may be persistently excreted and thus is communicable for long periods. Indeed, infants infected congenitally may excrete CMV for an average of 4 years and those acquiring the infection at the time of birth for 2 years [24]. In asymptomatic individuals, recurrent excretion may occur in several ways:

1. Following primary infection, a low grade chronic viraemia may be established in which viral excretion periodically reaches detectable levels.
2. Reinfection may occur in immune individuals owing to antigenetic and genetic disparity amongst the CMV strains.

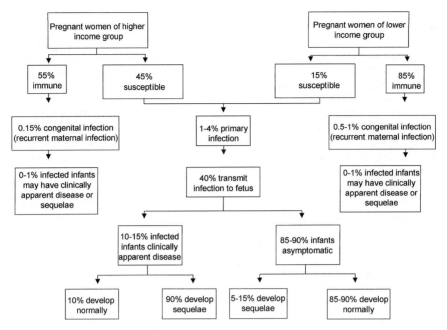

Fig. 3.1 An algorithm indicating the differential immunity and susceptibility rates in women of different socioeconomic groups (redrawn from [24]).

3. CMV may become latent and be reactivated when the host is immuno-suppressed.

The asymptomatic infection with excretion in pregnancy is common. Longitudinal studies have demonstrated that incidence of cervical excretion of the virus in pregnancy increases from 2.6 per cent (range 0–7.1%) in the first trimester to 7.6 per cent (range 2–28%) at term. These asymptomatic infections mainly occur in seropositive women and, therefore, reflect a recurrent infection [27].

The standard diagnostic test in the mother is viral culture in human fibroblasts to demonstrate cytopathic effects within these tissues. Although such cellular damage may be demonstrated within a few days, cultures need to be maintained for greater than 21 days to be certain that a result is negative. Maternal serological methods are available. Because maternal infection is almost always asymptomatic, the diagnosis is rarely suspected or confirmed in pregnancy. Even if there is a clinical suspicion of the disease, it is generally mild and CMV is usually overlooked as a diagnostic possibility. The complement fixation test is no longer a preferred method of diagnosis as it has considerable cross-reactivity with other herpes viruses. Although indirect haemagglutination and neutralisation tests have been used in epidemiological studies, fluorescent antibody tests and enzyme-linked immunoassays (ELISA) have the advantage of convenience and speed but have relatively poor sensitivities and specificities. PCR has been utilised to amplify CMV-specific DNA in donated blood [28] and may now be used to make the diagnosis from urine and amniotic fluid. Although PCR is highly sensitive, contamination from laboratory staff or the mother may contribute to a relatively high false positive rate. Also, failure to extract DNA from the body fluid sampled may cause false negative results. Occasionally, in the presence of symptoms, a diagnosis is made by the detection of specific anti-CMV IgM in maternal serum. However, anti-CMV IgM may persist for up to 16 weeks following a primary infection and detection of IgM in the first trimester may represent an infection that has occurred preconceptually [29]. The diagnosis is more certain if seroconversion is demonstrated. The use of a comparative assay taken early in pregnancy (as in a serum sample obtained for blood transfusion analysis) may well be extremely useful in prospectively demonstrating an acute infection.

Congenital CMV infection is generally the result of transplacental transmission of the virus, which causes in vitro infection [30]. Between 0.5 and 2.5 per cent of the neonatal population is infected by vertical transmission from the mother to the fetus during pregnancy and, in addition, 3–5% of live born infants acquires CMV peripartum. This latter infective process is presumably because of infected cervical secretions; maternal viraemia or infections through breast feeding [24]. These neonates who have perinatal CMV infection often have initial urine cultures that are negative but subsequently excrete CMV postnatally. Up to 50 per cent of neonates whose mothers have genital identifiable CMV infection at the time of birth will acquire the virus.

It is those infections transmitted in utero (i.e. transplacentally) that are of major concern, especially in relation to infant development. Congenital infections may occur following either a primary or a recurrent maternal infection. The occurrence of a demonstrably high rate (6 per cent) of congenital infection in infants born to previously immune mothers suggests that the current infection is an important cause of in utero transmission of CMV. The birth of one congenitally infected infant does not preclude the possibility of subsequent infection and fetal damage [31]. However, the rate of transmission is 40 per cent in primary infection and less than 1 per cent in reactivated infections [32]. In populations with a high rate of maternal seropositivity, reactivation accounts for a high proportion of the cases of congenital infection [33]. Ninety per cent of neonates with in utero acquired CMV infection are asymptomatic and 15 per cent of these asymptomatic congenitally infected neonates will develop later sequelae (Fig. 3.1) [32].

The timing of the infection during pregnancy and its effect on fetal outcome are debatable. Monif and colleagues [27] have shown that the more severely affected infants are those who acquire CMV infection during the first or second trimesters. In this series, babies in which third trimester maternal infection was noted were normal at birth and had anti-CMV IgM, suggesting silent congenital infection. Other studies [34] have shown that up to 50 per cent of mothers who develop primary infection during pregnancy have infants who excrete the virus after delivery; none of the babies of eight women in this study had reactivation of infection during pregnancy and were excreting the virus after delivery. Stagno's series [24] similarly noted that primary maternal CMV infection during the first 20 weeks of gestation was more likely to cause significant sequelae in the fetus than when infection occurred during the third trimester. However, it was of note that most women who excrete virus during pregnancy do so as a result of recurrent infection [35]. In utero CMV infection more often occurs following recurrent maternal infection than as primary infection.

The prognosis for babies who have clinically apparent disease either in utero or at birth is poor. Ultrasound findings include IUGR that may be symmetrical

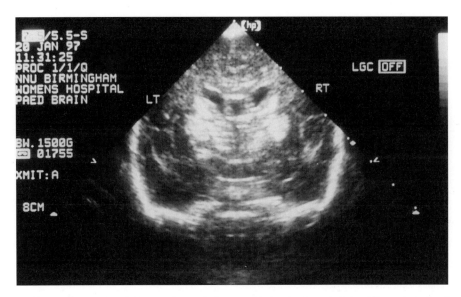

Fig. 3.2 A coronal view of a neonatal cranial ultrasound indicating hyperechogenic areas lateral and medial to the lateral ventricles (this ultrasound image was provided by Mrs Gillian Cattel, Senior Radiographer at Birmingham Women's Hospital, with permission).

or asymmetrical. There may also be microcephaly and cerebral calcification (Fig. 3.2) seen lateral to the ventricles [36] and around the basal ganglia [37,38]. Histologically, the viral encephalitis causes little if any inflammatory response but CMV inclusion may be visualised (Fig. 3.3). Other relatively common ultrasound findings include microcephaly, or ventriculomegaly, or both [39,40], hyperechogenic bowel [41] and, rarely, non-immune hydrops or fetal cardiac rhythm disturbance, or both [42]. Increased placental thickness may be noted on ultrasonography. This is because the transplacental passage of CMV may cause chronic villitis. This is composed almost entirely of plasma cells and there may also be focal necrosis of both trophoblasts and the microvasculature (Fig. 3.4). CMV has a predilection to infect and destroy trophoblast [43]. Occasionally, characteristic inclusion bodies of cytomegalic cells may be visualised. Certainly, retrospective PCR–DNA techniques have been utilised to elucidate the possible aetiology of severe fatal IUGR. Up to 35 per cent of all of these cases had evidence of CMV infection, which therefore, in this cohort, seems to indicate that CMV infection is a relatively common cause of fetal demise from IUGR [44]. Fetuses with congenital CMV as an aetiological cause of IUGR appear to have an abnormality of placental amino acid transport. In congenital CMV-infected fetuses, there was a decrease in valine and glycine levels compared with congenital CMV-infected fetuses with normal fetal growth. There was also a lower fetal concentration of these amnio acids compared with maternal levels in the intrauterine growth-restricted fetuses [45]. Thus, amino acid metabolic anomalies in the placenta of IUGR pregnancies may be further worsened by the presence of CMV infection.

The most common findings in the affected neonate include petechiae and thrombocytopenia, which occurs in up to 80 per cent of cases, hepatosplenomegaly, in 70 per cent, and jaundice, in 55 per cent. Up to 40 per cent of

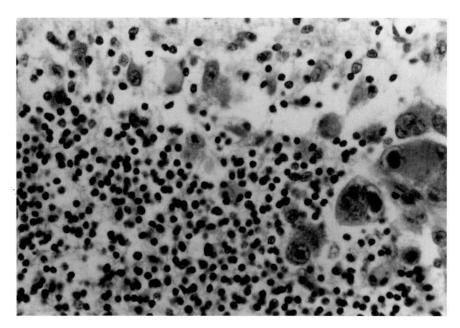

Fig. 3.3 Histological section of the fetal cerebral cortex indicating viral encephalitis with CMV inclusions.

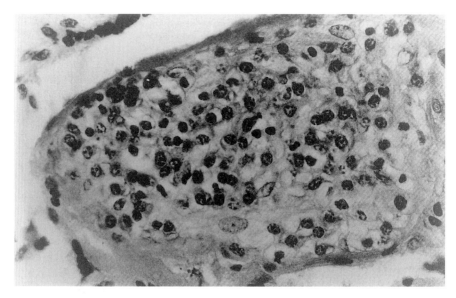

Fig. 3.4 Section of a placental villus indicating infiltration of the villus consisting almost entirely of plasma cells both within the stroma and perivascularly (reproduced from [6] by permission of Benirschke K, Kaufmann P).

fetuses are born SGA in the neonatal period, with 40 per cent of neonates having significant microcephaly and rarely associated seizures, interstitial pneumonias and congenital deafness [46]. As previously stated, the incidence of congenital infection varies between different populations depending upon the socio-economic distribution [35]. It may thus range between 0.3 and 3 per cent of live births. Of these, 5 per cent will be symptomatic at birth with a neonatal mortality of 30 per cent and long term handicap in many survivors. This includes neurodevelopmental delay in up to 90 per cent, hearing loss in 60 per cent and neurological deficits including abnormal and low IQ [24,47,48].

Many cases of congenital CMV infection are not diagnosed until the neonatal period. Prenatal diagnosis in the fetus is based upon prospective ultrasound findings or if there is some suspicion of maternal infection from serology. Isolation of CMV in amniotic fluid appears to be a reliable index of congenital infection, using PCR. Eight series reported 423 patients, in which the indication for prenatal testing was primary maternal CMV infection in the absence of fetal abnormalities on ultrasound [31,49–54]. One hundred and fifty-eight fetuses were found to be infected (37.4 per cent), and approximately 40–45% of infected fetuses had negative virus-specific IgM and 30 per cent had normal haematlogical and biochemical findings at blood sampling. These data highlight the difficulties in counselling patients in whom primary infection is suspected before viability. The rate of fetal infection is high but the sensitivity of prenatal diagnosis, even when multiple tests are performed and repeat amniocentesis is performed, is less than 90 per cent [55]. One study evaluating the PCR detection of CMV in amniotic fluid indicated that the sensitivity of the test was 69.2 per cent with one case being diagnosed at a second sampling. PCR was able to detect one additional infected fetus as compared with virus isolation from the amniotic fluid (sensitivity 76.9 per cent). Nested PCR (using more than one set of primers) did not increase the sensitivity of prenatal diagnosis. In this series three cases were not diagnosed at all using these techniques and the specificity of virus isolation from and DNA detection by PCR in amniotic fluid was 100 per cent. The negative predictive value of virus isolation from amniotic fluid was 76.5 per cent and for DNA detection by PCR it was 81.2 per cent. These results highlight that neither direct virus isolation nor PCR techniques are completely specific. The timing of prenatal diagnosis remains a crucial variable in dealing with women at risk of congenital CMV. It appears that amniocentesis for culture and PCR 4 to 6 weeks after documented primary infection allow early detection and the option for termination of pregnancy. However, the risk of a false negative diagnosis appears to increase with too short an interval from infection.

Fetal blood sampling (FBS) has been suggested as having a role in indicating which infected fetuses have organ damage in that those with normal haematological and biochemical indices are less likely to have serious sequelae because of the lack of fetal viraemia [51]. However, other groups [e.g. 50] have indicated that fetal haematological/biochemical changes may not concur with serological or microbiological confirmation of infection. In this series, serial prenatal testing using FBS may have a role in identifying which candidates may benefit from fetal therapy.

If primary CMV from transplacental transmission in pregnancy is confirmed, there is a 5 to 10 per cent chance of severe congenital disease. This, in association with ultrasound finding (including IUGR at an early gestational stage), therefore indicates a high probability of perinatal morbidity and mortality. It is in this

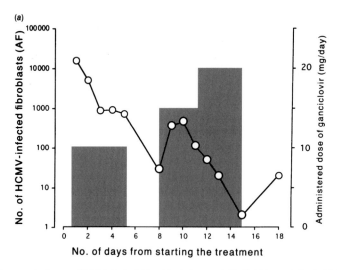

Fig. 3.5 Changes in human CMV-infected fibroblasts in amniotic fluid in an infected fetus in utero. Changes of CMV infectivity with number of days of treatment with Ganciclovir (reproduced from [58] Fisk NM, Moise KJ, editors, Fetal therapy: invasive and transplacental, Cambridge University Press, 1997, by permission).

group that termination of pregnancy should be considered. Recurrent disease carries a much lower risk of morbidity but, again, ultrasound evidence of disease may well put fetuses into a poor prognostic group. Attempts have been made to treat the infected fetus directly with antiviral agents, such as ganciclovir, either transplacentally [56] or directly into the fetus. In one case, ganciclovir has been reported to have been administered prenatally (given to the mother intra-vascularly) in a fetus with documented CMV infection, abnormal liver function tests and thrombocytopenia [57]. Two courses of treatment led to a dramatic reduction in viral load (as estimated by cytopathic effect in fibroblasts) with nor-malisation of platelet count and γ-glutamyl-transpeptidase concentrations (Fig. 3.5, [58]). However, ganciclovir has renal, hepatic and bone marrow toxicities and has a poor transplacental passage; therefore, treating the fetus via the mother presents problems. It should be noted that there are no randomised controlled trials indicating the efficacy of such therapy.

Other antiviral agents have been utilised, such as arabinoside (ara-A) and cyto-sine arabinoside (ara-C), in neonates with severe clinical infections although, again, these drugs have major cytotoxicity. Recent data in small series have indi-cated good results when ganciclovir is used to treat serious CMV infection (retinitis and oesophagitis) in AIDS patients [59] and as a prophylactic agent to prevent CMV after organ transplantation [60]. These data have lead to the hope that this therapy may be effective in the management of neonatal symptomatic disease.

The possibility of prevention seems remote. Routine screening for CMV posi-tivity in women is unlikely to be valuable since no vaccine is available and little can be done to prevent infection in those who are seronegative. Women in high risk groups of seroconversion, such as those who are immunosuppressed, may avoid intimate contact during their pregnancy [7]. Vaccines have been developed but are not useful because of concerns about the ontogenic potential and the risks of reactivation of the live attenuated viruses used [7].

Thus, congenital CMV may cause early onset IUGR that is commonly associated with other ultrasound findings. Such findings (along with a prospective diagnosis of fetal CMV viraemia) carry a high probability of perinatal morbidity and mortality.

Rubella

The rubella virus is an RNA-containing togavirus with only one identified serotype [8]. It consists of a single positive-stranded polyadenylated 40 S RNA of 9,756 nucleotides, enclosed in a nucleocapsid. The virus itself contains three structural proteins: two membrane-bound glycoproteins and a non-glycosylated capsid protein. In vertebrate cell cultures, the reproductive cycle of the rubella virus is longer than that of the alpha viruses. In Varo cells, virus production reaches a peak at 48 hours after infection and genomic and subgenomic RNA can be detected from 12 hours after infection [9].

Postnatally acquired infection occurs in a world-wide distribution. Before the introduction of vaccination, outbreaks usually occurred in the spring and early summer in temperate climate regions. Infection is uncommon in preschool children, but endemic outbreaks involving schoolchildren and young adults have been described. Occasionally, extensive world-wide pandemics have occurred and these have been responsible for high incidences reported in the United States, United Kingdom and Australia [9]. The augmentation of the rubella vaccination programme in 1988, in which the measles, mumps and rubella (MMR) vaccine was offered to preschool children of both sexes, resulted in a marked reduction in the incidence of rubella by increasing herd immunity and the lowest ever recorded number of cases in 1992 [61]. The rubella virus is transmitted by respiratory droplets and initially causes a nasopharyngeal infection that spreads to the cervical lymph nodes. It is then disseminated haematogenously and gives rise to constitutional symptoms including malaise and fever. A macular pinpoint rash appears on the face and trunk and then spreads to the extremities, with lesions coalescing to form an erythematous maculopapular rash. Lesions can also be seen on the soft palate. The rash lasts for a few days and is associated with occipital lymphadenopathy. It is primarily a mild disease of children, with a peak incidence at between 5 and 9 years of age and an incubation period of 13 to 20 days. Only on rare occasions have serious sequelae such as central nervous system involvement and thrombocytopenia developed. By reproductive age, about 75–85% of the population has had rubella, about half of whom have experienced subclinical infection. Once "wild" virus infection occurs, even if subclinical, immunity is lifelong. Infected individuals shed the virus from the nasopharynx several days before the onset of the rash and several days after its disappearance.

In the pregnant mother, most cases of suspected maternal infection present either as a contact with another affected individual (often a child) or a suspected rash. The clinical diagnosis is often difficult because it resembles a number of other exanthemas. Rubella virus can be isolated from the bloodstream and throat 7 to 10 days after exposure. Demonstration of a rise in IgM titres makes a

prospective diagnosis but a high antibody titre in a single sample is not diagnostic. For this reason, and because symptoms may not develop until after the
incubation period, a further maternal sample to detect anti-IgM rubella should
be measured 3 weeks after the first. Anti-rubella antibodies may be detected
using a haemagglutinating inhibition antibody (HIA) test. After wild virus infection, HIA titres usually remain positive for life. This IgG class of antibody has
been the most commonly used test for screening and a titre of more than one in
eight is conclusive evidence of immunity. Up to 15 per cent of women with
remote rubella infection have stable HIA titres of less than one in 256. If a repeat
titre shows a fourfold rise, the patient has acute rubella infection. Because of variations between laboratories and day to day variation, it is essential that paired
serum samples be tested on the same day in the laboratory. Antibody titres measured by other techniques such as the complement fixation test and ELISAs
become maximal several days later and many laboratories are switching to the
latter (ELISA) because of the rapidity with which the test can be done, its sensitivity and economy. Once detected, titres may remain elevated for years. Rubella-
specific IgM antibodies may be detected within a few days of development of the
rash and often remain elevated for a month or two after infection [62,63]. False
positives for anti-rubella IgM may occur in the presence of connective tissue diseases or infection with other viruses such as Epstein–Barr virus, CMV or parvovirus B19. Natural infection is followed by a very high order of protection
from reinfection. Initial reports have suggested that asymptomatic reinfection in
early pregnancy has been unlikely to be associated with fetal infection even
when a specific IgM response has been detected. However, there have been several
anecdotal cases described where rubella virus has been isolated from products
of conception when congenital rubella syndrome has been diagnosed in
patients with clinical reinfection [64]. It has been calculated that the risk of fetal
infection in a maternal reinfection is approximately 8 per cent in the first
16 weeks of pregnancy but that fetal malformations associated with the syndrome
are rare [65].

Gregg in Australia [66] first made the original description of congenital rubella
syndrome. Affected neonates had a classic triad of congenital anomalies comprising cataracts, deafness and congenital heart disease. In these classic series,
deafness was present in 70 per cent of patients, cataracts in 30 per cent and heart
defects that commonly affected the aortic and pulmonary outflow tracts in 20 per
cent of subjects. Central nervous system anomalies such as microcephaly have
also been described. Overall, the risk of congenital rubella syndrome is about
20 per cent for a primary maternal infection in the first trimester. The risk
ranges from 50 per cent in the first 4 weeks to 10 per cent at 12 weeks. Affected
neonates have a mortality of up to 20 per cent and survivors have significant
neurodevelopmental impairment.

Congenital infection occurs via transplacental transmission. Rubella virus is
also excreted via the cervix for at least 6 days after the onset of rash and may
multiply anywhere in the genital tract. Endothelial damage in the placenta and
fetus is extremely common with pathological lesions of "endangitis obliterans"
seen in many cases [67]. There is also evidence that cells may desquamate into the
lumen of the vessels and be transported into the fetal circulation and cause virus-
infected emboli to spread to various fetal organs. The marked absence of any
inflammatory cellular response is characteristic. In addition to virus-induced
tissue necrosis, the rubella virus itself induces retardation in cell division; this is

due to the presence of the rubella-specific protein, which reduces the rate of mitosis in infected cells. If this occurs at a critical phase of organogenesis, it is likely to cause major and multiple developmental defects. The cytopathic effects are also likely to be the aetiological cause of IUGR associated with this viral infection.

The risk of fetal damage is not just confined to the first trimester of pregnancy but after this time it decreases to less than 1 per cent [68].

The rubella also causes a viral villitis with focal trophoblastic necrosis, capillary endothelial damage, decidual perivascular round cell infiltration and enlarged Höfbauer cells [69].

Since virtually all cases of congenital rubella syndrome occur after infection in the first trimester of pregnancy, the detection of a growth-restricted baby with multiple congenital abnormalities is often visualised on ultrasound examination. In such circumstances, the only therapeutic option is termination of pregnancy. Indeed, in most patients who demonstrate a rising fourfold increase in anti-rubella IgM titres in the first trimester this finding would be sufficient grounds to consider ending the pregnancy. A late presentation after contact with rubella, or if a baby presents with ultrasound evidence of congenital malformations either suggestive of viral infection or where there is a history of viral infection, requires attempts to be made to confirm fetal infection directly. Viral isolation in amniotic fluid has been described but requires culture of the virus and has a high rate of false negatives. The use of PCR to detect virus in amniotic fluid should theoretically improve the sensitivity and specificity of diagnosis. Specific anti-rubella IgM may be demonstrated in a fetal blood sample but interpretation of such data, even after 22 weeks of gestation, is complex owing to the developing fetal immunity. Daffos [70] first described FBS to detect IgM titres but, despite this, one in six IgM-negative fetuses were infected at birth. Such information indicates the problems in interpreting fetal blood immunology when the immune system is undergoing major development.

The main therapeutic efforts in preventing congenital rubella syndrome have been aimed at vaccination programmes that are widely acceptable and readily implementable. The aim of the rubella vaccination programme is to prevent women acquiring rubella while pregnant. Seroconversion and lifelong immunity occur in 95 per cent of vaccinated individuals [65,71]. Two main vaccination policies have evolved:

1. Universal immunisation, which aims to interrupt transmission of the virus by vaccinating all preschool children (both boys and girls) and, therefore, to increase herd immunity. This policy requires a high uptake of vaccine among preschool children to be completely effective.
2. Selective vaccination has previously been employed in the United Kingdom, involves the selective vaccination of girls prior to reproductive age. Over the last 20 years, universal immunisation with herd immunity has been shown to reduce the prevalence of congenital rubella syndrome more markedly than the selective policies. Women of childbearing age who are seronegative should be offered immunisation, and contraception should be utilised for 3 months after vaccination. In a group of women who have been vaccinated inadvertently while pregnant, no congenital malformations have been described.

Varicella–Zoster Virus Infection

VZV, a member of the herpes virus family, is a DNA virus. Primary infection causes the childhood illness of "chicken pox" and may lead to latency of the virus in the sensory dorsal root ganglia. Reactivation of the virus later in life may give rise to "shingles". The common childhood disease is marked by typical skin lesions, which progress from a maculopapular to a vesiculopustular rash. The rash and VZV are highly contagious and have an incubation period of between 10 and 20 days.

Varicella is an unusual infection in adults and probably occurs with no greater frequency in pregnant women. The incidence of VZV infection during pregnancy has been estimated at up to 5 per 10,000 births [72]. Immunity once the subject has had an infection is then lifelong and "chicken pox" does not recur, although reactivation of VZV may occur in immunosuppressed individuals, giving rise to shingles. Ninety per cent of adults have immunity to VZV infection.

Infection in pregnancy may give rise to a fulminating varicella pneumonia, which has a reported maternal mortality of up to 25 per cent [73]. However, the vast majority of pregnant women who have an infection do not develop pulmonary signs. If this complication does occur, it begins on the 2nd to 6th day after the appearance of the rash and is associated with a non-productive cough. The patient may then develop pleuritic chest pain, haemoptysis, dyspnoea and frank cyanosis. Patients will need to be managed in a high dependency settling with full hospitalisation including availability of respiratory support.

A number of serological assays to detect antibodies to VZV infection have been utilised. These techniques include compliment fixation, immune adherence haemagglutination, fluorescent antibody against membrane antigen and ELISA. Because ELISA is the most readily available, it has become the method of choice for measuring antibodies. Both IgM and IgG antibodies appear with between 2 and 5 days after the rash and peak at 4 weeks. The acute IgM may remain elevated for 1 to 2 months after infection while IgG persists and confers lifelong immunity (present in 90 per cent of the adult population).

Transplacental VZV transmission before 20 weeks may be associated with a congenital varicella syndrome, but it is rare. The risk to the fetus of congenital infection differs with gestational age. Prevalences appear to be higher if infection occurs in the first trimester [74]. The virus when transmitted transplacentally infects the fetal tissues and is neurotrophic and denervates fetal structures. The VZV infection may cause multiple placental infarcts without viral inclusions. However, more commonly, no abnormality is seen at all (see below).

The congenital varicella syndrome of cutaneous scars, limb reduction defects, chorioretinitis and cataracts [75] has been found, in two cohort and three prospective studies, to occur with a cumulative rate of 2.8 per cent in first trimester infection. It is thus now appreciated that maternal VZV infection in the first 4 months of pregnancy rarely produces a congenital varicella syndrome.

The ultrasound findings associated with congenital varicella infection include ascites (with or without hydrops fetalis) and echogenic foci within the liver. There may also be associated polyhydramnios. Reduced fetal growth velocity and IUGR may also occur [76]. Sonographic monitoring for the detection of central nervous system abnormalities, including ventriculomegaly, carries a dismal prognosis.

Although the risk of congenital varicella syndrome is small, some authorities have recommended administration of varicella–zoster immunoglobulin (VZIG) to suspected pregnant women who have not had previous varicella but have been in contact with an infected individual within 96 hours. However, this treatment is expensive and there are no trials that have been conducted to establish benefit. The use of VZIG is, however, recommended in non-immune pregnant women who are in contact with the disease [77]. Acyclovir is also indicated in infected immunocompromised pregnant women and in pregnant women with varicella pneumonia. Treatment with VZIG is safe and does decrease maternal clinical manifestations of disease, such as pneumonia. The use of VZIG should thus be used to protect against maternal infection. Once sonographic evidence of infection occurs then morbidity may not be modified by antiviral therapy. There is some debate as to whether or not the congenital malformations associated with VZV infection are due to direct effects of the primary virus infection or whether they are a consequence of the VZV "scarring" in utero. Embryopathy may be the result of intrauterine reactivation of the virus and an inadequate cell-mediated fetal immune response being the cause for short latency between primary infection and the development of the herpes zoster infection. In women who have been infected by VZV infection in the first half of gestation, serial ultrasound is used to detect the more obvious structural abnormalities.

PCR using primers that define a 221 base pair (b.p.) region of the gene encoding for the 44 kilodalton (kDa) protein of VZV [77] has recently been used to diagnose prenatal infection in the first and second trimester [17]. This similar rate of maternal–fetal transmission has been documented by detecting VZV IgM antibodies in fetuses undergoing FBS after maternal infection in the first 20 weeks. Given the high frequency of transplacental passage and the low rate of malformations, any role for invasive prenatal diagnosis in the detection of the virus in fetal blood, amniotic fluid or chorionic villi would mainly be that of reassuring women whose fetuses tested negative.

Maternal infection at around the time of delivery may lead to neonatal chicken pox. In mothers whose rash appears between 5 days before and 2 days after delivery, the neonatal disease may be severe, with a fatality rate of up to 30 per cent. Prophylactic immunoglobulin is recommended for neonates delivering in this window.

Human Immunodeficiency Virus

HIV is one of five known human retroviruses. These organisms are single-stranded RNA-envelope viruses that have the ability to become incorporated into the host's cellular DNA. HIV-1, which used to be called human T-cell lymphotrophic virus III, has a diameter of about 100 nm. It contains principal core proteins (p18 and p24) and major surface proteins. There has been interest that the surface protein gp120 is a predictor of infectivity. Other retroviruses are much less common.

The HIV-1 virus attaches to host cells at the CD4 receptor and enters the cell. Most cells have a high density of CD4 on their surface and these include particularly lymphocytes, monocytes and neural cells. It is also of interest that some researchers have identified CD4 on Höfbauer cells in the placenta [79]. The virus uses a reverse transcriptase enzyme to produce double-stranded DNA that becomes circular and enters the nucleus [80]. Subsequently, when a cell becomes active, the DNA codes for the production of viral RNA and hence viral protein. The mechanism by which HIV-1 leads to immunodeficiency is by its effect on helper T lymphocytes (CD4). As these cells become progressively depleted, the host becomes susceptible to an increasing array of opportunistic infections. It is thus the peripheral CD4 count that confirms the overwhelming and fulminating HIV infection of AIDS (< 200 mm^2).

It is estimated that there are 4.5 million cases of AIDS and approximately 20 million people infected with HIV-1 virus world-wide. The prevalence of HIV infection in an obstetric population found antibodies only in patients with risk factors (7.1 per cent) whereas those without risk factors were HIV negative [81]. Since the beginning of the AIDS pandemic it has been clear that access to prevention and treatment would not be distributed equally. AIDS has occurred in some offspring and the vertical transmission rate of HIV is estimated to be 24 per cent [82,83]. There has been debate in the past as to whether infection occurs transplacentally or during delivery. However, high titres of HIV DNA have been described within 48 hours of birth, which suggests prenatal transmission in at least some cases [84]. The virus has been isolated from amniotic fluid [85] and placental tissue [86].

A morphological study of placentas by Jauniaux et al. [87] indicated microscopy changes as being minimal. Further ultrastructural studies showed "retrovirus-like particles" in the syncytiotrophoblast although such changes were sparse. Others have found the presence of "C-type particles" between the syncytiotrophoblast and the basement membranes of placenta [88].

In terms of screening, it has been recommended that prenatal HIV testing be offered to women who acknowledge a risk behaviour for HIV, but pilot studies have indicated that up to 40 per cent of HIV-positive women would be missed by such a policy. More recently, and perhaps more logically, the centres for disease control (1989) recommended that "all pregnant women are routinely counselled and encouraged to be tested for HIV infection" [89]. The offer of voluntary testing has repeatedly shown to yield high acceptance rates but, none the less, there have been calls in the medical literature for mandatory screening of all pregnant women, which causes bioethical dilemmas.

In HIV-1 infected women, the chance of vertical transmission to the child varies in different populations. In women in sub-Saharan Africa, rates appear to be as high as 30 per cent [82]. In these individuals, the presence of HIV antigenaemia beyond 18 months or the onset of AIDS or the detection of virus occurred in 16.2 per cent of mother–child pairs [83]. Vertical transmission appeared to be more common in the presence of:

- CD4 counts of less than 200 mm^2
- p24 antigenaemia
- breast feeding [82].

In the Western world, maternal age, parity and the use of intravenous drugs do not seem to be significantly related to vertical transmission, but in sub-Saharan Africa it is multiparity that seems to be the most significant risk factor [90]. Several prospective studies have indicated that the incidence of prematurity and IUGR are significantly higher in babies of HIV-seropositive mothers than in those of seronegative mothers (prematurity seropositive 12.7 per cent versus seronegative 3.8 per cent, $P < 0.01$; IUGR seropositive 7.7 per cent versus seronegative 4.4 per cent, $P < 0.05$) [14].

Also, experimental animal models (using the rhesus monkey *Macaca mulatta*) have indicated that maternal infection with a homologue of simian immunodeficiency virus (SIV) caused severe fetal growth restriction, associated oligohydramnios and altered CD4 counts. These effects were most pronounced when the fetus was infected in the mid-gestational phase (corresponding to the human early second trimester). Later infection appeared to cause less disruption of fetal growth. Interestingly, in this study, there seemed to be a major disruption of placental insulin growth factor (IGF) and IGF-binding protein function. It has been postulated that caesarean section delivery of such babies may significantly reduce the rate of vertical transmission [82]. However, it was estimated in this study that 12 caesarean sections needed to be performed to prevent one infected infant.

The ACTG076 study randomising women to placebo or active drug treatment enrolled 477 infected women with a CD4 count of > 200 per μl [91]. Women received zidovudine (AZT) antenatally (100 mg orally five times a day and intravascularly as a bolus of 2 mg/kg over an hour, followed by one mg/kg per hour infusion). Their children also received AZT (2 mg/kg four times a day for 6 weeks). This study demonstrated a 67.5 per cent (95% CI 40.7–82.1) reduction in the risk of HIV transmission compared with those women who received placebo. Previous studies have shown that zidovudine was well tolerated by pregnant women and was apparently in itself not associated with malformation, premature birth or fetal distress. There was also no evidence of haematological toxicity in newborns. Zidovudine is converted by intracellular kinases to form the active zidovudine triphosphate, which inhibits retroviral reverse transcriptase. This results in inhibition of HIV-1 replication in vitro and a reduction in viral load in vivo. However, the Concorde coordinating committee trial [92] did not show any long term benefit in single agent therapy. Thus, in these studies, AZT appears to work by reducing, in the short term, the viral load and therefore the risk of exposure of the fetus. Whether this would work in the long term is debatable. Recently, preliminary data from UNAIDS PETRA (PErinatal TRAnsmission) study showed that an abbreviated, more affordable regimen may be effective [93]. In the PETRA protocol, a combination of oral zidovudine/ lamivudine, given only during the intrapartum period and in the early neonatal period (mother and child), yielded a rate of perinatal transmission of only 10.8 per cent. It may be that a shorter course of pharmacoprophylaxis will be more affordable in developing countries and offer a significant reduction in perinatal transmission rates [93].

As with other transplacental viral infections of the fetus, the presence of IUGR in women with HIV-1 and/or AIDS is associated with first or second trimester infection and usually heralds increased perinatal morbidity and mortality.

Conclusion

Maternal viraemia (of several viral families) with transplacental infection to the fetus can lead to IUGR with or without significant structural fetal anomalies. In general terms, the earlier such infection occurs, the more likely an adverse outcome is to arise. Animal models have demonstrated that many viruses not associated with human infection may cause significant cytopathic effects during organogenesis and lead to multiple structural abnormalities and IUGR. Such viruses include alpha virus [94]) herpes simplex virus type 2 [95], blue tongue virus and bovine virus [96,97]. The association of IUGR and maternal/fetal viraemia often carries a poor prognosis. In most instances, perinatal morbidity and mortality are significantly increased and there is little evidence that therapeutic intervention may improve prognosis. In many instances, therefore, termination of pregnancy or delivery of a live neonate and evaluation in the newborn period is at present the only therapeutic option.

References

1. Ounsted M, Moar V, Scott WA. Perinatal morbidity and mortality in small-for-dates babies: the relative importance of some maternal factors. Early Hum Dev 1981;5:367–9.
2. Teberg AJ, Walther FJ, Pena IC. Mortality, morbidity and outcome of small for gestational age infants. Semin Perinatol 1988;11:84–9.
3. Lin C-C, Su S-J, River LP. Comparisons of associated high risk factors and perinatal outcome between symmetric and asymmetric fetal intrauterine growth retardation. Am J Obstet Gynecol 1991;164:1535–9.
4. Klein JO, Remington JS, Marcy SM. Current concepts of infection of the fetus and newborn. In: Remington JS, Klein JO, editors. Infectious disease of the fetus and newborn, 3rd edn, ch. 1. Philadelphia: WB Saunders, 1990;11–15.
5. Krebs C, Macara LM, Leiser R, Bowman AW, Greer IA, Kingdom JC. Intrauterine growth restriction with absent end diastolic flow velocity in the umbilical artery is associated with maldevelopment of the placental terminal villous tree. Am J Obstet Gynecol 1996;175:1534–42.
6. Benirschke K, Kaufmann P, editors. Pathology of the human placenta, 3rd edn. London: Springer-Verlag, 1995.
7. Alford CA, Stagno S, Pass RF, Britt WJ. Congenital and perinatal cytomegalovirus infection. Rev Infect Dis 1990;12:S745–53.
8. Banatavala JE, Best JM. Rubella in Topley and Wilson's principles of bacteriology, virology and immunology, 8th edn, vol 4. 1991.
9. Best JM, Banatvala JE. In: Zuckerman AJ, Banatvala JE, Patterson JR, editors. Principles and practice of clinical virology, 3rd edn, ch. 11. Chichester: John Wiley, 1995;363–400.
10. Alford CA Jr. Rubella. In: Remington JS, Klein JO, editors. Infectious diseases of the fetus and newborn. Philadelphia:WB Saunders, 1976;356–8.
11. Bart SW, Steller HC, Prebuld SR. Fetal risk associated with rubella vaccine: an update. Rev Infect Dis 1985;7:595–9.
12. Harrison CJ, Myers MG. Relation of maternal CMV viraemia and antibody response to the rate of congenital infection and intrauterine growth restriction. J Med Virol 1990;31:222–8.
13. Balducci J, Rodis JF, Rosengren S. Pregnancy outcome following first trimester varicella infection. Obstetr Gynaecol 1992;79:5–9.
14. Bulterys M, Chao A, Munyemana S, Kurawige JB, Nawrocki P. Maternal human immunodeficiency virus I infection and intrauterine growth: a prospective cohort study in Butare, Rwanda. Paediatr Infect Dis J 1994;13:94–100.
15. Creasy RK, Resnik R (1994) Intrauterine growth restriction. In: Maternal fetal medicine. Principles and practice, 3rd edn, ch. 36. Philadelphia: WB Saunders, 1994;561.
16. Branch DW, Scott JR. Immunology of pregnancy. In: Creasy RK, Resnik R, editors. Maternal-fetal medicine principles and practice, 3rd edn, ch. 6. Philadelphia: WB Saunders, 1994;115–27.
17. Bennett P, Nicolini U. Fetal infections: In: Fisk MN, Moise KJ, editors. Fetal therapy: invasive and transplacental, ch. 8. Cambridge: Cambridge University Press, 1997;92–116.
18. Morell A, Sidiropoulos D, Herrmann U. IgG sub-classes in antibodies to group B streptococci, pneumococci and tetanus toxoid in pre-term neonates after intravenous infusions of immunoglobulins to the mother. Paediatr Res 1986;20:933–6.
19. Weller TH. The cytomegaloviruses: the difficult years. J Infect Dis 1970;122:532–9.
20. Grose C, Weiner CP. Prenatal diagnosis of congenital cytomegalovirus infection: Two decades later. Am J Obstet Gynecol 1990;163:447–50.

21. Hanshaw JB. Congenital cytomegalovirus infection: a fifteen year prospective study. J Infect Dis 1971;123:555–9.
22. Hanshaw JB, Scheiner AP, Moxley AW. School failure and deafness after "silent" congenital cytomegalovirus infection. N Engl J Med 1976;295:468–71.
23. Ryan M, Miller E, Waight P. Public Health Laboratory Survey: Communicable disease report. Cytomegalovirus infection in England and Wales: 1992 and 1993. London: Public Health Laboratory, 1995; R74–6.
24. Stagno S, Pass RF, Cloud G, Britt WJ, Henderson RE, Walton PD, et al. Primary cytomegalovirus infection in pregnancy: Incidence, transmission to fetus and clinical outcome. JAMA 1986;256:1904–8.
25. Balfour CL, Balfour HH. Cytomegalovirus is not an occupational risk for nurses in renal transplant and neonatal units. JAMA 1986;256:1909–12.
26. Chandler SH, Alexander ER, Holmes HE. Epidemiology of cytomegalovirus infection in a heterogenous population of pregnant women. J Infect Dis 1985;152:249–54.
27. Monif GRG, Egan EA, Held B. The correlation of maternal cytomegalovirus infection during varying stages of gestation and neonatal involvement. J Paediatr 1972;80:17–21.
28. Stanier P, Kitchen AD, Taylor DL, Tyms AS. Detection of human cytomegalovirus in peripheral mononuclear cells and urine samples using polymerase chain reaction. Mol Cell Probes 1992;6:51–8.
29. Griffiths PD, Stagno S, Pass RF, Smith RJ, Alfred CA. Infection with cytomegalovirus in pregnancy: specific IgM antibodies as a marker of recent infection. J Infect Dis 1982;145:647–53.
30. Demmler GJ. Summary of a workshop on surveillance for congenital cytomegalovirus disease. Rev Infect Dis 1991;13:315–27.
31. Lamy ME, Mulongo KN, Gadisseux JF, Lyon G, Gaudey V, van Lierde M. Prenatal diagnosis of fetal cytomegalovirus infection. Am J Obstet Gynecol 1992;166:91–4.
32. Stagno S, Pass RF, Dworsky ME, Alford CA. Maternal cytomegalovirus infection and perinatal transmission. Clin Obstet Gynaecol 1982;25:563–76.
33. Tookey PA, Peckham CS. Cytomegalovirus. In: Greenhough A, Osbourne J, Sutherland S, editors. Congenital perinatal and neonatal infection. London: Churchill Livingstone, 1992;49–61.
34. Stern J, Tucker SM. Prospective study of cytomegalovirus infection in pregnancy. BMJ 1973;2:268–71.
35. Stagno S, Whitley RJ. Herpes virus infection in pregnancy. I: Cytomegalovirus and Epstein Barr Virus Infection. N Engl J Med 1985a;313:1270–4.
36. Ghidini A, Sirtori M, Regarni P, Marini S, Tucci E, Scola GC. Fetal intracranial calcifications. Am J Obstet Gynecol 1989;160:86–7.
37. Estroff JA, Parad RB, Teele RL. Echogenic vessels in the fetal thalami and basal ganglia associated with cytomegalovirus infection. J Ultrasound Med 1992;11:687–8.
38. Fakhry J, Khoury A. Fetal intracranial calcifications – the importance of periventricular hypoechogenic foci without shadowing. J Ultrasound Med 1991;10:51–4.
39. Twickler DM, Perlman J, Maeberry MC. Congenital cytomegalovirus presenting as cerebral ventriculomegaly on antenatal ultrasonography. Am J Perinatol 1993;10:404–6.
40. Drose JA, Dennis MA, Thickman D. Infection in-utero; ultrasound findings in 19 cases. Radiology 1991;178:369–74.
41. Forouzan I. Fetal abdominal echogenic mass: an early sign of intrauterine cytomegalovirus infection. Obstet Gynaecol 1992;80:535–7.
42. Monteagudo A, Matera C, Marx F. In-utero sonographic diagnosis of congenital cytomegalovirus infection. Society of Perinatal Obstetrics – 10th Annual Meeting, Houston, Texas, 1990;326 [abst].
43. Amirhessami-Aghili N, Manalo P, Hall MR, Tibbits FD, Ort CA, Afsari A (1987). Human CMV infection of human placental explants in culture. Am J Obstet Gynecol. 156:1365–74.
44. Liu B, Tao W, Liu D. The relationship between placental pathology and certain pathogens detected in paraffin embedded tissues in cases of intrauterine growth restriction. Chin J Obstet Gynaecol 1996;31:90–2.
45. Ljubic A, Cvetkovic M, Sulovic V, Novakov A, Kokai D, Bujko M, et al.Essential and non-essential amnio acids in appropriate and small for gestational age fetuses with congenital cytomegalovirus infection. Clin Exp Obstet Gynaecol 1997;24:207–8.
46. Pass RF, Stanno S, Myers GJ. Outcome of symptomatic congenital cytomegalovirus infection; results of long term longitudinal follow up. Pediatrics 1980;66:758–62.
47. Peckham CS, Johnson C, Ades A, Pearl K, Chin KS. Early acquisition of cytomegalovirus infection. Arch Dis Child 1987;62:780–5.
48. Preece PM, Pearl KN, Peckham CS. Congenital cytomegalovirus infection. Arch Dis Child 1984;59:1120

49. Lynch L, Daffos F, Emanuel D, Giovangrandi Y, Meisel R, Forestirer F, Cathomas G, Berkowitz RL. Prenatal diagnosis for cytomegalovirus infection. Am J Obstet Gynecol 1991;156:714–18.

50. Nicolini U, Kustermann A, Tassis B, Fogliani R, Fogliani R, Gamberti A, et al. Prenatal diagnosis of congenital human cytomegalovirus. Prenat Diagn 1994;14:903–6.

51. Hohlfeld P, Daffos F, Costa JM, Thulliez P, Forestirer F, Vidaud M. Prenatal diagnosis of congenital toxoplasmosis with a polymerase chain reaction test in amniotic fluid. N Engl J Med 1994;331:695–9.

52. Wen L, Wu S, Lu S. The epidemiological study of human cytomegalovirus infection of pregnant women and the maternal fetal transmission in 3 Chinese metropolis. Chin J Obstet Gynaecol 1996;31:714–17.

53. Ruellan-Eugene G, Barjot P, Campet M, Vabret A, Herlicoviez M, Muller G, et al. The evaluation of virological procedures to detect fetal human cytomegalovirus infection; avidity of IgG antibodies, virus detection in amniotic fluid and maternal serum. J Med Virol 1996;50:9–15.

54. Revello MG, Baldanti F, Furione M, Sarasini A, Percivalle E, Zavattoin M, et al. Polymerase chain reaction for prenatal diagnosis of human congenital cytomegalovirus infection. J Med Virol 1995;47:462–6.

55. Hagay ZY, Biran G, Ornoy A, Reece EA. Congenital cytomegalovirus infection: a longstanding problem still seeking a solution. Am J Obstet Gynecol 1996;174:241–5.

56. Einsele H, Eininger G, Steidle M, Vallbracht A, Mueller M, Schmidt H, et al. Polymerase chain reaction to evaluate antiviral therapy for cytomegalovirus. Lancet 1991;338:1170–2.

57. Revello MG, Percivalle E, Baldanti F. Prenatal treatment of congenital human cytomegalovirus infection by intravascular administration of Ganciclovir to the fetus. Clin Diagn Virol 1993;1:61–7.

58. Fisk NM, Moise KJ, editors. Fetal therapy: invasive and transplacental. Cambridge: Cambridge University Press, 1997.

59. Collaborative DHPG treatment study group: treatment of serious cytomegalovirus infection with 9-(1-3-dihydroxypropoxymethyl) quanine in a patient with AIDS and other deficiencies. N Engl J Med 1986;314:801–3.

60. Merigan TC, Runlund DG, Keay S. A controlled trial of Ganciclovir to prevent cytomegalovirus disease after heart transplantation. N Engl J Med 1992;326:1182–3.

61. Miller E, Maight PA, Vurdien JE. Rubella surveillance to December 1992: Second joint report from the PHLS and national rubella surveillance programme. CDR Rev 1993;3:R35–40.

62. Hermann KL. Available rubella serological tests. Rev Obstet Dis 1985;7:S109.

63. Sidle N. Rubella in pregnancy. London: SENSE, 1985.

64. Best JM, O'Shea S. Rubella virus. In: Schmidt N, Emmons RW, editors. Diagnostic procedures for viral rickettsial and chlamydial infections, 6th edn. Washington DC: American Public Health Association, 1989.

65. Morgan-Capner P, Miller A, Vurdien JE, Ramsay MEB. Outcome of pregnancy after maternal reinfection with rubella. CDR Rev 1991;1:R57–9.

66. Gregg NM. Cataract following German measles in the mother. Trans Ophth Soc Aust 1941;3:34–6.

67. Horn LC, Buttner W, Horn E (1993). Rotelnbedingte Plazentaveranderungen. Perinatal Med. 5:5–10.

68. Ender G, Nickerl-Pacher U, Muller E, Craddock-Watson JE. Outcome of confirmed preconceptual maternal rubella. Lancet 1988;i:1445–7.

69. Ornoy A, Segal S, Nishmi M, Simcha A, Polishuk W. Fetal and placental pathology in gestational rubella. Am J Obstet Gynecol 1973;116:949–56.

70. Daffos F, Forestier F, Grangeot-Keros L, Pavlovsky MC, Lebon P, Chartier M, et al. Prenatal diagnosis of congenital rubella. Lancet 1984;ii:1–3.

71. Morgan-Capner P. The detection of rubella specific antibody. Public Health Lab Serv Microbiol Dig 1983;1:6–11.

72. Stagno S, Whitney RJ. Herpes virus infection of pregnancy. 2. Herpes simplex virus and varicella zoster virus infection. N Engl J Med 1985b;313:1327–30.

73. Smego RA, Asperilla MO. Use of Acyclovir for varicella pneumonia during pregnancy. Obstet Gynaecol 1991;78:1112–15.

74. Pastuszak AL, Levy M, Schick B, Zuber C, Feldkamp M. Outcome after maternal varicella infection in the first 20 weeks of pregnancy. N Engl J Med 1994;330:901–5.

75. Alkalay AL, Pomerance JJ, Rimoin DL. Fetal varicella syndrome. J Pediatr 1987;111:320–3.

76. Pretorius DH, Haywood I, Jones KL. Sonographic evaluation of pregnancies with maternal varicella infection. J Ultrasound Med 1992;11:459–63.

77. Department of Health, Welsh Office, Scottish Home and Health Departments. Immunization against infectious disease. London: HMSO, 1990.

78. Davison AJ, Scott JE. The complete DNA sequence of varicella zoster virus. J Genet Virol 1986;67:1759–78.
79. Lewis SH, Reynolds-Kohler C, Fox HE, Nelson JA. HIV I in trophoblastic and villus Hofbauer cells and haematological precursors in the eight week fetus. Lancet 1990;335:565–8.
80. Sever JL. HIV biology and immunology. ClinObstet Gynaecol 1989;32:423–39.
81. Barton JJ, O'Connor TM, Cannon MJ, Weldon-Linne CM. Prevalence of human immunodeficiency virus in the general prenatal population. Am J Gynecol 1989;160:1316–24.
82. European Collaborative Study. Risk factors for mother to child transmission of HIV Lancet 31992;39:1007–12.
83. European Collaborative Study. Caesarean section and the risk of vertical tranmission of HIV I infection. Lancet 1994;343:1464–7.
84. Brandt CD, Rakusan TA, Sisson AV, Saxena ES, Ellaurie M, Sever JL. Human immunodeficiency virus infection in infants during the first two months of life: reliable detection and evidence of in-utero transmission. Arch Paediatr Adolesc Med 1994;148:250–4.
85. Mundey DC, Schinazi RF, Gerber AR, Nahmias AJ, Randle HW. The human deficiency virus isolated from amniotic fluid. Lancet 1987;2:459–60.
86. Hill RC, Bolton V, Carlson JR. Isolation of acquired immune deficiency syndrome virus from the placenta. Am J Obstet Gynecol 1987;157:10–13.
87. Jauniaux E, Nessmann C, Imbert MC, Meuris S, Puissant F, Hustin J. Morphological aspects of placenta in HIV pregnancies. Placenta 1988;9:633–42.
88. Kalter SS, Helmke RJ, Heberling RL, Panigel M, Fowler AK, Strickland JE, et al. C type particles in normal human placenta. J Natl Cancer Inst 1973;50:1081–3.
89. Horton R. Women as women with HIV. Lancet 1995;345:531–2.
90. Moodley D, Bobat RA, Cautsoudis A, Coovadia HM. Caesarean section and vertical transmission of HIV-1. Lancet 1994;334:338.
91. Connor EM, Sperling RS, Gelber R, Kiselev P, Scott G, O'Sullivan MJ, et al. Reduction of maternal–infant transmission of HIV type I with Zidovudin treatment. N Engl J Med 1994;331:1173–80.
92. Concorde Co-ordinating Committee, Concorde, MRC/ANRS. Randomised double-blind controlled trial of immediate and deferred Zidovudin in symptom free HIV. Lancet 1994;343:871–81.
93. [Anonymous]. A positive response to perinatal HIV. Lancet 1999;353:511–12.
94. Leonova ES, Karmysheva V, Siannikova NV. Characteristics of experimental alpha virus infection during pregnancy and in the early stages of ontogeny in mice. Vopr Virusol 1983;28:53–9.
95. Ando Y. Studies on the placental damage and intrauterine growth restriction caused by intra-vaginal inocculated herpes simplex virus type 2 during pregnancy. Acta Obstetr Gynaecol Japon 1981;33:681–9.
96. Duffell SJ, Sharp MW, Winkler CE, Terlecki S, Richardson C, Done JT, et al. Bovine virus diarrhoea – mucosal disease virus; induced fetopathy in cattle. Efficacy of prophylactic maternal pre-exposure. J Vet.Sci 1984;68:192–5.
97. Done JT, Terlecki S, Richardson C, Harkness JW, Sands JJ, Paterson DS, et al. Bovine virus, diarrhoea – mucosal disease virus: pathogenicity for fetal calf following maternal infection. Vet Rec 1980;106:473–9.

4 Therapeutic Drugs, Recreational Drugs and Lifestyle Factors

Frank D. Johnstone and David C. Howe

Introduction

Fetal growth is necessarily the result of genetic potential modified by exposure to environmental factors. The fetal environment is of course dictated entirely by maternal physiology, but this in turn is dependent upon the environment to which the mother is exposed. Drugs ingested by the mother are an obvious environmental agent with the potential to affect fetal growth either directly through toxic actions on proliferating cells, or indirectly by altering placental transfer of oxygen and metabolic substrate. In the broadest sense, however, environmental factors might encompass maternal lifestyle and a wide range of variables that are often difficult to precisely define and quantify. For example, low socioeconomic status is linked to many indices of poor health and it is perhaps not surprising that it has been suggested to be linked to low birthweight. Associated with low socioeconomic status there may be poor nutritional intake and higher rates of cigarette smoking, and of teenage pregnancy and high parity, all of which potentially influence fetal growth. Teasing out the important variables is often difficult. This chapter focuses on a number of therapeutic and recreational drugs linked with IUGR, and closes with a consideration of certain aspects of maternal lifestyle that have been suggested to be associated with it.

Therapeutic Drugs

Drugs are prescribed with caution in pregnancy and in many instances there is only limited experience of use in human pregnancy. Pre-existing or developing maternal illness is often associated with prematurity and low birthweight so that it is sometimes impossible to differentiate between the effects of the drugs and the condition for which the drugs were prescribed. We have chosen to concentrate on three particular agents (corticosteroids, cyclosporin A and beta adrenoreceptor antagonists) for which there is reasonable evidence of a specific drug effect in human and animal studies, and a plausible biological mechanism.

51

Corticosteroids

Evidence for an Effect of Corticosteroids on Fetal Growth

Corticosteroids are indicated in pregnancy for modulation of maternal inflammatory response in a number conditions complicating both maternal and fetal health, and specifically for the induction of fetal lung maturity. It is often difficult to avoid the use of steroids in such cases, but as a general principle, consideration should be given to minimise dosage and duration of treatment. The placenta normally presents a metabolic barrier to the transfer of biologically active corticosteroid from mother to fetus in late gestation due to the presence of 11 beta hydroxysteroid dehydrogenase [1,2]. Earlier in gestation there is probably greater transfer of unmetabolised corticosteroid [3,4]. Synthetic fluorinated corticosteroids are resistant to metabolism and have been used specifically to target the fetus for the induction of lung maturation and suppression of the fetal adrenal glands in cases of congenital adrenal hyperplasia [5–7]. Direct intrafetal injection may maximise fetal effects and minimize maternal side effects, but experience with this route of administration is limited. For treatment of maternal conditions, prednisone and prednisolone are the drugs of choice [8] since the placenta converts prednisolone to inactive predisone, and the fetal liver, in contrast to the maternal liver, is unable to convert prednisone back to the active metabolite.

Animal studies strongly suggests that exposure of the fetus to high doses of fluorinated corticosteroids results in intrauterine growth retardation. Because of species differences and differences in drug doses, however, it is not always possible to extrapolate the available data to human pregnancy. Surprisingly there is a paucity of data about the effects of corticosteroids on fetal growth in human pregnancy. Trials of antenatal steroids for lung maturation do not report birthweight controlled for fetal sex and maternal parity in those infants who were exposed to corticosteroid in utero, but were not delivered until term. There is good evidence for an effect of prolonged steroid administration to reduce birthweight from a retrospective analysis of 119 women (and 67 control cases) attending an infertility clinic who received 10 mg daily of prednisone prior to and throughout their pregnancy. It was noted that fetal weight was significantly less in prednisone treated women [9]. In this study all infants were born at term, but 13 per cent of those whose mothers received steroid were below 2.5 kg as opposed to 1.5 per cent in the control group. A case report suggested that even topical steroids when used over a prolonged time have the same effect [10].

Induction of fetal lung maturity exposes the fetus to supraphysiological doses of steroid over a short duration of time (recommendations in the United States of America are betamethasone 12 mg i.m. 24 hours apart, or dexamethasone 6 mg i.m. at 12 hour intervals for four doses [11]. It is calculated that two doses of 12 mg betamethasone 24 hours apart elevates glucocorticoid activity in fetal plasma for at least 72 hours, and that receptor occupancy may occur for even longer because of the high affinity of the synthetic steroid for the glucocorticoid receptor [12]. In non-human primates treated with doses of betamethasone similar to those used for lung maturation in human fetuses, significant reductions in fetal weight, placental weight, lung growth and head circumference have been reported by some [13–15] but not all authors [16]. In other non-primate species short courses of glucocorticoids have also been demonstrated to reduce fetal growth [17–20]. A single injection of 30 micrograms of dexamethasone into a guinea pig fetus markedly reduces cellular proliferation in many organs (as measured by radiolabelled thymidine uptake) for at least seven days [21]. The inhibition of cellular mitosis is dose related. Pregnant ewes given betamethasone at a dose of 0.5 mg/kg at 104 days of gestation (term is about 145 days) give birth to fetuses at term that are about 14 per cent lighter than control animals [20]. Repeated courses of corticosteroids produce an even larger decrease in fetal weight.

Corticosteroids: Mechanisms of Effect on Fetal Growth

In all species that have been investigated the concentrations of endogenous corticosteroids in the fetal circulation increase in late pregnancy and serve as an endocrine switch preparing the fetus for extra-uterine life [22]. It is presumed that the effects of synthetic fluorinated corticosteroids are mediated through premature activation of glucocorticoid and mineralocorticoid receptors in various fetal organs. Interestingly, recent research suggests that 11β hydroxysteroid dehydrogenase in the placenta is nutritionally regulated, and that maternal malnutrition may allow the fetus to be exposed to higher concentrations of endogenous maternal corticosteroids. In rats fed a protein deficient but isocalorific diet, there is a reduction in placental 11β hydroxysteroid dehydrogenase activity, increased transfer of maternal corticosteroid and a reduction in fetal weight [23]. This may be a mechanism by which such ill-defined variables as socioeconomic status and maternal stress influence fetal growth.

Glucocorticoids have an established effect on post-natal long bone growth in post-natal life, and its seems equally likely that they have a similar effect in utero. Corticosteroids slow axial growth in the ovine fetus [24] and inhibit osteoclast function in fetal rat calvarae in vitro [25]. In some cell types corticosteroids will induce apoptosis (programmed cell death) and if this occurred in stem cell pools during fetal organ growth it is easy to understand how there might be reductions in final organ size. Glucocorticoids appear to be important differentiation signals in several endocrine organs. For example, treatment of pregnant rats with dexamethasone in their drinking water from day 16–19 of pregnancy (normal gestation 21 days) leads to an increase in the expression of growth hormone in the fetal anterior pituitary [26]. Growth hormone has direct effects on tissues but also acts through stimulation of tissue insulin like growth factor (IGF) system. In fetal life IGF-2 is the predominant IGF in the circulation but post-natally IGF-1 is the major circulating growth factor [27]. Short term cortisol infusions administered to the late gestation ovine fetus result in a marked reduction in the expression of IGF-2 message in the liver and muscle [28]. Similarly, the increase in fetal plasma thyroid hormone concentrations at term is also dependent upon cortisol [29]. At present there is little information about how early in gestation premature exposure to corticosteroids can initiate these maturational changes.

Cyclosporin

Renal, cardiac and liver transplantation are becoming ever more common in women of reproductive age. About 1 in 50 women of childbearing age with a functioning renal transplant becomes pregnant [30], and growing numbers of pregnancies following heart, heart–lung and hepatic transplant are being reported [31, 32]. Organ rejection is prevented by maintenance immunosuppressive therapy and there have been concerns that cyclosporin A is associated with fetal growth restriction [33,34]. One series reported 24 pregnancies treated with prednisolone and azothiaprine and compared them with 11 treated with cyclosporin [34]. The mean birthweight in the cyclosporin group was lower than in the steroid/azothiaprine group (2464 g vs. 3056 g) but the gestation was also less (range 232–271 days vs. 257–284 days). Others have reported single patients with severe growth restriction with cyclosporin treatment [33]. It is worth remembering that renal transplant recipients are at risk of a number of complications that may result in growth restriction (hypertension, superimposed pre-eclampsia and congenital CMV infection) so that in the absence of large series controlling for such factors it is not possible to state categorically that cyclosporin A is associated with growth restriction [35]. For instance, in 154 pregnancies in renal transplant recipients treated with cyclosporin the incidences of prematurity (less than 37 weeks), low birthweight (under 2500 g) and pre-eclampsia were 56, 50 and 25 per cent respectively [36].

Cyclosporin A is a low molecular weight peptide (M.W. 1203) that crosses the placenta. Concentrations in the fetus are reported to be about 10–50 per cent of those in the maternal circulation [37–39]. Cyclosporin is a potent immunosuppressive agent that is active against T lymphocytes, and changes in the populations of T cells present during pregnancy have been documented [35]. It is theoretically possible that alteration of maternal T-cell responses may interfere with implantation and trophoblast invasion and so lead to growth restriction [40]. Cyclosporin has also been documented to decrease the production of prostaglandin E2 (PGE_2) from cultured amino cells from fetal membranes [41]. PGE_2 almost certainly has an immunosuppressive action within the decidua to help maintain pregnancy, but probably also functions as a vasodilator maintaining uterine blood flow [42]. Several animal studies have demonstrated an increase in circulating PGE_2 production during maternal food restriction, suggesting that another function of PGE_2 may be to direct maternal metabolism to maintain supply of metabolic substrate to the fetus [43,44].

Cyclosporin may be associated with IUGR, and there are plausible possible mechanisms. However, there has been no convincing evidence that this is a specific effect, for the reasons discussed. In any case, continuing cyclosporin in a patient with an allograft who is well maintained on this is obligatory.

Beta-adrenoreceptor Antagonists and other Antihypertensives

The Relationship Between Maternal Blood Pressure and Fetal Growth

The maternal cardiovascular system adapts to pregnancy with a progressive fall in diastolic blood pressure, reaching a nadir at about 18–20 weeks, some 10–15 mmHg lower than the non-pregnant state [45]. Blood pressure then rises to prepregnancy levels in the third trimester. Severe hypertension in pregnancy (diastolic persistently above 110 mmHg) increases the risks of maternal mortality, stroke, cardiovascular complications, stillbirth, abruption and fetal growth restriction [46]. The careful use of continuous ambulatory blood pressure monitoring reveals an inverse relationship between maternal blood pressure and birthweight. In a study of 209 consecutive nulliparous women specifically excluding those with chronic hypertension [47], the mean 24 hour ambulatory diastolic blood pressure at 28 weeks gestation was significantly inversely correlated with birthweight after correction for gestation at delivery. For every 5 mm increase in mean diastolic pressure there was a 68 g fall in birthweight. Similar correlation was found between birthweight and mean blood pressure at 36 weeks, but not with mean blood pressure at 18 weeks. The mechanism of this effect even at normal blood pressures is not understood.

Evidence for an Effect of Beta-adrenoreceptor Antagonists on Fetal Growth

Studies of antihypertensive treatment in pregnancy have not always included birthweight as a specific endpoint and often have insufficient power to make accurate statements [48]. The effects of treatment with a specific agent on birthweight are confounded by such factors as the degree of normalisation of blood pressure achieved, the duration of treatment, maternal age and parity (older multiparous women are more likely to start pregnancy with pre-existing hypertension) and the nature of the underlying pathology. None the less, the consensus of opinion is that cardioselective ($\beta1$) antagonists and the non-selective β-receptor antagonist propanolol are associated with a reduction in birthweight. In 30 women with diastolic blood pressure between 90 and 110 mmHg randomised at 16 weeks to either atenolol or placebo, there was a significant reduction in birthweight in the atenolol-treated group [49], although atenolol started at a later gestation for pregnancy-induced hypertension did not result in a reduction in birthweight [50]. A larger retrospective review of 76 women taking atenolol in early pregnancy compared with 91 women receiving other antihypertensives or 236 women with borderline hypertension not on treatment found that atenolol was associated with a significant reduction in birthweight [51].

Several studies have examined the effects of other α (prazosin), β (oxprenolol), metoprolol ($\beta1$ selective) or mixed α and β (labetalol) antagonists on birthweight. The use of oxprenolol after about 28 weeks' gestation for pregnancy-induced hypertension did not result in a significant prolongation of pregnancy or change in birthweight compared with placebo-treated women [52]. A recent study randomised 100 women with mild–moderate hypertension to nicardipine or metaprolol from a mean gestation of 29 weeks [53]. Drug dosages were fixed rather than titrated to blood pressure. At the doses used, the calcium channel antagonist lowered both systolic and diastolic blood pressure significantly more than the beta blocker, and resulted in a non-significant trend to increase birthweight. Sibai [54] randomised 300 women with chronic hypertension (mean diastolic at entry 90 mmHg) in the first trimester to no medication, or methyldopa, or labetalol adjusted to keep diastolic blood pressure below 90 mmHg. Although both agents were effective at lowering blood pressure, this was not associated with a significant increase in fetal birthweights. Similar findings have been reported comparing labetalol with methyldopa when treatment was initiated in the late second trimester and doses titrated to maintain diastolic blood pressure below 86 mmHg [55], or comparing labetalol with placebo [56]. Another randomised controlled trial in 200 women with proteinuric hypertension, however, found that labetalol did reduce birthweight compared with the placebo group [57].

Angiotensin-converting enzyme (ACE) inhibitors are often quoted as drugs causing fetal growth restriction. In a review of 25 publications documenting use of these drugs in 85 pregnancies, there was no evidence for an effect on fetal growth, though these agents do have powerful actions on fetal renal function [58]. Similarly, there is no evidence that diuretics cause IUGR [46].

Beta Adrenoreceptors: Mechanism of Effect on Fetal Growth

Hypertension maintains end-organ perfusion in the face of increased vascular resistance and it has been suggested that pregnancy-induced hypertension is a physiological response to help maintain placental perfusion. Antihypertensive treatment might reduce the maternal perfusion of the placental bed. Treatment may also have actions in the fetal circulation to reduce fetoplacental perfusion. Atenolol is reported to reduce Doppler flow velocity in the umbilical cord [59,60]. The action of labetalol on maternal and fetal circulations during pregnancy has also been examined and found to be without effect [61–64].

Pre-eclampsia, chronic hypertension and IUGR are associated with abnormal trophoblast invasion of maternal spiral arterioles and a subsequent failure of the development of maternal placental perfusion [62]. The endocrine and paracrine factors controlling migration of trophoblast are poorly understood. We know of no studies that have examined the effects of prolonged adrenoreceptor antagonism on the development of either the maternal or fetal placental vasculature. Beta adrenoreceptors also mediate metabolic effects. Neonates exposed to labetalol are more likely to be hypoglycaemic and hypoinsulinaemic.

Recreational Drugs

Drug use is common in contemporary Western society, and women are increasingly using nicotine and illicit drugs in the developing world. Several drugs appear to restrict fetal growth, but it is often difficult to control for confounding factors. For example, women who smoke are also more likely than non-smokers to indulge in other health risk behaviours, are more socially disadvantaged and have higher rates of emotional disturbance [66,67]. It is also difficult to ascertain and measure drug use. Even though smoking is legal, many women underreport the extent of their habit, presumably because of the opprobrium associated with putting the health of the unborn child at risk. Intuition suggests that women are even less likely to report accurately the use of illegal drugs. The impure nature of the drugs supplied makes it impossible to quantify exposure accurately and in addition there may have been exposure to several other drugs as well as to cigarette smoke. Drug misuse occurs in the context of other adverse personal, psychological and social circumstances that may have a bearing on pregnancy outcome. Furthermore, reviewer and editorial bias results in the preferential publication of studies showing harmful effects of drugs, as highlighted in the case of cocaine [68]. Much of this section is concerned with cigarette smoking because the enormous numbers of affected pregnancies make this a major issue at the population level. The quality of studies about smoking in pregnancy is good, huge numbers of pregnancies have been studied, and there are few remaining confounders. A comprehensive review of determinants of low birthweight carried out by Kramer for the WHO in 1987 [69] found that the overall methodological quality of studies on smoking was considerably higher than those or other factors. Forty studies satisfactorily met, and 33 partially met, the standards selected for further analysis. Nevertheless, one source of bias is particular to smoking. Undeclared conflict of interest seems common, as highlighted recently [70]. Characteristics that might determine the conclusion of review articles on passive smoking were examined [71]. Of 106 reviews, most concluded that passive smoking was harmful, but

37 per cent that it was not harmful. Three-quarters of the articles concluding that it was not harmful were written by tobacco industry affiliates.

Nicotine

Cigarette Smoking in Pregnancy

Of the 4,000 compounds in tobacco smoke, there is good evidence that nicotine is the key drug of addiction and nicotine; carbon monoxide and cyanide, however, are believed to be the compounds having the greatest adverse effects on the fetus. Nicotine causes dependence, with a recognised withdrawal syndrome, and indeed it is claimed to be the most powerful addictive agent known [72,73]. Most girls who smoke four cigarettes as adolescents will become dependent, with an average duration of dependence of 40 years [73]. Only 5 per cent of long term smokers trying to become abstinent will remain so at 1 year without help [74]. Sadly, having been recruited in adolescence, half of all smokers die because of the habit, one-third of them before the age of 65 years [74]. As one review cataloguing the illnesses caused by smoking concluded. "Twenty per cent of all deaths in developed countries are caused by smoking: an enormous human cost which can be completely avoided" [75]. There are large differences in smoking habit by country. For example, about a third of women in the UK smoke [76], whilst in the United States (in 1994) only 23 per cent of women, and 15 per cent of pregnant women, were smokers [77]. Because of the number of pregnancies affected, and the widespread effects on pregnancy complications, perinatal mortality, sudden infant death syndrome (SIDS) and long term infant development, smoking in pregnancy is a major public health issue.

Evidence for Effect on Intrauterine Growth Restriction

The evidence linking smoking with IUGR is unequivocal. Studies have consistently shown a reduction in overall birthweight by 150 to 330 g [78–83]. In one study, the overall smoking-related birthweight deficit of 292 g was reduced to 226 g after allowing for differences in the weights, ages, parity and gestation of the two groups [84]. Most of this reduction was due to the small but highly significant 2 day reduction in mean gestational age of babies born to smokers [84]. After controlling for possible confounders, including gestation, the odds ratio of giving birth to a low birthweight baby for smoking mothers compared with non-smoking mothers in New Zealand was 2.61 (95 per cent CI, 1.65–4.15) and in New South Wales was 2.12 (95 per cent CI, 1.93–2.32). Smoking as an independent risk factor for SGA babies is estimated to contribute 20–34 per cent of the risk [78,85,86].

It seems likely that the effects of smoking are dose and gestation dependent. Several studies have shown an inverse dose–response relationship where birthweight decreased as the number of cigarettes smoked per day increased. It is worth noting that the number of cigarettes smoked is not always an accurate guide to nicotine intake: the ratio of nicotine metabolites/creatinine in urine more accurately accounts for the birthweight deficits of babies born to mothers who smoke during their pregnancy than does reported daily cigarette consumption [84]. Indeed, smokers adjust the frequency and depth of inhalation to maintain constant nicotine levels [87].

Smoking seems to reduce birthweight by two mechanisms [84]. One apparently operates at very low levels of smoke intake and may be maximal at levels of smoke intake below those of the lightest active smokers. This has been noticed before in studies that used cotinine (a metabolite of nicotine) as a marker of cigarettes smoked [88,89]. This could be similar to the effect on birthweight noted with passive smoking [90–93]. The second mechanism exerts a seemingly linearly related effect over the whole range of nicotine intakes.

The effect of smoking on birthweight is confined to the second half of pregnancy, and particularly to the third trimester. This is important in terms of the scope for interventions that encourage cessation of smoking during pregnancy. One study of a hospital-based cohort of 11,177 women showed this effect nicely [94]. Women who stopped smoking by the third trimester were not at increased risk of SGA birth compared with non-smokers. Women who *began* smoking during the second or third trimester had an elevated risk of SGA birth, similar to that for women who smoked throughout pregnancy (odds ratio 2.20; 95 per cent CI, 1.90–2.54). Furthermore, several studies have shown that women who stop smoking in early pregnancy have infants of similar birthweight to those who did not smoke [82,95,96].

Smoking: Mechanisms of Effect on Fetal Growth

It is estimated that smoking 20 cigarettes per day delivers 20 mg of nicotine and 200–300 ng of carbon monoxide into the maternal lungs [97]. There are also numerous other potentially toxic components of tobacco smoke. Effects on fetal growth may be mediated through abnormal development of the maternal and fetal placental circulations, through the actions of nicotine to stimulate the secretion of vasoconstrictive catecholamines, or through the actions of carbon monoxide and other toxins on oxygen transport and oxidative metabolism.

Effects on Placental Morphology: The prevailing clinical view is that the placentas of women who smoke during pregnancy are small and gritty due to excessive infarction; however epidemiological studies indicate that smoking increases the median weight of the placenta at term [98]. Recent scanning electron microscopy studies suggest that this increased weight is due to adaptive angiogenesis in peripheral gas-exchanging capillaries [99] (see front cover of the book). Placental angiogenesis is stimulated by the hypoxia-sensitive gene vascular endothelial growth factor (VEGF) which in turn may be upregulated in the placentas of smokers due to displacement of oxygen in maternal blood by carbon monoxide (for review of growth factors on placental development see chapter by Dunk & Ahmed). Smoking may have significant and deleterious effects on early placental development [100]. It is possible that maternal smoking may result in either adaptive changes (to maintain flow-dependent transfer) or overwhelming pathology that leads to pregnancy loss. One mechanism for the latter pathway may be via the effect of smoking on programmed cell death (apoptosis) since it appears that smoking increases the incidence of apoptosis in the syncytiotrophoblast layer [101]. Further studies are required to resolve these issues, that integrate observations on cell turnover, villous development and vascular thrombosis.

Effects on Uteroplacental Blood flow: Maternal blood pressure and heart rate increase soon after smoking a cigarette, and there is an accompanying rise in fetal heart rate [102,103]. One study examining the washout of ^{133}Xe from over the placental site concluded that smoking a single cigarette acutely reduces intervillous blood flow [104]. Doppler ultrasound studies of the maternal and fetal circulations, however, suggest that smoking does not produce significant changes in the uterine artery resistance index, but does increase umbilical artery resistance index [105]. Unfortunately, these measurements may not be valid since Doppler assessment of flow and derived resistance index is sensitive to changes in fetal heart rate. Transdermal administration of nicotine in doses sufficient to raise salivary levels of nicotine into the range present in smokers does not alter umbilical artery resistance [106].

Carbon Monoxide: Carbon monoxide is the main component of the vapour phase of tobacco smoke [107]. Carbon monoxide interferes with oxygen delivery to the fetus by displacing oxygen from maternal haemoglobin, or by shifting the oxyhaemoglobin dissociation equilibrium to the left [69,108]. Binding to fetal haemoglobin diminishes the oxygen-carrying capacity of the fetal erythrocyte [109]. Fetal haemoglobin has a higher affinity for carbon monoxide than does adult haemoglobin [108] and carboxyhaemoglobin levels are higher in the newborn than in its smoking mother [110].

Miscellaneous Actions: Smoking in theory could blunt appetite and have an effect through reduced food intake, but this does not seem to be the explanation. One study suggested the negative effect of restricting fetal growth could not be prevented simply by increasing energy intake [86] and no protective effect can be demonstrated from higher maternal weight, pregnancy weight gain or body mass index (BMI) [111]. Low levels of zinc could theoretically contribute to low birthweight, as a side-effect of high levels of cadmium [112] though vitamin/mineral supplements do not seem to minimise the adverse effects of smoking [113].

Pregnancy Management: Smoking Cessation

Smoking in pregnancy has been calculated in a US study to be responsible for 10 per cent of all perinatal mortality [114]. Other studies confirm the serious impact on late intrauterine death [115,116]. This effect is mediated partly through IUGR, but also through increased rates of preterm delivery, and placental abruption. In addition to the pregnancy effects, there is a strong relationship with SIDS [117–119], a marked increase of respiratory disease and hospital admission in the first year of life [120] and an increase in respiratory disease in childhood and adulthood [121,122]. Strategies to encourage smoking cessation are therefore one of the main public health priorities in maternity care.

Some women stop smoking when they realise they are pregnant. By the time they attend the first antenatal clinic, approximately 20 per cent of smokers declare they have stopped smoking [81,123]. But this is not as impressive as it first seems. Some self-reported quitters are really continuing to smoke; others resume smoking later in pregnancy and it is likely that most of those who do successfully stop are non-dependent users [123]. One study [124] showed 22 per cent of cotinine-validated smokers denied smoking so objective testing is therefore necessary for any study. For those who do not stop in early pregnancy, there is usually little change in nicotine intake, even when self-reporting of cigarette smoking declines. Nicotine intake tends to be held constant, by alteration in frequency and depth of inhalation, even when the number of cigarettes is reduced or when cigarettes with lower nicotine yields are used [87]. For this reason, reduction in cigarettes smoked is probably not a useful aim and the target should be abstinence.

The success of different interventions to help people in general stop smoking has been examined in a meta-analysis of 188 randomised controlled trials [125]. Simple advice by the physician to stop smoking is significantly effective. However, only 2 per cent of smokers given this advice successfully stop and remain abstinent at 1 year. Supplementary intervention (follow-up visits, letters) has some additional but variable effect. Nicotine replacement also appears effective. Acupuncture is ineffective, the benefit of hypnosis is unproved and whether stopping is sudden or gradual seems to make no difference. Pregnant women are highlighted as a group more highly motivated to stop smoking and with higher success rates. A meta-analysis of 11 randomised controlled trials has shown that intervention in pregnancy does increase the rate of smoking cessation; in the two studies examining the risk of low birthweight, the odds ratio of this was only 0.6. There is therefore evidence that intervention programmes reduce the risk of low birthweight. In another study, smoking women randomly assigned to antismoking counselling had babies with higher birthweight [126]. Different studies have emphasised the importance of locally developed materials [127]. More intensive programmes do not always have higher cessation rates compared with less demanding systems [128].

Cessation rates may seem disappointing, but this needs to be kept in perspective. Nicotine is highly addictive and many women will be unable to become abstinent at that point in their life. Smoking is associated with depressive symptoms [67] and low socioeconomic class [129], and these factors work against successful intervention. However, smoking is the foremost cause of preventable perinatal mortality, and encouraging women to stop smoking is one of the few interventions in obstetrics that has been shown to be effective in randomised controlled trials. Every clinic should have a clear programme for encouraging cessation of smoking in women in early pregnancy, and this should include adequate information about the harms to the fetus, infant and child.

Ultimately, attempting acute interventions with highly addicted women will be of limited success. More important at a population level is to encourage efforts to stop recruitment of young girls. It is estimated that tobacco companies need to recruit 300 new users every day to make up for those smokers dying and more young girls than young boys are being recruited. Maternity workers should join other groups in encouraging community-based antitobacco programmes, increased taxation on cigarettes, restriction of advertising, limitation of sales outlets and an increase in smoke-free environments. "Additional research into effective prevention and smoking cessation programmes is urgently needed to forestall the ravaging of yet another generation by this preventable and deadly habit" [130].

Alcohol

Of all the recreational drugs, alcohol has the clearest association with teratogenesis. Although the adverse effects have been well documented with very high maternal intakes, mild or occasional use may be harmless. However, a safe level of maternal alcohol consumption has not been established and there may be less complete fetal effects with lesser intakes. Problem drinking is not common, but frequent alcohol use in pregnancy increased in the US from 0.9 per cent in 1991 to 3.5 per cent (95 per cent CI 20–5.1) by 1995 [131]. Problem drinking has longer term risks for mother and child, and is associated with 80 per cent of suicides, 40 per cent of road traffic accidents, 80 per cent of deaths from fire, one in three divorces, one in three cases of child abuse and 20–30 per cent of all hospital admissions [132]. In some Western countries, fetal alcohol syndrome is claimed to be the leading recognised cause of mental retardation [133].

Evidence for Effect on Intrauterine Growth Restriction

There is no doubt that there are fetotoxic effects at high maternal alcohol intakes. At its extreme form, this manifests as fetal alcohol syndrome. This diagnosis depends on three specific criteria (fetal growth restriction with a weight < 2 *sd* below the mean for the gestation, central nervous system involvement with neurological damage and characteristic facial dysmorphology). Whether this is truly specific to alcohol or represents a more general toxic effect is uncertain. It occurs at very high maternal alcohol intakes, and the average intake in one report was 17 units/day [134]. It is uncommon with a risk in high prevalence areas of about 1 per 1,000 pregnancies, but is devastating. Whether more moderate drinking in pregnancy is associated with IUGR is uncertain, but is important in population terms. Although many studies have reported no effect, prospective studies have tended to show a decrease in birthweight, though the effect of smoking is three times greater than that for alcohol [135]. Thus, at ≥ 3 units/day, alcohol was associated with an adjusted odds ratio of 2.3 (95 per cent CI 1.2–4.6) for IUGR [136], and other studies have also reported effects at these low intakes [137–139].

Mechanism of Effect on Fetal Growth

The fetotoxic nature of alcohol in very high doses is clear and has been confirmed in animal studies. The question of threshold of effect is one that has occupied public health specialists. The concern is less with fetal size *per se* but rather with fetal brain development. In animal models, alcohol can affect the brain at different times in pregnancy, with the greatest deficit in brain growth associated with exposure in the third trimester [140]. The effect is on developing cells and on baseline content of neurotransmitters [141]. Effects on brain development in humans have been claimed at a range of reported intakes. Threshold effects on subsequent reading, spelling and arithmetic abilities have been reported at intakes of only 1 unit/day [142,143].

Pregnancy Management

Excessive alcohol intake is such a potential risk for the developing fetal brain that detoxification, under very closely monitored hospital conditions, should be considered and usually advised at any gestation. This needs specialist supervision because of the potential dangers of alcohol withdrawal. It needs attenuation therapy, needs close fetal monitoring if in later pregnancy, and needs to be slow [132]. All women who are drinking heavily must be prescribed multivitamin preparations with particular attention to thiamine. Women should have liver function tests measured, to include prothrombin time. Disulfiram (Antabuse) is contraindicated in pregnancy. Moderate drinking is potentially a risk, and medical advice should be to reduce intake, with an explanation of current knowledge. It is not possible at present to give a level of consumption that is known to be without effect on the fetus.

Opiates

These are common drugs of misuse. Between 1 and 3 per cent of 18–25 year olds in the US have used opioids recreationally and about a third of users in most studies are women. These drugs do not appear to be teratogenic, but there is a high rate of neonatal abstinence syndrome and a definite increase in deaths from SIDS. Most studies report a high prevalence of IUGR, but these studies relate to hospital populations with all the problems of associated confounders [144–148]. It seems likely that opiates may have a small effect on inhibiting fetal growth, but that this is less than smoking [149].

There is support for an effect from animal experiments [149,150]. Opiates have been shown to retard fetal growth in rabbits [151] and young mice [152]. Unfortunately, in these species, maternal nutrition has a pronounced effect on fetal growth. This was examined in the rabbit, however, and the effect on fetal growth did not seem to be attributable to maternal nutrition [153]. It has been suggested [154] that the IUGR found was due mainly to a subnormal number of cells in the various organs.

Despite this, our population data do not suggest that opiates have a major specific effect on fetal growth. They are nevertheless an important consideration in the provision of antenatal care. Opiate abuse can carry the risks of non-sterile injecting, overdose, respiratory depression and maternal death [155–158]. The consequences of illicit drug use in an unstable, impoverished environment may affect access to care, or may complicate continuity of care.

Cocaine

This drug is widely used in the US and elsewhere in Europe. US studies based on sampling in the newborn (usually in inner cities) suggest prevalence rates of 5–31 per cent. There is a huge amount of descriptive evidence that cocaine has adverse effects on pregnancy outcome. There is also a plausible theoretical mechanism for its action. The central addictive action of cocaine is through inhibition of receptors of dopamine in the nucleus accumbens and prefrontal cortex, but it has important peripheral effects on inhibition of uptake of noradrenaline in presynaptic nerve terminals. The resulting high catecholamine levels cause vasoconstriction, tachycardia, hypertension and probably uterine contractility. Most pregnancy complications arise from this peripheral action. The mother is at risk from rare but dramatic events such as myocardial infarction, cerebrovascular accident, subarachnoid haemorrhage, hepatic rupture, cardiac arrhythmias, accidental injury and pre-eclamptic-like states [156,159–161]. Placental abruption, fetal cerebral injury and intrauterine death all seem to be events temporarily related to cocaine use. As far as IUGR is concerned, some studies suggest that birthweight deficits associated with cocaine use may be completely explained by covariables (nicotine, opiates, alcohol, low socio-economic status, lack of prenatal care) [162–164]. Nevertheless, a decrease in birthweight is plausible, based on animal studies that show a dose related decrease in uterine blood flow and decreased fetal size [165]. An excellent review also concluded that the consistency of the finding of impaired fetal growth in studies with quite different approaches suggested that this may be a true effect [166]. In a large study of 905 HIV-negative women with cocaine-exposed pregnancies, Burkette et al. [161] discuss the issues thoughtfully. They discuss the reports, including their own, showing much better perinatal outcome with comprehensive prenatal care [167–169]. Of course, selection bias may account for all the differences in outcomes. On the other hand, prenatal care is an implement for behavioural change. This gives access to support, drug rehabilitation and the opportunity for reduction in drug binges.

Benzodiazepines

These commonly used drugs have often been studied with low dose usage, whereas in some drug users very high doses are involved. There have been concerns about possible dysmorphic change, reduced growth and brain development and long term outcome, but it is difficult to be categorical about risks at the present time.

Cannabis

Some studies have reported lower birthweight but reports are not consistent. A meta-analysis of ten studies that adjusted for smoking [170], concluded that there was inadequate evidence that cannabis, at the doses typically consumed by pregnant women, caused IUGR.

Amphetamines

There are reports of reduced birthweight but data currently available do not allow any accurate estimate of risk. Since amphetamines and cocaine have similar central physiological effects, their impact on pregnancies may be similar. Both agents cause vasoconstriction and hypertension, which may result in acute or chronic fetal hypoxia, and large doses of amphetamines are associated with weight loss in adults. An excess of this drug could plausibly be associated with IUGR.

Designer Drugs

A number of analogues of fentanyl, mescalin, amphetamines and phenylcyclidine have been produced. The most widely used drugs at present are amphetamine analogues. Ecstasy (3,4-methyl-ne-dioxy-methylamphetamine, or MDMA) is one derivative related chemically to both amphetamines and hallucinogens. Complications of use are rare, but potentially devastating. There are some data suggesting this might be associated with congenital abnormality but there is no information on birthweight and, as this is a drug usually taken episodically, it is less likely to be an important cause of growth restriction.

Volatile Substances

This is an important cause of death in young people, with 605 people aged < 18 years dying in the UK of volatile substance abuse between 1981 and 1990. However, males are much more at risk than females. One study in rats [171] showed lower fetal weight gain and there is uncertainty about whether there is a discrete fetal solvent syndrome [172]. It is important to remember that, for every ecstasy death (which is widely reported in the media), 11 people die of inhaling volatile substances found in domestic consumer products.

Pregnancy Management and Illicit Drug Misuse

The underlying principle of management is a pragmatic approach emphasising rehabilitation with attention mainly paid to harm reduction, and obstetric and midwifery care focused on physical and psychological well-being in preparation for motherhood. These aims may be defined as normalisation and integration. Health care workers need to share the same aims and to have come to terms with the ethical issues involved [173]. Management is a complicated area that has been discussed in length elsewhere [150,173], also Johnstone PDU (in press)]. Some issues of support and help with living conditions are germaine to all drug users. In the case of opiate abuse, substitution therapy with methadone is possible, but for other drugs this is not the case. Once IUGR has occurred, subsequent monitoring and management may be hampered by inadequate or unreliable take-up of care. This is a challenge that is best resolved before the acute event. Although many different systems can be effective, one useful model is a community-based service along the lines described for Edinburgh [174].

Lifestyle Factors

Demographic studies have long related inequalities in health to economic and social variables, and complicated systems for grouping subjects by socioeconomic class have been devised. The artificial boundaries of socioeconomic class, however, obscure the individuality of behaviour, personal values, beliefs and opportunities that may affect maternal and fetal health. Not surprisingly, a whole range of lifestyle factors have been proposed as contributors to fetal growth restriction. These include the broad effects of low socioeconomic status, the particular effects of social deprivation, hard physical work or strenuous exercise, poor nutrition, inadequate social support, exposure to toxic waste and "stress".

Socioeconomic Status and Poverty

Socioeconomic status attempts to define a group of people with a common experience of wealth, work and housing who might be expected to have similar lifestyles. Associated with socioeconomic status there are multiple factors with an impact on fetal growth and these need to be taken in to account when assessing the effect of socioeconomic diversity on fetal growth. Kramer [175] has recently discussed the contribution of socioeconomic status to low birthweight, and starts by commenting, "one of the most robust findings in epidemiological research in the aetiology of low birthweight is the large socioeconomic disparities in both IUGR and preterm birth". This is found not only in the United States of America, where there are large differences in income across the population, but also in countries such as Canada, Sweden and Denmark, where there is a more even distribution of wealth [175]. Defining socioeconomic status in pregnancy is problematic however since many women cease employment, may be cohabiting rather than married, and may previously have been in a different socioeconomic grouping than would be assigned from their partner's occupation. For this reason, deprivation scores based on postcode area, using census variables, have been developed [176,177]. This approach has been used in a study in the East Midlands where it was concluded that there was an effect on birthweight of 47 g attributable to the Jarman index after the inclusion of known physiological and pathological factors in multivariate analysis [178]. Such small effects could equally well be explained by inaccurate data about cigarettes smoked, drug use or alcohol consumption. In fact, cigarette smoking alone can explain much of the disparity in birthweight associated with socioeconomic group [175,179]. Once known, or strongly suspected, confounding variables such as smoking are taken into account, socioeconomic disadvantage by itself is probably not an independent determinant of fetal growth. In an earlier review [69], Kramer located 113 studies that had a bearing on the effect of socioeconomic status on intrauterine growth and concluded that socioeconomic status had no independent effect on intrauterine growth. This was also the conclusion of a later series of papers from Australia [180].

Social Isolation and Support

Meta-analysis of clinical controlled trials shows little if any benefit of social support on IUGR. The pooled odds ratio was 1.06 (95 per cent CI 0.86–1.30) [181]. For example, a randomised controlled trial of support with a family worker found no significant difference in birthweight.

Physical Activity

Heavy work or intense exercise could contribute to the risk of IUGR by creating conflict between maternal energy demands and those of the growing fetus. This might be expected to be a particular problem in the developing world where women often continue prolonged strenuous work throughout pregnancy against a background of chronic borderline energy intake. This area has not been well investigated. Kramer [69] found no studies on physical activity that satisfactorily met the methodological criteria and 12 that partially did. His conclusion was that the effect of work on IUGR was uncertain. A review of the literature, published in 1997 [182], also did not find consistent results, but did highlight the possible risks of prolonged standing. A study of 349 sonographically defined growth restricted fetuses and 698 control pregnancies [183] did control well for potential confounders and found that the risk of IUGR was significantly higher (adds ratio (OR) = 2.4; 95 per cent CI 1.36–4.21) among women reporting moderate to heavy as opposed to light physical work.

Maternal exercise seems to have only minor changes in the fetus, with little effect on fetal metabolism, cardiovascular haemodynamics or blood catecholamine concentrations, and with little evidence of an effect on IUGR. However, most information concerning the fetus is derived from animal studies, and the upright posture of the human may affect fetal responses differently [184].

Other Environmental Factors

Concerns have been raised about refuse and possible toxins affecting fetal growth but there is little conclusive evidence. Reduced birthweight was reported in those near Love Canal during years of active dumping around the canal [185]. However, the study controlled poorly for potential confounding variables. Landfill sites have again come under scrutiny, but because of a possible association with non-chromosomal congenital abnormality [186].

A large literature has surrounded the potential effect of physiological factors and stress on birthweight. Kramer found only one study that satisfactorily met, and seven that partially met, his methodological criteria. He concluded that there was no link between psychological factors and intrauterine growth and no effect of stress could be found.

Conclusion

We have identified and discussed a number of specific drugs capable of altering maternal and/or fetal physiology in such a way as to restrict fetal growth. Whilst it is academically interesting to understand the pathophysiology involved, this is often not directly relevant to public health, or to the practising clinician. At a population level, cigarette smoking is by far the most important single factor we have considered, and strategies to reduce this are the overwhelming priority. Smoking, alcohol dependence and drug use should not be viewed in a vacuum. Some of the factors described are important not so much because of their effect on pathophysiology, but because of on their effect on access to care. Bad outcomes often arise because of the confluence of pathophysiology, lifestyle factors, lack of family support and inappropriate organisation of care. For example, the system of care may not respond well to women who are drug users, or who have very adverse social circumstances, and in turn these women may not access appropriately the care that is available. Although there have been many initiatives to improve care for the vulnerable, the inverse care law in maternity care remains true. Those at highest risk because of biological and social factors may get the least care. Once IUGR has been diagnosed, subsequent fetal monitoring and timing of delivery may be difficult to optimise. Programmes of care need to be flexible, and geared to woman herself. These considerations are more important than contemplation of the specificity of any drug effects.

References

1. Seckl JR, Miller WL. How safe is long-term prenatal glucocorticoid treatment? JAMA 1997;277:1077–9.
2. Sun K, Yang K, Challis JRG. Glucocorticoid actions and metabolism in pregnancy: Implications for placental function and fetal cardiovascular activity. Placenta, 1998;19:353–60.
3. Nathanielsz PW, Comline RS, Silver M, Paisey RB. Cortisol metabolism in the fetal and neonatal sheep. 1972 J Reprod Fertil Suppl;16:39–59.
4. Pepe GJ, Waddell BJ, Albrecht ED. Activation of the baboon fetal hypothalamic-pituitary-adrenocortical axis at midgestation by estrogen-induced changes in placental corticosteroid metabolism. 1990 Endocrinology;127:3117–3123.
5. Crowley P, Chalmers I, Keirse MJNC. The effects of corticosteroid administration before preterm delivery: an overview of the evidence from controlled trials. Brit J Obstet Gynaecol 1990;97:11–25.
6. Crowley PA. Antenatal corticosteroid therapy: a meta-analysis of the randomised trials, 1972 to 1994. Am J Obstet Gynecol 1995;173:322–35.
7. Forest MG, Morel Y, Dard M. Prenatal treatment of congenital adrenal hyperplasia. Trends Endocrinol Metab 1998;9:284–9.
8. Ostesen M. Optimisation of antirheumatic drug treatment in pregnancy. 1994 Clin Pharmacokinetics; 27:486–503.
9. Reinisch JM, Simon NG, Karow WG. Prenatal exposure to predisone in humans and animals retard intrauterine growth. Science, 1978;202:436–8.
10. Katz VL, Thorp JM, Bowes WA. Severe symmetric intrauterine growth retardation associated with the topical use of triamcinolone. Am J Obstet Gynecol 1990;162:396–7.
11. [Anonymous]. NIH Consensus Conference: Effect of corticosteroids for fetal maturation on perinatal outcomes. J A M A 1995;273:413–18.
12. Ballard PL, Ballard RA, Scientific basis and therapeutic regimes for uses of antenatal glucocorticoids. Am J Obstet Gynecol 1995;173:254–62.
13. Johnson JWC, Mitzner W, London WT, Palmer AE, Scott R, Kearney K. Glucocorticoids and the rhesus fetal lung. Am J Obstet Gynecol 1978;130:905–15.
14. Johnson JWC, Mitzner W, London WT, Palmer AE, Scott R. betamethasone and the rhesus fetus: multisystemic effects. Am J Obstet Gynecol 1979;133:677–84.
15. Bunton TE, Plopper CG. Triamcinolone-induced structural alterations in the development of the lung of the fetal rhesus macaque. Am J Obstet Gynecol 1984;148:203–15.
16. Epstein MF, Farrell PM, Sparks JW, Pepe G, Driscoll SG, Chez RA. Maternal betamethasone and fetal growth and development in the monkey. Am J Obstet Gynecol 1977;127:261–3.
17. Benediktsson R, Lindsay RS, Noble J, Seckl JR, Edwards CRW. Glucocorticoid exposure in utero: new model for adult hypertension. Lancet, 1993;341:339–41.
18. Ikegami M, Polk DH, Jobe AH, Newnham J, Sly P, Kohan R, Kelly R. Effect of interval from fetal corticosteroid treatment to delivery on postnatal lung function of preterm lambs. J Appl Physiol 1996;80:591–7.

19. Dodic M, May CN, Wintour EM, Coghlan JP. An early prenatal exposure to excess glucocorticoid leads to hypertensive offspring in sheep. Clinical Science 1998;94:149–155.
20. Jobe AH, Wada N, Berry IM, Ikegami M, Ervin MG. Single and repetitive maternal glucocorticoid exposures reduce fetal growth in sheep. Am J Obstet Gynecol 1998;178:880–5.
21. Sanfacon R, Possmayer F, Harding PGR. Dexamethasone treatment of the guinea pig fetus: its effects on the incorporation of 3H-thymidine into deoxyribonucleic acid. Am J Obstet Glynecol 1977;127:745–52.
22. Liggins GC. Adrenocortical-related maturational events in the fetus. Am J Obstet Gynecol 1976;126:931–9.
23. Langley-Evans SC, Phillips GJ, Benediktsson R, Gardner DS, Edwards CRW, Jacobs AA, Seckl JR. Protein intake in pregnancy, placental glucocorticoid metabolism and the programming of hypertension in the rat. Placenta, 1996;17:169–72.
24. Fowden AL, Szemere J, Hughes P, Gilmour RS, Forhead AJ. The effects of cortisol on the growth rate of the sheep fetus during late gestation. J Endocrinol 1996;151:97–105.
25. Dietrich JW, Canalis EM, Maina DM, Raisz LG. Effects of glucocorticoids in fetal rat bone collagen synthesis in vitro. Endocrinology, 1979;104:715–9.
26. Nogami H, Tachibana T. Dexamethasone induces advanced growth hormone expression in the fetal rat pituitary gland *in vivo*. Endocrinology 1993;132:517–23.
27. Sara VR, Hall K. Insulin-like growth factors and their binding proteins. Physiol Rev 1990;707:591–614.
28. Li J, Saunders JC, Gilmour RS, Silver M, Fowden A. Insulin-like growth factor-II messenger ribonucleic acid expression in fetal tissues of the sheep during late gestation: effects of cortisol. Endocrinology, 1993;132:2083–9.
29. Sensky PL, Roy CH, Barnes RJ, Heath MF. Changes in fetal thyroid hormone levels in adrenalectomised fetal sheep following continuous cortisol infusion 72 h before delivery. J Endocrinol 1994;140:79–83.
30. Davison JM. Pregnancy in renal allograft recipients: problems, prognosis and practicalities. Bailliere's Clin Obstet Gynaecol 1994;8:501–25.
31 Baxi, JV, Rho, BB. Pregnancy after cardiac transplantation. Am J Obstet Gynecol 1993;169:33–4.
32. Vile Y, Fernandez H, Samuel D, Bismuth H, Frydman R. Pregnancy in liver transplant recipients: course and outcome in 19 cases. Am J Obstet Gynecol 1993;168:896–902.
33. Pickerell MD, Sawers R, Michael J. Pregnancy after renal transplantation: severe intrauterine growth retardation during treatment with cyclosporin A. BMJ 1988;296:825.
34. Haugen G, Fauchald P, Sodal G, Leivestad T, Moe N. Pregnancy outcome in renal allograft recipients, influence of cyclosporin A. Eur J Obstet Gynaecol 1991;39:25–9.
35. Davison JM, Redman CWG. Pregnancy post-transplant: the establishment of a UK registry. Br J Obstet Gynaecol 1997;104:1106–7.
36. Armenti VT, Ahlswede KM, Ahlswede BA, Jarrell BE, Moritz MJ, Burke JF. National transplantation pregnancy registry-outcomes of 154 pregnancies in cyclosporin-treated female kidney transplant recipients. Transplantation, 1994;57:502–6.
37. Fletchner SM, Karz AR, Rogers AJ, Van Buren C, Kahan BD. The presence of cyclosporin in body tissues and fluids during pregnancy. Am J Kidney Dis 1985;5:60–3.
38. Derfler K, Schaller A, Herold C, Balcke P, Nowotny C, Walter R, Kopsa H, Endler M, Stockenhuber F, Kletter K. Successful outcome of a complicated pregnancy in a renal transplant recipient taking cyclosporin A. Clin Nephrol 1988;29:96–102.
39. Biesenbach G, Zazgornik J, Kaiser W, Stoger H, Derfler K, Balcke P, Hauser CH. Cyclosporin requirement during pregnancy in renal transplant recipients. Nephrol Dial Transplant 1989;4:667–9.
40. Piccinni MP, Beloni L, Livi C, Maggi E, Scarselli G, Romasnani S. Defective production of both leukemia inhibitory factor and type 2 T-helper cytokines by decidual T cells in unexplained recurrent abortions. Nat Med 1998;4:1020–4.
41. Edwin SS, Branch DW, Scott JR, Silver RM, Dudley DJ, Mitchell MD. Cyclosporin A inhibits prostaglandin E2 production by fetal amnion cells in response to various stimuli. Prostaglandins, 1996;52:51–61.
42 Kelly RW. Pregnancy maintenance and parturition: The role of prostaglandins in manipulating the immune and inflammatory response. Endocr Rev 1994;15:684–706.
43. Fowden AL, Harding R, Ralph MM, Thorburn GD. The nutritional regulation of plasma prostaglandin E concentrations in the fetus and pregnant ewe during late gestation. J Physiol 1987;3094:1–12.
44. Thorburn GD. The placenta, prostaglandins and parturition: A review. Reprod Fertil Dev 1991;3:277–94.
45. MacGillivray I, Rose GA, Rowe D. Blood pressure survey in pregnancy. Clin Sci 1969;37:395.
46. Sibai BM. Treatment of hypertension in pregnant women. N Engl J Med 1996;335:257–65.

47. Churchill D, Perry IJ, Beevers DG. Ambulatory blood pressure in pregnancy and fetal growth. Lancet, 1997;349:7–10.
48. Henriksen T. Hypertension in pregnancy: use of antihypertensive drugs. Acta Obstet Gynecol Scand 1997;76:96–106.
49. Butters L, Kennedy S, Rubin PC. Atenolol in essential hypertension during pregnancy. BMJ 1990;301:587–9.
50. Rubin PC, Butters L, Clark DM, Reynolds B, Summer DJ, Steedman D, Low RA, Reid JL. Placebo-controlled trial of atenolol in treatment of pregnancy-associated hypertension. Lancet, 1983;I:431–44.
51. Lip GYH, Beevers M, Churchill D, Shaffer LM, Beevers DG. Effect of atenolol on birthweight. Am J Cardiol 1997;15:1436–8.
52. Plouin PE, Breart G, Ilado J, Dalle M, Keller ME, Goujon H, Berchel C. A randomised comparison of early with conservative use of antihypertensive drugs in the management of pregnancy-induced hypertension. Brit J Obstet Gynaecol 1990;97:197–204.
53. Jannet D, Carbonne B, Sebban E, Milliez J. Nicardipine versus metoprolol in the treatment of hypertension during pregnancy. A randomised comparative trial. Obstet Gynecol 1994;84:354–9.
54. Sibai BM, Mabie WC, Shamsa F, Vllar MA, Anderson GD. A comparison of no medication versus methyldopa or labetalol in chronic hypertension during pregnancy. Am J Obstet Gynecol 1990;162:960–7.
55. Plouin PF, Breart G, Maillard F, Papiernik E, Relier JP. Comparison of antihypertensive efficacy and perinatal safety of labetalol and methyldopa in the treatment of hypertensive patients in pregnancy; a randomised controlled trial. Brit J Obstet Gynaecol 1988;95:868–76.
56. Pickels CF, Syminds EM, Broughton Pipkin F. The fetal outcome in a randomised double blind controlled trial of labetalol versus placebo in pregnancy induced hypertension. Brit J Obstet Gynaecol 1989;96:38–43.
57. Sibai BA, Gonazalez AR, Mabie WC, Morietti M. A comparison of labetalol plus hospitalisation versus hospitalisation alone in the management of preeclampsia remote from term. Am J Obstet Gynecol 1987;70:323–7.
58. Hanssens M, Keirse MJNC, Vankelecom F, Van Assche FA. Fetal and neonatal effects of treatment with angiotensin-converting enzyme inhibitors in pregnancy. Obstet Gynecol 1991;78:128–35.
59. Montan S, Ingermarsson I, Marsal K, Sjoberg N-O. Randomised controlled trial of atenolol and pindolol in human pregnancy: effects on fetal hemodynamics. BMJ 1992;304:946–9.
60. Rasanen J, Jouppila P. Uterine and fetal hemodynamics and fetal cardiac function after atenolol and pindolol infusion – a randomised study. Eur J Obstet Gynecol Reprod Biol 1995;62:195–201.
61. Jouppila P, Rasanen J. Effect of labetalol infusion on uterine and fetal hemodynamics and fetal cardiac function. Eur J Obstet Gynecol Reprod Biol 1993;51:111–7.
62. Mahmoud TZK, Bjornsson S, Calder AA. Labetalol therapy in pregnancy-induced hypertension – the effects on fetoplacental circulation and fetal-outcome. Eur J Obstet Gynecol Reprod Biol 1993;50:109–13.
63. Morgan MA, Silavin SL, Dormer KJ, Fishburne BC, Fishburne JI. Effects of labetalol on uterine blood-flow and cardiovascular hemodynamics in the hypertensive gravid baboon. American J Obstet Gynecol 1993;168:1574–9.
64. Petersen OB, Skajaa K, Svane D, Gregersen H, Forman A. The effects of dihydralazine labetalol and magnesium-sulfate on the isolated, perfused human placental cotyledon. British J Obstet Gynaecol 1994;101:871–8.
65. Fox H. Placentation in untrauterine growth retardation. Fetal Matern Med Rev 1997;9:61–73.
66. Stewart DE, Streiner DL. Cigarette smoking during pregnancy. Can J Psychiatry 1995;40:603–7.
67. Pritchard CW. Depression and smoking in pregnancy in Scotland. J Epidemiol Community Health 1994;48:377–82.
68. Koren G, Shear H, Graham K, Einarson T. Bias against the null hypothesis: The reproductive hazards of cocaine. Lancet 1989;2:1440–2.
69. Kramer MS. Determinants of low birth weight. Methodological assessment and meta-analysis. Bull World Health Organ 1987;65:633–737.
70. Smith R. Beyond conflict of interest. Br M J 1998;317:291–2.
71. Barnes DE, Bero LA. Why review articles on the health effects of passive smoking reach different conclusions. JAMA 1998;279:1566–70.
72. Benowitz NL. Pharmacologic aspects of cigarette smoking and nicotine addiction. N Engl J Med 1988;319:1318–30.
73. Russell MAH. The nicotine addiction trap: A 40-year sentence for four cigarettes. Br J Addiction 1990;85:293–300.
74. Sell L, Finch E, Farrell M, Strang J. Addiction. Br J Hosp Med 1996;56:136–40.

75. Wald NJ, Hackshaw AK. Cigarette smoking: an epidemiological overview. Br Med Bull 1996;52:3–11.
76. Bevan R, Kenney A. Smoking and women's health. The Diplomate 1996;3:274–9.
77. Kendrick JS, Merritt RK. Women and smoking: an update for the 1990s. Am J Obstet Gynecol 1996;175:528–35.
78. Wong PPL, Bauman A. How well does epidemiological evidence hold for the relationship between smoking and adverse obstetric outcomes in New South Wales? Aust N Z J Obstet Gynaecol 1997;37:168–73.
79. Ellard GA, Johnstone FD, Prescott RJ, Ji-Xian W, Jian-Hua M. Smoking during pregnancy: the dose dependence of birthweight deficits. Br J Obstet Gynaecol 1996;103:806–13.
80. US Department of Health and Human Services. The health consequences of smoking for women. A report of the Surgeon General. DHHS, 1980.
81. US Department of Health and Human Services. The health benefits of smoking cessation. A report of the Surgeon General. DHHS, 1990.
82. Rush D, Cassano P. Relationship of cigarette smoking and social class to birthweight and perinatal mortality among all births in Britain, 5–11 April 1970. J Epidemiol Community Health 1983;37:249–55.
83. Malloy MH, Kleinman JC, Land GH, Schramm W. The association of maternal smoking with age and cause of infant death. Am J Epidemiol 1988;128:46–55.
84. Ellard GA, Johnstone FD, Prescott RJ, Ji-Xian W, Jian-Hua M. Smoking induced birthweight deficits. Br J Obstet Gynaecol 1996;103:806–13.
85. Thompson MJD, Wright SP, Mitchell EA, Clements MS, Becroft DMO, Scragg RKR. Risk factors for small for gestational age infants: a New Zealand study. NZ Med J 1994;107:71–3.
86. Muscati SK, Koski KG, Gray-Donald K. Increased energy intake in pregnant smokers does not prevent human fetal growth retardation. J Nutr 1996;126:2984–9.
87. Withey CH, Papacosta AO, Swan AV, Fitzsimons BA, Ellard GA, Burney PG, et al. Respiratory effects of lowering tar and nicotine levels of cigarettes smoked by young male middle tar smokers: II Results of a randomised controlled trial. J Epidemiol Community Health 1992;46:281–5.
88. Haddow JE, Knight GJ, Palomaki GE, Kloza EM, Wald NJ. Cigarette consumption and serum cotinine in relation to birth weight. Br J Obstet Gynaecol 1987;94:678–81.
89. Haddow JE, Knight GJ, Palomaki GE, McCarthy JE. Second-trimester serum cotinine levels in nonsmokers in relation to birthweight. Am J Obstet Gynecol 1988;159:481–4.
90. Martinez FD, Wright AL, Taussig LM, Group Health Medical Associates. The effect of paternal smoking on the birthweight of newborns whose mothers did not smoke. Am J Public Health 1994;84:1489–91.
91. Lazzaroni F, Bonassi S, Manniello E, Morcaldi L, Repetto E, Ruocco A, et al. Effect of passive smoking during pregnancy on selected perinatal parameters. Int J Epidemiol 1990;19:960–6.
92. Rubin DH, Krasilnikoff PA, Leventhal JM, Weile B, Berget A. Effect of passive smoking on birth-weight. Lancet 1986;ii:415–7.
93. Ogawa H, Tominaga S, Hori K,. Noguchi K, Kanea I, Matsubara M. Passive smoking by pregnant women and fetal growth. J Epidemiol Community Health 1991;45:164–8.
94. Lieberman E, Gremy I, Lang JM, Cohen AP. Low birthweight at term and the timing of fetal exposure to maternal smoking. Am J Public Health 1994;84:1127–31.
95. Papoz L, Eschwege E, Pequignot G, Barrat J, Schwartz D. Maternal smoking and birth weight in relation to dietary habits. Am J Obstet Gynecol 1982;142:770–86.
96. Naeye RL. Influence of maternal cigarette smoking during pregnancy on fetal and childhood growth. Obstet Gynecol 1981;57:18–21.
97. Benowitz NL. Nicotine replacement therapy during pregnancy. JAMA 1991;266:3174–7.
98. Williams LA, Evans SF, Newnham J. Prospective cohort studies of factors influencing the relative weights of the placenta and the newborn infant. BMJ 1997;314:1864–8.
99. Pfarrer C, Macara L, Leiser R, Kingdom J. Adaptive angiogenesis in placentas of heavy smokers. Lancet 1999;354:303.
100. Jauniaux E, Burton GJ. The effect of smoking in pregnancy on early placental morphology. Obstet Gynecol 1992;79:645–8.
101. van der Veen F, Fox H. The effects of cigarette smoking on the human placenta: a light and electron microscopic study. Placenta 1982;3:243–56.
102. Kelly J, Mathews KA, O'Conor M. Smoking in pregnancy: effects on mother and fetus. Br J Obstet Gynaecol 1984;91:111–17.
103. Lambers DS, Clark KE. The maternal and fetal physiological effects of nicotine. Semin Perinatol 1996;20:115–26.

104. Lehtovirta P, Forss M, Kariniemi V, Rauramo I. Acute effects of smoking on fetal heart rate variability. Br J Obstet Gynaecol 1983;90:3–6.

105. Morrow RJ, Ritchie JWK, Bull SB. Maternal cigarette smoking: the effects on umbilical and uterine blood flow velocity. Am J Obstet Gynecol 1988;159:1069–71.

106. Wright LN, Thorp JM, Kuller JA, Shrewsbury RP, Ananth C, Hartmann K. Transdermal nicotine replacement in pregnancy: maternal pharmacokinetics and fetal effects. Am J Obstet Gynecol 1997;176:1090–4.

107. Mactutus CF. Developmental neurotoxicity of nicotine, carbon monoxide and other tobacco smoke constituents. Ann NY Acad Sci 1989;562:105–22.

108. Longo LD. The biological effects of carbon monoxide on the pregnant woman, fetus and newborn infant. Am J Obstet Gynecol 1977;129:69–103.

109. Longo LD. Carbon monoxide: effects on oxygenation of the fetus in utero. Science 1976;194:523–5.

110. Visnjevac V, Mikov M. Smoking and carboxyhaemoglobin concentrations in mothers and their newborn infants. Hum Toxicol 1986;5:175–7.

111. Zaren B, Cnattingius S, Lindmark G. Fetal growth impairment from smoking – is it influenced by maternal anthropometry? Acta Obstet Gynecol Scand 1997;76:30–3.

112. Jensen OH, Foss OP. Smoking in pregnancy. Effects on the birth weight and on thiocyanate concentrations in mothers and baby. Acta Obstet Gynecol Scand 1981;60:177–81.

113. Wu T, Buck G, Mendola P. Can regular multivitamin/mineral supplementation modify the relation between maternal smoking and select adverse birth outcomes? Ann Epidemiol 1998;8:175–83.

114. Kleinman JC, Pierre MB, Madans JH, Land GH, Schramm W. The effects of maternal smoking on fetal and infant mortality. Am J Epidemiol 1988;127:274–82.

115. Meyer MB, Tonascia JA. Maternal smoking, pregnancy complications and perinatal mortality. Am J Obstet Gynecol 1977;128:494–502.

116. Cnattingius S, Haglund B, Meirik O. Cigarette smoking as risk factor for late fetal and early neonatal death. Br M J 1988;297:258–61.

117. Alm B, Milerad J, Wennergren G, Skaerven R, Oyen N, Norvenius G, et al. A case-control study of smoking and sudden infant death syndrome in the Scandinavian countries, 1992 to 1995. Arch Dis Child 1998;78:329–34.

118. Mitchell EA, Tuohy PG, Brunt JM, Thompson JMD, Clements MS, Stewart AW, et al. Risk factors for sudden infant death syndrome following the prevention campaign in New Zealand: A prospective study. Pediatrics 1997;100:835–40.

119. MacDorman MF, Cnattingius S, Hoffman HJ, Kramer MS, Haglund B. Sudden infant death syndrome and smoking in the United States and Sweden. Am J Epidemiol 1997;146:249–57.

120. Tager IB, Ngo L, Hanrahan JP. Maternal smoking during pregnancy. Effects on lung function during the first 18 months of life. Am J Respir Crit Care Med 1995;152:977–83.

121. Upton MN, Watt GCM, Smith GD, McConnachie A, Hart CL. Permanent effects of maternal smoking in offspring's lung function. Lancet 1998;352:453.

122. Hu FB, Persky V, Flay BR, Zelli A, Cooksey J, Richardson J. Prevalence of asthma and wheezing in public schoolchildren: Association with maternal smoking during pregnancy. Ann Allergy 1997;79:80–4.

123. Panjari M, Astbury J, Bishop SM, Dalais , Rice GE. Women who spontaneously quit smoking in early pregnancy. Australian and New Zealand Journal of Obstetrics and Gynaecology 1997;37:271–8.

124. Ford RPK, Tappin DM, Schluter PJ, Wild CJ. Smoking during pregnancy: How reliable are maternal self reports in New Zealand? J Epidemiol Community Health 1997;51:246–51.

125. Law M, Tang JL. An analysis of the effectiveness of interventions intended to help people stop smoking. Arch Intern Med 1995;155:1933–41.

126. Sexton M, Hebel JR. A clinical trial of change in maternal smoking and its effect on birth weight. JAMA 1984;251:911–5.

127. Lowe JB, Balanda KP, Clare G. Evaluation of antenatal smoking cessation programs for pregnant women. Aust N Z J Public Health 1998;22:55–9.

128. Valbo A, Thelle DS, Kolas T. Smoking cessation in pregnancy: A multicomponent intervention study. J Matern Fetal Med 1996;6:3–8.

129. Najman JM, Lanyon A, Andersen MA, Williams G, Bor W, O'Collaghan M. Socioeconomic status and maternal cigarette smoking before, during and after a pregnancy. Aust N Z J Public Health 1998;22:60–6.

130. Woolf AD. Smoking and nicotine addiction: A pediatric epidemic with sequelae in adulthood. Curr Opin Pediatr 1997;9:470–7.

131. Ebrahim SH, Luman ET, Floyd RL, Murphy CC, Bennett EM, Boyle CA. Alcohol consumption by pregnant women in the United States during 1988–1995. Obstetr Gynecol 1998;92:187–92.

132. Ashworth M, Gerada C. Addiction and dependence. II alcohol. B M J 1997;315:358–60.
133. Abel EL, Sokol RJ. Fetal alcohol syndrome is now leading cause of mental retardation. Lancet 1986;1:222 [editorial].
134. Oulellette EM, Rosett HL, Rosman NP, Weiner L. Adverse effects in offspring of maternal alcohol abuse during pregnancy. N E J Med 1977;297:528–30.
135. Abel EL, Hannigan JH. 'J-shaped' relationship between drinking during pregnancy and birth weight: Reanalysis of prospective epidemiological data. Alcohol Alcohol 1995;30:345–55.
136. Windham GC, Fenster L, Hopkins B, Swan SH. The association of moderate maternal and paternal alcohol consumption with birthweight and gestational age. Epidemiology 1995;6:591–7.
137. Passaro KT, Little RE, Savitz DA, Noss J. The effect of maternal drinking before conception and in early pregnancy on infant birthweight. Epidemiol 1996;7:377–83.
138. Lazzaroni , Bonassi S, Magnani M, Calvi A, Repetto E, Serra G, et al. Moderate maternal drinking and outcome of pregnancy. Eur J Epidemiol 1993;9:599–606.
139. Larroque B, Kaminski M, Lelong N, Subtil D, Dehaene P. Effects on birth weight of alcohol and caffeine consumption during pregnancy. Am J Epidemiol 1993;137:947–50.
140. Maier SE, Chen W-JA, Miller J, West JR. Fetal alcohol exposure and temporal vulnerability: Regional differences in alcohol-induced microencephaly as a function of the timing of binge-like alcohol exposure during rat brain development. Alcohol Clin Exp Res 1997;21:1418–28.
141. Maier SE, Chen W-JA, West JR. Prenatal binge-like alcohol exposure alters neurochemical profiles in fetal rat brain. Pharmacol Biochem Behav 1996;55:521–9.
142. Goldschmidt L, Richardson GA, Stoffer DS, Geva D, Day NL. Prenatal alcohol exposure and academic achievement at age six: A non-linear fit. Alcohol Clin Exp Res 1996;20:763–70.
143. Konovalov HV, Kovetsky NS, Bobryshev YV, Ashwell KWS. Disorders of brain development in the progeny of mothers who used alcohol during pregnancy. Early Hum Dev 1997;48:153–66.
144. Zelson C, Lee SJ, Casalino M. Neonatal narcotic addiction: comparative effects of maternal intake of heroin and methadone. N Engl J Med 1973;289:1216–20.
145. Connaughton JF, Reeser D, Schut J, Finnegan LP. Prenatal addiction: outcome and management. Am J Obstet Gynecol 1977;129:679–85.
146. Ostrea EM, Chavez CJ. Perinatal problems (excluding neonatal withdrawal) in maternal drug addiction: a study of 830 cases. J Pediatr 1979;94:292–5.
147. Ellwood DA, Sutherland P, Kent C, O'Connor M. Maternal narcotic addiction: pregnancy outcome in patients managed by a specialised drug-dependency antenatal clinic. Aust NZJ Obstet Gynaecol 1987;27:92–8.
148. Alroomi LG, Davidson J, Evans TJ, Galea P, Howat R. Maternal narcotic abuse and the newborn. Arch Dis Child 1988;63:81–3.
149. Johnstone FD, Raab GM, Hamilton BA. The effect of human immunodeficiency virus infection and drug use on birth characteristics. Obstet Gynecol 1996;88:321–6.
150. Johnstone D. Drug abuse in pregnancy. Contemp Rev Obstet Gynaecol 1990;2:96–103.
151. Taeusch HW, Carson SH, Wang NS, Avery ME. Induction of lung maturation and growth retardation in fetal rabbits. J Pediatr 1972;82:869–75.
152. Crofford M, Smith AA. Growth retardation in young mice treated with methadone. Science 1973;181:947–9.
153. Raye JR, Dubin JW, Blechner JN. Fetal growth retardation following maternal morphine administration: nutritional or drug effect. Biol Neonate 1977;32:222.
154. Naeye KL, Blanc W, Leblanc W, Khatamee MA. Fetal complications of maternal heroin addiction: abnormal growth, infections, and episodes of stress. J Pediatr 1973;83:1055–61.
155. Tardiff K, Marzuk PM, Leon AC, Portera L, Hartwell N, Hirsch CS, et al. Accidental fatal drug overdoses in New York City: 1990–1992: Am J Drug Alcohol Abuse 1996;22:135–46.
156. Marzuk PM, Tardiff K, Leon AC, Hirsch CS, Stajic M, Portera L, et al. Poverty and fatal accidental drug overdoses of cocaine and opiates in New York City: An ecological study. Am J Drug Alcohol Abuse 1997;23:221–8.
157. Woodburn KR, Murie JA. Vascular complications of injecting drug misuse. Br J Surg 1996;83:1329–34.
158. Robertson JR, Ronald PJM, Raab GM, Ross AJ, Parpia T. Deaths, HIV infection, abstinence, and other outcomes in a cohort of injecting drug users followed up for 10 years. BMJ 1994;309:369–72.
159. Cregler LL, Mark H. Medical complications of cocaine abuse. N Eng J Med 1986;315:1495–1500.
160. Marzuk PM, Tardiff K, Leon AC, Hirsch CS, Stajic M, Portera L, et al. Fatal injuries after cocaine use as a leading cause of death among young adults in New York City. N Eng J Med 1995;332:1753–7.

161. Burkett G, Gomez-Marin O, Yasin SY, Martinez M. Prenatal care in cocaine-exposed pregnancies. Obstet Gynecol 1998;92:193–200.

162. Strauss RS. Effects of the intrauterine environment on childhood growth. Br Med Bull 1997;53:81–95.

163. Miller Jr JM, Boudreaux MC, Regan FA. A case-control study of cocaine use in pregnancy. Am J Obstet Gynecol 1995;172:180–5.

164. Shiono PH, Klebanoff MA, Nugent RP, Cotch MF, Wilkins DG, Rollins DE, et al. The impact of cocaine and marijuana use on low birth weight and preterm birth: A multicenter study. Am J Obstet Gynecol 1995;172:19–27.

165. Morris P, Binienda Z, Gillam MP, Klein J, McMartin K, Koren G, et al. The effect of chronic cocaine exposure throughout pregnancy on maternal and infant outcomes in the rhesus monkey. Neurotoxicol Teratol 1997;19:47–57.

166. Holzman C, Paneth N. Maternal cocaine use during pregnancy and perinatal outcomes. Epidemiol Rev 1994;16:315–34.

167. MacGregor SN, Keith LG, Bachicha JA, Chasnoff IJ. Cocaine abuse during pregnancy: Correlation between prenatal care and perinatal outcome. Obstet Gynecol 1989;74:882–5.

168. Racine A, Joyce T, Anderson R. The association between prenatal care and birthweight among women exposed to cocaine in New York City. JAMA 1993;270:1581–6.

169. Broekhuizen FF, Utrie J, Van Mullem C. Drug use or inadequate prenatal care? Adverse pregnancy outcome in an urban setting. Am J Obstet Gynecol 1992;166:1747–56.

170. English DR, Hulse GK, Milne E, Holman CDJ, Bower CI. Maternal cannabis use and birth weight: A meta-analysis. Addiction 1997;92:1553–60.

171. Jones HE, Kunko PM, Robinson SE, Balster RL. Developmental consequences of intermittent and continuous prenatal exposure to 1,1,1-trichloroethane in mice. Pharmacol Biochem Behav 1996;55:635–46.

172. Medrano MA. Does a discrete fetal solvent syndrome exist? Alcohol Treat Quart 1996;14:59–76.

173. Johnstone FD. Drug addiction and obstetric practice. In: Bewley S, Ward H, editors. Ethics in Obstetrics and Gynaecology. London: RCOG Press, 1994;237–49.

174. Greenwood J. Creating a new drug service in Edinburgh. BMJ 1990;300:587–9.

175. Kramer MS. Socioeconomic determinants of intrauterine growth retardation. Eur J Clin Nutr 1998;52:S29–33.

176. Carstairs V, Morris R. Deprivation: explaining differences in mortality between Scotland and England and Wales. BMJ 1989;299:886—9.

177. Jarman B. Jarman index 1991;302:527.

178. Wilcox MA, Smith SJ, Johnson IR, Maynard PV, Chilvers CED. The effect of social deprivation on birthweight, excluding physiological and pathological effects. Br J Obstet Gynaecol 1995;102:918–24.

179. Najman JM, Morrison J, Williams GM, Keeping JD, Anderson MJ. Unemployment and reproductive outcome: an Australian study. Br J Obstet Gynaecol 1989;96:308–13.

180. Morrison J, Najman JM, Williams GM, Keeping JD, Anderson MJ. Socio-economic status and pregnancy outcome. An Australian study. Br J Obstet Gynaecol 1989;96:298–307.

181. Hodnett ED. Support from caregivers during at-risk pregnancy – Pregnancy and Childbirth Module: In: Cochrane database of systematic reviews – Review no: 04169. Oxford: Cochrane Updates on Disk – Update Software, 1994;27 April.

182. Gabbe SG, Turner LP. Reproductive hazards of the American lifestyle: Work during pregnancy. Am J Obstet Gynecol 1997;176:826–32.

183. Spinillo A, Capuzzo E, Baltaro F, Piazzi G, Nicola S, Iasci A. The effect of work activity in pregnancy on the risk of fetal growth retardation. Acta Obstet Gynecol Scand 1996;75:531–6.

184. Lotgering FK, Gilbert RD, Longo LD. Maternal and fetal responses to exercise during pregnancy. Physiol Rev 1985;65:1–36.

185. Vianna NJ, Polan AK. Incidence of low birth weight among Love Canal residents. Science 1984;226:1217–19.

186. Dolk H, Vrijheid M, Armstrong B. Risk of congenital anomalies near hazardous-waste landfill sites in Europe: the EUROHAZCON study. Lancet 1998;352:423–7.

5 Studies of Fetal Growth in Animals

Clare Steyn and Mark Hanson

Introduction

Fetal growth is influenced by environmental factors such as maternal size and health, nutrient availability, altitude and ambient temperature. Internal factors such as genetics (see Ch. 2) and the growth potential of the different organs and tissues also determine fetal size at various stages of differentiation. Thus there are so-called "critical periods" of development for each organ system. Influences that interfere with development during one of these critical periods in the early development of an organism may lead to a permanent change in the physiology of that system, resulting in what has come to be called "programming". Thus, diseases that manifest themselves during neonatal and adult life may have been programmed during the in utero life of an individual (see [1] for review).

Determinants of Fetal Growth

Nutrient supply, endocrine status, genetic make-up and various environmental factors all influence fetal growth. It is difficult to quantify the extent to which these different factors independently determine the growth rate of the fetus; however, it is possible to indicate their relative importance. For example, without oxygen the fetus would die, therefore oxygen is essential for growth. However, adrenalectomised fetuses are able to survive [2], therefore cortisol is not *essential* for growth and survival of the fetus. Likewise, thyroidectomised fetuses survive but are growth restricted [3], which suggests that the pituitary–thyroid axis facilitates, though is not essential for, fetal growth.

Nutrients

Nutrient supply to the fetus is the major regulator of fetal growth. There are three different sources from which the fetus may receive nutrients:

1. Transport from the maternal circulation.
2. Synthesis by the placenta and transport to the fetus.
3. Endogenous production by the fetal tissues.

Under normal circumstances the maternal pool is the primary source of nutrients for the fetus [4]. The main nutrients required for fetal growth are oxygen, glucose, lactate, amino acids and lipids (Table 5.1).

Table 5.1 Relative importance of the various factors that determine fetal growth. (*** > ** > *)

Requirements for fetal growth	Importance
oxygen	***
glucose	***
lactate	***
fructose	*
amino acids	***
lipids	***
insulin	***
thyroid hormones	**
cortisol	*
growth hormone	*
IGFs	***
other growth factors	**
genetic	*
maternal size	*

Oxygen

P_aO_2 values in the mother are higher (aorta: 95 mmHg) than those of the fetus (umbilical vein: 35 mmHg); this steep gradient facilitates diffusion of oxygen from mother to fetus. However the rate of oxygen uptake by the placenta is about 50 per cent greater, per gram of tissue, than that of the fetus, which significantly reduces the amount of oxygen that eventually reaches the fetus [4,5]. Oxygen affinity is higher in fetal than in the maternal blood and tissue perfusion is also relatively high, thus ensuring that an adequate supply of oxygen reaches the fetal tissues. The fetal carcass (skin, bone, muscle) has the highest (50 per cent of total) consumption of absolute oxygen, followed by the heart, brain and liver, which together make up a further 35–40% of total oxygen consumption. The heart consumes almost double the amount of oxygen as does brain or liver on a weight-specific basis [5].

Carbohydrates

Glucose and lactate are the major carbohydrates metabolised by the fetus, though some species (ruminants, pig, horse) also utilise fructose [5].

Glucose: Glucose is the main substrate for oxidative metabolism in utero. Maternal and fetal blood glucose concentrations, and the ratio between the two, vary from species to species. Typical values measured in the sheep are 2.25–3.00 mmol/l in the mother and 0.75–1.25 mmol/l in the fetus. The low maternal to fetal concentration gradient means that facilitated diffusion of glucose across the placenta must occur. As with oxygen, a large amount of the glucose leaving the maternal circulation is consumed by the placenta: in late gestation this is 60–75% of the total uterine glucose uptake [4]. Glucose taken up by the placenta may either be oxidised or may be used for lipogenesis, glycogenesis and conversion to lactate, fructose or amino acids, some of which may be subsequently released into the umbilical circulation. The fetus can also produce glucose endogenously by glucogenesis in the liver and kidneys, though this usually only occurs in adverse conditions such as IUGR. The carcass utilises most of the glucose supplied to the fetus, though the brain also consumes fairly large amounts (15 per cent) [4,5].

Lactate: The second most important carbohydrate fuel in the fetus is lactate. It is produced in large quantities by the placenta as a result of the breakdown of glucose (both maternal and fetal in origin) and fructose (fetal), and is released into both maternal and fetal circulations. Its production is affected by fetal, but not placental, metabolism. Fetal tissues produce lactate at approximately twice the rate of the placenta.. Most of this endogenous lactate is derived from glucose, though some may be formed from fructose and amino acids; 70 per cent of the lactate consumed by the fetus is oxidised to CO_2 and the rest contributes to the fetal carbon pool. A large proportion (30 per cent) of the lactate taken up by the fetal organs is utilised by the heart and liver. Although some lactate is produced anerobically, generally this does not imply anerobic metabolism in the fetus. In stressful conditions, however, lactate may be a substrate for glucogenesis by the liver [4,5].

Fructose: Fructose is not an important carbohydrate for metabolism in the fetus. It is produced at a very low rate from glucose in the placenta of the sheep. Only very small amounts are oxidised and it may be converted to lactate [5].

Amino Acids

In the fetus amino acids are essential for oxidation, protein accretion, and as a source of carbon and nitrogen. Concentrations are higher in the fetal than in the maternal circulation – and are higher in the placenta than in either circulation. Thus amino acid transport is an active process. Essential amino acids by definition must come from the mother, whilst non-essential amino acids may be synthesised either by the placenta or endogenously by the fetus. Therefore, the supply of some amino acids to the fetus is dependent on placental metabolism as well as transplacental transport [4–6].

Lipids

Lipids are essential for fetal growth and they may play a minor role in oxidative metabolism. The source of free fatty acids may be maternal, de novo synthesis by the fetoplacental tissues, or the breakdown of triglycerides and phospholipids. It is thought that the triglycerides are produced endogenously [4,5].

Endocrine and Paracrine Factors

Fetal growth not only involves supply of substrates to the fetus, but is a complex interaction between nutrition and various endocrine and paracrine regulators. Growth during childhood is known to be dependent on a wide variety of hormones, in particular GH and the family of IGFs, thyroid hormone, insulin, glucocorticoids and the sex steroids. However, the endocrine regulation of growth in the fetus is much less clearly defined. Maternal hormones that are involved in the regulation of growth (e.g. GH, thyroid hormones, insulin, and steroid hormones) do not cross the placenta in concentrations that are sufficient to influence fetal growth. Therefore, the hormones regulating fetal growth seem to be contained within the fetus itself [7–9].

Insulin

Insulin is essential for fetal growth. It is first detected at 11 weeks' gestational age (GA) in the human fetus, 42 days' GA in the sheep, and 18 days' GA in the rat (see [10] for review). The action of insulin in allowing the cellular uptake of glucose and amino acids in part explains the role of insulin in fetal growth. However, it is also thought to modulate growth by its actions on the IGFs (see [11]). It enhances IGF-I secretion and at high concentrations can bind to IGF-1R, as well as having an inhibitory effect on IGFBP-1 production. Thus, it is likely that insulin does not have a direct effect on fetal growth, but regulates other factors that do [8,9,12,13]. Undernutrition throughout pregnancy in the rat has been seen to result in decreased levels of insulin in offspring at birth, as well as IUGR [14].

Thyroid Hormones

The hypothalamic–pituitary–thyroid axis is active from 10 weeks' GA in the human fetus [13], 50 days' GA in the sheep and 19 days' GA in the rat (see [10]). Tri-iodothyronine (T4), the active form of thyroid hormone, promotes fetal growth by increasing protein synthesis, and by its synergistic action with growth hormone-releasing hormone (GHRH) in the secretion of GH and the IGFs. It has been suggested that increased thyroxine (T4) levels may cause an increase in IGF-I and asymmetrical growth retardation is observed in hypothyroid sheep [9]. Fetal thyroid function is significantly affected by nutrient availability. Reduced substrate supply, (e.g. from maternal starvation or uterine artery occlusion) leads to a decrease in plasma T4 concentration and IUGR [15].

Cortisol

Cortisol concentrations are low (about 10 ng/ml) for most of gestation in fetal sheep, then start to rise gradually 10–15 days before birth (up to about 20 ng/ml), with a final surge 3–5 days before birth (up to about 70 ng/ml) [7]. Fetal cortisol has maternal and placental origins, as well as being produced from the fetal adrenal. It is thought to be a modulator of fetal growth because there is a decline in fetal growth concomitant with the rise in cortisol towards the end of gestation. In addition, adrenalectomised fetuses are heavier than intact fetuses. However, the mechanisms by which cortisol may affect growth are not known. Postnatally, cortisol has an antagonistic effect on insulin and downregulates IGF gene expression.

Cortisol is involved in the maturation of various organs during the perinatal period. In the lung it is involved in the manufacture of pulmonary surfactant [9,13]. In the gut it is important for proliferation of microvilli and the induction of digestive enzymes [7]. In the liver it is involved in the maturation of glycogen synthase, an enzyme essential for accumulation of hepatic glycogen during the last trimester. Cortisol also induces beta receptors and hepatic gluconeogenic activities important for the supply of glucose to the neonate following birth [2,4,7,16]. These effects on tissue maturation may in part be due to the effects of cortisol on IGF production. In the ovine fetus, liver and adrenal gene expression of IGF-II is depressed, expression of IGF-I is enhanced in the liver, and hepatic GH receptor mRNA is increased following cortisol administration [7].

One recent study in sheep showed that excess glucocorticoid exposure during early pregnancy programmed hypertension in the offspring, an effect that persisted into adult life [17], despite the fact that there was no reduction in fetal or neonatal growth. In rats, treatment with dexamethasone during the last week of pregnancy resulted in reduced birthweight and elevated blood pressure of the adult offspring, via mechanisms thought to involve glucocorticoid and mineralo-corticoid receptors in the hippocampus [18]. Langley-Evans [19] showed in rats that exposure to maternal low protein diet in utero increased hypothalamic glycerol-3-phosphate dehydrogenase activity, which he suggested may indicate hypersensitivity to the actions of glucocorticoids. The above findings, taken together, suggest a mechanism involving the glucocorticoids, as a result of under-nutrition during pregnancy, in the programming of hypertension in later life.

Pituitary Hormones

GH is found in the fetal circulation from at least 12 weeks' gestation in the human. It reaches levels of around 100 ng/ml during mid gestation, which is higher than at any other time during life [9,13]. Until recently it was thought that GH was not a major determinant of fetal growth. However, it is now thought to be involved in the control of fetal growth through its actions on the IGFs. GH deficiency is accompanied by a decrease in IGF-I levels, and GH is thought to be responsible for the production of IGFBP-3 during late gestation [13].

Insulin-like Growth Factors

The IGFs, IGF-I and -II, are polypeptide hormones that structurally and func-tionally are similar to insulin. They have both anabolic and mitogenic effects by which they promote growth. The primary source of fetal IGF-I is the liver, but all tissues produce both IGF-I and -II [11,20]. Their actions are modulated through IGFBP, to which they are bound in the plasma. Six have thus far been identified: numbered IGFBP-1–IGFBP-6. IGF-II binds specifically to IGFBP-2 and IGFBP-6, and the other IGFBPs show similar affinity for either IGF-I or -II [20]. The IGFs also have specific cell membrane receptors, IGF-1R and IGF-2R. IGF-I binds to IGF-1R, and IGF-II can bind to both IGF-1R and -2R. The IGFs also interact with two other receptor types, the so-called "hybrid receptor" and the insulin receptor [11]. The principal sites of IGF-I synthesis are muscle and liver, however, all tissues express mRNA for both IGF-I and -II.

Regulation of the IGF-signalling pathway is complex and evolving. The most potent regulator of IGF-I is GH, though prolactin, thyroid-stimulating hormone (TSH), luteinising hormone (LH) (or hCG) and follicle-stimulating hormone (FSH) have also been found to stimulate IGF-I production. Low doses of oestro-gens increase plasma IGF-I, whereas pharmacological doses cause a decrease, except in the uterus where IGF-I expression is stimulated by high oestrogen doses. The glucocorticoids also have an effect on IGF-I. They do not affect IGF-I expression, but seem to inhibit its effects. There are a number of other hormones that influence IGF-I synthesis. Parathyroid hormone causes an increase in IGF-I concentration in bone, but not in plasma, and insulin has a permissive effect on GH-stimulated IGF-I production. Platelet-derived growth factor (PDGF), epider-mal growth factor (EGF), transforming growth factor β (TGFβ) and basic fibro-blast growth factor (bFGF) stimulate local IGF-I production, whilst TGFβ is both stimulatory and inhibitory. After GH, nutritional status is the second most important regulator of IGF-I concentration. Both protein and calorie intake have an influence, and a decrease in intake results in a decrease in IGF-I. Less is known about the regulation of IGF-II stimulation than about IGF-I. However, it has been observed that GH causes an increase in brain, skeletal and cardiac muscle, but not hepatic levels of IGF-II. Adrenocorticotrophic hormone (ACTH) and FSH have also been seen to stimulate IGF-II production [20]. Reduced nutrient intake causes a decrease in IGF-II, but to a lesser degree than IGF-I [11].

It appears that early during fetal development IGF-II is critical for the regulation of growth, but in later gestation IGF-I is important [11]. "Knockout" models have provided evidence for the roles played by the IGFs in fetal growth. Mice that have had the *IGF-I* gene knocked out by homologous recombination have severe growth restriction, which becomes evident around 13.5 d GA when the chorioallantoic placenta is functional. The data support the idea that IGF-I is important for growth only in late gestation. IGF-II knockout mice display growth restriction (and reduced placental growth) from 11 days' GA, resuming a normal growth rate after 18 days' GA. In combination these data suggest that IGF-II plays a role in early fetal growth but that IGF-I takes over at a later stage [11,13]. Clearly then the IGFs have a substantial impact on placental and fetal growth and development; however, their regulation of growth is complex and is not fully understood. The growth-promoting actions of both IGF-I and -II are probably mediated via IGF-1R, while the actions of IGF-II are mediated by another as yet unknown receptor type. IGF-1R is important in mediating the actions of IGF-I and IGF-II. The evidence comes from IGF-1R knockout mice, who are more growth restricted than the IGF-I or IGF-II knockout phenotypes. IGFBP-1 is associated with reduced fetal growth via a reduction in the availability of IGF-I. The actions (endocrine and paracrine) of the IGFs are somatogenic, anabolic and anticatabolic, and generally IGF-I is more potent than IGF-II. Their roles during fetal development are many, including regulation of embryogenesis, placental growth, fetal and placental metabolism, and organ growth and differentiation [11].

During the last 2 weeks of gestation there is a marked rise in cortisol in the fetus. There is also a decrease in fetal growth during this period, as well as a decrease in plasma levels of IGF-II. Cortisol has been shown to suppress hepatic IGF-II mRNA expression during late gestation, by a mechanism that involves alterations in the transcriptional regulation of the *IGF-II* gene [21]. It therefore follows that if fetal glucocorticoid levels are affected there may well be alterations in levels of IGF-II, which may affect the further growth and development both during fetal life and postnatally. Indeed it has been demonstrated in rats that chronic maternal undernutrition for the duration of pregnancy results in IUGR that is accompanied by postnatal growth failure, altered allometric growth patterns and changes in postnatal levels of IGF-I and IGFBP-1 and -2 [14].

Other Growth Factors

Most growth factors act in an autocrine or paracrine fashion, though some may be endocrine, intracrine or juxtacrine [9]. Apart from the IGFs there are a plethora of other growth factors that are involved in the regulation of fetal growth. EGF, TGFβ and PDGF are mitogenic in mesenchymal cells, while EGF also has proliferative effects on epithelial tissues. There are various fibroblast growth factors, the most abundant of which is bFGF. This is a potent mitogen and angiogenic growth factor in connective tissues. TGFβ exists in various isomeric forms. It inhibits epithelial cell proliferation, but is also involved in the formation of basal membranes where it causes fibroblasts to increase their production of fibronectin and collagen. Nerve growth factor (NGF) promotes axonal growth, differentiation and survival of sympathetic ganglia [9,22,23]. Together these factors promote cellular proliferation, differentiation, induction, migration, aggregation, maintenance, regeneration and apoptosis.

Other Influences

Plurality

It is well known that plurality influences the size of the fetus at birth. Pregnancies where there is more than one conceptus result in competition between fetuses for space and nutrients, which results in a reduced growth rate compared with singleton pregnancies.

Infection

Infection of the fetus during gestation can result in impaired fetal growth (see Ch. 3). This effect is seen clearly in cases of bovine viral diarrhoea (BVD) in cattle (see [24] where the calf may be born alive, but severely growth restricted. In addition, the induction of cytokines (especially interleukins) by infection (e.g. after premature rupture of the membranes) can induce preterm labour [25] and they may interact with growth factors.

Temperature

Chronic hyperthermia has an adverse affect on fetal and placental development, resulting in reduced growth [26].

Genetic Factors

Growth is in part genetically determined and this is illustrated by the fact that any given species has a typical mean birthweight and adult height, or length, attainment (e.g. in humans birthweight is about 3500 g and adult height is around 1.7 m). However, the variation from one individual to another is not only due to genetic variation, but also reflects environmental influences [27]. There is interaction between maternal and paternal genetic contribution, which is necessary for normal fetal growth. For example, the *IGF-II* gene is paternal and the *IGFR-2* gene maternal. Over- and underexpression of the *IGF-II* gene result in o vergrowth and dwarfism respectively [13].

Environmental Factors

Maternal Size

During life in utero, growth is strongly influenced by the mother, while the paternal genotype is relatively unimportant. However, following birth the genetic make-up of the offspring usually becomes more important than environmental influences. The influence of maternal size during pregnancy was very elegantly demonstrated by the experiments of Walton and Hammond [28], in which Shire horses were crossed with Shetland ponies. They found that when either a Shire or a Shetland stallion was crossed with a Shire mare the newborn foals were of similar size and were quite large. When the mare was a Shetland, again the newborn foals were similar in size, regardless of whether the stallion was Shire or Shetland, but were small. Recently, these findings were corroborated by similar experiments carried out in pony and thoroughbred mares [29]. In these experiments within-breed pregnancies were established by artificial insemination and between-breed pregnancies were established by embryo transfer. It has been suggested that, in the case of the horse, which has a diffuse epitheliochorial placenta, maternal size affects fetal growth as a result of the area of uterine endometrium available for placentation.

Maternal Nutrition

Maternal nutrient intake primarily determines the nutrient supply to the fetus. It follows, therefore, that if maternal nutrient supply is restricted it will result in fetal nutrient restriction also. The effect of maternal undernutrition on fetal growth depends on the specific nutrients that are in short supply, timing, duration, and severity. The fetus requires 95 kcal/kg.day, of which 40 are required for growth and 55 are oxidised (Milner & Gluckman, 1996).

Experimental Measurement of Fetal Growth Rate

Technological limitations mean that it is difficult to measure fetal growth in early gestation, owing to the small size of the fetus. In experimental animals fetal growth can be measured cross-sectionally by sacrificing animals at different gestational ages, but this approach suffers from a lack of longitudinal measurements of growth. Mellor and Matheson [30] developed a technique for measuring fetal growth during late gestation using a CRL-measuring device. This consisted of a nylon monofilament threaded through a sleeve of transparent polyethylene tubing, which was sealed at one end. The open end of the device was attached at the rump and the monofilament was tunnelled subcutaneously along the spine of the fetus to the crown where it was secured. The tubing was then brought to the skin surface through the ewe's flank. Growth of the fetus caused the nylon to be drawn out of the polyethylene tube and could then be measured. Using this device, curves of growth in the fetal sheep between 100 and 140 days' gestation can be obtained. This technique has also been implemented more recently to look at the effect of various factors (e.g. cortisol) on fetal growth during late gestation (see [7]). Longitudinal measurements of fetal growth are also available for the human fetus by serial ultrasound measurements from 6 weeks' gestation [31]. The method is now being applied to large animals, for example Anjari et al. [32] have successfully measured growth of alpaca fetuses from as early as 33 days' GA (term = 345 days) using ultrasound.

This measurement of body growth ignores the importance of measuring the growth of individual fetal organs. Discussion of this is beyond the scope of this chapter, but has been the focus of several recent reviews and books [33–35].

Animal Models for Studying Fetal Growth

Species

There has been much animal research directed at investigating the mechanisms involved in IUGR and programming. A number of different species have been used, including: sheep, rats, guinea pigs, chick embryos, non-human primates, llamas and alpacas, pigs, goats and horses. Apart from cost and availability, the choice of species is determined by the specific question being addressed.

1. Do we know enough about the comparative physiology of the species in question with respect to the human to make valid comparisons?
2. Is the fetus of the species of choice big enough for us to be able to perform the manipulations that are required by the study?
3. Would a species with a particular specialist adaptation better enable us to investigate a certain phenomenon?

So the types of things that we would consider when choosing our animal model include availability, cost, size, precocity, placentation, development and physiology of individual organ systems, and rate of reproduction.

Programming and Critical Periods of Development

McCance and Widdowson [36] and Osofsky [37] reviewed data from the preceding 50 years or so in an attempt to gain insight into the factors that are important for growth and development of the fetus and child. Whilst they both concluded that the factors determining growth are complex and multifactorial, it was clear that the development of growth restriction depends not only upon the type of insult, but also on its severity, duration and the time of exposure during development.

A recent review [38] discussed our current understanding of nutrition during pregnancy and its importance during critical periods for cardiovascular and endocrine development of the fetus. It highlighted the complexity of the mechanisms involved, discussing not only the effects of different nutrients, but also their importance for the development of the various different organ systems, in both animal and human studies. It also highlights the fact that altered development as a result of inadequate intrauterine nutrition is not necessarily accompanied by a reduction in birthweight. The fact that birthweight need not be significantly reduced for there to be physiological effects of reduced nutrition in pregnancy is further emphasised by studies in sheep [39]. In these studies it has been shown that moderate maternal undernutrition during the first half of pregnancy results in altered placental development and disturbed development of the hypothalamic–pituitary–adrenal (HPA) axis, blood pressure and small resistance vessels of the fetus and neonate. Furthermore, it has been shown that dietary deprivation during pregnancy, whether global undernutrition or a low protein diet, results in changes in vascular function of adult offspring that may become hypertensive (see Ch. 20, also [40,41]), although this may depend on the timing of the challenge [42].

Type of Insult

The particular nutrient that the fetus is deprived of is also an important factor in determining body and organ growth. McCance and Widdowson [36] found that pigs kept on an energy-deficient diet were asymmetrically growth restricted and skinny, whilst protein-deficient animals were also asymmetrically growth restricted but tended to become fat. Osofsky [37] described decreased brain weight, as a consequence of protein deprivation, as being more severe than if the diet was purely caloric restriction. Prenatal protein deprivation produced a permanent stunting of growth. Osofsky indicated that brain growth and development are particularly affected by protein deficiency. Recent experiments in rats have shown that a maternal diet low in protein (50 per cent reduction in casein compared with controls) during pregnancy results in hypertensive offspring, an effect that is suggested to be the result of altered corticosteroid exposure to the fetus [19]. Reduced caloric intake (rather than just that of a specific nutrient) during intrauterine life has also been shown to affect cardiovascular development of the fetus, while restrictions in both caloric and protein intake result in alterations in endocrine function [38].

During both early and mid gestation, decreased caloric intake has either no effect on fetal growth [43,45,46] or causes a reduction [47]. Placental weight is either unaffected [43] or increased [45,46]. Caloric deprivation in mid to late gestation causes primary IUGR [48] with reduced placental weight, but with an increased placental to birthweight ratio. However, uterine artery ligation over a similar period of gestation, which results in decreased CaO_2, evokes secondary IUGR and reduced placental growth, but the ratio of placental to fetal weight remains unchanged from that of controls [49]. Undernutrition in late gestation results in asymmetrical growth [43,45,50] and appears to have little effect on placental growth [43]. Oxygen deprivation in late gestation causes either secondary [51–54] or primary [48] growth restriction: placental weight is also reduced, thus placental to fetal body weight ratio is unaffected [53,54]. Block et al. [48] found that placental weight was reduced, but this is not surprising as they were embolising the placenta. Reduced oxygen supply for most of pregnancy causes growth restriction [55–59] but has varying effects on placental growth, but decreased weight [57,58] or increased weight [55,56,59] have been reported.

Timing of Insult

McCance and Widdowson [36] made the statement that "there is a metabolic clock in every animal that determines when each organ shall begin and end its growth or its function, how the animal will behave at every age and when its life is getting near its end". It therefore follows that the outcome of an interruption in growth and/or function is determined by exactly when during the development of the animal that interruption occurs. The effect on an organ or system will be dependent upon the stage of development of the organ/system. This is defined by what has come to be known as "critical" periods of development.

It has been suggested that primary growth restriction is the result of factors acting early in gestation, and that secondary growth restriction is a consequence of events later on in development [1,60].

Studies of human pregnancies [37,43,61] are extremely inconsistent. One observation was made of babies born to mothers who were subjected to near-starvation by the Nazis during the siege of Leningrad, which took place during World War II from August 1941 to January 1943 [62]. This study showed no effect of early nutritional deprivation on fetal growth but a decline in birthweight with undernutrition in late gestation. Similarly, Stein and Susser [43] reported that early nutritional deprivation was not associated with impaired fetal growth, whereas nutritional deprivation in late gestation resulted in secondary growth restriction. Contrary to this, however, is the report that maternal weight gain prior to 28 weeks' gestation affects anthropometric measurements at birth [37]. To add to the discrepancies already seen, some studies carried out in the 1940s related maternal nutritional supplementation during pregnancy to improved fetal growth whilst others did not [37]. It may be possible to account for the disagreements between studies on the basis of geography. Those studies that saw a benefit from supplementation were carried out in Toronto, England, Wales and Glasgow, and those that did not were carried out in Chicago, Philadelphia and Nashville. Another complicating factor is the food supplements that were used. In the study carried out in England and Wales a multivitamin milk supplement was used. The study in Chicago gave a protein supplement, whilst that in Philadelphia split the women into three groups: some receiving vitamin, some protein and some vitamin and protein supplements. Another factor that may be significant is that food intake was self-recorded. Further observations have been carried out in Santiago, Chile on infants whose mothers were severely undernourished during pregnancy, resulting in fetal or neonatal death from malnutrition [63]. Severe IUGR resulted, and there was up to a 40 per cent reduction in brain cell number, which was also associated with reduced head circumference. Kramer et al. [61] challenged the view that early onset of growth restriction leads to symmetrical growth failure; in their study asymmetrical growth restriction was more common with taller mothers, pre-eclampsia and male offspring.

McCance and Widdowson [36] described studies conducted in neonatal rats from which it was concluded that undernutrition for a brief period *earlier*, rather than later, in neonatal life restricted both birthweight and the subsequent rate of growth, despite unlimited access to food postnatally. Body proportionality was not affected. Osofsky [37] agreed with the idea that growth was more profoundly and irreversibly affected the earlier following birth at which nutritional deprivation occurred. He also cited studies in pregnant rats that showed that both protein and caloric restriction resulted in fetal growth restriction with decreased brain weight (brain to body weight ratios were not given so it is not clear whether growth was symmetrical or not). Furthermore, and somewhat contrary to the data in neonatal animals, he described effects of a protein-free diet during pregnancy where the effects on brain growth were more severe the *later* in pregnancy deprivation occurred; presumably body weights were affected similarly.

A number of more recent studies in rats [14,54,64] guinea pigs [49] and sheep [45,48,50–53,60,65,66] describe the effects of gestation-specific substrate deprivation on fetal body proportionality (Table 5.2). DeBarro et al. [47] restricted maternal nutritional intake in sheep during early pregnancy, by altering grazing stock rates in pastures, and found a reduction in fetal growth. They did not specify the type of growth restriction observed – symmetrical or asymmetrical. Undernutrition in mid gestation (food intake regulated to achieve a loss of 8 kg liveweight between 30 days' and 96 days' GA) has been reported not to result in growth restriction [46]. Some workers have investigated the effects of nutrient deprivation throughout mid and late gestation [49,66]. Detmer et al. [49], found that uterine artery ligation in the guinea pig, which tended to result in decreased CaO_2, produced fetuses that were asymmetrically growth retarded. Bauer et al. [66] found that mid to late gestation nutritional insult (25 per cent of the recommended energy and protein requirements) caused symmetrical growth restriction. Nutrient deprivation in late gestation, whether in the sheep [45,50–53] or rat [54], and whether due to undernutrition [45,50], placental embolisation [51,52], hypobaric hypoxaemia [53], or uterine artery ligation [54] always resulted in asymmetrical growth retardation. The only exception to this was the study of Block et al. [48], which produced symmetrical growth retardation following placental embolisation. This inconsistency, so far as fetal growth is concerned, may arise because the last study embolised for only 9 days, as opposed to 21 days or more in the other embolisation studies [51,52]. Finally, restricted nutrient supply for the whole of or most of gestation always caused secondary IUGR, regardless of species or method of nutrient restriction employed (Table 5.2).

The complexities surrounding the issue of timing are further emphasised by recent experiments in sheep [45,50]. Periconceptual undernutrition that caused a slowing of fetal growth was not affected by a further nutritional insult in late gestation, although the added insult in late gestation did produce asymmetrical growth (small brains, and big hearts and kidneys). These findings suggest that the

Table 5.2 Summary of the growth patterns observed in different species as a result of various insults

	Early	Mid	Mid and late	Late	Throughout
IUGR	none[ab]	none[o]	primary[k] secondary[e]	primary[j] secondary[abcdir]	secondary[dfgq]
Growth	↓[h]			↓[p]	↓[lmn]
Species	human[a] sheep[bh]	sheep[o]	sheep[k] guinea pig[e]	human[a] rat[i] sheep[bcdfjpr]	human[lm] rat[g] sheep[dfg] guinea pig[n]
Pl.:BW	⇔[a] ↑[h]	↑[o]	⇔[e] ↑[k]	⇔[adi] ↓[j]	⇔[dn] ↑[lm] ↓[q]
Duration: – absolute	30 d[bh] 3 m[a]	66 d[o]	24 d[k] 30 d[e]	60 min[i] 9 d[j] 10 d[br] 21 d[d] 28 d[c] 3m[a]	
Duration – % gestn	20[bh] 30[a]	40[o]	20[k] 50[e]	0.2[i] 10[bdjr] 20[c] 30[a]	
Insult	undernutrition[abh]	undernutrition[o]	undernutrition[k] uterine artery ligation[e]	undernutrition[abr] uterine artery ligation[i] embolisation[jc] hypobaric hypoxia[d]	hypobaric hypoxia[dn] carunclectomy[q] high altitude[m] anaemia[l]

The data are drawn from: [a][43], [b][45], [c][51,52], [d][53], [e][49], [f][65], [g][64], [h][47], [i][54], [j][48], [k][66], [l][56,59], [m][55], [n][57], [o][46], [p][30,68], [q][69], [r][50], [s][14].

early nutritional insult increases susceptibility to a second nutritional insult, perhaps via an alteration in growth sequence or function of specific organs [45].

It is clear that the timing of a reduction in substrate supply is critical in influencing fetal body and organ growth. However no clear-cut rule exists from which we can say that an insult at a particular time will result in a particular pattern of fetal and placental growth. Perhaps the evidence so far is clouded by differences species and in the duration and severity of exposure.

Duration and Severity of Insult

McCance and Widdowson [36] showed that severe prolonged undernutrition of pigs in the early postnatal period resulted in severe asymmetrical growth retardation, regardless of whether or not the diet was deficient in energy or protein. Rehabilitation to a normal diet resulted in spectacular catch-up growth, though full size was never attained. They also quoted similar results in undernourished rats. Osofsky [37] cited a study where the decrease in brain weight was greater the longer the duration of protein deprivation. Thus, it would appear that the longer the period of stress the greater is the degree of IUGR, though it is unclear whether longer duration produces symmetrical or asymmetrical growth.

Undernutrition in early pregnancy for 20 per cent of gestation in sheep did not affect fetal growth in one study [45] but caused reduced growth in another [47]. The discrepancy between these two studies may be because DeBarro et al. [47] recorded fetal weight at 90 days' GA, whereas Harding and Johnston [45] measured fetal body and organ weights at 125 days' GA. Undernutrition for 30 per cent of gestation in humans [43] did not affect fetal growth. Similarly, in the sheep, undernutrition for 40 per cent of gestation did not produce growth restriction of the fetus [46]. Nutrient restriction for a period during both mid and late gestation resulted in primary IUGR when imposed for 20 per cent of gestation [66] and secondary IUGR when it lasted for 50 per cent of gestation [49]. This pattern is in keeping with the suggestion that the longer the duration of insult the more severe is the outcome. However, the fact that the 20 per cent duration was in the sheep and the 50 per cent duration in the guinea pig means that any differences may be simply due to species differences rather than duration per se. Growth restriction occurs in late gestation irrespective of the duration of insult or species (Table 5.2). Secondary IUGR resulted in all but one study where the insult lasted for 10 per cent of gestation [48]. The latter finding may be related to severity of insult. Perhaps the degree of hypoxaemia (P_aO2 about 17 mmHg), produced for a period of only 9 days, was not sufficient to cause secondary IUGR. Nutrient deprivation throughout pregnancy always produced asymmetrical growth restricted fetuses (where growth pattern was reported). It seems, therefore, that greater duration of deprivation does indeed have more profound effects on growth. Certainly duration of deprivation does affect outcome in terms of blood pressure. Gagnon et al. [67] found no alteration in blood pressure in fetuses that were exposed to repeated placental embolisation over a period of 10 days. However, when the period of embolisation was extended to 21 days, fetuses became hypertensive [52].

The data in Table 5.2 summarise the effects on fetal growth that are produced in various species. It illustrates the importance of timing, severity and duration of insult in determining the degree of growth restriction that results. It also serves to illustrate the complexity of the issues surrounding growth restriction in utero.

References

1. Barker DJP. Mothers, babies and health in later life, 2nd edn. Edinburgh: Churchill Livingstone, 1998.
2. Fowden AL, Coulson RL, Silver M. Endocrine regulation of tissue glucose-6-phosphotase activity in the fetal sheep during late gestation. Endocrinology 1990;126:2823–30.
3. Fowden AL, Apatu RSK, Silver M. The glucogenic capacity of the fetal pig: developmental regulation by cortisol. Exp Physiol, 1995;80:457–67.
4. Fowden AL. Endocrine regulation of fetal growth. Reprod Fertil Dev, 1995;7:351–63.
5. Fowden AL. Fetal metabolism and energy balance. In: Thorburn GD, Harding R, editors, Textbook of fetal physiology. Oxford: Oxford University Press, 70–82.
6. Battaglia FC. New concepts in fetal and placental amino acid metabolism. J Animal Sci 1992;70:3258–63.
7. Fowden AL. Nutrient requirements for normal fetal growth and metabolism. In: Hanson, MA, Spencer, JAD, Rodeck, CH, editors, Fetus and neonate: physiology and clinical applications, vol 3: Growth. Cambridge: Cambridge University Press, 1995;31–56.
8. Han VKM, Hill DJ. Growth factors in fetal growth. In: Thorburn G.D. & Harding R, editors, Textbook of Fetal Physiology, Oxford: Oxford University Press, 1994;48–69.
9. Han VKM & Fowden AL. (1994). Paracrine regulation of fetal growth. In: Ward RHT, Smith SK, Donnai D. editors, Early fetal growth and development. London: RCOG Press, 1994;275–91.
10. Parkes M. (1988). Endocrine factors in fetal growth. In: Fetal and Neonatal Growth, ed. Cockburn F. pp. 33–48. John Wiley & Sons.
11. Gluckman PD. Insulin-like growth factors and their binding proteins. In: Hanson MA, Spencer JAD, Rodeck CH, editors, Fetus and neonate. Physiology and clinical applications, vol 3: Growth Cambridge: Cambridge University Press, 1995; 97–115.
12. Bassett JM. Glucose and fetal growth derangement. In: Hanson MA, Spencer JAD, Rodeck CH, editors, Fetus and Neonate. Physiology and cinical applications, vol 3: Growth. Cambridge: Cambridge University Press, 1995;223–54.
13. Milner RDG, Gluckma PD. Regulation of intrauterine growth. In: Gluckman PD, Heymann MA, editors, Pediatrics and Perinatology. The Scientific Basis. London: Arnold, 1996;284–9.
14. Woodall SM, Breier BH, Johnston BM, Gluckman PD. A model of intrauterine growth retardation caused by chronic maternal undernutrition in the rat: effects on the somatotrophic axis and post-natal growth. J Endocrinol. 1996;150:231–42.
15. Symonds ME. Pregnancy, parturition and neonatal development: interactions between nutrition and thyroid hormones. Proc Nutr Soc. 1995;54:329–43.
16. Fowden AL, Mijovic J, Silver M. The effects of cortisol on hepatic and renal gluconeogenic enzyme activities in the sheep fetus during late gestation. J Endocrinol, 1992;137:213–22.
17. Dodic M, May CN, Wintour EM, Coghla, JP. An early prenatal exposure to excess glucocorticoid leads to hypertensive offspring in sheep. Clin Sci, 1998;94(2):149–55.
18. Levitt NS, Lindsay RS, Holmes MC, Seckl JR. Dexamethasone in the last week of pregnancy attenuates hippocampal glucocorticoid receptor gene expression and elevates blood pressure in the adult offspring in the rat. Neuroendocrinology, 1996;64(6):412–18.
19. Langley-Evans SC. Hypertension induced by fetal exposure to maternal low protein diet, in the rat, is prevented by pharmacological blockade of maternal glucocorticoid synthesis. J Hyperten, 1997;15(5):537–44.
20. Blum WF, Gluckman PD. Insulin-like growth factors. In: Gluckman, PD, Heymann MA, editors, Pediatrics and perinataology. The scientific basis. London: Arnold, 1996;314–23.
21. Li J, Saunders JC, Fowden AL, Dauncey MJ, Gilmour RS. Transcriptional regulation of insulin-like growth factor-II gene expression by cortisol in fetal sheep during late gestation. J biol Chem, 1998;273(17):10586–593.
22. Engström W, Heath JK. Growth factors in early embryonic development. In: Cockburn F, editors, Fetal and Neonatal Growth, Chichester: John Wiley, 1998;11–32.
23. Hill DJ, Han VKM. Role of growth factors in tissue development. In: Gluckman PD, Heymann MA, editors, Pediatrics and Perinatology. The scientific basis, London: Arnold, 1996;279–83.

24. Brownlie J, Hooper LB, Thompson I, Collins ME. Maternal recognition of fetal infection with bovine virus diarrhaea virus (BVDV) – the bovine pestivirus. Clin Diagn Virol, 1998;10:141–50.

25. Yoon BH, Romero R, Jim JK, Maymon E, Gomez R, Mazor M, et al. An increase in fetal plasma cortisol but not dehydroepiandosterone sulfate is followed by the onset of preterm labor in patients with preterm premature rupture of the membranes. Am J Obstet Gynecol, 1988;179:1107–114.

26. Bell AW, McBride BW, Slepatis R, Early RJ, Currie WB. Chronic heat stress and prenatal development in sheep: I. Conceptus growth and maternal plasma hormones and metabolites. J Am Sci, 1989;67:3289–299.

27. Yates JRW. Genetics of fetal and postnatal growth. In: Cockburn F, editors, Perinatal practice, vol 5. Fetal and neonatal growth. Chichester: John Wiley & Sons, 1998;1–10.

28. Walton A, Hammond J. (1938). The maternal effects on growth and confirmation in Shire horse-Shetland pony crosses. J of Proceedings of the Royal Society of London, Series B, 125:311–335.

29. Allen WR, Steward M, Ball M, Fowden A, Ousey JC, Rossdale PD. (1998). The influence of maternal size on fetal and postnatal development in the horse. Proceedings of the Dorothy Russel Havemeyer Foundation; Sidney, Australia, 9.

30. Mellor DJ, Mathieson IC. (1979). Daily changes in the curved crown-rump length of individual sheep fetuses during the last 60 days of pregnancy and effects of different levels of maternal nutrition. Quarterly Journal of Experimental Physiology. 64:119–131.

31. Robson SC, Chang TC. Measurement of human fetal growth. In: Hanson MA, Spencer JAD, Rodeck CH, editors, Fetus and neonate: Physiology and clinical applications, Vol 3: Growth Cambridge: Cambridge University Press, 1995;297–325.

32. Anjari JE, Del Campo CH, Guerra FA, Del Campo MR. (1996). Ultrasonographic estimation of gestational age in alpaca. Proceedings of 23rd Annual Meeting of Fetal and Neonatal Physiological Society, Africa, Chile.

33. Hanson MA. (1986). Peripheral chemoreceptor function before and after birth. In: Respiratory Control and Lung Development in the Fetus and Newborn. Eds. BM Johnston & P Gluckman. Perinatology Press, pp. 311–330.

34. Gluckman PD, Heyman M. (1996) Pediatrics and perinatology: the scientific basis. E. Arnold.

35. Ward RHT, Smith SK, Donnai D. In: editors. Early fetal growth and development. London: RCOG. 1975;

36. McCance RA, Widdowson EM. (1974). The determinants of growth and form. Proceedings of the Royal Society of London (Biological), 185:1–17.

37. Osofsky HJ. Relationships between nutrition during pregnancy and subsequent infant and child development. Obstetrl and Gynecol Survey, 1975;30(4):227–41.

38. Hoet JJ, Hanson MA. (1999). Intrauterine nutrition: Its importance during critical periods for cardiovascular and endocrine development. J. Physiol. (in press).

39. Hanson MA, Hawkins P, Ozaki T, Steyn C, Mathews SG, Noakes D, Poston L. (1999). Effects of experimental dietary manipulation during early pregnancy on cardiovascular and endocrine function in fetal sheep and young lambs. In: Fetal Programming: Influences on development and disease in later life, 36th RCOG Scientific Study Group, RCOG Press (in press).

40. Langley, Jackson, (1994). Increased systolic blood pressure in adult rats induced by fetal exposure to maternal low protein diets. Clin Sci, 1994;86(2):217–22.

41. Hanson MA, Ozaki T, Nishina H, Poston L (1999). In: editors, Barker DJP, Lenfant C, Marcel Dekker, Fetal Origins of Cardiovascular Disease. New York:

42. Holemans K, Gerber R, Meurrens K, Spitz B, Declerck F, Poston L, et al. (1999). Maternal malnutrition in the rat affects vascular function but not blood pressure of adult offspring. Br J Nutr (in press).

43. Stein Z, Susser M (1975a). The Dutch famine, 1944–1945, and the reproductive process. I. Effects on six indices at birth. Pediatr Res. 9:70–6.

44. Stein Z, Susser M (1975b). The Dutch famine, 1944–1945, and the reproductive process. II. Interrelations of caloric rations and six indices at birth. Pediatrc Res. 9:76–83.

45. Harding JE, Johnston BM. (1995). Nutrition and fetal growth. Reproduction, Fertility and Development 7:539–547.

46. McCrabb GJ, Egan AR, Hosking BJ (1991). Maternal undernutrition during mid-pregnancy in sheep. Placental size and its relationship to calcium transfer during late pregnancy. Br J Nutr. 65:157–68.

47. DeBarro TM, Owens JA, Earl CR, Robinson JS (1992). Mating weight influences the effect of mid-pregnancy nutrition on placental growth in the sheep. Proc Austr Nutr Soc, pp. 7403

48. Block BS, Schlafer DH, Wentworth RA, Kreitzer LA, Nathanielsz PW. (1990). Regional blood flow distribution in fetal sheep with intrauterine growth retardation produced by decreased umbilical placental perfusion. J Dev Physiol 13:81–85.

49. Detmer A, Gu W, Carter AM (1991). The blood supply to the heart and brain in the growth retarded guinea pig fetus. Deve Physiol 15:153–60.
50. Harding JE. (1994). The role of nutrition and pre-natal growth development. Proceedings of the 4th International Conference on Veterinary Perinatology. Cambridge, UK.
51. Creasy RK, Barrett CT, Deswiet M, Kahanpää KV, Rudolph AM (1972). Experimental intrauterine growth retardation in the sheep. Am J Obstet Gynecol 112(4):566–73.
52. Murotsuki J, Challis JRG, Han VKM, Fraher LJ, Gagnon R (1997). Chronic fetal embolization and hypoxemia cause hypertension and myocardial hypertrophy in fetal sheep. Am J Physiol 272:(1 pt 2): R201–7.
53. Jacobs R, Robinson RS, Owens JA, Falconer J, Webster MED (1988a). The effect of prolonged hypobaric hypoxia on growth of fetal sheep. J Dev Physiol 10:97–112.
54. Tanaka M, Natori M, Ishimoto H, Miyazaki T, Kobayashi T, Nozawa S. (1994). Experimental growth retardation produced by transient period of uteroplacental ischemia in pregnant Sprague-Dawley rates. Am J Obstet & Gynecol 171:1231–1234.
55. Krüger H, Arias-Stella J (1970) The placenta and the newborn infant at high altitudes. Am J Obst Gynecol 106(4):586–91.
56. Beischer NA, Sivasamboo R, Vohra S, Silpisornkosal S, Reid S (1970). Placental hypertrophy in severe pregnancy anaemia. Obstetr Gynaecol Br Common 77:398–409.
57. Bacon BJ, Bilbert RD, Kaufmann P, Smith AD, Trevino FT, Longo LD. (1984). Placental anatomy and diffusing capacity in guinea pigs following long-term maternal hypoxia. Placenta 5:475–488.
58. Jacobs R, Owens JA, Falconer J, Webster MED, Robinson JS (1988). Changes in metabolite concentration in fetal sheep subjected to prolonged hypobaric hypoxia. Deve Physiol 10:113–21.
59. Godfrey KM, Redman CWG, Barker DJP, Osmond C (1991). The effect of maternal anaemia and iron deficiency on the ratio of fetal weight to placental weight. Br Obstetr Gynaecol 98:886–91.
60. Owens JA, Owens PC, Robinson JS (1995). Experimental restriction of fetal growth. In: editors, Hanson MA, Spencer JAD, Rodeck CH. Fetus and neonate: physiology and clinical applications. vol 3: Growth Cambridge: Cambridge University Press, 1995;139–75.
61. Kramer MS, Olivier M, McLean FH, Dougherty GE, Willis DM, Usher RD. (1990). Determinants of fetal growth and body proportionality. Pediatrics, 86:18–26.
62. Antonov AN. Children born during the siege of Leningrad in 1942. Pediatr 1947;30:250–59.
63. Winick M (1969). Malnutrition and brain development. Pediatr 74(5):667–679.
64. Desai M, Crowther NJ, Ozanne SE, Lucas A, Hales CN. (1995). Adult glucose and lipid metabolism may be programmed during fetal life. Biochem Soc Trans 23(2):331–335.
65. Kamitomo M, Alonso JG, Okai T, Longo LD, Gilbert RD. Effects of long-term, high-altitude hypoxaemia on ovine fetal cardiac output and blood flow distribution. Am Obstetr Gynaecol 1993;169:701–7.
66. Bauer MK, Breier BH, Harding JE, Veldhuis JD, Gluckman PD. (1995). The fetal somatrophic axis during long term maternal undernutrition in sheep: evidence for nutritional regulation in utero. Endocrinology 136:1250–1257.
67. Gagnon R, Challis J, Johnston L, Fraher L (1994). Fetal endocrine responses to chronic placental embolization in the late-gestation ovine fetus. Am Obstetr Gynaecol 1994;170:929–38.
68. Mellor DJ, Murray L (1981). Effects of placental weight and maternal nutrition on the growth rates of individual fetuses in single and twin bearing ewes during late pregnancy. Res Veterin Sci 1981;30:198–204.
69. Owens JA, Falconer J, Robinson JS. (1986). Effect of restriction of placental growth on umbilical and uterine blood flows. Am. J. Physiol 250:R427–434.
70. Wheeler T, O'Brien PMS (Eds.) (1999). Fetal Programming: Influences on development and disease in later life. RCOG Press London (in press).

6 The Uteroplacental Circulation: Extravillous Trophoblast

Fiona Lyall and Peter Kaufmann

Introduction

In this chapter we review extravillous trophoblast (EVT) and the mechanisms that control their invasion into the decidua and myometrium. EVT is a highly migratory, proliferative and invasive population of cells that emerge from tips of anchoring villi. Like tumour invasion, trophoblast invasion of the uterus involves attachment of the cells to the extracellular matrix (ECM), degradation of the matrix and subsequent migration through it. However, in contrast to tumour invasion, trophoblast invasion is a tightly controlled process that is regulated by decidual cells, the trophoblast cells themselves and many diffusable factors within the placental bed itself. The literature reviewed will be mainly confined to humans and will focus primarily on the trophoblast cells themselves. Particular emphasis has been placed on topics that, in the authors' opinion, have been where the most exciting developments have been. While several investigators have also studied extravillous trophoblast in pre-eclampsia, the literature on intrauterine growth restriction is sparse.

Extravillous Trophoblast

Trophoblast is present in the areas overlying chorionic villi, in the columns that anchor the placenta to the decidua, in the trophoblastic shell that surrounds the implanted blastocyst early in gestation, in the decidua in the basal plate and the myometrium of the placental bed, in spiral arteries below the placenta and underlying the chorioamnion that invests the endometrial cavity later in gestation. EVT is made up of all trophoblast found outside the villi. EVT are primarily mononuclear cells, although syncytial or multinucleated cells are also found mainly in the deeper parts of the junctional zone. EVT are found in several places: in the chorionic plate, the smooth chorion, cell islands, cell columns, the basal plate, the placental septa and in the walls and lumen of uteroplacental vessels (Fig. 6.1). Kurman suggested the term "intermediate trophoblast" for a distinctive form of trophoblast, localised outside the villi, with specific morphological, biochemical and functional features based on immunocytochemical studies with hCG, human placental lactogen (hPL) and pregnancy-specific beta 1-glycoprotein (SP1–)[1]. It is our view that this population is identical to that defined by the term "extravillous trophoblast".

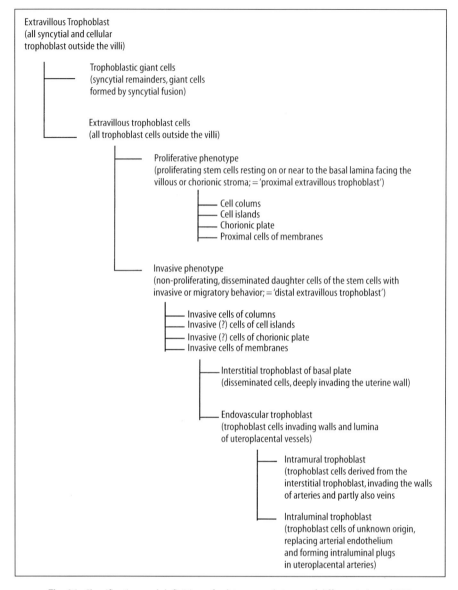

Fig. 6.1 Classification and definition of subtypes and stages of differentiation of EVT.

Proliferation Markers

Staining of first and second trimester placentas with proliferation markers such as Ki-67, MIB-1, antibodies against proliferating cell nuclear antigen (PCNA) or [³H]thymidine have shown that only cells close to the basal lamina of the anchoring villus are positive [2–6]. The proliferation markers show characteristic differences in their staining patterns, which can result in misinterpretations [6,7].

[^{3}H]thymidine uptake experiments must be performed on fresh tissue and incomplete diffusion of the incubation medium, particularly in the compact cell columns, can lead to false negative results.

Ki-67 and MIB-1 are both directed against the same nuclear antigen, which is expressed in all stages of the cell cycle except G_o and G_i. As a result, this marker shows higher staining indices. With this marker, immunoreactivity is found in two to six proximal layers of columns. The deep invasive and intravascular trophoblast cells are always negative for Ki-67, MIB-1 and [^{3}H]thymidine. PCNA is expressed throughout the cell cycle; however, it has a half-life of about 20 hours. This has led to problems in interpreting data; for example, PCNA expression was found in intravascular trophoblast [8], which suggests that these cells were replicating. However, a later study by the same group using Ki-67 concluded that the immunoreactivity seen with PCNA was in fact due to the long half-life of the antigen [5]. In conclusion, the cells close to the villous basal lamina represent the stem cells whereas all other EVT are derived from the closest proliferation site by migration or invasion.

Other Markers

Cytokeratins are related to differentiation and proliferation of epithelial cells and this appears to include trophoblast cells. EVTs in cell islands and cell columns are positive for cytokeratin 13 only in cell layers proximal to the villous stroma, whereas distal and more differentiated cells do not stain [9]. All trophoblasts are cytokeratin 7 positive in cell islands and columns; however, cells deep within the decidua are negative. These observations, along with those on villous trophoblast, show that populations of human trophoblast express different cytokeratins according to their state of differentiation and development.

Cell Adhesion Molecules and the Extracellular Matrix

Cell adhesion molecules (CAMs) and the ECM have been extensively studied in relation to trophoblast invasion and thus a background to the ECM and CAMs precedes this topic.

The ECM

The ECM of tissues is composed of a variety of proteins and polysaccharides assembled into an organised meshwork and is mainly produced by cells within the matrix [10–12]. In most connective tissues, matrix molecules are secreted by fibroblasts or overlying epithelial sheets. The two main classes of molecules that make up the matrix are: (i) polysaccharide chains of the glycosaminoglycan (GAG) class, usually found linked to proteins in the form of proteoglycans, and (ii) fibrous proteins of two functional types: those that are mainly structural (e.g. collagen and elastin) and those that mainly play a role in attachment (e.g. fibronectin and laminin). The main groups of GAGs are hyaluronan, chondroitin sulphate, dermatan sulphate, heparan sulphate, heparin and keratan sulphate. GAGs form a gel structure, containing large amounts of water, allowing the matrix to withstand compression forces (in contrast to collagen fibres, which resist stretching forces). However, proteoglycans not only provide hydrated space around and between cells, but can also act as coreceptors with conventional cell surface receptor proteins in binding cells to the ECM and in altering the response of some cells to growth factors such as TGFβ.

Collagens are long, stiff, triple-stranded helical structures [13,14]. About 15 types of collagen molecules have been identified. The main types of collagen fibres found in connective tissues are types I, II, III, V and XI and are assembled into fibrils. Types IX and XII decorate the surface of collagen fibrils and are thought to link the fibrils to one another and to other components in the ECM. Types IV and VII are network-forming collagens: type IV forms a meshwork that constitutes a major part of the basal lamina, whereas type VII assembles into anchoring fibrils helping to attach the basal lamina of multilayered epithelia to the underlying connective tissue.

The ECM contains a number of non-collagen "adhesive proteins" each with specific binding sites for other matrix molecules and for receptors on the surface of cells. Thus they help organise the matrix and help cells attach to it. Fibronectin, a large glycoprotein, is a member of this group [15]. Individual domains within the molecule bind to collagen, heparin or to specific receptors on the surface of various cell types. The major region in fibronectin responsible for cell binding is known as the RGD (Arg-Gly-Asp) sequence. The RGD sequence is also found in a number of ECM proteins and is recognised by several members of the integrin family of cell surface matrix receptors. Produced by a single gene as a result of alternative splicing of mRNAs, three different types of homology regions (type I, type II and type III domains) as well as several special domains (ED-A, ED-B and III-CS) are expressed in humans. The ED-B domain is expressed only in oncofetal fibronectins that are specific for invasive trophoblast and tumour cells [16,17]. Apart from plasma fibronectin, all other fibronectin forms assemble on the cell surface and are released into the ECM as fibronectin filaments. Fibronectin is not only important for cell adhesion to the matrix but also guides cell migration. Another ECM molecule, tenascin, is abundant in the ECM of embryonic tissues [18]. This large glycoprotein complex, in contrast to fibronectin, can both promote and inhibit cell adhesion depending on the cell type.

Laminins are a family of ECM glycoproteins [19,20]. Laminin is a large protein complex of three long polypeptide chains held together by disulphide bonds assembled to form a cruciform molecule with one long and three short arms comprised of an α, β and γ subunit. It too, like many other ECM proteins, has a number of functional domains: one binds to type IV collagen, one to heparan sulphate, one to the sulphated glycoprotein entactin and two or more to laminin receptors on cell surfaces. Laminin, along with entactin, the proteoglycan per-lecan and type IV collagen, make up the basement membrane, that is, the area of ECM that underlies all epithelial sheets. There are two distinct layers in the base-ment membrane: the basal lamina is the area immediately adjacent to the cells and is a product of the epithelial cells themselves, whereas the reticular lamina is produced by fibroblasts of the underlying connective tissue and contains fibrillar collagen. Eleven laminins have been identified to date (alternative names and subunits are shown in brackets): laminin 1 (EHS laminin, $\alpha1b1\gamma1$), laminin 2 (merosin, $\alpha2\beta1\gamma1$), laminin 3 (S laminin, $\alpha1\beta2\gamma1$), laminin 4 (S merosin, $\alpha2\beta2\gamma1$), laminin 5 (kalinin/nicein, $\alpha3\beta3\gamma2$), laminin 6 (K laminin, $\alpha3\beta1\gamma1$), laminin 7 (K-S laminin, $\alpha3\beta2\gamma1$) and laminins 8 ($\alpha4\beta1\gamma1$), 9($\alpha4\beta2\gamma1$), 10($\alpha5\beta1\gamma1$) and 11 ($\alpha5\beta2\gamma1$). Some of the subunits discussed in this article were previously known as: A (α1), M (α2), S(β2), B1(β1) and B2(γ1). In contrast to fibronectin, laminins are found mainly in basal laminae. Specific laminins are present in each basement membrane; for example, laminins 1–4 have been reported in human placental villous basement membrane [21]. Laminin binding to cells is important in adhesion, polarisation and migration of many cells and, indeed, both choriocarcinoma [22] and human cytotrophoblast (CTB) [23] attach to substrates that contain laminin 1.

CAMs

The Cadherin Family

The cadherins are a family of calcium-dependent adhesion molecules found both within and outside the nervous system [23–27]. A schematic representation of the structure of the cadherins is shown in Fig. 6.2. Most cadherins are single pass transmembrane glycoproteins of about 700–750 amino acids and contain an extracellular domain containing 3–5 repeats of approximately 110 amino acids. Repeats 1–3 contain putative Ca^{2+}-binding site motifs. In the absence of calcium, cadherins undergo a conformational change and are rapidly degraded. The biological significance of this striking calcium dependency is unknown. The N terminal 113 amino acids are important in ligand binding and specificity. The extracellular domain is anchored to the cell membrane by a transmembrane domain of approximately 24 amino acids. The short cytoplasmic domain is the most highly conserved region of homology between cadherins and is particularly important for cadherin function. The first three cadherins discovered were named after the tissues where they were found: E cadherin is present on many types of epithelial cells, N cadherin on nerve, muscle and lens cells,, and P cadherin in placenta and epidermis. All are also found transiently on various other tissues during development. Subclasses of cadherins also include R, B and VE cadherins. At least a dozen cadherins are known. Cadherins usually mediate homophilic cell–cell adhesion, although binding between different cadherin molecules is possible. Cadherins are responsible for holding cells together, segregating cell collectives into discrete tissues during development and maintaining tissue integrity, and are expressed in a temporal and spatial manner during embryonic development. On the cell surface cadherins tend to be concentrated at cell–cell junctions (zonula adherens junctions). The demonstration that addition of anticadherin antibodies to embryonic tissues leads to dissociation of the tissue into single cells emphasises the importance of these CAMs. Most cadherins function as transmembrane linker proteins with the cytoplasmic domain interacting with the cytoskeleton of the cells they join together. This is achieved by the cytoplasmic tail interacting with intracellular attachment proteins, such as catenins, which couple the cadherin to the cytoskeleton [28].

The Immunoglobulin Family

The immunoglobulin family has over 70 members and can act as calcium-independent intercellular adhesion molecules, signal transducing receptors, or both [29]. The immunoglobulin family includes a number of cell membrane glycoproteins with structural homology to antibodies. This family, which includes platelet endothelial CAM (PECAM-1), vascular cell adhesion molecule-1 (VCAM-1) and intercellular adhesion molecule-1, 2 and 3 (ICAM-1, 2 and 3), shares the

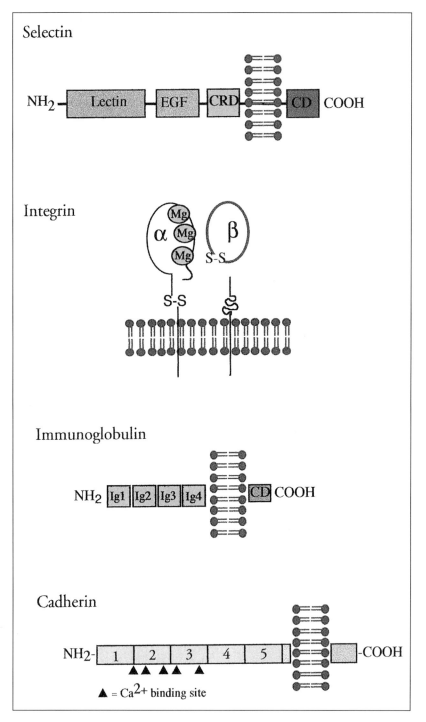

Fig. 6.2 Schematic representation of the four major cell adhesion molecule families.

immunoglobulin domain composed of 970–1100 amino acids arranged in a sandwich of two sheets of antiparallel β strands stabilised by a central disulphide bond. Sequence homology suggests that immunoglobulins, major histo-compatibility molecules, some CAMs and cytokine receptors belong to this multigene family. There is enormous variation in the primary structure of the immunoglobulins but their tertiary structure is remarkably similar (Fig. 6.2). Although interactions between identical and non-identical family members are common amongst members of the immunoglobulin superfamily, non-immunoglobulin superfamily members have also been identified as ligands. These include LFA-1 and Mac-1, which bind ICAM-1, and VLA-4 and $\alpha 4\beta 7$, which bind VCAM-1. Additional receptors include components of the ECM including collagen, heparin and heparan sulphate. Unlike hormones and growth factors, which bind their receptor with high affinity, receptors that bind to molecules on cell surfaces of the ECM do so with relatively low affinity and rely on binding strength by simultaneous binding of multiple receptors to multiple ligands on opposing cells or matrix. Just like cadherins, this is not enough to ensure cell adhesion and integrins must also attach, via attachment proteins, to the cytoskeleton. This not only allows the stabilisation and clustering of adhesion molecules to allow multipoint binding but also allows the adhering cell to exert traction on the ECM, or vice versa. It has become increasingly apparent that an exclusive role in cell adhesion is the exception rather than the rule, with most adhesion molecules also serving as signal transducers. Probably the best studied member of this family is N (neural)-CAM, which is expressed by many cell types including nerve cells. NCAM binds other cells via homophilic interactions. Multiplicity of function is well illustrated by NCAM [30]. Immunoglobulins are widely used during development and in the regulation of the immune system.

The Selectin Family

Selectins are a group of CAMs that bind to carbohydrates via a lectin-like domain on the cells that they bind to [29]. They are integral membrane glycoproteins with an N-terminal, C-type lectin domain followed by an EGF-like domain, a number of units homologous to complement binding proteins (CRD), decay-accelerating factor, a transmembrane domain and a short cytoplasmic tail (CD) (Fig. 6.2). The three members of this family, E, P and L selectin, are involved in the inflam-matory response. Each member of the selectin family may recognise a number of ligands, and binding depends on the cell type and context in which they are pre-sented; for example, sialyl Lewisx is a major legend found on neutrophils that binds E selectin. This ligand is absent on T cells, yet T cells can bind E selectin through a separate antigen. Specificity can also be controlled by induced alter-ations in affinity. Variations in post- translational modifications of selectins may also affect specificity. Selectins have been named after the cell type in which each molecule was first described: L selectin (leucocyte), E selectin (endothelial) and P selectin (platelets). Selectins are involved in the early stages of a series of events leading to leucocyte extravasation when leucocytes move towards the edge of the capillary and roll along the endothelium.

The Integrin Family

The integrins are made up of a family of heterodimeric membrane glyco-proteins and bind to ECM proteins (fibronectin, fibrinogen, laminin, collagen, thrombospondin, vitronectin and von Willebrand factor) and to members of the immunoglobulin superfamily such as ICAM-1, 2 and 3, and VCAM [31–33]. The name "integrin" comes from the fact that integrins *integrate* the organisation of the cytoskeleton with the ECM. All integrins are made upof two non-covalently associated subunits, α and β (Fig. 6.2). The β chain contains a large loop stabilised by disulphide bonds and the α chain contains divalent cation binding sites. The α–β pairing determines the legend-binding specificities. The major vertebrate integrins and their corresponding ligands are shown in Table 6.1. To date about 20 integrins made from 14 α and 9 β subunits have been identified. Although some integrins, such as the classical fibronectin receptor, interact with only one ECM molecule, it is more common for an individual integrin to recognise several matrix molecules with their specificity depending on in which cell type they are expressed [34]. Ligand binding is cation dependent. The cytoplasmic domain of both subunits appears to be required for binding to cytoskeletal components, thus linking the ECM to the cytoskeleton. Two integrins may bind the same region of a ligand but may have different functions; the cytoplasmic domains, particularly of the α subunits, have highly divergent sequences, which suggests that each may have its own specialised function [35].

As adhesion molecules, integrins play an important role in many biological functions including inflammation, immune function, platelet aggregation, wound healing, tumour metastasis and tissue migration during embryogenesis. In con-

Table 6.1 Vertebrate integrins and their ligands

Integrin pairing	Synonyms	Ligand
$\beta 1\alpha 1$	(VLA-1)	collagens, laminin
$\beta 1\alpha 2$	(VLA-2)	collagens, laminin
$\beta 1\alpha 3$	(VLA-3)	collagens, fibronectin, laminin
$\beta 1\alpha 4$	(VLA-4)	fibronectin, VCAM-1**
$\beta 1\alpha 5$	(VLA-5)	fibronectin
$\beta 1\alpha 6$	(VLA-6)	laminin
$\beta 1\alpha 7$		laminin
$\beta 1\alpha 8$		?
$\beta 1\alpha v$		vitronectin, fibronectin
$\beta 2\alpha_L$	(LFA-1)	ICAM-1*, ICAM-2*
$\beta 2\alpha_M$	(MAC-1)	fibrinogen, factor X, ICAM-1*, C3b component of complement
$\beta 2\alpha_x$	gp150,95,CR4	fibrinogen, C3b component of complement
$\beta 3\alpha_{IIb}$	platelet glycoprotein IIb/IIIa, CD41,CD61	fibronectin, fibrinogen vitronectin, thrombospondin von Willebrand factor
$\beta 3\alpha_v$	vitronectin receptor	collagen, fibronectin, fibrinogen osteopontin, thrombospondin vitronectin, von Willebrand factor
$\beta 4\alpha_6$		laminin
$\beta 5\alpha_v$		vitronectin, fibronectin, osteopontin
$\beta 6\alpha_v$		fibronectin, tenascin
$\beta 7\alpha_4$		fibronectin, VCAM-1**
$\beta 8\alpha_v$		laminin

* Intercellular adhesion molecule.
** Vascular cell adhesion molecule.

trast to the $\beta1$ integrins, which are expressed on almost all vertebrate cells, the $\beta2$ integrins such as $\alpha L\beta2$ (LFA-1) and $\alpha M\beta2$ (MAC-1) are expressed only on the surface of white blood cells and interact with members of the immunoglobulin superfamily expressed on cells such as endothelial cells. They play a key role in inflammatory responses by mediating firm attachment of white blood cells to the endothelium. However, integrins are also involved in cellular signalling pathways transmitting signals both in and out of cells [35,36]. Adhesion mediated by integrins requires activation of the receptor by specific signals resulting in a conformational change that enables it to bind the ligand. This in turn may then trigger a series of intracellular events. Unlike the β subunit [37], the α subunit cytoplasmic domain does nor appear to regulate ligand binding but it does appear to be important after ligand binding in subsequent cellular events [36]. Multiple integrins, all of which bind the same ligand, can be coexpressed in the same cell type; this can be explained by the fact that different cell responses can be mediated by different integrin cytoplasmic domains in response to a common extracellular ligand. Integrins can function as receptors that can transduce signals to the inside of the cell [35,38]. This is achieved by triggering specific biochemical signals or by interacting directly with the cytoskeleton thus influencing adhesiveness, shape and motility. The clustering of integrins that occurs during the formation of adhesive contacts on cells spread on fibronectin results in tyrosine phosphorylation of a complex of proteins of 120 to 130 kDa. A 125 kDa protein that has been shown to accumulates in focal adhesive contacts has been identified as a substrate for the src family of tyrosine kinases and been termed pp^{125} focal adhesion kinase (pp^{125}FAK) [39]. Thus integrin–ligand interaction followed by integrin clustering and cytoskeletal reorganisation leads to increased tyrosine phosphorylation of pp^{125}FAK, resulting in signal transduction from the ECM to inside the cell.

Adhesion Molecules in Trophoblast Invasion

Normal human placental development depends on two pathways of CTB differentiation, resulting in two populations of cells that are functionally and morphologically distinct [40]. In the first trimester, CTB cells in "floating villi" exist as polarised epithelial monolayers anchored to a basement membrane and surrounded by a stromal core that contains fetal blood vessels. In the first trimester these CTB cells are highly proliferative and differentiate by fusing to form the syncytiotrophoblast layer, which covers the villous tree. Floating villi do not come in contact with the uterine wall and are bathed in maternal blood supplied by maternal spiral arteries; their function is to exchange gas, nutrients and waste products for the fetus [40].

In contrast, CTB cells of the anchoring villi can fuse to form a syncytium; however, at selected sites they break through the syncytium and form multilayered columns of non-polarised cells as a result of local proliferation. It is only the proximal CTB that proliferate (proliferative phenotype of the extravillous trophoblast, see Fig. 6.1). It is these columns that physically connect the placenta to the uterine wall and give rise to the most highly invasive and migratory CTB. These EVT follow two different pathways [40–45]. In one pathway (interstitial trophoblast, see Fig. 6.3) the cells invade the placental bed, which comprises the

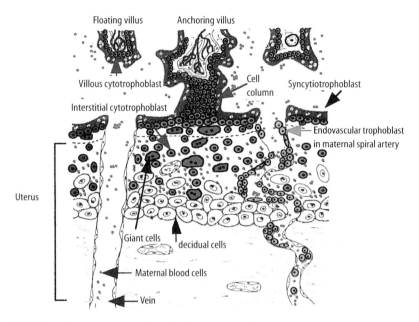

Fig. 6.3 Schematic representation of trophoblast invasion of spiral arteries showing both interstitial and endovascular pathways. Two different waves of endovascular invasion occur: the first into the decidual segments and the second into the myometrial segments of the spiral arteries.

decidualised endometrium and the first third of the myometrium; finally, some infiltrating cells differentiate further to become giant cells of the placental bed and myometrium. In the other pathway (endovascular trophoblast) the cells also invade the uteroplacental vessels. The origin of the endovascular trophoblast is still under debate [40]; it is very unlikely that those cells infiltrating the vascular walls of arteries, and partly also of the veins (intramural trophoblast), are final stages of the interstitial pathway. In contrast, the intraluminal cells replacing arterial endothelium and forming intraluminal plugs within the arteries tend to spread migration along the arterial lumina, but it is still unclear how they enter the lumina. It has been reported that the endovascular pathway occurs in two waves, the first at 8–10 weeks' gestation into the decidual segments of spiral arteries and the second wave at 16–18 weeks' gestation extending into the myometrial segments [42]. Trophoblast cultures have not been able to differentiate between these two different invading cells. During the first trimester the formation of anchoring villi and trophoblast invasion leads to rapid placental expansion. Anchoring villi thus, by attaching the placenta to the uterus, allow flow of oxygenated maternal blood to the intervillous space [46–48].

Migrating CTB is able to invade basement membranes as well as interstitial matrices. This leads to the physiological changes of pregnancy, that is, loss of the endothelial and muscular layer of the spiral arteries [49–51]. Similar findings have been found in primates where placentation is similar to humans [52–54]. These changes convert the blood supply through the spiral arteries from a low flow–high resistance circuit to a high flow–low resistance circuit to meet the needs of the growing fetus and placenta. Moreover, loss of contractility results in loss of maternal vasomotor control of the intervillous circulation [55]. Although it is not known exactly when CTB invasion takes place in humans, in Rhesus monkeys spiral arteries are invaded by CTB 5 days after implantation [45].

CTB invasion of the uterine wall and spiral arteries requires that the cells take on an invasive phenotype, a process analogous to tumour progression, and this is accompanied by a reduction in their proliferative capacity as well as expression of specific proteinases [56,57]. All highly invasive cells also have altered expression of CAM phenotypes and matrix-degrading enzymes [58] and therefore, as we will see, it is not surprising that this is also the case for invasive CTB.

Understanding the molecular processes that occur during trophoblast invasion is important because insufficient trophoblast invasion is thought to contribute to several pathological states in women including the development of pre-eclampsia [59–64], IUGR [50,61,65,66] and miscarriage [67], whereas unrestricted invasion can lead to premalignant conditions such as hydatidiform moles, placenta accreta and choriocarcinoma.

In Vivo Studies Suggest CTB Invasion is Associated with Switching of Integrin Repertoires

Much of the information on the mechanisms of human placentation has come from studies on placental bed biopsies; these contain basal decidua and under-lying myometrium containing uteroplacental (spiral) arteries. Immuno-histochemical approaches have been used to study adhesion molecules and ECM components on first trimester implantation sites and, although these studies may provide useful information, it is important to note that adhesion by integrins can also be mediated by switching from high to low affinity states [68]. Immuno-cytochemical studies performed on first trimester placenta and placental bed samples suggest that marked changes in the expression of adhesion molecules and ECM components occur in parallel to the spatial distribution of CTB from the chorionic villi to the uterine wall; however, the exact timing of these changes is unknown.

These and other studies suggest the following changes in CAM occur. In the villous compartment, where CTB exists as a polarised epithelial monolayer anchored to the trophoblast basement membrane, trophoblast cells express integrin ECM receptors typical of many polarised epithelia such as the basal layer of the skin [69,70]; $\alpha6/\beta4$ is the major integrin expressed by CTB in villi [23,71–74], whereas about a third of villous CTB cells weakly express $\alpha3/\beta1$. The basement membrane to which the trophoblast are anchored in the first trimester also expresses collagen and laminins 1–4 and 8–11 and heparan sulphate [19,20,73,75–78]. Whereas fibronectin and collagen IV immunostaining is strong in the villous stroma fibronectin, immunostaining of the basement membrane is weak, and collagen immunostaining is intense [73].Changes in the distribution of laminin and fibronectin isoforms during the differentiation of villus into EVT have been described [79]. Whereas the villous trophoblastic membrane contains laminin $\alpha1$, $\alpha2$, $\beta1$, $\beta2$ and $\gamma1$ chains, no $\alpha2$ or $\beta2$ chains have been detected in association with EVT cells.

Within the cell columns, where CTB cells are no longer associated with the basement membrane but are still proximal to the villous area a number of changes have been noted: fibronectin, collagen IV and laminins S (β2) and M (α2) are no longer expressed [20,73,76,80], which suggests that as the CTB migrate from the villous basement membrane they continue to secrete laminin into the matrix but the laminins produced are selectively downregulated. Also in this area the α3 integrin is no longer detectable on CTB or distal to the villous area; however, α6/β4 remains intense on the CTB [73]. It is worth noting that absence of immunocytochemically detected matrix proteins does not rule out their being secreted but may also be due to activity of matrix-degrading enzymes.

In the distal regions of the column, cellular fibronectin (A^+B^+) and collagen IV expression increases [73]; moreover, oncofetal fibronectin can be found [16,80,81]. Since there are no other cell types present in the columns the source of these ECM molecules is probably the CTB themselves. Matching the increase in fibronectin is a marked increase in the α5/β1 subunits of the fibronectin receptor on CTB cells [73]. Finally, in this region the expression of the laminin receptor α6/β4 decreases [71,73], although one study [23] identified α6 in at least some CTB infiltrating the decidua.

Within the placental bed itself the column structure is lost and CTB cells can be seen as either single cells or clusters of cells. Here the CTB cells express α1/β1 and α5/β1 integrins [73]. Also, in this area, decidual cells express α1/β1 and α6/β1 integrins [73]; these cells were reported to interact primarily with matrix associated with maternal cells i.e. fibronectin A^+B^+, collagen IV and laminins A (α1), B1 (β1), B2 (γ1) and M (α2). In contrast to the basal layer of stem cells, secretion of the ECM is not polarised but appears all over the surface of the cells [17,80]. The matrix is no longer homogenous but showsa patchy mosaic pattern. The above group reported detection of collagen IV laminin, heparan sulphate, fibronectins and vitronectins but no collagens I, III or VI or fibrin.

The ECM component tenascin, although absent from villous CTB, is abundant in stroma at sites of CTB column formation, at the periphery of some maternal blood vessels and in the myometrium [73]. This, along with the observation that tenascin is found not only at areas of CTB proliferation (i.e. beneath columns) but also under degenerative syncytiotrophoblast [82], suggests that tenascin's antiadhesive properties would promote trophoblast migration [83].

CAM expression by interstitial and endovascular trophoblast may also differ. Burrows et al. [84] noted expression of N-CAM by endovascular trophoblast but only by isolated cells of the CTB shell. Similar findings have been reported by others [85].

The ECM of the EVT at the histological level has a staining behaviour that is similar to that of blood-derived fibrin. Both can be found in the human placenta in huge amounts and they often mix with each other. Since it can be problamatic discriminating between them, the term "fibrinoid" covering both came into use [40]. Using refined histological techniques and immunohistochemistry, however, discrimination between them is straightforward. Parts of the fibrinoid are coarsely fibrillar and do not encase EVT cells. This subtype of fibrinoid is immunoreactive for fibrin and some fibronectin epitopes and is likely to be a blood clot product; this has been called fibrin-type fibrinoid and can be identified by orange staining in PAF-Halmi-stained sections (a modified par-aldehyde [17,80] fuchsin stain) [86]. The remaining fibrinoid is histologically more glossy or granular in nature and stains violet to green with PAF-Halmi stain. It is also specifically stained with the lectin from lycopersicon esculentum [86]. This is different from fibrin-type fibrinoid and encapsulates non-proliferating invasive EVT cells that have not yet reached the uteroplacental arteries. Immunohistochemically it lacks fibrin and is reactive for basal lamina molecules [80]. It has thus also been called pseudobasement membrane [87], basement membrane-like layer [88] and matrix-type fibrinoid [89].

In Vitro Studies also Suggest that CTB Invasion is Associated with Switching of Integrin Repertoires

In vitro models have also been used to study the role of CAMs in regulating CTB invasion [57,90]. Studies have been performed on CTB cells isolated from first trimester human placentas; in these experiments CTB are plated on to a porous filter coated with a reconstituted basement membrane material, matrigel. The isolated CTB cells attach as a monolayer, migrate and form aggregates and then penetrate the matrigel [74,91]. CTBs within matrigel produce ECM molecules characteristic of those produced by cells about to enter the uterine wall (i.e. fibronectin, type IV collagen and laminins A (α1), B1 (β1) and B2 (γ1)). The integrin pattern also generally matches that seen in vivo, that is, strong immunostaining for β1, α1 and α5 subunits while β4 and α6 immunostaining is markedly reduced [74].

Antibody perturbation studies suggest that CTB–fibronectin and CTB–collagen/laminin interactions appear to have opposing effects [74,92]: antibody perturbations of interactions involving laminin or collagen IV and their integrin α1/β1 inhibited invasion by CTB, suggesting α1/β1-laminin/collagen interactions promote invasion, whereas perturbations between fibronectin and the α5/β1 receptor accelerated invasion, suggesting that α5/β1–fibronectin interactions restrain invasion. Late gestation CTB cells, which have a greatly decreased invasive capacity, are unable to upregulate α1/β1, which provides further evidence that α1/β1 is important for invasion. Studies to identify mechanisms involved in CTB invasion have also been performed on placental villous tissues cocultured with decidua parietalis [93]. In this model, contact with the decidua stimulates local breakdown of the syncytium, CTB proliferation and formation of columns. These columns also show similar alterations in adhesion molecules to those seen in vivo, including induction of α5/β1 and loss of α6/β4. However, not all studies agree; there is a report that blocking α5/β1 inhibits trophoblast invasion in vitro [94]. Differences in findings may reflect unknown differences in experimental conditions. Tumour necrosis factor (TNF), a cytokine secreted from decidua, has also been reported to upregulate expression of α1/β1 [95].

Expression of α6 by extravillous CTB also positively correlates with gelatinase secretion, with secretion stopping when α5 expression is switched on [96]. The observation that decidua-derived IGFBP-1 binding to α5/β1 promotes invasion also suggests that IBFBP-1 may be involved in these processes [96]. Thus, although there are some inconsistencies in the literature, overall the evidence from in vivo and in vitro studies suggests that CTB changes in adhesion phenotype have the net effect of enhancing CTB invasiveness and motility.

Invading CTB Expresses Endothelial CAMs

More recent studies have suggested that CTB cells that invade spiral arteries switch their adhesion molecules repertoire so as to mimic the endothelial cells they replace [97]. Chorionic villi and placental bed biopsies immunostained for integrin, cadherin and immunoglobulin adhesion molecules characteristic of endothelial cells and leucocytes demonstrated the following. In second trimester tissue, of the αv integrins, $\alpha v/\beta 5$ was detected only on CTB on chorionic villi and $\alpha v/\beta 6$ was detected only at sites of column formation and on the first layers of cell columns. However, $\alpha v/\beta 3$ expression was enhanced on CTB that had invaded the uterine wall and maternal vasculature but was weak on villous CTB or initial layers of the cell columns. Interestingly the expression of $\alpha v/\beta 3$ expression is stimulated on endothelial cells during angiogenesis [98].

E-cadherin expression is intense on the surface of CTB in contact with one another and with the overlying syncytiotrophoblast layer; however, it is reduced on CTB in cell columns near the uterine wall and on CTB that is within the decidua or has colonised maternal blood vessels [97,99,100]. These findings are more pronounced in the second trimester compared with the first. Paradoxically E-cadherin expression is intense in CTB in all locations in term placentas, a time when CTB invasion is reported to be minimal [97]. In contrast to these studies on tissues, in vitro studies by the same group did not demonstrate significant changes in E-cadherin protein expression in invasion assays [97], although in vitro migration assays used by others [101] have been able to demonstrate down-regulation of E-cadherin by invasive CTB. The differences in these findings may be related to the culture conditions since the latter study used placental villi rather than isolated CTB.

E-cadherin expression appears to change during differentiation of CTB in vitro since a marked reduction in expression occurs during fusion to form a syncytium [102]. Furthermore, antibodies against E cadherin blocked formation of the syncytium [102]. Cadherin expression changes during embryonic development; however, first and second trimester placental tissues do not express P cadherin [97]. In contrast, VE cadherin is present on endothelium of fetal blood vessels, absent on villous CTB but present on CTB on cell columns, in the decidua and on unmodified maternal vessels [97]. Following endovascular invasion CTB cells lining maternal blood vessels express VE cadherin strongly. Parallel in vitro studies largely support these findings [97] with function-perturbing antibodies being used to shown that, in vitro, $\alpha v/\beta 3$ and VE cadherin enhance whereas E cadherin inhibits CTB invasion [97]. Additional studies on cadherins [103] have shown that cadherin-11 is expressed on syncytiotrophoblast and cell columns while cadherin-6 was reported to be the main cadherin expressed on the highly invasive EVT.

Studies on VCAM-1, PECAM-1 and E-selectin expression during CTB invasion have shown that E selectin is expressed in all first and second trimester CTB cells; however, there are no reports on third trimester material [97]. Neither VCAM-1, which is usually only expressed on activated endothelium, or PECAM-1, which is constitutively expressed on endothelium, are expressed on villous CTB [97]; however, they are expressed on CTB within the uterine wall, on endovascular CTB and on maternal endothelium [97]. Studies by Coukos et al. [104] have shown on first trimester implantation sites that only interstitial EVT and endovascular trophoblast immunostain positively for PECAM-1. CTB cells in cell columns express the $\alpha4$ subunit of the VCAM-1 receptor and in vitro data support the possibility that this pair could be involved in CTB–CTB or CTB–endothelial interactions during endovascular invasion [97]. Thus there is a tendency for CTB cells to express adhesion molecules that are more similar to those expressed on endothelial cells. It has been hypothesised that this allows the CTB cells to replace the endothelial cells in the spiral arteries and this had been likened to a vasculo/angiogenic response by the invading CTB [105–107].

N-CAM is responsible for cell–cell and cell–matrix adhesion. In early pregnancy N-CAM-positive EVT cells are abundant in all parts of the basal plate including intraluminal trophoblast cells in the rhesus monkey [108]. These findings have been confirmed in humans [108]. It is the unique form of the polysialylated form of N-CAM that is responsible for cell adhesion within the intraluminal trophoblastic plugs in uteroplacental arteries and within trophoblastic aggregates in the neighbourhood of uteroplacental arteries. Adhesion of the trophoblast cells to the maternal endothelium may occur via expression of the cell surface carbohydrate sialyl-Lewis^x [109], their receptors being E and P selectins. These are expressed only by maternal endothelial cells at the implantation site [110]; thus one possibility is that trophoblastic invasion of the arterial walls activates the endothelium resulting in selectin expression and intraluminal trophoblast adhesion. Interestingly the sialyl-Lewis^x/E-selectin interaction is also involved in adhesion of human cancer cells to human umbilical vein endothelial cells in vitro [111]. ICAM-1 is expressed on maternal endothelial cells, large granular lymphocytes, macrophages, interstitial trophoblast around uteroplacental vessels and intravascular trophoblast [110]. This group, however, did not find VCAM expression on EVT, in contrast to the studies above.

CTB Invasion, CAMs and Pre-eclampsia

Pre-eclampsia is one of the major causes of maternal death in the Western world and is responsible for considerable perinatal morbidity and mortality [112]. In this condition trophoblast invasion of the uteroplacental arteries is reduced and does not extend beyond the decidual portions of the spiral arteries. As a result, the diameter of the myometrial spiral arteries is much reduced compared with those of a normal pregnancy [60,61,113,114]. Furthermore the number of vessels invaded by trophoblast is reduced [63]. The ultimate consequence of this is a reduction in uteroplacental blood flow [115].

Immunocytochemical studies have shown that pre-eclampsia is associated with abnormal expression of CAMs by invasive CTB cells [116]. In a study of placental bed samples obtained from the late second trimester to term, CTB invasion was reported to be confined to the superficial portions of the decidua [116]. No cytokeratin-positive CTB cells were found by these authors in the deeper decidua and myometrium of three of the nine samples studied and, when present in the myometrium, only a few cells were found. None of the uterine blood vessels in the pre-eclamptic samples showed evidence of CTB invasion or physiological change. Integrin expression studies revealed that CTB cells in floating villi expressed $\alpha6\beta4$, just as in normal pregnancy; however, in pre-eclampsia $\alpha6\beta4$ was not downregulated in columns and in the uterine wall as previously reported for normal pregnancy. Again, in contrast to normal pregnancy, in pre-eclampsia CTBs in the uterine wall also failed to upregulate expression of $\alpha1\beta1$. However, expression patterns of integrins $\alpha3\beta1$ and $\alpha5\beta1$ were not different in pre-eclampsia when compared with normal pregnancies. In contrast to the different pattern of integrin switching in pre-eclampsia, no major changes in ECM molecules were noted between normal and pre-eclamptic pregnancies, with the exception that CTB-associated laminin A and B2 tended to be stronger in pre-eclamptic placental beds.

More recent studies have also shown that pre-eclamptic CTB cells do not express the same repertoire of endothelial CAMs reported for normal pregnancy [117]. Pre-eclampsia was associated with differences in all three αV family members. Fewer CTB stem cells were positive for $\beta5$; $\beta6$ immunostaining was much stronger in pre-eclamptic tissue and also extended beyond the columns to include superficial decidua; $\beta3$ immunostaining was weak on all CTB cells including cells that had invaded the uterine wall. In contrast to normal pregnancies, E-cadherin immunostaining was not only strong on CTB cells in villi and decidua but was also strong on CTB cells that had invaded the superficial portions of the spiral arteries.

In contrast to the data published by Zhou et al. [116], other groups have shown that invasion along the interstitial route is not restricted in pre-eclampsia [45,60] but rather only endovascular trophoblast invasion is restricted. Indeed, in contrast to the above observations, in a study of integrin expression in amniochorion and placental basal plate no differences in CAM expression could be demonstrated between normal and pre-eclamptic pregnancies [118]. Thus although there are several pieces of evidence linking aberrant CAM expression with abnormal CTB invasion in pre-eclampsia, further studies are required before this can be unequivocally resolved.

In a recent study of EVT on placentas collected from normal and IUGR pregnancies, VCAM-1, $\alpha2\beta1$, $\alpha3\beta1$ and $\alpha5\beta1$ expression were reported to be reduced in the IUGR group when compared with the controls [119]. ICAM-3 was also expressed on EVT and expression was upregulated in the EVT of IUGR placentas. No differences were noted for ICAM-1, ICAM-2, $\alpha4\beta1$ and $\alpha6\beta1$.

Oxygen Tension, CTB Proliferation and Adhesion Molecules

The oxygen content at the fetomaternal interface changes with gestation. Before week ten of pregnancy the placenta is relatively hypoxic since there is little blood flow into the intervillous space. At this time CTB invasion is mainly interstitial and physiological adaptation of the arteries has not yet taken place. Studies with oxygen electrodes [120] have shown that the oxygen pressure in the intervillous space rises from 17.9 ± 6.9 mmHg at 8–10 weeks' gestation to 60.7 ± 8.5 mmHg at 12–13 weeks' gestation as a result of remodelling of the spiral arteries by invading CTB. The CTB lining the spiral arteries would be expected to be exposed to arterial blood oxygen pressures of 95–100 mmHg. Pre-eclampsia and IUGR have been reported to be associated with placental hypoxia, although this is not valid for all cases [121]. Variations in oxygen concentrations can alter expression of many different proteins [122–124] and, because of its possible involvement in pre-eclampsia, the effects of oxygen tension have also been tested on CTB invasion and CAM expression [125]. CTB from first and second trimester placentas grown in hypoxic (2 per cent oxygen) and normoxic oxygen conditions on matrigel-coated wells or on decidual explants express different CAMs depending on the oxygen levels in the culture medium. Hypoxic culture conditions increase the proliferative capacity of the cells whilst inhibiting invasion, whereas in normoxic conditions invasion proceeds whilst proliferation is reduced. This in vitro behaviour is in agreement with in vivo data obtained from severely anaemic mothers [7] and it would make biological sense, since enhanced proliferation with associated migration occurs in tumour progression, a clearly undesirable scenario. Thus for invasion to proceed a mechanism must allow for CTB to have a minimal invasion capacity at the onset to overcome the hypoxic barrier. This invasive capacity would then increase since a positive feedback process might be envisaged whereby, as some cells invade blood vessels and begin to transform vessels, the oxygen tension would increase to eventually overcome the inhibitory effect and allow invasion to proceed. The concept has also arisen that blood flow to the intervillous space is blocked by endovascular trophoblast plugs in early pregnancy [126]. However, it is unlikely that this block is complete, totally preventing maternal perfusion of the intervillous space. From 12 weeks on intervillous blood flow would be increased by gradual dissolving of the plugs [126]. Studies on CAM expression in relation to oxygen pressure have shown that, when exposed to 2 per cent oxygen, CTB failed to upregulate the integrin $\alpha1\beta1$, a feature of pre-eclampsia, but continued to upregulate $\alpha5\beta1$, which suggests that hypoxia results in initiation but not completion of the integrin switching seen in normal pregnancy. Thus the similarity between some aspects of integrin switching in pre-eclampsia and in vitro models of hypoxic CTB invasion lends support to the idea that low oxygen levels may be involved in abnormal integrin switching in pre-eclampsia, although this clearly requires further investigation.

Proteinases, Inhibitors and Activators

Trophoblast invasion requires degradation of the endometrial ECM. This involves several proteinases, activators and their inhibitors.

Proteinases

The best-studied proteinases are the metalloproteinases (MMPs). MMPs are thought to play an important role in invasion processes (normal or pathological) by degrading basement membranes and ECM components. The studies below strongly support a role for proteinases, their activators and their inhibitors in trophoblast degradation of the ECM. Most studies have involved cell culture and/or decidual samples. Thus the information available is on the early stages of invasion into the decidua.

MMP-1 (interstitial collagenase)

MMP-1 can degrade several collagens including collagens 1 and IV, which are abundant in endometrium. Invasive EVT expresses MMP-1 both in vivo and in vitro [81,127,128]. Studies on early human placenta and decidua have demonstrated both protein and mRNA for MMP-1 on CTB of trophoblast columns and infiltrating intermediate trophoblast in decidual membranes [129], which also suggests a role for this enzyme in trophoblast invasion.

MMP-2 (72 kD type IV collagenase, gelatinase A)

MMP-2 mainly degrades collagen IV. MMP-2 mRNA and protein are expressed in EVT [130–134]. The in situ hybridisation studies of Polette [134] demonstrated that MMP-2 is not expressed by proliferating trophoblast but is expressed by invasive cells throughout pregnancy. A different study reported colocalisation and high expression of MMP-2, its putative activator, the membrane type 1 matrix metalloproteinase (MT1-MMP) and type IV collagen in EVT of anchoring villi, in CTB that have penetrated the placental bed and in CTB cell islands [135]. The coexpression of MT1-MMP and MMP-2 mRNA in some of the decidual cells indicates that these cells are also actively involved in the placentation process.

MMP-3 (stromelysin-1)

MMP-3 causes degradation of fibronectins, laminin, various collagens and core proteins of proteoglycans. It was reported to be weakly expressed in the proximal proliferating layers, early invasive stages did not express MMP-3 and expression increased with increasing depth, being strongest in intravascular trophoblast and decidual cells [81].

MMP-7 (matrilysin)

MMP-7 degrades several extracellular molecules including fibronectins, collagens, laminin and proteoglycans. MMP-7 is strongly expressed during trophoblast invasion and its expression is increased in pre-eclampsia [136]

MMP-9 (92 kD type IV collagenase, gelatinase B)

MMP-9, like MMP-2, mainly degrades collagen IV but it has a different expression pattern. It is expressed by proximal, proliferating EVT [134]. Expression is downregulated in invasive stages and then upregulated in the deeper later stages of invasion in vitro. In vitro, trophoblast invasion is completely inhibited by preincubation with an antibody that recognises MMP-9 [137]. Expression also decreases towards term [56,134,137]. The stage of trophoblast differentiation has been shown, in vitro, to be linked to MMP production. During invasion EVT cells expressing the α6 integrin represent the invasive population and express high gelatinase and low fibronectin, whereas when the integrin α5 is turned on their invasive behaviour ends and they secrete low amounts of gelatinases and high amounts of fibronectin [138]. In vitro studies also suggest that MMP-9 secretion may be regulated in an autocrine manner by trophoblast-derived interleukin-1β acting on receptors on the trophoblast cells themselves [91].

MMP-11 (stromelysin-3)

MMP-11 degrades laminin, collagen and proteoglycans. Immunocytochemical studies have shown that it is expressed only by invasive trophoblast and expression decreases with advancing gestation [134,139].

MT-MMP

MT-MMP-1 activates MMP-2 and is expressed by proliferating and invasive trophoblast in the first and third trimester [140] with strongest expression in the first trimester. The expression of gelatinase A and MT1-MMP by the EVT suggests that these cells may use the MT-MMP pathway to activate progelatinase A. The observed decline in MT1-MMP expression at term in EVT despite an abundance of gelatinase A in EVT may thus contribute to the decline in trophoblast invasiveness at term.

Tissue Inhibitors

MMPs are regulated by their tissue inhibitors (TIMPs). Trophoblast proteases and their inhibitors are intimately associated. Both interstitial collagenase and gelatinase B can also be directly activated by plasmin, which in turn arises by activation of plasminogen by plasminogen activators, urokinasePA being the major contributor in trophoblast.

TIMP-1

Messenger RNAs for 92 kDa type IV collagenase, TIMP-1, TIMP-2 and TIMP-3 have been identified in CTB columns [141].

TIMP-2

TIMP- 2 appears to be important in both activating as well as inhibiting gelatinase A [142]. Interestingly, both TIMP-1 and TIMP-2 are additionally expressed by decidual cells: TIMP-2 being constantly expressed throughout pregnancy whereas TIMP-1 activity increases towards term [143]. These results suggest that decidual cells limit trophoblast invasion. The importance of TIMP-1 and TIMP-2 in invasion is shown by the fact that both completely inhibit CTB invasion in vitro [137].

TIMP-3

Studies using protease–substrate gel electrophoresis have shown human CTB to express primarily TIMP-3. TIMP-3 expression is coexpressed with MMP-9. The highest levels of mRNA and protein of both were found after differentiation to a fully invasive phenotype and during early gestation when invasion peaks [144]. In decidua TIMP-3 mRNA is expressed in EVT and maternal decidual cells. MMPs may also involved in separation of the placenta from the uterine wall. During spontaneous labour MMP-3 and MMP-9 mRNA levels increase, and after delivery tPA (see below) and TIMP-1 levels are increased [145].

Activators

Plasminogen activators are serine proteases that convert plasminogen to plasmin, which activates other proteases. Two plasminogen activators are known: urokinase-type plasminogen activator (uPA) and tissue-type PA (tPA). Expression of uPA [146] and expression of saturable uPA-binding sites by first trimester trophoblast cells in vitro [147] are believed to correlate with their invasive ability.

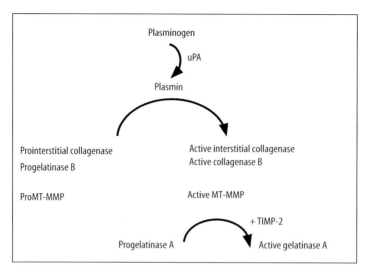

Fig. 6.4 Trophoblast protease interactions lead to the activation of intersitial collagenase, collagenase B, MT-MMP and gelatinase A. Trophoblast uPA converts plasminogen to plasmin. Plasmin can in turn activate interstitial collagenase, gelatinase B and MT-MMP. Gelatinase A is activated when progelatinase A binds to a complex of active MT-MMP and TIMP-2.

The polarised expression of a high affinity uPA receptor at the invasion front of human EVT cells suggests that the receptor may aid in determining the direction of invasion [148]; however, knockout mouse studies have shown, at least in this species, that knocking out uPA [149] or its receptor [150] has no effect on fertility or implantation. Fig. 6.4 shows the trophoblast protease interactions leading to the activation of proteinases as suggested by Lala and Hamilton [142].

Inhibitors of uPA and tPA (i.e. PAI-1 and PAI-2) have been identified in human trophoblast [132,151]. Corresponding with uPA expression, only PAI-1 is expressed by invasive CTB of cell islands and cell columns [152], whereas tPA and PAI-2 were identified only in villous syncytiotrophoblast where they are thought to regulate fibrinolysis [152]. In vitro antibodies against PAI-1 or uPA only partially inhibit trophoblast invasion [137]. There are limited studies on other serine protease inhibitors such as $\alpha 1$ antichymotrypsin, $\alpha 1$ antitrypsin and inter-α-trypsin inhibitor. None are detected on EVT but rather in areas of surrounding matrix-type fibrinoid and basal plate [153]. This is largely consistent with another study [154] except that $\alpha 1$ antichymotrypsin and $\alpha 1$ antitrypsin were found in trophoblast within uteroplacental arteries.

Another possible step in the regulation of trophoblast invasion is at the level of the low density lipoprotein-related protein/α_2 macroglobulin receptor (LRP). LRP is expressed by trophoblast [155]. This cell surface receptor binds pro-uPA as well as complexes between uPA and PAI-1 and also mediates their internalisation. Placentas obtained from patients with pre-eclampsia exhibit reduced cell surface-associated PA activity [156]. It is possible that reduced PA is due to altered expression of LRP. Bischof et al. [157] have reported that leukaemia inhibitory factor (LIF) inhibits the gelatinolytic activity secreted by CTBs. Since LIF is produced by the human endometrium and placenta, it was suggested that it may also inhibit trophoblast invasion in vivo.

Although from the above literature there appears to be very good evidence to support a role for proteinases, their activators and their inhibitors in trophoblast degradation of the ECM, it is clear that further work, particularly in pathological pregnancies, is still required.

Growth Factors, their Receptors and Proto-oncogenes

Transforming Growth Factors

TGFβs are members of a large superfamily of cytokines that includes activins, inhibins, bone morphogenic proteins and others [158]. TGFβs are composed of three related dimeric proteins, that is, TGFβ-1, 2 and 3. TGFβs exert their biological effects through binding to cell surface receptors designated types I (ALK-1), II and III. Endothelial cells also express another TGFβ-binding protein, endoglin, which has structural homology to the type III receptor. Endoglin is an integral membrane protein that binds TGFβ-1 and TGFβ 3 but not TGFβ-2. TGFβ also binds to decorin, which neutralises its activity. TGFβ has a pronounced inhibitory effect on endothelial proliferation and migration. The mechanisms of inhibition include downregulation of the type II receptor and interaction with other cytokines. There is also substantial evidence that TGFβ can regulate trophoblast invasion.

TGFβ immunoreactivity has been demonstrated in first and second trimester syncytiotrophoblast [159–161]. Lysiak [160] showed that immunoreactive TGFβ-1 is present in villous syncytiotrophoblast and EVT of the CTB shell throughout gestation and is abundant in decidua. Subsequent studies on placental tissue have shown strong immunoreactivity for TGFβ-3 at 5–9 weeks of pregnancy that was markedly reduced by 12–13 weeks and 29–34 weeks. TGFβ-1 was absent at 5 weeks and transiently expressed at 8 weeks. Staining for TGFβ receptors I and II was strong at 5–8 weeks but absent at 12–13 weeks and 29–34 weeks [162]. The altered expression of TGFβ and its receptors at the time of the first wave of trophoblast invasion is consistent with these molecules having an important role in placentation. Endoglin is upregulated in the transition from polarised undifferentiated CTB cells to non-polarised intermediate CTBs as the cells align in columns. This occurs in parallel to the upregulation of $\alpha5\beta1$ and precedes the loss of $\alpha6\beta4$ [163]. Decorin, a natural inhibitor of TGFβ, was not identified in villous or EVT [160]. However, an association between decorin and TGFβ in ECM and decidual cells in decidual tissue suggests decorin may limit the effects of TGFβ in the ECM. Studies on placentas from pregnancies complicated by pre-eclampsia have also shown that there is strong staining of TGFβ-3 and its receptors on syncytiotrophoblast and stromal cells at 27–34 weeks' gestation; at this gestation staining was absent from normal villous tissue [162].

In vitro studies have also provided evidence that TGFβ produced by decidual cells and to a minor extent by trophoblast cells themselves limits trophoblast invasion. TGFβ may also inhibit trophoblast invasion by increasing adhesion to the ECM through stimulation of oncofetal fibronectin production [164,165]. TGFβ can also regulate expression of integrin subunits [164] and indeed has been shown to increase $\alpha5/\beta1$ integrin expression with concomitant reduced migratory ability of invasive CTB [94]. TGFβ suppressed invasion of first trimester trophoblast in an amnion invasion assay; the anti-invasive effect was mediated by induction of TIMP-1 by trophoblasts themselves and to some extent by decidual cells [161,166] and downregulation of trophoblast-derived uPA [167]. Interestingly Bass et al. [168] failed to demonstrate of TGFβ on trophoblast invasion, which again perhaps reflects differences in the cells used. Antisense disruption of endoglin triggers invasion of trophoblast from first trimester villous explants in vitro, suggesting that this receptor plays a crucial role in invasion [169]. Human villous explants of 5–7 weeks' gestation (no invasion in vivo at this time) cultured in matrigel have been shown to remain viable but do not invade the surrounding matrigel. In contrast, trophoblast cells from 9–13 week explants (a time when invasion takes place in vivo) spontaneously invade the matrigel with an up-regulation of fibronectin and integrin switching. However, trophoblast invasion of explants at 5–7 weeks can be induced by incubation with antisense TGFβ-3, TGFβ receptor I or TGFβ receptor II. Antisense to TGFβ-1 led to minimal invasion whereas antisense to TGFβ-2 failed to induce invasion. These in vitro data suggest that TGFβ-3 via the ALK-1 receptor complex is a major regulator of trophoblast invasion in vitro. Flow cytometric analysis of integrin and an in vitro cell migration assay have revealed that exogenous TGFβ upregulates integrin expression and reduces migratory ability of invasive trophoblast [94].

Vascular Endothelial Growth Factor

Vascular endothelial growth factor (VEGF) is a secreted growth factor composed of two identical subunits linked by disulphide bonds [170]. VEGF action is mediated through the tyrosine kinase receptors flt-1 (fms-like tyrosine kinase) and KDR (kinase insert-domain-containing receptor). Ahmed et al. [171] reported that first, second and third trimester CTB and syncytiotrophoblast expressed VEGF with the intensity of staining being much stronger on CTB. EVT associated with the placental tissues did not express VEGF. In the same study flt-1 was identified in first trimester syncytiotrophoblast and CTB, with staining being more intense in CTB. EVT stained intensely for flt-1 and this was reduced in the early third trimester. Maternal decidual cells expressed VEGF throughout pregnancy. It was suggested that VEGF released from these cells may act as a chemoattractant for trophoblast. Sharkey et al. [172] identified VEGF in villous CTB and syncytiotrophoblast in the first trimester and in decidual macrophages but not in EVT. At term VEGF was expressed in syncytiotrophoblast and in EVT. Maternal macrophages within the decidua also expressed VEGF. Cooper et al. [173] showed that, in the first trimester, VEGF immunoreactivity was localised to placental macrophages (Höfbauer cells), and, in decidua, to glandular epithelium and maternal macrophages. In the term placenta, VEGF immunoreactivity was present in EVT and in extracellular material; flt immunoreactivity was demonstrated on EVT in first trimester and term, and on Höfbauer cells within placental villi [173]. In situ hybridisation studies have shown flt mRNA expression in villi from mid-gestational placenta, while low levels were found in term villi [174]. EVT was found to contain both mRNA encoding flt and flt-like immunoreactivity throughout pregnancy, In contrast, KDR mRNA was found only on endothelial cells. The decidua contained multiple flt immunopositive cell types during the first trimester but only EVT trophoblast were positive later in gestation. VEGF immunoreactivity tended to colocalise with the staining for flt. The authors concluded that VEGF may exert an important role within both the placental villi and the maternal decidua in relation to the growth, differentiation and migration of trophoblast and that this is mediated primarily through the spatial and temporal regulation of the flt receptor rather than the KDR receptor.

The complex pattern of both VEGF and flt-like immunoreactivity suggests that VEGF may be involved not only in the regulation of placental angiogenesis, but also in trophoblast invasion and regulating vascular permeability.

Insulin-like Growth Factors

IGFs and their specific binding proteins (IGFBPs) are believed to be important regulators of fetal growth. IGFBP protease, which proteolyses IGFBPs, is also thought to be involved in fetal growth. IGF-I is found in decidual cells and EVT [175,176]. IGFBP-1 and 2 are both found in decidual cells; expression of IGFBP-1 mRNA is most abundant in decidual cells close to adjacent invading EVT that express IGF-II mRNA [177]. IGFBP-1 contains an RGD sequence recognising certain integrins and stimulates trophoblast invasion in vitro [178]. Furthermore IGFBP-1 trophoblast migration can be blocked by $\alpha 5$- and $\beta 1$-blocking antibodies. In contrast, IGF-II had no effect on integrin expression but stimulated migration [94]. IGF-II has been shown to be broadly distributed in first and third trimester. These data suggest that IGF produced by invasive trophoblast and IGF-binding proteins produced by decidua interact to regulate trophoblast invasion.

Epidermal Growth Factor Receptor

Epidermal growth factor receptor (EGF-R) is expressed on the same layers of cells in columns that express proliferation markers [4,179,180]. However, one study [179] also described some immunoreactivity in the deeply invasive multinucleated CTB cells. EGF is a potent epithelial mitogen and has also been reported to stimulate trophoblast invasion [168]; however, others have reported that EGF and other EGF-R ligands including TGFα and amphiregulin promote proliferation without stimulating invasion in vitro [178]. Differences in vitro studies may be partly due to the use of different subpopulations of trophoblast used in the experiments. EGF is also secreted by EVT [181] and has also been localised to uterine epithelial and decidual cells [182]. The erb-B2 oncogene has been shown to be a deleted version of the EGF receptor gene [183]. In some cells these mutations cause a constitutive activation of the receptor and uncontrolled growth; erb-B2 shows a reciprocal expression pattern when compared with EGF-R and is expressed at the surface of all EVT cells that are negative for the EGF-R [4,179]. It therefore characterises all differentiated and invasive stages. Studies on first trimester trophoblast cells showed that, as cells aggregated to form a syncytium, expression of the EGF-R increased while invasive CTB expressed colony-stimulating factor receptor (c-fms/CSR-1R) and c-erbB2 proteins but low levels of EGF-R [184]. Studies have been performed on the effects of human trophoblast-induced interferon alpha/beta on the expression of c-fms/CSF-1R, EGF-R and c-erbB2 (ligands are thought to be important in the growth and differentiation of invasive and non-invasive trophoblast). Human trophoblast-induced interferon alpha/beta reduced the expression of EGF-R in both invasive and non-invasive cells and reduced the expression of c-fms/CSR-1R and c-erbB2 protein in invasive trophoblast cells.

Fibroblast Growth Factor

FGFs are a family of heparin-binding polypeptide growth factors [185]. FGFs exert their effects through specific receptors that have intrinsic tryosine kinase activity. They can be either acidic (FGF-1) or basic (FGF-2). Codistribution of basic fibroblast growth factor (βFGF) and heparan sulphate proteoglycan (HSPG) has been shown in the growth zones of first trimester human placentas [186]. In cell islands and columns βFGF was detected in cytoplasm of extravillous CTB cells, whereas HSPG was localised between extravillous CTB cells and in their cytoplasm. Ferriani et al. [187] reported that FGF-1 and FGF-2 were colocalised in decidua to EVT and endothelial cells. In vitro studies also suggest that heparin or heparan sulphate present in the ECM surrounding the invasive trophoblast play a role in trophobast invasion and differentiation by enhancing the effects of heparin-binding growth factors such as basic FGF [188].

Hemopoietic Colony-stimulating Factors

Hemopoietic colony-stimulating factors (CSFs) are glycoprotein growth factors that control cell proliferation and differentiation and survival. CSF-1 binds to the CSF-1 receptor (*c-fms* proto-oncogene product), which has intrinsic tyrosine kinase activity; *fms* is reported to be strongly expressed in early invasive stages but weaker during deeper invasion including endovascular trophoblast [189,190]. CSF itself is secreted from villous CTB [191], from endometrial cells [192] and from invasive EVT cells [193]. Thus neighbouring cells as well as EVT themselves may influence proliferation and migration of these cells.

Endothelin

Endothelin (ET) is a potent vasoconstrictor and growth factor. Three forms of ET (ET-1, ET-2 and ET-3) exist. ET-1 immunoreactivity has not only been demonstrated in endothelium of placental blood vessels and syncytiotrophoblast but is also found in decidual cells and EVT of the basal plate and chorionic plate. These results support a role for trophoblastic origin of ET and indicate that ET may also be involved in trophoblast physiology.

Angiotensin II

Angiotensin II is a potent vasoconstrictor and growth promoter. In situ and immunocytochemical studies have revealed the angiotensin AT (I) receptor mRNA and protein are present on CTB, syncytiotrophoblast and EVT as well as in blood vessels of placental villi. The intensity of staining of the receptor mRNA was reported to be reduced in the syncytiotrophoblast of IUGR pregnancies in this study [194].

Tumour Necrosis Factor α

TNFα has been demonstrated within proliferating cytotrophoblastic cell columns [195]. More recent studies have shown that, in early pregnancy, TNFα is expressed on proliferating tips of anchoring villi, invasive interstitial trophoblast (but not giant cells) and endovascular trophoblast invading spiral arteries. At term weak staining is found in endovascular trophoblast [196]. Moreover, TNFα is a macrophage cytokine [197,198] that is likely also to be expressed by decidual macrophages. The TNF receptor 1 (p55-receptor) is expressed by trophoblast cells, and in vitro TNFα induced apoptosis in the latter [199]. Taken together, these data suggest that TNFα, by means of autocrine and/or paracrine loops, is involved in the control of trophoblast invasion by induction of apoptosis.

Other Proto-oncogenes

The Vav proto-oncogene is a signal-transducing molecule. Its expression is thought to be highly specific for haematopoietic cells. In situ hybridisation studies have demonstrated Vav mRNA in the CTB shell and columns in first trimester through to third trimester placentas [200]. The same study showed that antisense oligonucleotides to the Vav mRNA significantly inhibited growth of BeWo cells. These results suggest that Vav also plays a role in trophoblast migration.

C-kit, also known as stem cell factor, is a blood cell mitogen also expressed by EVT cells [201]. The receptor for this growth factor is expressed by villous macrophages and by large granular lymphocytes (natural killer or NK cells) of the junctional zone.

The c-Ets1 proto-oncogene codes for a transcription factor and is associated with neovascularisation and invasion processes. In situ hybridisation studies have identified Ets-1 mRNA in first trimester EVT invading uterine vessels [202]. It was suggested that Ets-1 may be linked to the regulation of metalloproteinase gene transcription since this gene family is known to be a target for Ets protein.

Other Cytokines

Granulocyte macrophage colony-stimulating factor (GM-CSF) is a cytokine that has been implicated in placental growth and development. In the first trimester GM-CSR receptor was expressed in all extravillous cytotrophoblast cells, which suggests GM-CSF may regulate trophoblast function [203].

Nitric Oxide

Nitric oxide (NO) is a small molecular weight mediator with diverse functions that include vasodilatation, inhibition of platelet aggregation and vascular remodelling [204]. NO results from the enzymatic action of nitric oxide synthase (NOS), which converts L-arginine, in the presence of oxygen, to L-citrulline and NO. Three NOS enzymes have been cloned and sequenced: bNOS (type I NOS), iNOS (type II NOS) and eNOS (type III NOS). Human placental syncytiotrophoblast cells express eNOS but not iNOS; eNOS is also expressed on villous endothelial cells, and NO produced from these cells is believed to be an important vasodilator within the placental vasculature [205–210]. Spiral artery transformation is thought to result from the loss of normal musculoelastic structure by CTB action [42,49,50,54,63,65]. However, vascular changes have been reported as early as 8–10 weeks' gestation, before endovascular CTB invasion has occurred [43,211]. Pijnenborg et al. [196] have related these vascular changes to the presence of interstitial CTB, suggesting these cells may produce vasoactive mediators. Furthermore one of us (P.K.) has shown that, in the guinea pig, in which maternal arterial vasodilatation also precedes endovascular trophoblast invasion [212], interstitial trophoblast expresses eNOS and iNOS. Thus local production of NO by invading CTB may be an important mediator of spiral artery transformation in this species. The other author of this chapter (F.L.) has tested the hypothesis that, in the human placental bed, invading CTB express eNOS or iNOS and therefore have the potential to influence spiral artery transformation directly. This hypothesis was tested in placental bed biopsies obtained from normal human pregnancies between 8 and 19 weeks' gestation [213]. At no time during invasion did CTB express eNOS or iNOS. The latter study underscores the limitations of extrapolating animal data to the human situation. Human placentation differs from the guinea pig, and cell columns do not exist in rodents. Furthermore, it appears that the NOS isoforms in guinea pig differ from those in humans [214]. If NO is not responsible for vessel structural changes then the question remains of what other factors could be involved. Although it is possible that trophoblast releases an as-yet unidentified vasodilator, another possibility is that the initial changes are brought about by a factor or factors circulating in the maternal spiral arteries and not from the trophoblast cells themselves. Further investigation into identifying such factors is required.

Gap Junctions and Connexins

Gap junctions are junctions between cells and consist of many pores that allow the passage of molecules up to 900 Da in size. Each pore is formed by a hexagonal array (connexon) of six transmembrane proteins (connexins, or Cx) in each plasma membrane. Only Cx-40 has been identified in EVT. Expression is in the proximal proliferative parts of columns and cell islands where the cells are still in contact with each other [99,215,216]. Some CTB cells express Cx-40. With increasing invasiveness Cx-40 is downregulated but is then upregulated in deep aggregated cells. Furthermore transfection of JEG 3 choriocarcinoma cells with various connexin genes showed that while these cells do not normally express Cx-40, transfection with Cx-40 did not reduce the highly proliferative activity of the cells. In contrast transfection with Cx-43 markedly reduced proliferation [216].

Human Chorionic Gonadotrophin

Receptors for hCG have been demonstrated on invasive trophoblast as well as choriocarcinoma cells. In trophoblast invasion models hCG has been shown to stimulate invasion of JEG 3 cells through matrigel-coated chambers but had no effect on proliferation [217]. The endogenous production of hCG by the trophoblast suggests an autocrine or paracrine control of invasion by hCG. Furthermore, hCG can increase the activity of MMP-9 in a extended-lifespan first trimester trophoblast cell line [218], which supports the idea that hCG might alter trophoblast invasion by altering the activity of MMP-9.

Activins and Inhibins

Both activin and inhibin, as well as the activin-binding protein follistatin, are produced by various trophoblast cells throughout pregnancy. In studies of cultured explants of first trimester chorionic villi [219], addition of activin-A, but not inhibin-A, stimulated the outgrowth of trophoblast into the surrounding matrix and this was blocked by the activin-binding protein follistatin. The outgrowth was characteristic of that observed in extravillous CTB cells in vivo; it was accompanied by synthesis of fibronectin, expression of human leucocyte antigen G (HLA-G) and MMP-9. Thus activin may play a role on CTB column formation by regulating differentiation of villous CTB into extravillous CTB cells.

The Major Histocompatibility Complex

Human implantation is particularly invasive compared with other species since trophoblast cells invade the inner third of the myometrium. This means that fetal cells come in intimate contact with maternal cells, which are genetically different. In fact the fetus has been likened to an allograft and in the past it was assumed that the interaction of fetal cells with the maternal uterine cells would be controlled by the mechanisms of classical transplantation immunology, which control transplanted organs (i.e. a maternal T-cell response would be initiated in response to the non-self histocompatibility antigens expressed by the fetal cells). However, there is now a great deal of evidence to suggest that a unique immune system that involves NK cells exists in the maternal decidua [220]. In support of the idea that maternal decidua modulates trophoblast invasion, overinvasion of trophoblast in placenta percreta usually occurs where decidua is deficient, such as at sites of scar tissue from a previous caesarean section. Similarly, in hydatidiform mole, where the blastocyst contains two paternal sets of chromosomes, over-invasion of trophoblast occurs. This has led to the concept of a "tug-of war" between the maternal and paternal genes, with the invading fetal cells being restrained by the mother [221].

The highly polymorphic major histocompatibility complex (MHC) antigens, known as the HLA system in humans [222], is responsible not only for presenting antigens to T cells but also for recognition of non-self in graft rejection. The HLA system is made up of three classical loci (HLA-A, HLA-B and HLA-C) and three non-classical loci (HLA-E, HLA-F and HLA-G). Villous CTB and syncytio-trophoblast express neither class 1 or class 2 antigens. CTB cells in cell columns are also negative for these antigens; however, EVT are known to express HLA-C [223] and HLA-G [224–226]. The balance of evidence suggests that, although the mRNA for HLA-G is expressed in a variety of cell types, the distribution of the protein appears to be restricted to EVT. It has been suggested that this may be due to the limited availability of antibodies directed against HLA-G [220]. Using antibodies generated by different methods two studies [226–228] have reported that HLA-G is restricted to EVT whereas one study [229] showed that other placental cells, including chorionic villous mesenchyme and macrophages, expressed HLA-G. Although Chumbley [227] found HLA-G in all populations of EVT, McMaster et al. and others [230,231] did not find any in the proliferating subset. The expression of HLA-E in placenta has also been reported [232]. The development of HLA-E antibodies is awaited to elucidate the expression profiles of the protein.The functions of HLA-G and HLA-C on trophoblast are still not understood although there is evidence that HLA-G may present antigens (nine-residue peptides derived from cellular proteins) to T cells in the same way as the classical HLA molecules [233,234] and can inhibit NK cell-mediated lysis [235].

Analysis of leucocyte populations in the uterus has shown that T cells are sparse. In addition there is lack of evidence that they demonstrate any immune reactivity to invading trophoblast. NK cells are the predominant population and their numbers are under the control of the menstrual cycle; they are sparse during the proliferative phase and the numbers peak at the early stages of pregnancy [220]. It is generally accepted that NK cells preferentially kill target cells with low or absent HLA-1 antigens. This had been the basis of the "missing self" hypothesis that, in contrast to T cells, means that the presence of class 1 molecules on T cells prevents NK-mediated cell lysis [236]. The paucity of T cells but the accumulation of NK cells at the implantation site has led to the proposal that interaction of NK cells with invading trophoblast may provide the basic mechanism that controls recognition of the placenta [220]. NK cells express receptors that can recognise HLA class 1 molecules. These are known to express killer inhibitory receptors (KIRs), which on interaction with HLA class 1 molecules inhibit cytolysis or cytokine production. They also express killer activatory receptors (KARs), which activate killing or cytokine production. HLA-C appears to be the most important in influencing NK function [237]. However, it also appears that two KIRs that are specific for HLA-C alleles also recognise HLA-G, which suggests that HLA-G may be a universal inhibitor of NK cell killer activity [235]. More recently, a second class of NK cell receptors for class 1 HLA molecules, CD94, has also been identified. It recognises HLA-C and possibly HLA-G [238]. CD94 forms heterodimers with NKG2, another NK lectin. Thus the evidence to date suggests that decidual NK cells express KIRs, KARs and CD94, which recognise HLA-C and HLA-G expressed by invading trophoblast. This results in positive and negative signals regulating killer activity and cytokine production (Fig. 6.5). Since NK cells can secrete several cytokines that trophoblasts have

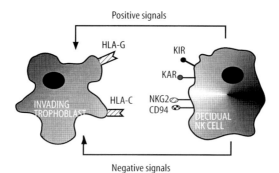

Fig. 6.5 Diagramatic representation of class 1 (HLA) antigens expressed by invading human trophoblasts. Also shown are the receptors thought to be expressed in decidual NK cells (KAR, KIR, CD94). Interaction of the two cells may be led to positive or negative signals from the NK cells and, associated with this, changes in their cytotoxic effects or production of cytokines (adapted from [220]).

receptors for, NK cells may influence trophoblast migration and function. Furthermore, since it is known that the repertoire of KIRs expressed by women can differ in different women, the possibility arises that certain combinations of receptors may favour a good outcome whereas others may lead to conditions involving poor control of trophoblast invasion such as IUGR. This clearly is an area that requires future study.

A recent study identified a single base pair (bp) deletion at position 1597 in exon 3 of HLA-G in 7.4 per cent of African Americans, 3 per cent of Hispanics and in no Caucasians. Individuals homozygous for this allele do not make HLA-G; however, HLA-G expression has been shown not to be necessary for fetal survival and development into adulthood [239].

Clearly this is an exciting area that is under intensive research. With the development of specific antibodies to other HLA molecules being close to completion, we suspect that new insights into the immunology of trophoblast invasion are not far away.

Blood Group Antigens

Carbohydrate epitopes are a subgroup of oncofetal antigens that are related to normal adult blood group antigens. Blood group antigen "i" is the most primitive precursor of the ABO system of blood groups. It is expressed by immature red blood cells and by all stages of EVT but not by proliferating cells [240]. It may be that this immature blood group antigen prevents immune recognition of EVT cells by the maternal immune system. The slightly more mature blood group antigen "I" can be detected on human trophoblast, but only after sialidase treatment, indicating that not "I" but sialyl-"I" is present [240]. Sialyl-"I" was found on villous syncytiotrophoblast and only in a few cases on the surfaces of EVT, where it was coexpressed with "I". The cell surface carbohydrate sialyl-Lewis^x is expressed by intra-arterial trophoblast cells, which form huge trophoblastic plugs [109]. Since it acts as a ligand for E and P selectin, which are expressed by endothelium, it probably plays a role in trophoblast adhesion to the vessel walls (see section on adhesion molecules) [110].

Proliferative EVT

Cell Islands

Cell islands are roundish or irregularly shaped accumulations of EVT cells, at least partly embedded in fibrinoid, attached to free floating tips of larger villi. The main difference between cell islands and cell columns is that the latter are attached to the basal plate [40]. When cell islands are stained with the proliferation marker MIB-1, proliferating cells were found only close to the basal lamina, just as for cell columns [89]. Explants from first trimester placentas cultured in vitro have shown that EVT cells from cell islands behave like those derived from cell columns [241].

Chorionic Plate

The chorionic plate is also rich in EVT [40,242–244]. There are few immuno-histochemical studies; however, expression patterns of collagen type IV, laminin and fibronectins in the macaque chorionic plate are similar to that described for cell columns [245]. Only cells resting on the basal lamina facing the chorionic mesoderm proliferate [40,89] and in term placenta it is difficult to find any pro-liferating trophoblast cells in the chorionic plate. Thus it appears that there are no obvious differences in these EVT compared with cell columns.

Smooth Chorion

Only cells resting on the basal lamina proliferate [Kaufmann, unpublished data]. The ECM surrounding the EVT cells has been studied in more detail [87,246]. It appears that there are no major immunohistochemical differences between them, compared with other locations of EVT.

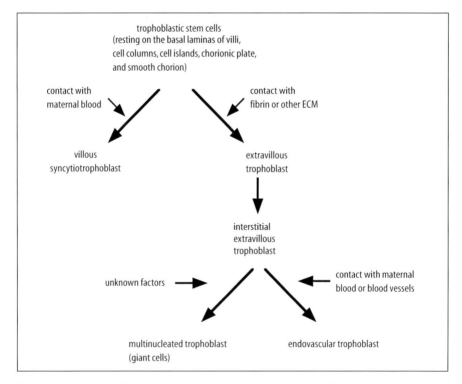

Fig. 6.6 The routes of differentiation from trophoblastic stem cells to villous or different subsets of EVT are controlled by exogeneous factors, the exact nature of which is still largely a mystery. Environmental conditions such as exposition to ECM molecules and presence or absence of contact with maternal blood seem to be decisive.

Routes of Trophoblast Differentiation

The routes of trophoblast differentiation from trophoblastic stem cells to villous or different subsets of extravillous trophoblast are controlled by exogenous factors, the exact nature of which is still a mystery (Fig. 6.6). Experimental conditions such as exposition to ECM molecules and presence of absence of contact with maternal blood seem to be decisive.

Conclusions

The establishment of the human haemochorial placenta is dependent on the proliferation, migration and invasion of trophoblast into the maternal decidua and myometrium. Although some aspects of trophoblast invasion resemble tumour invasion, the striking difference between the two is that trophoblast invasion of the uterus is tightly controlled by a plethora of factors expressed within the decidua and on the trophoblasts themselves. As outlined in this chapter, these include CAMs and the ECM, proteinases and their inhibitors, growth factors, cytokines and others. Abnormalities in any one of these mechanisms may well lead to pathological conditions associated with shallow invasion of trophoblast, for example pre-eclampsia/IUGR or overinvasion of trophoblast (in tubal pregnancy, placenta increta, molar pregnancies, or choriocarcinoma). The precise mechanisms that are abnormal in IUGR pregnancies are still poorly understood and urgently require further investigation. Only by understanding these pathological mechanisms can future strategies for therapeutic targets be developed.

References

1. Kurman RJ, Main CS, Chen H-C Intermediate trophoblast: a distinctive form of trophoblast with specific morphological, biochemical and functional features. Placenta 1984;5:349–70.
2. Bulmer JN, Morrison L, Johnson PM. Expression of the proliferation markers Ki67 and transferrin receptor by human trophoblast populations. J Reprod Immunol 1988;14:291–302.
3. Kohnen G, Kosanke G, Korr H, Kaufmann P. Comparison of various proliferation markers applied to human placental tissue. Placenta 1993;14:A38.
4. Mühlhauser J, Crescimanno C, Kaufmann P, Höfler H, Zaccheo D, Castellucci M. Differentiation and proliferation patterns in human trophoblast revealed by c-erbB-2 oncogene product and EGR-R. J Histochem Cytochem 1993;41:165–73.
5. Blankenship TN, King BF. Developmental expression of Ki-67 antigen and proliferating cell nuclear antigen in macaque placentas. Dev Dynam 1994;201:324–33.
6. Kosanke G. Proliferation, Wachstum und Differenzierung der Zottenbäume der menschlichen Placenta. Aachen, FRG: Verlag Shaker, 1994.
7. Kosanke G, Kadyrov M, Korr H, Kaufmann P. Maternal anemia results in increased proliferation in human placental villi. Troph Res 1997;11:339–57.
8. King BF, Blankenship TN. Expression of proliferating cell nuclear antigen (PCNA) in developing macaque placentas. Placenta 1993;14:A36.
9. Mühlhauser J, Crescimanno C, Kasper M, Zaccheo D, Castellucci M. Differentiation of human trophoblast populations involves alterations in cytokeratin patterns. J Histochem Cytochem 1995;43:579–89.
10. Kreis T, Vale R. Guidebook to the extracellular matrix and adhesion proteins. Oxford: Oxford University Press, 1993.

11. Birk DE, Silver FH, Trelstad RL. Matrix assembly. In Hay E, editor. Cell biology of extracellular matrix. New York: Plenum, 1991;221–54.
12. Alberts B, Bray D, Lewis J, Raff M, Roberts K, Watson J. Molecular biology of the cell. New York: Garland, 1994.
13. Linsenmayer TF. Collagen. In: Hay E, editor. Cell biology of extracellular matrix. New York: Plenum, 1991;7–44.
14. Van der Rest M, Garrone R. Collagen family of proteins. FASEB J 1991;5:2814–23.
15. Hynes RO. Fibronectins. Sci Am 1986;254:42–51.
16. Feinberg RF, Kliman HJ. Tropho-uteronectin (TUN): A unique oncofetal fibronectin deposited in the extracellular matrix of the tropho-uterine junction and regulated in vitro by cultured human trophoblast cells. Troph Res 1993;7:167–81.
17. Huppertz B, Kertschanska S, Frank HG, Gaus G, Funayama H, Kaufmann P. Extracellular matrix components of placental extravillous trophoblast: immunocytochemistry and ultrastructural distribution. Histochem Cell Biol 1996;106:291–301.
18. Erickson HP. Tenascin-C, tenascin-R and tenascin-X; a family of talented proteins in search of functions. Curr Opin Cell Biol 1993;5:869–76.
19. Tryggvason K. The laminin family. Curr Opin Cell Biol 1993;5:877–82.
20. Church HJ, Richards AJ, Aplin JD Laminins in decidua, placenta and choriocarcinoma cells. Troph Res 1997;10:143–62.
21. Engvall E, Earwicker D, Haaparanta T, Ruoslahti E, Sanes JR. Distribution and solation of four laminin variants; tissue restricted distribution of heterotrimers assembled from five different subunits. Cell Regul 1990;1:731–40.
22. Aplin JD, Charlton AK, Ayad S. The role of matrix macromolecules in the invasion of decidua by trophoblast. Troph Res 1990;4:139–58.
23. Burrows TD, Enders AC, Loke YW. Expression of integrins by human trophoblast and differential adhesion to laminin and fibronectin. Hum Reprod 1993;8:475–84.
24. Geiger B, Ayalon O. Cadherins. Annu Rev Cell Biol 1992;8:307–92.
25. Takeichi M. Morphogenetic roles of classic cadherins. Curr Opin Cell Biol 1995;7:619–27.
26. Kemler R. Classical Cadherins. Semin Cell Biol 1992;3:149–55.
27. Okada TS. The pathway leading to the discovery of cadherin: In retrospect. Dev Growth Different 1996;38:583–96.
28. Tsukita S, Tsulita S, Nagatuchi A, Yonemura S. Molecular linkage between cadherins and actin filaments in cell-cell adherins junctions Curr Opin Cell Biol 1992;4:834–9.
29. Harlan JM, Liu DY. Adhesion. Its role in inflammatory disease. New York: WH Freeman, 1992.
30. Doherty P, Ashton SV, Moore SE, Walsh FS. Morphoregulatory activities of NCAM and N-cadherin can be accounted for by G protein-dependent activation of L-type and N-type neuronal Ca2+ channels. Cell 1991;67:21–33.
31. Hynes RO. Integrins: a family of cell surface receptors Cell 1987;48:549–54.
32. Ruoslahti E. Integrins as receptors for extracellular matrix. In: Hay ED, editor. Cell biology of extracellular matrix. New York: Plenum, 1991;343–59.
33. Ruoslahti E. Integrins. J Clin Invest 1991;87:1–5.
34. Albelda SM, Buck CA. Integrins and other cell adhesion molecules. FASEB J 1990;4:2868–80.
35. Juliano RL, Haskill S. Signal transduction from the extracellular matrix. J Cell Biol 1993;120:577–85.
36. Hynes RO. Integrins – versatility, modulation, and signaling in cell-adhesion. Cell 1992;69:11–25.
37. Hibbs ML, Xu H, Stacker SA, Springer TA. Regulation of adhesion to ICAM-1 by the cytoplasmic domain of LFA-1 integrin beta subunit. Science 1991;251:1611–13.
38. Sastry SK, Horwtiz AF. Integrin cytoplasmic domains: mediators of cytoskeletal linkages and extra and intercellular initiated transmembrane signalling. Curr Opin Cell Biol 1993;5:819–31.
39. Schaller MD, Borgman CA, Cobbs BS, Vines RR, Reynolds AB, Parsons JT. pp125FAK, a structurally unique protein kinase assocaiated with focal adhesions. Proc Natl Acad Sci USA 1992;89:5192–6.
40. Benirschke K, Kaufmann P. Pathology of the human placenta, 3rd edn. New York: Springer, 1995.
41. Pijnenborg R, Bland JM, Robertson WB, Dixon G, Brosens I. Trophoblast invasion and the establishment of hemochorial placentation in man and laboratory animals. Placenta 1981;2:303–15.
42. Pijnenborg R, Dixon G, Robertson WB, Brosens I. Trophoblastic invasion of human decidua from 8 to 18 weeks of pregnancy. Placenta 1980;1:3–19.
43. Pijnenborg R, Bland JM, Robertson WB, Brosens I. Uteroplacental arterial changes related to interstitial trophoblast migration early human pregnancy. Placenta 1983;4:397–414.
44. Pijnenborg R. Trophoblast invasion and placentation: morphological aspects. Troph Res 1990;4:33–50.

45. Pijnenborg R. The placental bed. Hypertens Preg 1996;15:7–23.
46. Cross JC, Werb J, Fisher SJ. Implantation and the placenta; key pieces of the development puzzle. Science 1994;266:1508–18.
47. Brosens I, Dixon HG. The anatomy of the maternal side of the placenta. J Obstet Gynaecol Br Commonwlth 1966;73:357–63.
48. Boyd JD, Hamilton WJ. Development and structure of the human placenta from the end of the third month of gestation. J Obstet Gynaecol Br Cmwlth 1967;74:161–226.
49. Brosens I, Robertson WB, Dixon HG. The physiological response of the vessels of the placental bed to normal pregnancy. J Pathol Bacteriol 1967;93:569–79.
50. De Wolf F, De Wolf-Peeters C, Brosens I. Ultrastructure of the spiral arteries in human placental bed at the end of normal pregnancy. Am J Obstet Gynecol 1973;117:833–48.
51. Sheppard BL, Bonnar J. The ultrastructure of the arterial supply of the human placenta in early and late pregnancy. J Obstet Gynaecol Br Cmwlth 1974;1:497–511.
52. Enders AC, King BF. Early stages of trophoblastic invasion of the maternal vascular system during implantation in the macaque and baboon. Am J Anat 1991;192:239–46.
53. Blankenship TN, Ender AC, King BF (1993) Trophoblastic invasion and the development of uteroplacental arteries in the macaque: immunohistochemical localizaton of cytokeratins, desmin, type IV collagen, laminin and fibronectin. Cell Tissue Res 1993;272:227–36.
54. Blankenship TN, Enders AC, King BF Trophoblastic invasion and modification of uterine veins during placental development macaques. Cell Tissue Res 1993;274:135–244.
55. Moll W, Nienartowicz A, Hees H, Wrobel K-H, Lenz A. Blood flow regulation in the uteroplacental arteries. Troph Res 1988;3:83–96.
56. Fisher SJ, Cui TY, Zhang L, Hartman L, Grahl K, Zhang GY, et al. Adhesive and degradative properties of human placental cytotrophoblast cells in vitro. J Cell Biol 1989;109:891–902.
57. Vicovac L, Aplin J. Epithelial–mesenchymal transition during trophoblast differentiation. Acta Acta Anat 1996;156:202–16.
58. Alexander C, Werb Z. Extracellular matrix degradation. In: Hay E, editor. Cell biology of the extracellular matrix. New York: Plenum, 1991;255–302.
59. Roberston WB. Discussion. Pathology of the uteroplacental bed. In: Sharp F, Symonds E, editors. Hypertension in pregnancy. New York: Perinatology Press, 1987;115.
60. Brosens IA, Robertson WB, Dixon HG. The role of the spiral arteries in the pathogenesis of pre-eclampsia. In: Wynn RM, editor. Obstetrics and gynecology annual. New York:Appleton-Century-Crofts, 1972;177–91.
61. Brosens IA. Morphological changes in the utero-placental bed in pregnancy hypertension. Clin Obstet Gynaecol 1977;4:573–93.
62. Khong TY, Sawyer IH, Heryet AR. An immunological study of endothelialization of utero-placental vessels in human pregnancy–evidence that the endothelium is focally disrupted by trophoblast in pre-eclampsia. Am J Obstet Gynecol 1992;167:751–6.
63. Khong TY, De Wolf F, Robertson WB, Brosens I. Inadequate maternal vascular response to placentation in pregnancies complicated by pre-eclampsia and by small-for-gestational age infants Br J Obstet Gynaecol 1986;93:1049–59.
64. Robertson WB, Brosens I, Dixon HG. The pathological response of the vessels of the placental bed to hypertensive pregnancy. J Pathol Bacteriol 1967;93:589–92.
65. Sheppard BL, Bonnar J.The ultrastructure of the arterial supply of the human placenta in pregnancy complicated by fetal growth retardation. J Obstet Gynaecol Br Cmwlth 1976;83:948–59.
66. Sheppard BL, Bonnar J. An ultrastructural study of utero placental arteries in hypertensive and normotensive pregnancy and fetal growth retardation. Br J Obstet Gynaecol 1981;88:695–705.
67. Khong TY, Liddell HS, Robertson WB. Defective haemochorial placentation as a cause of miscarriage: a preliminary study. Br J Obstet Gynaecol 1987;94:649–55.
68. Mould P, Garratt AN, Askari JA, Akiyama SK, Humphries MJ. Identification of a novel anti-integrin monoclonal antibody that recognises a ligand-induced binding site epitope on the $\beta 1$ subunit. FEBS Letters 1995;363:118–22.
69. Larjava H, Peltonen J, Akiyama S, Gralnik H, Uitto J, Yamada KM. Novel functions for $\beta 1$ integrins in keratinocyte cell–cell interactions. J Cell Biol 1990;111:803–15.
70. Carter WGP, Kaur SG, Gil PJ, Wayer EA. Distinct functions for a3b1 in focal adhesions and $\alpha 6/\beta 4$ bullous pemphigoid antigen in a new stabilising anchoring contact (SAC) of keratinocytes:-relation to hemidesmosomes. J Cell Biol 1990;111:3141–54.
71. Aplin JD. Expression of integrin $\alpha 6 \beta 4$ in human trophoblast and its loss from extravillous cells. Placenta 1993;14:203–15.
72. Korhonen M, Ylanne J, Laitnen L, Cooper HN, Quaranta V, Virtanenen I.. Distribution of the $\alpha 1$–$\alpha 6$ integrin subunits in human developing and term placenta. Lab Invest 1991;65:347–56.

73. Damsky CH, Fitzgerald ML, Fisher SJ. Distribution patterns of extracellular matrix components are intricately modulated during first trimester cytotrophoblast differentiation along the invasive pathway, in vivo. J Clin Invest 1992;89:210–22.

74. Damsky CH, Librach C, Lim K-H, Fitgerald ML, McMaster MT, Janatpour M, et al. Integrin switching regulates normal trophoblast invasion. Development 1994;120:3657–66.

75. Leivo I, Laurila, P, Wahlström T, Engvall E. Expression of merosin, a tissue specific basement membrane protein, in the intermediate trophoblast cells of choriocarcinoma and placenta. Lab Invest 1989;60:783–90.

76. Castellucci M, Crescimanno C, Schöter CA, Kaufmann P, Mühlhauer J. Extravillous trophoblast: immunohistochemical localization of extracellular matrix molecules. In: Genazzani F, Petraglia F, Genazzani A, editors. Frontiers in gynecologic and obstetric investigation. New York: Parthenon, 1993;19–25.

77. Rukosuev VS. Immunofluorescent localization of collagen types I, II, III, IV, V, fibronectin, laminin, entactin and heparan sulphate proteoglycan in human immature placenta. Experientia 1992;48:285–7.

78. Ohno M, Martinez-Hernandez Ohno A, Kelfalides NA. Laminin M is found in placental basement membranes but not in basement membranes of neoplastic origin. Connect Tissue Res 1986;15:199–207.

79. Korhonen M, Virtanen I. The distribution of laminins and fibronectins is modulated during extravillous trophoblastic cell differentiation and decidual cell response to invasion in the human placenta. J Histochem Cytochem 1997;45:569–81.

80. Frank HG, Malekzadeh F, Kertschanska S, Crescimanno C, Castellucci M, Lang I, et al. Immunohistochemistry of two different types of placental fibrinoid. Acta Anat 1994;150:55–68.

81. Huppertz B, Kertschanska S, Demir A, Frank HG, Kaufmann P (1998) Immunohistochemistry of matrix metalloproteinases (MMP), their substrates and their inhibitors (TIMP) during trophoblast invasion in the human placenta. Cell Tissue Res 1988;291:133–48.

82. Castellucci M, Classen-Linke I, Munlhauser J, Kaufmann P, Zardi L, Chiquet-Ehrismann R. The human placenta: a model for tenascin expression. Immunol Histochem 1991;95:449–58.

83. Aufderheide E, Ekblom P. Tenascin during gut development: appearance in the mesenchyme, shift in molecular forms and dependence on the epithelial–mesenchymal interactions. J Cell Biol 107:2341–9.

84. Burrows TD, King A, Loke YW. Expression of adhesion molecules by endovascular trophoblast and decidual endothelial cells – implications for vascular invasion during implantation. Placenta 1994;15:21–33.

85. Pröll J, Blaschitz M, Hartmann J, Thalhamer J, Dohr G. Human first-trimester placenta intra-arterial trophoblast cells express the neural cell adhesion molecule. Early Pregnancy: Biol Med 1996;2:271–5.

86. Lang I, Hartmann M, Blaschitz A, Dohr GA, Kaufmann P, Frank-HG, et al. Differential lectin binding to the fibrinoid of human full-term placenta: correlation with a fibrin antibody and the PAF-Halmi method. Acta Anat 1994;150:170–7.

87. Aplin JD, Campbell S. An immunofluorescence study of extracellualar matrix associated with cytotrophoblast of the chorion laeve. Placenta 1985;6:469–79.

88. King BF, Blankenship TN. Ultrastructure and development of a thick basement membrane-like layer in the anchoring villi of macaque placentas. Anat Rec 1994;238:489–506.

89. Kaufmann P, Castellucci M. Extravillous trophoblast in the human placenta. Troph Res 1997;10:21–65.

90. Yagel S, Casper RF, Powell P, Parhar RS, Lala PK. Characterisation of pure human 1st-trimester cytotrophoblast cells in long-term culture-growth-pattern, markers, and hormone production. Am J Obstet Gynecol 1989;160:938–45.

91. Librach CL, Feigenbaum SL, Bass KE, Cui TY, Verastas N, Sadovsky Y, et al. Interleukin-1 beta regulates human cytotrophoblast invasion in vitro. J Biol Chem 1994;269:125–31.

92. Librach CL, Fisher SJ, Fitgerald ML, Damsky CH. Cytotrophoblast–fibronectin and cytotro-phoblast–laminin interactions have distinct roles in cytotrophoblast invasion. J Cell Biol 1991;115:6a.

93. Vicovac L, Jones CS, Aplin JD. Trophoblast differentiation during formation of anchoring in a model of the early human placenta in vitro. Placenta 1995;16:41–56.

94. Irving JA, Lala PK. Functional role of cell surface integrins on human trophoblast cell migration: Regulation by TGFβ, IGF-II and IGFBP-1. Exp Cell Res 1995;217:419–27.

95. Delfilippi P, Silengo L, Tarone G. Alpha 6 beta 1 integrin (laminin receptor) is down regulated by tumour necrosis factor alpha and interleukin 1 beta in human endothelial cells. J Biol Chem 1992;267:18303–7.

96. Irving JA, Lala PK. Decidua-derived IGFBP-1 stimulates human intermediate trophoblast invasion by binding to the alpha5/beta1 integrin subunits. Placenta 1994;16:413–33.

97. Zhou Y, Fisher SJ, Janatpour M, Genbacev O, Dejana E, Wheelock M. Human cytotrophoblasts adopt a vascular phenotype as they diferentiate. A strategy for successful endovasular invasion? J Clin Invest 1997;99:2139–51.

98. Brooks FC, Clark RAF, Choresh DA. Requirement of integrin $\alpha v \beta 3$ for angiogenesis. Science 1994;264:569–71.

99. Winterhager E, von Ostau C, Grümmer R, Kaufmann P, Fisher SJ. Connexin and E-Cadherin Expression während der Differenzierung des humanen Trophoblasten. Versamm Anat Ges 1996:March:91.

100. MacCalman CD, Omigbodum A, Bronner MP, Struass JF. Identification of the cadherins present in human placenta. J Soc Gynecol Invest 1995;2:146.

101. Babawale MO, van Noorden S, Pignatelli M, Stamp GWH, Elder MG, Sullivan MHF. Morphological interaction of human first trimester placental villi co-cultured with decidual explants. Human Reprod 1996;1:444–50.

102. Coutifaris C, Kao LC, Sehdev HM, Chin U, Babalola GO, Blaschuk OW, et al. E-cadherin expression during the differentiation of human trophoblasts. Development 1991;113:767–77.

103. MacCalman CD, Chen GTC. Type 2 cadherins in the human endometrium and placenta: their putative roles in human implantation and placentation. Am J Reprod Immunol 1998;39:96–107.

104. Coukos G, Makrigiannakis A, Amin K, Albelda SM, Coutifaris C. Platelet endothelial cell adhesion molecule-1 is expressed by a subpopulation of human trophoblasts: a possible mechanism for trophoblast-endothelial interaction during haemochorial placentation. Mol Hum Reprod 1998;4:357–67.

105. Vittet D, Prandini M-H, Perthier R, Schweitzer A, Martin-Sisteron G, Uzan G. Embryonic stem cells differentiate in vitro to endothelial cells through successive maturation steps. Blood 1996;88:3424–31.

106. Risau W, Flamme I. Vasculogenesis. Ann Rev Cell Dev Biol 1995;11:73–91.

107. Heyward SA, Dubois-Stringfellow N, Rapoport R, Bautch VL. Expression and inducibility of vascular adhesion receptors in development. FASEB J 1995;9:956–62.

108. King BF, Blankenship TN. Neural cell adhesion molecule is present on macaque intra-arterial cytotrophoblast. Placenta 1995;16:A36.

109. King A, Loke YW. Differential expression of blood-group-related carbohydrate antigens by trophoblast subpopulations. Placenta 1988;9:513–21.

110. Burrows TD, King A, Loke YW. Expression of adhesion molecules by endovascular trophoblast and decidual endothelial cells – implications for vascular invasion during implantation. Placenta 1994;15:21–33.

111. Takada, Ohmori K, Yoneda T, Tsuyoka K, Hasegawa A, Ksio M, et al. Contribution of carbohydrate antigens sialyl Lewisa and sialyl Lewisx to adhesion of human cancer cells to vascular endothelium. Cancer Res 1993;53:354–61.

112. Roberts JM, Redman CW. Pre-eclampsia: more than pregnancy-induced hypertension. Lancet 1993;341:1447–51.

113. Moodley J, Ramsaroop R. Placental bed morphology in black women with eclampsia S Afr Med J 1989;75:376–8.

114. Gerretsen G, Huisjes HJ, Elema JD. Morphological changes of spiral arteries in the placental bed in relation to pre-eclampsia and fetal growth retardation. Br J Obstet Gynaecol 1981;88:876–81.

115. Lunell NO, Nylund LE, Lewander R, Sarby B. Uteroplacental blood flow in pre-eclampsia. Measurements with indium-113m and a computer-linked gamma camera. Clin Exp Hypertens 1982;B1:105.

116. Zhou Y, Damsky CH, Chiu K, Roberts JM, Fisher SJ. Preeclampsia is associated with abnormal expression of adhesion molecules by invasive cytotrophoblasts. J Clin Invest 1993;91:950–60.

117. Zhou Y, Damsky CH, Fisher SJ. Preeclampsia is associated with failure of human cytotrophoblasts to mimic a vascular adhesion phenotype. J Clin Invest 1997;99:2152–64.

118. Divers MJ, Bulmer JN, Miller D, Lilford RJ. Beta 1 integrins in third trimester human placentae: no differential expression in pathological pregnancy. Placenta 1995;16:245–60.

119. Zygmunt M, Boving B, Wienhard J, Munstedt K, Braems G, Bohle RM, et al. Expression of cell adhesion molecules in the extravillous trophoblast is altered in IUGR. Am J Reprod Immunol 1997;38:295–301.

120. Rodesch F, Simon P, Donner C, Jauniaux E. Oxygen measurements in endometrial and trophoblastic tissues during early pregnancy. Obstet Gynecol 1992;80:283–5.

121. Kingdom JCP, Kaufmann P. Oxygen and placental villous development: origins of fetal hypoxia. Placenta 1997;18:613–21.

122. Shweiki D, Itin A, Soffer D, Keshet E. Vascular endothelial growth factor induced by hypoxia may mediate hypoxia-initiated angiogenesis. Nature 1992;359:843–5.
123. Kourembanas S, Marsden PA, McQuillan LP, Faller DV. Hypoxia induces endothelin gene expression and secretion in cultured endothelium. J Clin Invest 1991;6:670–4.
124. Heacock CS, Sutherland RM. Induction characteristics of oxygen related proteins. Int J Oncol Biol Phys 1986;81:4843–7.
125. Genbacev O, Joslin R, Damsky CH, Polliotti BM, Fisher SJ. Hypoxia alters early gestation human cytotrophoblast differentiation/invasion in vitro and models the placental defects that occur in preeclampsia. J Clin Invest 1996;97:540–50.
126. Hustin J, Schapps JP. Echocardiographic and anatomic studies of the maternotrophoblastic border during the 1st trimester of pregnancy. Am J Obstet Gynecol 1987;157:162–8.
127. Moll UM, Lane BL. Proteolytic activity of first trimester human placenta: Localisation of interstitial collagenase in villous and extravillous trophoblast. Histochemistry 1990;94:555–60.
128. Emonard HP, Christiane Y, Smet M, Grimaud JA, Foidart JM. Type IV and interstitial collagenolytic activites in normal and malignant trophoblast cells are specifically regulated by the extracellular matrix. Invasion Metastasis 1990;10:170–7.
129. Hurskainen T, Seiki M, Apte SS, SyrjakallioYlitalo M, Sorsa T, Oikarinen A, et al. Production of membrane-type matrix metalloproteinase-1 (MT-MMP-1) in early human placenta: a possible role in placental implantation. J Histochem Cytochem 1998;46:221–9.
130. Blankenship TN, King BF. Identification of 72-kilodalton type-IV collagenase at sites of trophoblast invasion of macaque spiral arteries. Placenta 1994;15:177–87
131. Autio-Harmainen H, Hurskainen T, Niskasaari K, Hoyhtya M, Tryggvason K. Simulataneous expression of 70 kilodalton type IV collagenase and type IV collagen alpha 1 (IV) chain genes by cells of early human placenta and gestational endometrium. Lab Invest 1992;67:191–200.
132. Fernandez PL, Merino MJ, Nogales FF, Charonis AS, Stetler Stevenson WG, Liotta L Immunohistochemical profile of basement membrane proteins and 72-kilodalton type-IV collagenase in the implantation placental site – an integrated view. Lab Invest 1992;66:572–9.
133. Graham CH, Hawley TS, Hawley RG, MacDougall JR, Kerbel RS, Khoo N, et al. Establishment and characterization of first trimester human trophoblast cells with extended lifespan. Am J Obstet Gynecol 1993;206:204–11.
134. Polette M, Nawrocki B, Pintiaux A, Massenat C, Maquoi E, Volders L, et al. Expression of gelatinases A and B and their tissue inhibitors by cells of early and term human placenta and gestational endometrium. Lab Invest 1994;71:838–46.
135. Bjorn SF, Hastrup N, Lund LR, Dano K, Larsen JF, Pyke C. Co-ordinated expression of MMP-2 and its putative activator, MT1-MMP in human placentation. Mol Hum Reprod 1997;3:713–23.
136. Vettraino IM, Roby J, Tolley T, Parks WC. Collagenase-1, stromelysin-1 and matrilysin are expressed within the placenta during multiple stages of human pregnancy. Placenta 1996;17:557–63.
137. Librach CL, Werb Z, Fitzgerald ML, Chui K, Corwin NM, Esteves RA, et al. 92-kD type IV collagenase mediates invasion of human trophoblasts. J Cell Biol 1991;113:437–49.
138. Bischof P, Haenggeli L, Capana A. Gelatinase and oncofetal fibronectin secretion is dependent on integrin expression on human cytotrophoblasts. Hum Reprod 1995;10:734–42.
139. Maquoi E, Polette M, Nawrocki B, Bischof P, Noel A, Pintiaux A, et al. Expression of stromelysin-3 in the human implantation placental site. Placenta 1995;16:A46.
140. Nawrocki B, Polette M, Marchand V, Maquoi E, Beorchia A, Tournier JM, et al. Membrane-type matrix metalloproteinase-1 expression at the site of human implantation. Placenta 1996;17:565–72.
141. Hurskainen T, Hoyhtya M, Tuuttila A, Oikarinen A, AutioHarmainen H. mRNA expressions of TIMP-1, -2 and -3 and 92-kD type IV collagenase in early human placenta studied by in situ hybridization. J Histochem Cytochem 1996;44:1379–88.
142. Lala PK, Hamilton GS. Growth factors, proteases and protease inhibitors in the maternal–fetal dialogue. Placenta 1996;17:545–55.
143. Ruck P, Marzusch K, Kaiserling E, Horny HP, Dietl J, Geiselhart A. The distribution of cell-adhesion molecules in decidua of early pregnancy – an immunohistochemical study. Lab Invest 1994;71:94–101.
144. Bass KE, Li HX, Hawkes SP, Howard E, Bullen E, Vu TKH, et al. Tissue inhibitor of metalloproteinase-3 expression is upregulated during human cytotrophoblast invasion in vitro. Dev Genet 1997;21:61–7.
145. Bryant-Greenwood GD, Yamanoto SY. Control of peripartal collagenolysis in the human chorion-decidua. Am J Obstet Gynecol 1995;172:63–70.
146. Yagel S, Parhar RS, Jeffrey JJ, Lala PK. Cell Physiol 1988;136:455–62.

147. Zini JM, Murray SC, Graham CH, Lala PK, Kariko K, Barnathan ES, et al. Characterisation of urokinase receptor expression by human placental trophoblasts. Blood 1992;79:2917–29.

148. Multhaupt HAB, Mazar A, Cines DB, Warhol MJ, McCrae KR. Expression of urokinase receptors by human trophoblast, a histochemical and ultrastructural analysis. Lab Invest 1994;71:392–401.

149. Carmeliet P, Schoonjans L, Ream B, Degen J, Bronson R, Devos R, et al. Physiological consequences of loss of plasminogen activator gene function in mice. Nature 1994;368:419–24.

150. Bugge TH, Suh TT, Flick MJ, Daugherty CC, Romer J, Solberg H, et al. The receptor for urokinase-type plasminogen activator is not essential for mouse development or fertility. J Biol Chem 1994;270:16886–94.

151. Astedt B, Hagerstrand I, Lecander I. Cellular localisation in placenta of placental type plasminogen activator inhibitor. Thromb Haemost 1986;56:63–5.

152. Feinberg RF, Kao LC, Haimowitz JE, Queenan JTJ, Wun TC, Strauss JF, et al. Plasmonogen activator inhibitor types 1 and 2 in human trophoblasts. PAI-1 is an immunocytochemical marker of invading trophoblasts. Lab Invest 1989;61:20–26

153. Castellucci M, Theelen T, Pompili E, Fumagalli L, Derenzis G, Mühlhauser J (1994) Immunohistochemical localization of serine-protease inhibitors in the human placenta. Cell Tissue Res 278:283–289

154. Earl UM, Morrison L, Gray C, Bulmer JN. Proteinase and proteinase inhibitor localization in the human placenta. Int J Gynecol Pathol 1989;8:114–24.

155. Coukos G, Gafvels ME, Wisel S, Ruelaz EA, Strickland DK, Strauss III JF, et al. Expression of a2 macroglobulin receptor/low density lipoprotein receptor-related protein and the 39-kd receptor-associated protein in human trophoblasts. Am J Patho 1994;144:383–92.

156. Graham CH, McCrae KR. Altered expression of gelatinase and surface-associated plasminogen activator activity by trophoblast cells isolated from placentae of preeclamptic patients. Am J Obstet Gynecol 1996;175:555–62.

157. Bischof P, Haenggeli L, Campana A. Effect of leukemia inhibitory factor on human cytotrophoblast differentiation along the invasive pathway. Am J Reprod Immunol 1995;34:225–30.

158. Pepper MS. Transforming growth factor beta: vasculogenesis and vessel wall integrity. Cytokine Growth Factor Rev 1997;8:21–4.

159. Vuckovic M, Genbacev O, Kumar S. Immunolocalization of transforming growth factor beta in 1st and 3rd trimester human placenta. Pathobiol 1992;60:149–50.

160. Lysiak JJ, Hunt J, Pringle GA, Lala PK. Localization of transforming growth factor beta and its natural inhibitor decorin in the huaman placenta and decidua throughout gestation. Placenta 1995;16:221–31.

161. Graham CH, Lysiak JJ, McCrae KR, Lala PK. Localization of transforming growth factor-B at the human fetal–maternal interface: role in trophoblast growth and differentiation. Biol Reprod 1992;46:561–72.

162. Grisaru_Granovsky S, Post M, Lye S, Caniggia I. Preeclampsia is associated with a failure to downregulate TGF-b3 and its receptors. J Soc Gynecol Invest 1997;4:96A.

163. St Jacques S, Forte M, Lye SJ, Letarte M. Localization of endoglin, a transforming growth factor binding protein, and of CD44 and integrins in placenta during the first trimester of pregnancy. Biol Reprod 1994;51:405–13.

164. Janat MF, Argraves WS, Liau G. Regulation of vascular smooth muscle cell integrin expression by transforming growth factor beta-1 and by platelet-derived growth factor- Br J Cell Physiol 1992;151:588–95.

165. Feinberg RF, Kliman HJ, Wang CL. Transforming growth factor beta stimulates trophoblast oncofetal fibronectin synthesis in vitro – implications for trophoblast implantation in vivo. J Clin Invest 1994;78:1241–8.

166. Graham CH, Lala PK. Mechanism of control of trophoblast invasion in situ. J Cell Physiol 1991;148:228–34.

167. Graham CH. Effect of transforming growth factor-β on the plasminogen activator system in cultured first trimester human cytotrophoblasts. Placenta 1997;18:137–43.

168. Bass KE, Morrish DW, Roth I, Bhardwaj D, Taylor R, Zhou Y, et al. Human cytotrophoblast-invasion is upregulated by epidermal growth factor. Evidence that paracrine factors modify this process. Dev Biol 1994;164:560–1.

169. Cannigia I, Taylor CV, Ritchie JWK, Lye SJ, Letarte M. Endoglin regulates trophoblast differentiation along the invasive pathway in human placental villous explants. Endocrinology 1997;138:4977–88.

170. Ferrara N, Houck K, Jakeman L, Leung D. Molecular and biological properties of the vascular endothelail growth factor family of proteins. Endocr Rev 1992;13:18–32.

171. Ahmed A, Li XF, Dunk C, Whittle MJ, Rushton DI, Rollason T. Colocalization of vascular endothelial growth factor and its Flt-1 receptor in human placenta. Growth Factors 1995;12:235–43.

172. Sharkey AM, Charnock-Jones DS, Boocock CA, Brown KD, Smith SK. Expression of mRNA for vascular endothelial growth factor in human placenta. J Reprod Fertil 1993;99:609–15.

173. Cooper JC, Sharkey AM, McLaren J, CharnockJones DS, Smith SK. Localization of vascular endothelial growth factor and its receptor flt in human placenta and decidua by immunohistochemistry. J Reprod Fertil 1995;105:205–13.

174. Clark DE, Smith SK, Sharkey AM, CharnockJones DS. Localization of VEGF and expression of its receptors Flt and KDR in human placenta. Hum Reprod 1996;11:1090–8.

175. Ohlsson R, Homgren I, Glaser A, Specht A, Pfeifer-Ohlsson S. Insulin like growth factor 2 and short range stimulatory loops in control of human placental growth. EMBO J 1993;8:1993–9.

176. Thomsen BM, Clausen HV, Larsen LG, Nurberg L, Ottesen B, Thomsen HK. Patterns in expression of insulin-like growth factor-II and of proliferative activity in the normal human first and third trimester placenta demonstrated by non-isotopic and in situ hybridization and immunohistochemical staining for MIB-1. Placenta 1997;18:145–54.

177. Han VKM, Bassett N, Walton J, Challis JRG. The expression of insulin-like growth factor (IGF) and IGF-binding protein (IGFBP) genes in the human placenta and membranes: evidence for IGF–IGFBP interaction at the feto-maternal interface. J Clin Endocrinol Metabol 1996;81:2680–.

178. Lala PK, Lysiak JJ. Role of locally produced growth factors in human placental growth and invasion with special reference to transforming growth factors. In: Hunt J, editor. Immunology of reproduction. New York: Springer-Verlag, 1994;57–81.

179. Jokhi PP, King A, Loke YW. Reciprocal expression of epidermal growth factor receptor (EGF-R) and c-erbB2 by non-invasive and invasive human trophoblast populations. Cytokine 1994;6:433–42.

180. Duello TM, Bertics BJ, Fulgham DL, Vaness P (1994) Localization of epidermal growth factor receptors in first- and third-trimester human placentae: No differential expression in pathological pregnancy. J Histochem Cytochem 42:907–915

181. Hofmann P, Drews MR, Scott RTJ, Navot D, Heller DS, Deligdisch L. Epidermal growth factor and its receptor in human implantation trophoblast: immunohistochemical evidence for autocrine/paracrine function. J Clin Endocrinol Metabol 1992;74:981–8.

182. Hoffman GE, Scott Jr RT, Bergh PA. Immunochemical localization of epidermal growth factor in human endometrium, decidua and placenta from early, mid and late gestation. Am J Obstet Gynecol 1991;73:882–7.

183. Hayman MJ. erb-B: growth factor receptor turned oncogene. In: Bradshaw R, Prentis S, editors. Oncogenes and growth factors. Amsterdam: Elsevier, 1987;84–9.

184. Aboagye Mathiesen G, Zdravkovic M, Toth FD, Ebbesen P. Effects of human trophoblast-induced interferons on the expression of cfms/CSF-1R, EGF-R and c-erbB2 in invasive and non-invasive trophoblast. Placenta 1997;18:155–61.

185. Mason IJ. The ins and outs of fibroblast growth factors. Cell 1994;78:547–52.

186. Mühlhauser J, Marzioni D, Morroni M, Vuckovic M, Crescimanno C. Codistribution of basic fibroblast growth factor and heparan sulfate proteoglycan in the growth zones of the human placenta. Cell Tissue Res 1996;285:101–7.

187. Ferriani RA, Ahmed A, Sharkey A, Smith SK. Colocalization of acidic and basic fibroblast growth factor (FGF) in human placenta and the cellular effects of bFGF in trophoblast cell line JEG-3. Growth Factors 1994;10:259–68.

188. Lim KH, Damsky CH, Fisher SJ. Basic fibroblast growth factor and heparin stimulate integrin-alpha-1 expression by cytotrophoblasts. J Soc Gynecol Invest 1995;2:287.

189. Jokhi PP, Chumbley G, King A, Gardner L, Loke YW. Expression of the colony stimulating factor-1 receptor (c-fms product) by cells at the human uteroplacental interface. Lab Invest 1993;68:308–20.

190. Daiter E, Pampfer S, Yeung YG, Barad D, Stanley ER, Pollard JW. Expression of colony-stimulating factor-1 (CSF-1) in the human uterus and placenta. J Clin Endocrinol Metabol 1992;74:850–8.

191. Shorter SC, Clover LM, Starkey PM. Evidence for both an autocrine and paracrine role for colony-stimulating factors in regulating placental growth and development. Placenta 1992;12:A58.

192. Shorter SC, Vince GS, Starkey PM. Production of granulocyte colony-stimulating factor at the materno-foetal interface in human pregnancy. Immunology 1992;5:468–74.

193. Hamilton GS, Lysiak JJ, Watson AJ, Lala PK. Colony-stimulating factor-1 provides an autocrine signal for first trimester extravillous trophoblast cell proliferation. Placenta 1995;16:A24.

194. Li X, Shams M, Zhu J, Khalig A, Wilkes M, Whittle M, et al. Cellular localization of AT(1) receptor mRNA and protein in normal placenta and its reduced expression in intrauterine growth retardation – angiotensin II stimulates the release of vasorelaxants. J Clin Invest 1988;101:442–54.
195. Yang Y, Yelavarthi KK, Chen HL, Pace JL, Terranova PF, Hunt JS. Molecular, biochemical, and functional characteristics of tumor necrosis factor-alpha produced by human placental cytotrophoblastic cells. J Immunol 1993;150:5614–24.
196. Pijnenborg R, Mclaughlin PJ, Vercruysse L, Hanssens M, Johnson PM, Keith Jr. JC, et al. Immunolocalization of tumour necrosis factor-a (TNF-α) in the placental bed of normal and hypertensive pregnancies. Placenta 1998;19:231–9.
197. Hunt JS. The role of macrophages in the uterine response to pregnancy. Placenta 1990;11:467–75.
198. Steinborn A, VonGall C, Hildenbrand R, Stutte HJ, Kaufmann M. Identification of placental cytokine-producing cells in term and preterm labor. Obstet Gynecol 1998;91:329–35.
199. Yui J, Hemmings D, GarciaLoret M, Guilbert LJ. Expression of the human p55 and p75 tumor necrosis factor receptors in primary villous trophoblasts and their role in cytotoxic signal transduction. Biol Reprod 1996;55:400–9.
200. Higuchi T, Kanzaki H, Fujimoto M, Hatayama H, Watanabe H, Fukumoto M, et al. Expression of Vav protooncogene by non hematopoietic trophoblast. Biol Reprod 1995;53:840–6.
201. Sharkey AM, Jokhi PP, King A, Loke YW, Brown KD, Smith SK. Expression of c-kit and kit ligand at the human maternofetal interface. Cytokine 1994;6:195–205.
202. Luton D, Sibony O, Oury JF, Blot P, DieterlenLievre F, Pardanaud L. The c-ets 1 protooncogene is expressed in human trophoblast during the first trimester of pregnancy. Early Hum Dev 1997;47:147–56.
203 Jokhi PP, King A, Jubinsky P, Loke Y-W. Demonstration of the low affinity alpha subunit of the granulocyte macrophage colony stimulating factor receptor (GM-CSF-R-alpha) on human trophoblast and uterine cells. J Reprod Immunol 1994;26:147–64.
204. Knowles RG, Moncada S. Nitric oxide synthases in mammals. Biochem J 1994;298:249–58.
205. Myatt L, Brewer AS, Brickman DE. The action of nitric oxide on the perfused fetal-placental circulation. Am J Obstet Gynecol 1991;164:687–92.
206. Myatt L, Brewer A, Langdon G, Brockman DE. Attenuation of the vasoconstrictor effects of thromboxane and endothelin by nitric oxide in the human fetal–placental circulation. Am J Obstet Gynecol 1992;166:224–30.
207. Myatt L, Brockman DE, Langdon G, Pollock JS. Constitutive calcium dependent isoform of nitric oxide synthase in the human placental villous vascular tree. Placenta 1993;14:373–83.
208. Myatt L, Brockman DE, Eis ALW, Pollock JS. Immunohistochemical localization of nitric oxide synthase in the human placenta. Placenta 1993;14:487–95.
209. Eis ALW, Brockman DE, Pollock JS, Myatt L. Immunohistochemical localization of endothelial nitric oxide synthase in human villous and extravillous trophoblast populations and expression during syncytiotrophoblast formation *in vitro*. Placenta 1995;16:113–26.
210. Lyall F, Jablonka-Shariff A, Johnson RD, Olson LM, Nelson DM. Gene expression of nitric oxide synthase in cultured human term placental trophoblast during in vitro differentiation. Placenta 1998;17:253–60.
211. Craven CM, Morgan T, Ward K (1998) Decidual spiral artery remodelling begins before cellular interaction with cytotrophoblasts. Placenta 19:241–252.
212. Nanaev AK, Chwalisz K, Frank-H.G., Kohnen G, Hegele-Hartung C, Kaufmann P (1995) Physiological dilation of uteroplacental arteries in the guinea pig depends on nitic oxide synthase of extravillous trophoblast. Cell Tissue Res 282:407–421.
213. Lyall F, Bulmer JN, Kelly H, Duffie E, Robson SC. Human trophoblast invasion and spiral artery transformation. The role of Nitric Oxide. Am J Pathol 1999;154:1105–14.
214. Zarlingo TJ, Eis ALW, Brockman DE, Kossenjans W, Myatt L. Comparative localization of endothelial and inducible nitric oxide synthase isoforms in haemochorial and epitheliochorial placenta. Placenta 1997;18:511–20.
215. von Ostau C, Grümmer P, Kohnen G, Kaufmann P, Winterhager E. Expression verschiedener Connexine während der Entwicklung der humanen Plazenta. Ann Anat 1995;2:A102/103.
216. Hellmann P, von Ostau C, Grümmer R, Winterhager E. Connexin-40 expression in the human trophoblast: Implicator for proliferation and invasive properties. Placenta 1995;16:A26.
217. Zygmunt M, Hahn D, Münstedt K, Braems G, Bischof P, Lang U. hCG stimulates trophoblast invasion in vitro. J Soc Gynecol Invest 1998;5:118A.
218. El-Hendy UA, Wei KA, Subramanian MG, Diamond MP, Yelian FD. hCG modulates MMP-9 activity in first trimester trophoblast cells. J Soc Gynecol Invest 1998;5:118A.

219. Caniggia I, Lye SJ, Cross JC. Activin is a local regulator of human cytotrophoblast cell differentiation. Endocrinology 1997;138:3976–36.

220. Loke YW, King A. Immunology of human placental implantation: clinical implications of our current understanding. Mol Med Today 1997;April:153–9.

221. Haig D. Genetic conflicts in human pregnancy. Quart Rev Biol 1993;68:495–532.

222. Janeway CA, Travers P. Immunobiology: the immune system in health and disease. London: Current Biology, 1996.

223. King A, Boocock C, Sharkey AM, Gardner L, Beretta A, Siccardi AG, et al. Evidence for the expression of HLA-C class 1 mRNA and protein by human first trimester trophoblast. J Immunol 1996;156:2068–76.

224. Kovats SC, Librach P, Fisch EK, Main PM, Sondel SJ, Fisher SJ, et al. Expression and possible function of the HLA-G chain in human cytotrophoblasts. Science 1990;248:220–2.

225. Ellis SA, Palmer MS, McMichael J Human trophoblast and the choriocarcinoma cell line BeWo express a truncated HLA class 1 molecule. J Immunol 1990;144:731–5.

226. McMaster MT, Librach CL, Zhou Y, Lim KH, Janaipour MJ, Demars R, et al. Human placental HLA-G expression is restricted to differentiated cytotrophoblasts. J Immunol 1995;154:3771–8.

227. Chumbley G, King A, Gardner L, Howlett S, Holmes N, Loke YW. Generation of an antibody to HLA-G in transgenic mice and demonstration of tissue reactivity of this antibody. J Reprod Immunol 1994;27:173–86.

228. Bensussan A, Mansur IG, Mallet V, Rodriguez AM, Girr M, Weiss EH, et al. Detection of membrane-bound HLA-G translated products with a specific monoclonal antibody. Proc Natl Acad Sci USA 1995;92:10292–6.

229. Yang Y, Chu W, Geraghty DE, Hunt JS. Expression of HLA-G in human mononuclear phagocytes and selective induction by IFN-g. J Immunol 1996;156:4224–31.

230. Shorter SC, Starkery PM, Ferry LM, Clover LM, Sargent IL, Redman CWG. Antigenic hetero-geneity of human cytotrophoblast and evidence for the transient expression of MHC class 1 antigens distinct from HLA-G. Placenta 1993;14:571–82.

231. Butterworth BH, Khong TY, Loke YW, Roberston WB. Human cytotrophoblast populations studied by monoclonal antibodies using single and double botin-avidin-peroxidase immuno-cytochemistry. J Histochem Cytochem 1985;33:977–83.

232. Le Bouteiller P, Lenfant F. Antigen-presenting function(s) of the non-classical HLA-E, -F and -G class 1 molecules: the begining of a story. Res Immunol 1996;147:301–13.

233. Diehl M, Munz C, Keilholz W, Stevanovic S, Holmes N, Loke YW, et al. Non-classical HLA-G molecules are clasical peptide presenters. Curr Biol 1995;6:305–14.

234. Lee N, Malacko AR, IshitaniI A, Chen MC, Bajorath J, Marquardt H, et al. The membrane-bound and soluble forms of HLA-G bind identical sets of endogenous peptides but differ with respect to TAP association. Immunity 1995;3:591–600.

235. Pasmany L, Mandelboim O, Vales-Gomez M, Davis DM, Reyburn HT, Strominger JL. Pro-tection from natural killer cell-mediated lysis by HLA-G expression on target cells. Science 19966;274:792–5.

236. Ljunggren S, Main EK, Librach C, Stubblebine M, Fisher SJ, DeMars R. In search of the"missing self": MHC molecules and NK cell recognition. Immunol Today 1990;11:237–44.

237. Colonna M, Borsellino G, Falco M, Ferrara GB, Strominger JL. HLA-C is the inhibitory ligand that determines dominant resistance to lysis by NK1- and NK2-specific natural killer cells. Proc Natl Acad Sci USA 1993;90:12000–4.

238. Phillips JH, Chang CW, Mattson J, Gumperz JE, Parham P, Lanier LL. CD94 and a novel associ-ated protein (94AP) form an NK cell receptor involved in the recognition of HLA-A, HLA-B and HLA-C allotypes. Immunity 1996;5:163–72.

239. Ober C, Aldrich C, Rosinsky B, Robertson A, Walker MA, Willadsen S, et al. HLA-G1 protein is not essential for fetal survival. Placenta 1998;19:127–32.

240. Frank H-G, Huppertz B, Kertschanska S, Blanchard D, Roelcke D, Kaufmann P. Anti-adhesive glycosylation of fibronectin-like molecules in human placental matrix-type fibrinoid. Histochem Cell Biol 1995;104:317–29.

241. DeMesy Jensen K, Genbacev O, Penney D, Maltby K, Miller RK. Human cytotrophoblast cell islands – morphological characteristics in vitro. Placenta 1993;14:A14.

242. Bourne GL. The human amnion and chorion. London: Lloyd-Luke, 1962.

243. Wiese KH. Licht- und elektronenmikroskopische untersuchungen an der Chorionplatte der reifen menschlichen Plazenta. Arch Gynecol 1975;218:243–59.

244. Weser H, Kaufmann P. Lichtmikroskopische und histochemische Untersuchungen an der Chorionplatte der reifen menschlichen Plazenta. Arch Gynecol 1978;225:15–30.

245. King BF, Blankenship TN. Differentiation of the chorionic plate of the placenta. Cellular and extracellular matrix changes during development in the macaque. Anat Rec 1994;240: 267–76.
246. Malak TM, Ockleford CD, Bell SC, Dalgleish R, Bright NA, MacVicar J. Confocal immuno-fluorescence localization of collagen type-1, type-III, type-IV, type-IV, type-V and type-VI and their ultrastructural organization in term human fetal membranes. Placenta 1993;14:385–406.

7 Villous Development and the Pathogenesis of IUGR

Gaby Kohnen and John Kingdom

Introduction

Successful human pregnancy depends upon a coordinated series of events in developmental biology – not only of the embryo, but also of the placenta. The initial events in placentation involve the formation of a spheroidal trophoblastic shell that functions as a barrier to the diffusion of oxygen during embryogenesis until the end of the first trimester (see Chs 6, 12 and [1]). By contrast the embryonic placental circulation perfuses the placental villi from 7 postmenstrual weeks of gestation. Diffusion of oxygen to the embryo appears less important in these circumstances, which is in marked contrast to the situation in the third trimester when adequate oxygen transfer to the fetus depends on well-developed uteroplacental and fetoplacental vascular beds. This chapter describes the development of placental villi during normal pregnancy, leading to a discussion of the evidence supporting the concept of villous maldevelopment in IUGR. For more detailed discussion of this topic the reader is referred to one of the following specialised texts [2–4].

Development of Placental Villi

Early Events Following Implantation

The trophoblastic shell forms from the blastocyst, which encloses the developing embryo (Fig. 7.1) [4]. Following attachment and penetration through the endometrium, cells from the blastocyst proliferate and surround the embryo. This comprises an outer syncytiotrophoblast, which expands via syncytial fusion of proliferating cytotrophoblast beneath. The syncytial layer develops a series of lacunae, which coalesce to become the forerunner of the intervillous space. Cytotrophoblast cells grow out radially in the central parts of the trabeculae, where they advance beyond the leading edge of syncytium to proliferate around the entire conceptus to form the trophoblastic shell.

Initial Villous Development

Cytotrophoblast proliferation gives rise to side branches of the trabeculae (Fig. 7.1) [4]. These protrude into the lacunae to begin development of the villous tree. The distal parts of these so-called *primary villi* are formed from

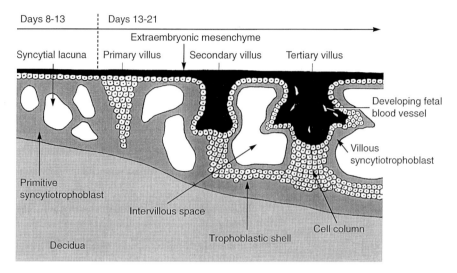

Fig. 7.1 Simplified diagram illustrating early placental development (modified from [4], by permission of W. B. Saunders and Professor Harold Fox, Manchester).

cytotrophoblast. At 5 weeks of gestation the primary villi are invaded centrally by allantoic mesenchyme, derived from the embryoblast [5], transforming them into *secondary villi*. The mesenchyme is the central stroma of the villi from which the fetoplacental blood vessels form. The de novo formation of blood vessels is termed *vasculogenesis* and is discussed in Ch. 8. The first fetoplacental capillaries are evident at 5 weeks of gestation [6,7] transforming them into *tertiary villi*. The

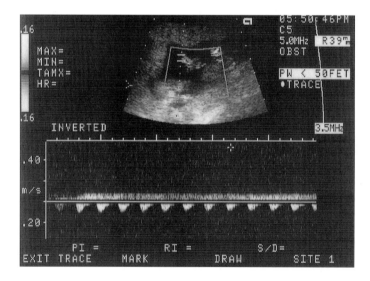

Fig. 7.2 Pulsed Doppler examination of umbilical cord at 10 weeks of gestation. (Note absent EDF in the lower channel.)

nomenclature of villous development is important to appreciate, since some authors writing on the pathology of IUGR use the term "tertiary stem villi". The second part of this chapter will explain the placental pathology of IUGR in relation to the development of these villi.

Hematopoiesis occurs within the villous capillaries, which become connected with the invading branches of the chorionic plate vessels. A formal fetoplacental circulation is established by 7 weeks of gestation [3] since umbilical arterial and venous flow velocity can be demonstrated using Doppler ultrasound (Fig. 7.2). The umbilical artery waveform shows only systolic peaks of flow velocity, suggesting high fetoplacental vascular impedance [8]. Fig. 7.3 [9] illustrates the exter-

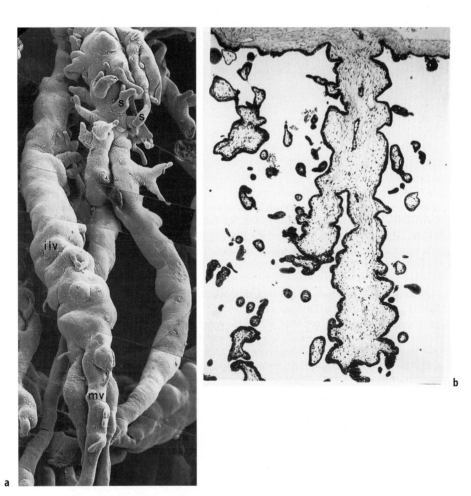

Fig. 7.3 a Scanning electron micrograph of several long villi, which illustrate developmental stages from immature intermediate villi (iiv) into mesenchymal villi (mv). Several trophoblastic sprouts (s) originate from the surface of the villi. They show a broad base and slender syncytial tips (× 105). **b** Methacrylate section corresponding to **a**. Centrally a branching villus arises from the chorionic plate (above) and illustrates the developmental stage of an immature intermediate villus to a mesenchymal villus. Numerous trophoblastic sprouts are seen in close vicinity (6 weeks of gestation, × 75; from [9], courtesy of Professor Peter Kaufmann, Aachen, Germany).

nal and internal structure of early first trimester villi, which comprise trophoblast sprouts and poorly vascularised villi. Perfusion is thus poor, but of no consequence since maternal–placental blood flow is underdeveloped and embryogenesis takes place in a hypoxic environment (see Ch. 6 and [10]).

The following section will discuss the anatomical development of the villous tree from tertiary villi to terminal villi. This covers the period from around 10 weeks' gestation until term. In essence this process is divided into two phases: formation of the proximal muscularised vessels and differentiation of stem villi followed by production and differentiation of terminal villi. A simple, though entirely accurate, corollary is the production of branches, followed by leaves, on a tree. Over the past 5–10 years a considerable knowledge has been gained regarding the molecular events that control growth and differentiation of placental villi. Dunk and Ahmed present this information in Ch. 8.

The Second Trimester: Differentiation and Development of Tertiary Villi

As will become evident, the principal anatomical site of maternal–fetal exchange is the terminal villus, illustrated by transmission electron microscopy (see Fig. 9.1 in Ch. 9). Successful placentation depends upon the exponential evolution of these structures, which by term provide a surface area of 15 m^2 for diffusional exchange [11,12]. This can only occur following the production of sufficient numbers of branches, the so-called stem villi.

At the outset of the second trimester, stem villi are beginning to form, but 8–16 generations of dichotomous branches are required for optimal development of the tree. This evolution is made possible because tertiary villi continue to form from primary mesenchymal villous sprouts, as outlined in Fig. 7.4 [9]. (For detailed review see [3].) The key structure during this phase of placental development is the *immature intermediate villus (IIV)*, predominating between 14 and 20 weeks when formation of stem villi is most intense. IIV are characterised by a loose expanded stroma, containing macrophages and numerous newly differentiated capillaries [13]. Placental macrophages and trophoblast provide growth factors for growth and remodelling of the stromal capillaries (see Ch. 8). Central vessels expand and develop a surrounding stroma containing smooth muscle (see below) while peripheral capillaries regress. New mesenchymal sprouts form (Fig. 7.3) [9] to continue this cycle. IIV are thus far poorly studied structures in placental pathology. However, their position in development makes them good candidates for controlling the final size of the villous tree, which is relevant to the pathology of IUGR [14,15]. Future villus-specific studies of growth factor signalling will no doubt unravel their importance.

The cycle of villous development in the second trimester is geared towards formation of stem villi. These are characterised by a condensed fibrous stroma that contains arteries and veins with a light-microscopically-identifiable media (Fig. 7.5) [16,17]. Primary stems connect the villous trees with the chorionic plate. A further four generations of thick branches are followed by several more generations (8–16 in total) of unequal dichotomous branches leading into the gas-exchanging villi (Fig. 7.6) [18].

Contractile smooth muscle cells surround the lumen of the stem arteries. These presumably are involved in the regulation of fetoplacental blood flow (for

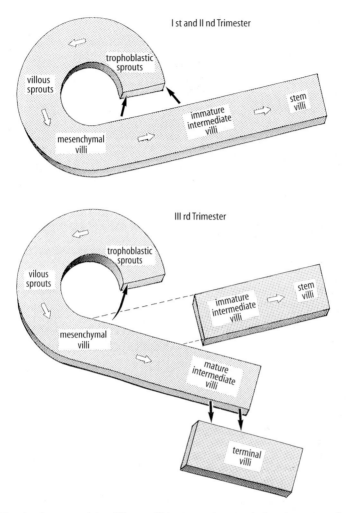

Fig. 7.4 The development of the different villous types changes during the course of gestation. In the first and second trimester production of new sprouts occurs on the surface of mesenchymal and immature intermediate villi. These transform initially into new mesenchymal villi and subsequently into immature intermediate villi. The latter finally differentiate into stem villi. During the third trimester, however, mesenchymal villi no longer differentiate into immature intermediate villi but into mature intermediate villi that will eventually give rise to terminal villi. Remaining immature intermediate villi will continue to transfom into stem villi but the decreasing number of newly formed immature intermediate villi will ultimately decrease the actual number of stem villi. As a consequence of the gestational changes the actual number of stem villi is determined during the first and second trimester (white arrows: differentiation of villous types, dark arrows: production of new villi; from [9], courtesy of Professor Peter Kaufmann, Aachen).

detailed review see [19]. A layer of longitudinally arranged cells lie outside the circular layer of the vascular smooth muscle cells. Some of these extravascular cells have differentiated into a secretory phenotype with cytoskeletal features of myofibroblasts and demonstrate immunoreactivity for several vasoactive substances [17,18,20,21]. A paracrine dialogue may exist between these two layers

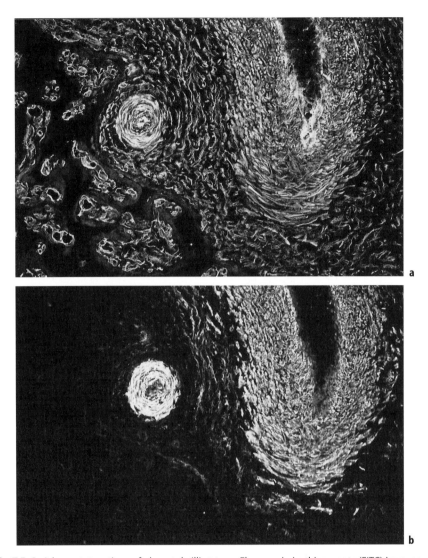

Fig. 7.5 Serial cryostat sections of placental villi at term. Fluorescein isothiocyanate (FITC) immuno-histochemistry shows binding of: **a** vimentin, an intermediate filament expressed in cells of mesenchymal origin, and **b** GB42, an antibody directed against a cytoskeletal antigen that is closely related to γ-smooth muscle actin and expressed in myofibroblasts and smooth muscle cells [16]. A tangential section of a large stem villus (right) is surrounded by numerous terminal villi. Vascular smooth muscle cells coexpress vimentin (**a**) and GB42 (**b**). All extravascular stromal cells in placental villi express vimentin (**a**). A subpopulation of extravascular stromal cells in stem villi close to the fetal vessel wall coexpresses GB42 (**b**) thus illllustrating that extravascular stromal cells in placental stem villi have characteristics of smooth muscle cells and myofibroblasts [16,17] (× 180).

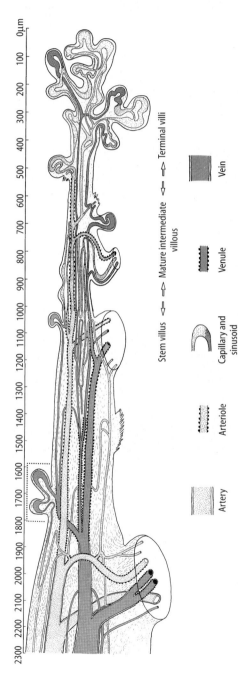

Fig. 7.6 Simplified drawing from a peripheral part of the villous tree at term reconstructed from serial semithin sections [18]. Vessel length and calibre are drawn on the same scale while the vessel diameter is reduced to two-thirds. Immature intermediate villi are missing in this drawing by chance. The localisation of the vessels is simplified owing to the two-dimensional representation of the original three-dimensional arrangement (from [18], courtesy of Professor Peter Kaufmann, Aachen Germany).

[22], which may be relevant to intervillous space volume regulation where contraction of anchoring villi will reduce placental volume or the regulation of stem artery vessel tone [17,20,21,23–26].

The Third Trimester: Formation of Gas-exchanging Villi

As the pregnancy approaches fetal viability, from 24 weeks of gestation, there is a gradual switch in emphasis from formation of conductance vessels in stem villi to the formation of gas- and nutrient-exchanging villi. This is illustrated in Fig. 7.4 [9]. The key step is the differentiation of IIV into their mature counterparts, the *mature intermediate villi (MIV)*. As can be seen in Fig. 7.4 [9], MIV do not self-replicate: rather they elongate and produce terminal villi by "intussusception" as outlined in Fig. 7.6 [18]. Note that the intussusceptive process requires that the capillaries within MIV elongate faster than the growth of MIV themselves – that way, terminal villi form from the outpouching of capillary loops from the trophoblast surface. This second and final phase in villous development is one of capillary growth in a longitudinal manner. It is qualitatively different from angiogenesis in IIV [27,28], and thus presumably influenced by different growth factors, the most favoured of which is placenta-like growth factor (PlGF – see

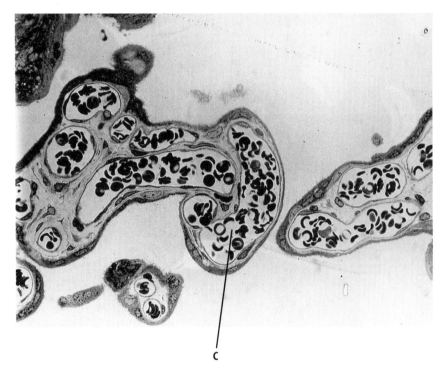

c

Fig. 7.7 Semithin section illustrating the transition of a mature intermediate villus into a terminal villus located close to another terminal villus. The dilated fetal capillary (c) of the terminal villus bulges against the villous surface where the adjacent villous syncytiotrophoblast appears attenuated and very thin corresponding to a vasculosyncytial membrane: (× 770; from [29], courtesy of Professor Peter Kaufmann, Aachen).

Ch. 8). The reader can imagine the active outgrowth of capillaries, displacing cytotrophoblast cells and leaving only a thin layer of syncytiotrophoblast between maternal and fetal blood – the *vasculosyncytial membrane* – illustrated in Fig. 7.7 [29]. This arrangement is ideal for the transfer of diffusion-limited substances such as carbon dioxide and oxygen (see Ch. 9).

In summary, successful development of the villous tree of the human placenta takes place in two interdependent phases. First the co-ordinated formation of generations of stem villi, followed by a developmental switch to the production of terminal villi. As will be seen in the next section, IUGR arising from "placental insufficiency" may have its origins at different stages of villous development.

Villous Maldevelopment in IUGR

Recent progress in our understanding of placental pathology in IUGR has resulted from two developments: first, from an appreciation of the developmental biology of the normal villous tree, and, secondly, from ultrasound techniques, which allow the obstetrician to identify growth-restricted fetuses from within a population of SGA pregnancies (see Chs 11 and 13). As the reader will appreciate in Ch. 1, a broad distinction can be made between early onset IUGR, typically presenting at < 30 weeks of gestation, and the more common milder forms towards term. Undoubtedly the majority of placentas included in SGA studies before 1980 were from deliveries in the late third trimester [30]. The first reports of umbilical artery Doppler studies identifying preterm SGA fetuses at high risk of perinatal death appeared in the early 1980s [31]. They stimulated the use of this technique to identify a "focused" group of pregnancies with IUGR. Furthermore, since the abnormal Doppler waveforms suggested a significant impairment of fetoplacental blood flow [32], researchers could focus on providing explanations for this observation.

Umbilical Cord

In the sheep fetus, whose cord is shorter than the human, the cord arteries contribute a significant portion of fetoplacental vascular resistance [33] and thus in the human this effect is likely to be greater. Single [34] and discordant [35,36] umbilical artery diameters have been reported in association with IUGR. The mediae of these vessels are hypoplastic [37] and contract poorly to pressor agents [38]. Reduced volume flow, and thus vascular pressure, may render these thin vessels susceptible to extrinsic compression, thereby influencing fetoplacental vascular impedance [39]. Pulsatile flow in the umbilical vein is an ominous sign in IUGR [40], though no studies have reported the cord histology in these circumstances. The cord venous endothelium contains a number of vasoactive peptides, which may influence arterial tone in a paracrine manner [41], but to date these methods have not yet been applied to the IUGR cord.

Stem Arteries

These vessels are not innervated, and thus the branching pattern of the arterial tree and the paracrine interactions of endothelium and smooth muscle govern vascular impedance. Since the fetoplacental circulation is characterised by low impedance to flow, it probably operates at near-maximal vasodilatation under normal circumstances (for reviews see [19] and [22]).

Reduced Density of Stem Arteries

The landmark paper in this field was from Australia, which reported reduced stem artery density in preterm IUGR placentas with abnormal umbilical artery Doppler waveforms [42]. Others found similar findings [43,44]. Despite the consistency of these reports, others have criticised their validity from several technical angles: lack of perfusion–fixation to try and preserve the in vivo situation, suboptimal sampling methods thus introducing selection bias [45], and lack of immunohistochemical localisation of vessels. Systematic random block sampling of the placenta [46] implies that all – generally excluding areas of obvious infarction – parts of the organ have an equal chance of being sampled. When applied to the preterm IUGR placenta with impaired cord flow before delivery, no specific differences in stem arterial development could be found [14]. When immunohistochemical methods were employed – albeit without random sampling – again no differences in vascular tree elaboration could be found [47]. More recently, we have combined immediate perfusion–fixation with systematic random block sampling of the placenta, restricting fixation to 16 hours in order that conventional immunohistochemical methods can be applied to paraffin-embedded sections. It is hoped this approach will clarify the issue of stem arterial anatomy in due course.

Alterations in Stem Artery Structure

Part of the confusion in the previous section relates to artefactual alterations in the placenta following delivery. Unless the cord is clamped immediately, or worse if the cord vessels are inadvertently ruptured during delivery, a significant degree of capillary collapse, and arterial constriction, will occur [48]. Fetoplacental arterial vasoconstriction is an intense "end response" designed to prevent neonatal exsanguination and is mediated primarily by contractile prostaglandins [49]. These effects will appear even more dramatic at high magnifications. With this background information, it becomes difficult to interpret the significance of papers addressing the anatomy of stem arteries using immersion-fixed material (where the time from delivery to initial fixation is unspecified). Las Heras and Haust [50] reported endothelial cell swelling, and herniation of the basal cytoplasm through the basal lamina. Fok and colleagues [51] reported stem artery hypertrophy, which correlated with the degree of cord flow abnormality, and finally Salafia and colleagues [52] reported further observations on "endarteritis obliterans" in early onset IUGR, showing increased intra-luminal thromboses. Todros and colleagues [15] reported reduced stem artery branching in preterm IUGR, though no differences in vessel wall thickness. As outlined in the previous section, in our recent studies with combined immediate perfusion-fixation, restricted fixation and random block sampling we found no evidence of intra-luminal thrombosis, vessel wall hypertrophy or of reduced stem artery measurements in similar cases with absent/reversed end-diastolic flow (EDF) in the umbilical arteries before delivery.

The chronically instrumented ovine fetal model has been used to demonstrate that microsphere embolisation induces alterations in umbilical artery Doppler waveforms comparable to those seen in the preterm IUGR human fetus [32,53]. Whilst it is accepted that stem artery thrombosis/embolisation can occur, at the present time there is no convincing proof that this mechanism underscores the placental pathology of early onset IUGR.

Gas-exchanging Villi

A wider appreciation of the development of gas exchanging villi in the early 1990s, together with an understanding that these small structures could be studied quantitatively by stereological tools, led investigators to study the more distal parts of the villous tree. Furthermore, the knowledge from fetal blood sampling studies [54,55] that the preterm IUGR fetus is typically hypoxic and acidotic focused attention on terminal villi.

Stereological examination of immersion-fixed tissues recently found a significant reduction in the volume of terminal villi in preterm IUGR with abnormal umbilical artery Doppler [56], consistent with earlier findings [14]. Recently Todros and colleagues [15] compared subgroups of such pregnancies with absent or positive EDF in the umbilical arteries, and found evidence of adaptive angiogenesis where EDF remained at delivery. Three-dimensional studies of gas-exchanging villi in preterm IUGR have revealed reduced numbers of elongated and malformed villi (Fig. 7.8) [57]. Parallel immunohistochemical and electron microscopic studies revealed stromal fibrosis, reduced cytotrophoblast proliferation [58] and reduced expression of VEGF [59], all of which suggested that intraplacental oxygenation in preterm IUGR was closer to arterial values than under normal circumstances (where high fractional extraction of oxygen exists) [60]. This scenario was termed "placental hyperoxia" [27] and is illustrated in Fig. 7.9. As will become apparent in the following chapter, the reduced volume of gas-exchanging villi in preterm IUGR appears to be due to an arrest of normal angiogenesis within mature intermediate villi. Placental growth in the third trimester is primarily due to angiogenesis, which in turn is driven by oxygen-sensitive growth factors.

In clinical terms, however, preterm IUGR is very much the exception to the rule since most IUGR pregnancies deliver in late gestation. The first ultrasound evidence that the fetus may be at risk of IUGR is the detection of bilateral notching/high impedance in the uterine arteries at 20–24 weeks of gestation [61]. Recent embolisation studies, in the ovine model, demonstrate that this waveform abnormality is associated with a 50 per cent reduction in uteroplacental blood flow [62], implying ischaemia of the intervillous space. Normally the placenta compensates for this by increased fractional extraction of flow-limited substances. Adaptive angiogenesis within the peripheral villi allows the placenta to increase this further [63,64]. These anatomical changes may result from the effects of villous ischaemia upon the local expression of angiogenic growth factors and their receptors (see Ch. 8).

From a clinical perspective, we know that the majority of pregnancies in otherwise healthy women with abnormal uterine artery Doppler flow are successful [65], which suggests that the placenta is capable of evoking compensatory changes to sustain fetal growth and well-being. This pathway represents the classic histological changes of pre-eclampsia, often coexisting with IUGR in late gestation. Trophoblast proliferation is increased in pre-eclampsia [66], which is consistent with observed findings in vitro [67]. This increased villous angiogenic

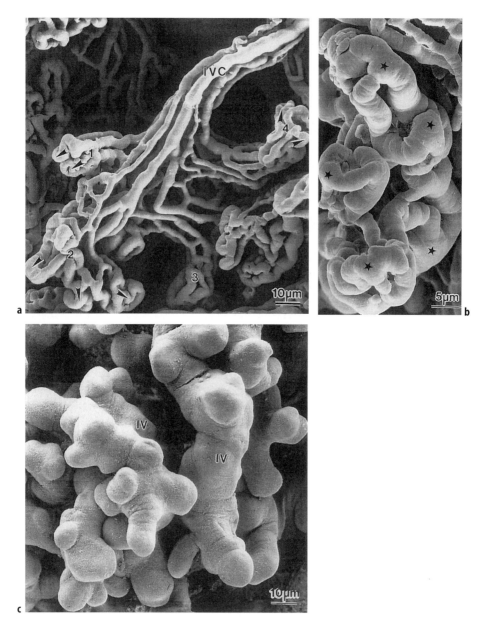

Fig. 7.8 Scanning electron micrographs illustrating: **a–c** Vascular casts and the villous surface from a preterm control placenta; **d–f** IUGR placenta with absent end-diastolic flow velocity. Both cases are 32 weeks gestation. **a** The vascular cast from the preterm control shows the intermediate villous capillaries (IVC) branch into four terminal capillary convolutions (1–4) with numerous loops (arrowheads). **b** The capillaries show typically coiling, branching and sinusoidal dilations (stars). **c** The scanning micrograph of the villous surface shows the distal part of mature intermediate villi (IV) with typical bud-like projections of multiple terminal villi.

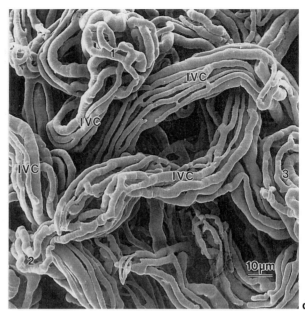

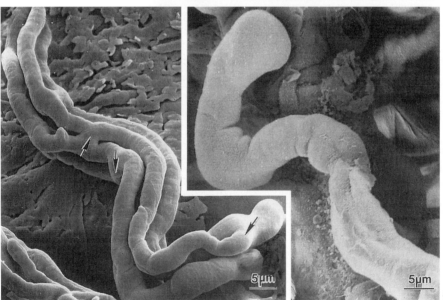

Fig. 7.8 (*continued*) **d** The vascular cast of the IUGR case shows that the bundles of intermediate villous capillaries (IVC) are extremely elongated. The terminal convolutions (1–3) are sparse with inconspicuous loops. **e** Higher magnification shows that the terminal capillary loops are uncoiled with only few branches (arrows). **f** The surface of a terminal villus is simple and devoid of branching (original magnifications **a** × 1,000, **b** × 2,400, **c** × 1,000, **d** × 1,000, **e** × 2,300, **f** × 2,350; from [57], by permission of Am J Obstet Gynecol and Dr Christane Krebs, Giessen Germany).

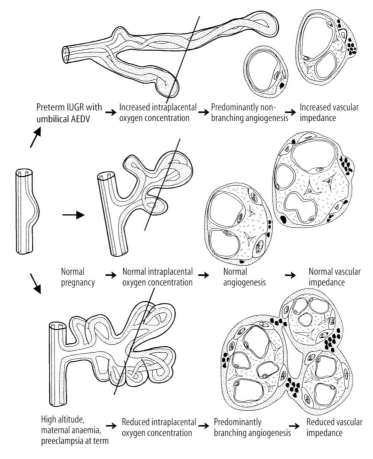

Preterm IUGR with → **Increased intraplacental** → **Predominantly non-** → **Increased vascular**
umbilical AEDV   **oxygen concentration**   **branching angiogenesis**   **impedance**

Normal → **Normal intraplacental** → **Normal** → **Normal vascular**
pregnancy   **oxygen concentration**   **angiogenesis**   **impedance**

High altitude, → **Reduced intraplacental** → **Predominantly** → **Reduced vascular**
maternal anaemia,   **oxygen concentration**   **branching angiogenesis**   **impedance**
preeclampsia at term

Fig. 7.9 Villous angiogenesis according to villous oxygenation. The capillarisation pattern of placental hyperoxia (above), normal pregnancy (middle) and preplacental as well as uteroplacental hypoxia (below) are illustrated to the left. The oblique lines illustrate the typical histological features of terminal villi on the right (from [27], by permission of W.B. Saunders and Professor Peter Kaufmann, Aachen Germany).

response will in turn confer lower vascular impedance, which explains why the majority of late gestation IUGR pregnancies have normal umbilical artery Doppler waveforms [68], or even reduced impedance, compared with normal [69].

Summary

Modern ultrasound techniques, including Doppler flow measurement, have refined the diagnosis of IUGR, thus providing more homogeneous groups of placentas for pathological study. Whilst debate continues as to the relevance of stem arteries, largely because of suboptimal methodology, much progress has been made in relating villous maldevelopment to the process of IUGR. The underlying process of placental development is angiogenesis, which will be considered in the following chapter.

References

1. Jaffe R, Jauniaux E, Hustin J. Maternal circulation in the first-trimester human placenta – myth or reality? Am J Obstet Gynecol 1997;176:695–705.
2. Boyd JD, Hamilton WJ. The human placenta. Cambridge: W Heffer, 1970.
3. Benirschke K, Kaufmann P. The pathology of the human placenta,. 3rd edn. New York, Berlin, Heidelberg: Springer-Verlag, 1995.
4. Fox H. Pathology of the placenta, 2nd edn. London: WB Saunders, 1997.
5. Luckett WP. Origin and differentiation of the yolk sac and extraembryonic mesoderm in presomite human and rhesus monkey embryos. Am J Anat 1978;152:59–97.
6. King BF. Ultrastructural differentiation of stromal and vascular components in early macaque placental villi. Am J Anat 1987;178:30–44.
7. Demir R, Kaufmann P, Castellucci M, Erbengi T, Kotowski A. Fetal vasculogenesis and angiogenesis in human placental villi. Acta Anat (Basel) 1989;136:190–203.
8. Fisk NM, MacLachlan N, Ellis C, Tannirandorn Y, Tonge HM, Rodeck CH. Absent end-diastolic flow in first trimester umbilical artery. Lancet 1988;2:1256–7.
9. Castellucci M, Scheper M, Scheffen I, Celona A, Kaufmann P. The development of the human placental villous tree. Anat Embryol 1990;181:117–28.
10. Rodesch F, Simon P, Donner C, Jauniaux E. Oxygen measurements in endometrial and trophoblastic tissues during early pregnancy. Obstet Gynecol 1992;80:283–5.
11. Jackson MR, Mayhew TM, Boyd PA. Quantitative description of the elaboration and maturation of villi from 10 weeks of gestation to term. Placenta 1992;13:357–70.
12. Luckhardt M, Leiser R, Kingdom J, Malek A, Sager R, Kaisig C, et al. Effect of physiologic perfusion-fixation on the morphometrically evaluated dimensions of the term placental cotyledon. J Soc Gynecol Invest 1996;3:166–71.
13. Kadyrov M, Kosanke G, Kingdom JCP, Kaufmann P. Increased fetoplacental angiogenesis during first trimester in anaemic women. Lancet 1998;52:1747–9.
14. Jackson MR, Walsh AJ, Morrow RJ, Mullen JB, Lye SJ, Ritchie JW. Reduced placental villous tree elaboration in small-for-gestational-age pregnancies: relationship with umbilical artery Doppler waveforms. Am J Obstet Gynecol 1995;172:518–25.
15. Todros T, Sciarrone A, Piccoli E, Guiot C, Kaufmann P, Kingdom J. Umbilical Doppler waveforms and placental villous angiogenesis in pregnancies complicated by fetal growth restriction. Obstet Gynecol 1999; 93:499–503.
16. Kohnen G, Castellucci M, Hsi BL, Yeh CJ, Kaufmann P. The monoclonal antibody GB 42 – a useful marker for the differentiation of myofibroblasts. Cell Tissue Res 1995;281:231–42.
17. Kohnen G, Kertschanska S, Demir R, Kaufmann P. Placental villous stroma as a model system for myofibroblast differentiation. Histochem Cell Biol 1996;105:415–29.
18. Leiser R, Luckhardt M, Kaufmann P, Winterhager E, Bruns U. The fetal vascularisation of term human placental villi. I. Peripheral stem villi. Anat Embryol 1985;173:71–80.
19. Kingdom JC, Burrell SJ, Kaufmann P. Pathology and clinical implications of abnormal umbilical artery Doppler waveforms. Ultrasound Obstet Gynecol 1997;9:271–86.
20. Graf R, Langer JU, Schonfelder G, Oeney T, Hartel-Schenk S, Reutter W, et al. The extravascular contractile system in the human placenta. Morphological and immunocytochemical investigations. Anat Embryol 1994;190:541–8.
21. Graf R, Schoenfelder G, Muhlberger M, Gutsmann M. The perivascular contractile sheath of human placental stem villi: its isolation and characterization. Placenta 1995;16:57–66.
22. Kingdom JCP, Poston L. Stem villous arteries as regulators of fetal placental blood flow. Troph Res 1998;12:403–8.
23. Krantz KE, Parker JC. Contractile properties of the smooth muscle in the human placenta. Clin Obstet Gynecol 1963;6:26–38.
24. Castellucci M, Kaufmann P. A three-dimensional study of the normal human placental villous core: II. Stromal architecture. Placenta 1982;3:269–85.

25. Graf R, Neudeck H, Gossrau R, Vetter K. Elastic fibres are an essential component of human placental stem villous stroma and an integrated part of the perivascular contractile sheath. Cell Tissue Res 1996;283:133–41.

26. Demir R, Kosanke G, Kohnen G, Kertschanska S, Kaufmann P. Classification of human placental stem villi: review of structural and functional aspects. Microsc Res Tech 1997; 38:29–41.

27. Kingdom JC, Kaufmann P. Oxygen and placental villous development: origins of fetal hypoxia. Placenta 1997;18:613–21.

28. Ahmed A, Kilby MD. Hypoxia or hyperoxia in placental insufficiency? Lancet 1997;350:826–7.

29. Kaufmann P, Bruns U, Leiser R, Luckhardt M, Winterhager E. The fetal vascularisation of term human placental villi. II. Intermediate and terminal villi. Anat Embryol 1985;173:203–14.

30. Sandstedt B. The placenta and low birth weight. Curr Top Pathol 1979;66:1–55.

31. FitzGerald DE, Stuart B, Drumm JE, Duignan NM. The assessment of the feto-placental circulation with continuous wave Doppler ultrasound. Ultrasound Med Biol 1984;10:371–6.

32. Trudinger BJ, Stevens D, Connelly A, Hales JR, Alexander G, Bradley L, et al. Umbilical artery flow velocity waveforms and placental resistance: the effects of embolization of the umbilical circulation. Am J Obstet Gynecol 1987;157:1443–8.

33. Adamson SL, Morrow RJ, Langille BL, Bull SB, Ritchie JW. Site-dependent effects of increases in placental vascular resistance on the umbilical arterial velocity waveform in fetal sheep. Ultrasound Med Biol 1990;16:19–27.

34. De Catte L, Burrini D, Mares C, Waterschoot T. Single umbilical artery: analysis of Doppler flow indices and arterial diameters in normal and small-for-gestational age fetuses [see comments]. Ultrasound Obstet Gynecol 1996;8:27–30.

35. Dolkart LA, Reimers FT, Kuonen CA. Discordant umbilical arteries: ultrasonographic and Doppler analysis. Obstet Gynecol 1992;79:59–63.

36. Raio L, Ghezzi F, Di Naro E, Gomez R, Saile G, Bruhwiler H. The clinical significance of antenatal detection of discordant umbilical arteries. Obstet Gynecol 1998;91:86–91.

37. Bruch JF, Sibony O, Benali K, Challier JC, Blot P, Nessmann C. Computerized microscope morphometry of umbilical vessels from pregnancies with intrauterine growth retardation and abnormal umbilical artery Doppler. Hum Pathol 1997;28:1139–45.

38. Templeton AG, Kingdom JC, Whittle MJ, McGrath JC. Contractile responses of the human umbilical artery from pregnancies complicated by intrauterine growth retardation. Placenta 1993;14:563–70.

39. Adamson SL, Whiteley KJ, Langille BL. Pulsatile pressure–flow relations and pulse-wave propagation in the umbilical circulation of fetal sheep. Circ Res 1992;70:761–72.

40. Rizzo G, Capponi A, Talone PE, Arduini D, Romanini C. Doppler indices from inferior vena cava and ductus venosus in predicting pH and oxygen tension in umbilical blood at cordocentesis in growth-retarded fetuses. Ultrasound Obstet Gynecol 1996;7:401–10.

41. Sexton AJ, Loesch A, Turmaine M, Miah S, Burnstock G. Electron-microscopic immunolabelling of vasoactive substances in human umbilical endothelial cells and their actions in early and late pregnancy. Cell Tissue Res 1996;284:167–75.

42. Giles WB, Trudinger BJ, Baird PJ. Fetal umbilical artery flow velocity waveforms and placental resistance: pathological correlation. Br J Obstet Gynaecol 1985;92:31–8.

43. Bracero LA, Beneck D, Kirshenbaum N, Peiffer M, Stalter P, Schulman H. Doppler velocimetry and placental disease. Am J Obstet Gynecol 1989;161:388–93.

44. McCowan LM, Mullen BM, Ritchie K. Umbilical artery flow velocity waveforms and the placental vascular bed. Am J Obstet Gynecol 1987;157:900–2.

45. Jauniaux ER, Burton GJ. Correlation of umbilical Doppler features and placental morphometry: the need for uniform methodology. Ultrasound Obstet Gynecol 1993:3;233–5.

46. Mayhew TM, Burton GJ. Stereology and its impact on our understanding of human placental functional morphology. Microsc Res Tech 1997;38:195–205.

47. Macara L, Kingdom JC, Kohnen G, Bowman AW, Greer IA, Kaufmann P. Elaboration of stem villous vessels in growth restricted pregnancies with abnormal umbilical artery Doppler waveforms. Br J Obstet Gynaecol 1995;102:807–12.

48. Bouw GM, Stolte LAM, Baak JPA, Oort J. Quantitative morphology of the placenta. 1. Standardization of sampling. Eur J Obstet Gynecol Reprod Biol 1976;6:325–31.

49. Templeton AG, McGrath JC, Whittle MJ. The role of endogenous thromboxane in contractions to U46619, oxygen, 5- HT and 5-CT in the human isolated umbilical artery. Br J Pharmacol 1991;103:1079–84.

50. Las Heras J, Haust MD. Ultrastructure of fetal stem arteries of human placenta in normal pregnancy. Virchows Arch A, 1981;393:133–44.

51. Fok RY, Pavlova Z, Benirschke K, Paul RH, Platt LD. The correlation of arterial lesions with umbilical artery Doppler velocimetry in the placentas of small-for-dates pregnancies. Obstet Gynecol 1990;75:578-3.
52. Salafia CM, Pezzullo JC, Minior VK, Divon MY. Placental pathology of absent and reversed end-diastolic flow in growth-restricted fetuses. Obstet Gynecol 1997;90:830-6.
53. Morrow RJ, Adamson SL, Bull SB, Ritchie JW. Effect of placental embolization on the umbilical arterial velocity waveform in fetal sheep. Am J Obstet Gynecol 1989;161:1055-60.
54. Nicolaides KH, Bilardo CM, Soothill PW, Campbell S. Absence of end diastolic frequencies in umbilical artery: a sign of fetal hypoxia and acidosis. BMJ 1988;297:1026-7.
55. Nicolini U, Nicolaidis P, Fisk NM, Vaughan JI, Fusi L, Gleeson R, et al. Limited role of fetal blood sampling in prediction of outcome in intrauterine growth retardation. Lancet 1990;336:768-72.
56. Hitschold TP. Doppler flow velocity waveforms of the umbilical arteries correlate with intra-villous blood volume. Am J Obstet Gynecol 1998;179:540-3.
57. Krebs C, Macara LM, Leiser R, Bowman AW, Greer IA, Kingdom JC. Intrauterine growth restriction with absent end-diastolic flow velocity in the umbilical artery is associated with maldevelopment of the placental terminal villous tree. Am J Obstet Gynecol 1996;175:1534-42.
58. Macara L, Kingdom JC, Kaufmann P, Kohnen G, Hair J, More IA, et al. Structural analysis of placental terminal villi from growth-restricted pregnancies with abnormal umbilical artery Doppler waveforms. Placenta 1996;17:37-48.
59. Lyall F, Young A, Boswell F, Kingdom JC, Greer IA. Placental expression of vascular endothelial growth factor in placentae from pregnancies complicated by pre-eclampsia and intrauterine growth restriction does not support placental hypoxia at delivery. Placenta 1997;18:269-76.
60. Pardi G, Cetin I, Marconi AM, Bozzetti P, Buscagli M, Makowski EL et al. Venous drainage of the human uterus: respiratory gas studies in normal and fetal growth-retarded pregnancies. Am J Obstet Gynecol 1992;166:699-706.
61. Bower S, Bewley S, Campbell S. Improved prediction of preeclampsia by two-stage screening of uterine arteries using the early diastolic notch and color Doppler imaging. Obstet Gynecol 1993;82:78-83.
62. Ochi H, Matsubara K, Kusanagi Y, Taniguchi H, Ito M. Significance of a diastolic notch in the uterine artery flow velocity waveform induced by uterine embolisation in the pregnant ewe. Br J Obstet Gynaecol 1998;105:1118-21.
63. Jackson MR, Mayhew TM, Haas JD. On the factors which contribute to thinning of the villous membrane in human placentae at high altitude. I. Thinning and regional variation in thickness of trophoblast. Placenta 1988;9:1-8.
64. Kingdom J. Adriana and Luisa Castellucci Award Lecture 1997. Placental pathology in obstetrics: adaptation or failure of the villous tree? Placenta 1998;19:347-51.
65. Geary M, Kingdom J, Persaud M, Wilshin J, Hindmarsh P, Rodeck C. Incidence of uterine notching in the third trimester and association with obstetric outcome. J Obstet Gynaecol 1998;18 Suppl 1:S58.
66. Fox H. The villous cytotrophoblast as an index of placental ischaemia. J Obstet Gynaecol Br Commonwlth 1964;71:885-93.
67. Fox H. Effect of hypoxia on trophoblast in organ culture. A morphologic and autoradiographic study. Am J Obstet Gynecol 1970;107:1058-64.
68. Olofsson P, Saldeen P, Marsal K. Association between a low umbilical artery pulsatility index and fetal distress in very prolonged pregnancies. Eur J Obstet Gynecol Reprod Biol 1997;73:23-9.
69. Hitschold T, Muentefering H, Ulrich S, Berle P. Does extremely low fetoplacental impedance as estimated by umbilical artery Doppler velocimetry also indicate fetuses at risk? Ultrasound Obstet Gynecol 1996;8:S39.

8   Growth Factor Regulators of Placental Angiogenesis

Caroline Dunk and Asif Ahmed

Introduction

The human placenta is a highly vascularised organ that mediates gas and nutrient exchange between the maternal and fetal circulations. In this chapter we discuss the processes of vasculogenesis, angiogenesis and the factors influencing them in the formation of the placental vasculature. Also described are the effects of growth factors on the specialised structures of the mature intermediate and terminal villi, which are the main site of gas exchange. We have identified VEGF to be a key agent in early placental angiogenesis, acting in concert with a related factor, placenta growth factor (PlGF) via two high affinity receptors VEGFR-1 and VEGFR-2 to stimulate endothelial cell proliferation and vessel formation. A second class of receptor tyrosine kinases includes the Tie-2 receptor. Its newly identified ligands angiopoietin-1 and a natural antagonist angiopoietin-2 are thought to play a role in vessel maturation, acting downstream to VEGF.

This chapter describes the localisation of these proteins in the placenta throughout gestation, and discusses some of their in vitro effects on trophoblast and endothelium. The role of the local oxygen environment during gestation and its effect on the expression of VEGF and PlGF, perturbations of which are thought to contribute to IUGR, are also considered. Babies born SGA are at high risk of cardiovascular disease in adult life. A better molecular understanding of the factors regulating placental angiogenesis may lead to novel therapeutic intervention that leads to healthier babies.

Vasculogenesis

Vascularisation of the placental villi starts at day 21 postconception [1]. It is the result of local de novo formation of capillaries rather than protrusion of embryonic vessels into the placenta. The villous trees at this stage are made up of solid trophoblastic or primary villi, and secondary villi, which are characterised by a outer trophoblastic surface surrounding a loose mesenchyme derived from the extraembryonic coelomic cavity in the centre of the embryonic sac. Prior to the formation of the first vessels, mesenchyme-derived macrophages (Höfbauer cells) [1] appear in the mesenchyme of the secondary villi. The early appearance of these macrophages and the observation that they express angiogenic growth factors suggest a paracrine role in the initiation of vasculogenesis [1,2]. The maternal decidua and maternal macrophages also express angiogenic growth factors and it has been suggested that a paracrine mechanism mediating trophoblast invasion also exists. Current information on the production, secretion and action of angiogenic factors in early placental development is of a preliminary nature and will be discussed later in this chapter.

Immunohistochemistry and ultrastructural studies in early fetal villi have demonstrated the existence of the precursors of fetal endothelium, the mesenchymally derived haemangioblastic cell cords. These cells form long string-like aggregates and are densely packed; the intercellular spaces are bridged by spot-like junctions resembling desmosomes, or by band-like junctions resembling tight junctions [1]. The endothelial clusters begin to form into tubes as early as day 21 postconception. Here the development of fetoplacental capillary lumens differ from that observed in any other organs where lumens are formed by fusion of intracellular vacuoles. In contrast, fetoplacental lumina always seem to form by acquisition of a junctionally defined extracellular compartment within the haemangioblastic cell cords through focal enlargement of centrally located clefts that later fuse to become larger lumina (guinea pig: [3]; rhesus monkey: [4]; human: [1]. No observation of basal lamina material has been reported at this stage of development of the vasculature.

Branching Angiogenesis

From day 21 of development until the end of the first trimester the villous vasculature increases in number rather than type of vessels. The number of fetal red blood cell-containing capillaries increases, and sprouting and branching angiogenesis from the existing capillaries give rise to a primative capillary network surrounded by an incomplete layer of pericytes [5].

Basal lamina begins to form around the placental capillaries from the 6th week postconception. These mechanisms result in a web-like arrangement of the capillaries within the stroma of smaller (mesenchymal) villi, while in larger villi (immature intermediate) most of the capillaries are located superficially beneath the trophoblast covering the villous surface [6]. In these larger villi a few centrally located endothelial tubes (early villous arteries and veins) have larger diameter (> 100 μm) and become surrounded by cells expressing alpha, gamma smooth muscle actins, vimentin and desmin [7]. In larger villi from the 15th week onwards the adventitia of these central vessels fuse, forming a fibrosed stromal core in the centre of the villus, and the contractile cells concentrate around the lumina acquiring the full spectrum of cytoskeletal antigens including smooth muscle action in addition to those listed above [7,8] forming a stem villus (see Ch. 7).

Non-branching Angiogenesis

From 26 weeks' gestation until term the villous vascular growth undergoes a change from branching to non-branching angiogenesis owing to the formation of the mature intermediate villi that specialise in gas exchange. These form at the tips of the villous trees and are long (> 100 μm) and slender (80–120 μm diameter) containing one or two long, poorly branched capillary loops. These arise as a result of a decease in trophoblast proliferation and an increase in endothelial proliferation along the entire length of the capillary giving a final capillary loop exceeding 4000 μm in length [9]. As these capillaries grow in excess of the villi they coil and bulge through the trophoblastic surface forming the terminal villi.

Angiogenic Growth Factors and their Receptors

The human placenta is a rich source of angiogenic growth factors. To date studies have reported the expression and localisation of acidic and basic FGF [10,11,12], VEGF [2,13–17], the related PlGF [16–18] and hepatocyte growth factor (HGF) [19–21]. In addition, several receptors have been localised within human placental tissues, including VEGFR-1 (flt-1) and VEGFR-2 (flk-1/KDR) [12,14,16,22] and the HGF receptor, c-met [21].

VEGF, PlGF, flt-1 and KDR

Many studies have identified VEGF as a key angiogenic factor in both physiological and pathological conditions. Originally identified as a potent permeability factor (VPF) [23,24], it is now known that VEGF exists in five isoforms, generated by alternate splicing of the mRNA, to give proteins of 121, 145, 165, 189 and 206 amino acids in length (for review see [25]). VEGF exerts its effect by binding with high affinity to two tyrosine kinase receptors VEGFR-1/flt-1 [26] and VEGFR-2/KDR [27] that are present on endothelial cells [28]. Recent studies in mouse embryos have given some understanding of the early development events mediated by VEGF. Deletion of the VEGF allelles results in abnormal blood vessel development and mid-gestational death [29], while null mutation of KDR in results in defects in differentiation of haemangioblasts to form angioblastic and haematopoetic cell lineages [30]. After differentiation KDR is downregulated in haematopoetic but not in endothelial cells [30], which is indicative of an early role for VEGF via KDR in differentiation of stem cells of Fetoplacental capillaries. VEGF's other receptor VEGFR-1/flt-1 appears to have a later role, as mouse embryos lacking flt-1 develop angioblasts but blood vessel assembly and tube formation is impaired [31].

In the human placenta, VEGF expression has been analysed by in situ hybridisation and immunohistochemical studies and has been demonstrated to be localised to the villous trophoblast and macrophages of both fetal and maternal origin [2, 13, 17] (Fig. 8.1). A more recent addition to the VEGF family, PlGF, was originally isolated from a placental cDNA library. PlGF shares 53 per cent homology with VEGF [32] and is expressed both in villous syncytiotrophoblast [16,17] and in the media of larger stem vessels [18] in the human placenta (Fig. 8.2). It has also been demonstrated that trophoblast secretes VEGF in vitro in cell culture [16, 33]. As VEGF is known to act in a paracrine manner on endothelial cells, it seems likely that in the placenta the macrophage and trophoblast cells play a role in the initiation of placental vasculogenesis. However, further data on the expression of both ligands and their receptors in early placental development is needed.

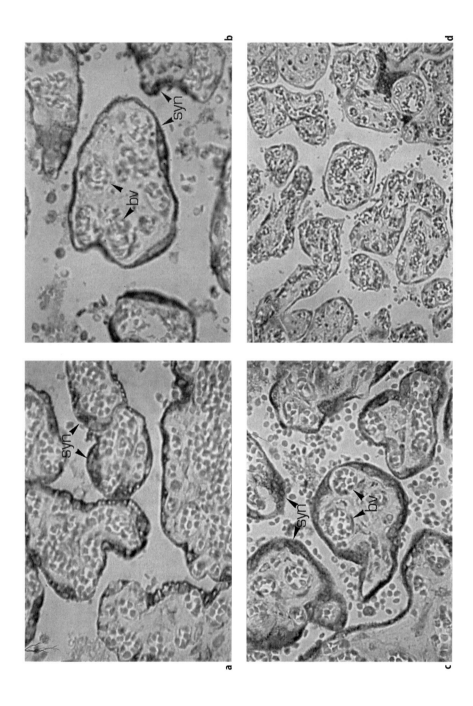

Fig. 8.1 VEGF immunostaining in paraffin sections of: **(a)** normal, **(b)** PE and **(c)** IUGR placentas. **a** Intense to very intense immunostaining for VEGF is demonstrated in the vasculosyncytial membrane (syn), whereas vascular capillary endothelial cells and Höfbauer cells within placental villi are negative (bv = blood vessel). **b, c** There is no change in immunostaining intensity or distribution for VEGF in PE or IUGR sections. **d** Control sections incubated without the primary antibody to VEGF showed no immunostaining.

◄───

The two tyrosine kinase receptors, VEGFR-1/flt-1 and VEGFR-2/KDR, were originally thought to be endothelial cell specific. However, in the placenta both endothelial and non-endothelial cells express the VEGF receptors. Both flt-1 and KDR are expressed by human placental villous endothelium [12,22,34], and flt-1 mRNA has also been demonstrated to be highly expressed in the cytotrophoblast shell and columns [35] while the protein localises to the trophoblast bilayer and EVT [2] (Fig. 8.3). These data, together with the observation that maternal macrophage and decidual cells express VEGF whilst the EVT express flt-1, have led to the hypothesis that VEGF acts as a chemoattractant stimulating trophoblast invasion. This view has been further supported by the observation that flt-1 immunoreactivity decreases at 24 weeks of gestation when the migration of trophoblast is complete [2]. However, recent functional studies have reported that EVT in culture do not migrate or invade in response to VEGF [36]. These results are questionable as VEGF was used as a direct trophoblast agonist in the upper well of the migration chamber and not as a chemoattractant in the lower well. Monocyte chemotaxis and migration have been demonstrated to be mediated through activation of flt-1 by both VEGF and PlGF [37]. Therefore, further research is required to determine whether VEGF is a true chemotactic agent for trophoblast. To date the localisation of KDR within human placenta has been reported to be restricted to the fetoplacental endothelial cells [38]. However, in mid-gestational mice the homologous receptor flk-1 is strongly expressed by trophoblast [28] and RT-PCR has demonstrated the presence of KDR both in human choriocarcinoma cell line, BeWo [35] and in the non-transformed first trimester trophoblast cell line [14]. We have also demonstrated an increase in tyrosine phosphorylated KDR in trophoblast cultured under hypoxic conditions [33]. To date, many studies have focused on VEGF's action on endothelial cells and VEGF has been demonstrated to be a potent stimulator of endothelial cell proliferation [39–42], migration [43] and production of the plasminogen activators required for proteolytic degradation of the ECM, both in vitro and in vivo [44]; all are markers of angiogenic activity. In contrast, PlGF has been demonstrated to be a very weak stimulator of endothelial cell chemotaxis and proliferation [45] at physiological (< 100 ng/ml) concentrations [46] VEGF also induces microvascular permeability in the Miles assay [23,47] while PlGF has no effect alone but potentiates the action of low doses of VEGF [48]. These different effects may be explained by the fact that PlGF binds flt-1 but not KDR [48]. In vitro studies on the chorioallantoic membranes of the chicken have demonstrated that VEGF binding to both flt-1 and KDR mediates branching angiogenesis while PlGF binding to flt-1 alone results in non-branching angiogenesis [49,50]. In the human placenta VEGF, PlGF and the two receptors are differentially expressed throughout gestation; VEGF and KDR are most intense during early gestation and decline as pregnancy advances [35,51,52], whereas PlGF and flt-1 increase towards term [12,22]. Correlation of these growth factor effects and their expres-

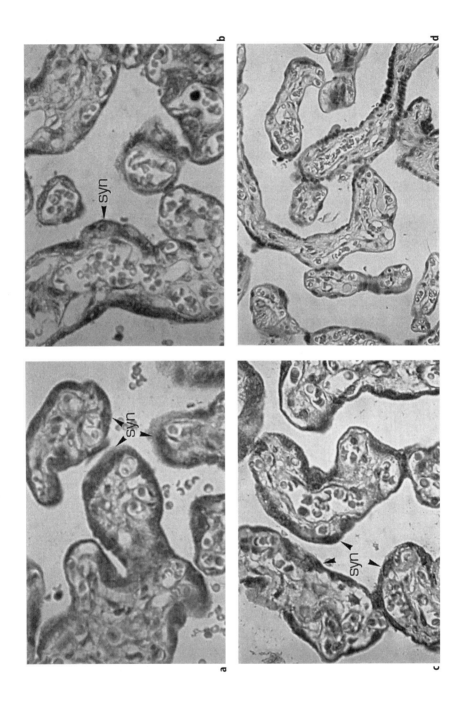

Fig. 8.2 PlGF immunostaining in paraffin sections of: **(a)** normal, **(b)** PE and **(c)** IUGR placentas. **a** Moderate to intense immunostaining for PlGF is demonstrated in the vasculosyncytial membrane (syn) whilst weak/no immunostaining for PlGF was demonstrated in vascular capillary endothelial cells and Höfbauer cells within placental villi. **b, c** There is no change in immunostaining intensity or distribution for PlGF in PE or IUGR sections. **d** Control sections incubated without the primary antibody to PlGF showed no immunostaining.

sion patterns throughout gestation with the development of the villous angioarchitecture [9,53] suggests that VEGF and KDR are involved in the first two trimesters of pregnancy in the establishment of the richly branched capillary beds of the mesenchymal and immature intermediate villi, whereas PlGF and flt-1 are more likely to be involved in the formation of the long poorly branched terminal capillary loops in the last trimester (see Fig. 8.7).

More recently VEGF has been implicated to act as an endothelial survival factor by promoting scaffold formation and cell attachment in microvascular endothelial cells [54]. As VEGF declines throughout gestation these data suggest a possible mechanism for the regression of the capillary nets during stem villus formation.

Many of VEGF's observed actions have been attributed to be almost exclusively mediated by activation of the KDR receptor [25]; transfection of porcine aortic endothelial cells with either KDR or flt-1 demonstrated that, though both receptors undergo phosphorylation, only KDR-transfected cells displayed migratory and proliferative responses in response to VEGF [55]. The colocalisation of VEGF, PlGF, KDR and flt-1 in the trophoblast, together with the fact that the outer syncytiotrophoblastic surface of the placental villi is in direct contact with maternal blood, must imply that trophoblast cells have some endothelial functions. It also suggests an autocrine role for VEGF in trophoblast cell function in addition to its paracrine action on endothelial cells. Indeed, VEGF has been reported to stimulate BeWo [35], first trimester trophoblast [56] and EVT cell proliferation [36]. In addition to its mitogenic and chemotactic activities, VEGF also stimulates fluid and protein extravasation from blood vessels [25], and mediates calcium influx [57,58] and the release of NO in HUVEC [14,59]. We have recently demonstrated that a first trimester trophoblast cell line (ED27) expresses VEGF, KDR and flt-1 and that stimulation of a trophoblast cell line with 10 ng/ml exogenous VEGF resulted in release of NO through phosphorylation of flt-1 (Fig. 8.4) [14]. As NO is a potent vasodilator and prevents platelet aggregation, we have proposed that trophoblast-derived NO may regulate the haemodynamics of the maternal fetal interface and aid dilation of the maternal arteries that supply the intervillous space. This view is in agreement with data obtained in the guinea pig placenta where dilation of uteroplacental arteries is initiated by trophoplast-derived NO [60]. We have also demonstrated that flt-1 and NO are capable of suppressing trophoblast and endothelial cell DNA synthesis [14]. It has also been demonstrated that NO can inhibit vascular smooth muscle cells (VSMC) [61] and endothelial [62] cell proliferation. These data have led us to hypothesise that flt-1 functions as a growth regulatory receptor counteracting the proliferative actions of KDR through NO release in both trophoblast and endothelial cells [14]. In addition, it has recently been demonstrated that NO dephosphorylates the transcription factor AP-1 in cardiac endothelium via a protein kinase C (PKC)-dependent mechanism, preventing its action on the VEGF promoter, resulting in a

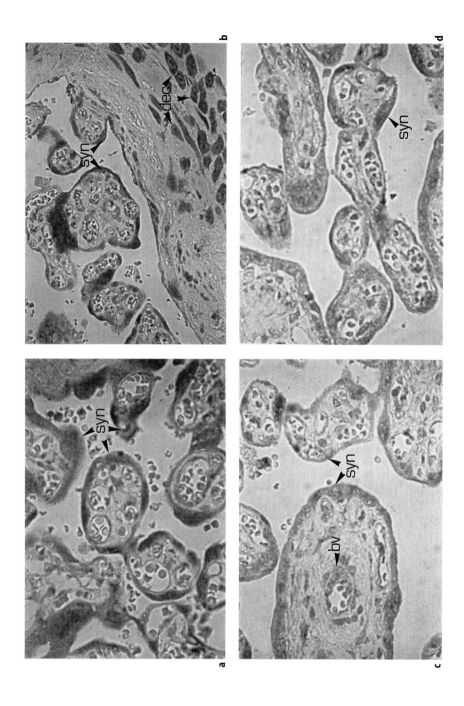

Fig. 8.3 Immunostaining of flt-1 in paraffin sections of: **(a)** normal, **(b)** PE and **(c)** IUGR placentas. **a** Moderate to weak immunostaining for flt-1 is demonstrated in the vasculosyncytial membrane (syn), vascular capillary endothelial cells and Höfbauer cells of placental villi. **b** Intense immunostaining is demonstrated in the material decidual cells (dec). **c, d** There is no change in immunostaining intensity or distribution for flt-1 in PE or IUGR sections. Control sections incubated without the primary antibody to PIGF showed no immunostaining (results not shown).

◀───

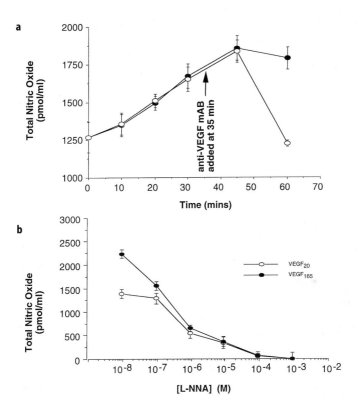

Fig. 8.4 VEGF stimulates NO release from trophoblast through flt-1. **(a)** Time-dependent NO release in response to 10 ng/ml $VEGF_{165}$ (solid circle) or in the presence of 50 ng/ml anti-VEGF-neutralising monoclonal antibody (anti-VEGF mAb) added after 35 min of stimulation with 10 ng/ml $VEGF_{165}$ (open circle). **b** Effect of inhibition of NO synthesis by N^G-monomethyl-L-arginine (L-NNA) on $VEGF_{165}$ (solid circle) and $VEGF_{20}$ (open circle) induced NO release. D-NNA has no inhibitory effect of VEGF-induced nitric oxide release (data not shown). **c** Inhibition of $VEGF_{165}$ stimulated NO release by 30 ng/ml of a polyclonal anti-flt-1 antibody. 10 ng/ml $VEGF_{165}$ alone (solid column) stimulates NO release above basal value (open column), which is inhibited by preincubation with 30 ng/ml anti-flt-1 antibody (hatched column). The anti-flt-1 antibody is displaced by increasing concentrations of $VEGF_{165}$. Cells were stimulated for maximum period of 30 min (or as indicated) with the agonist in the presence or in the absence of the above agents. The reaction was terminated by the removal of supernatant, which was immediately stored at –80 °C for NO analysis using a Sievers NOA chemiluminesence analyser. All results shown have been corrected for background levels of NO present in the media (data are expressed in picomoles of NO per ml; the results are expressed as mean ± $s_{\bar{x}}$ of a typical experiment (quadruplicate determinations per experiment of three similar experiments)).

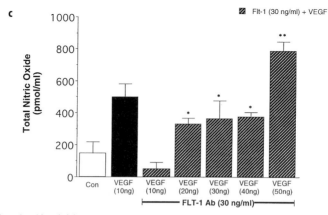

Reproduced from Lab Invest. 76;6, 779-79: Ahmed et al 1997

Fig. 8.4 (*continued*)

downregulation of VEGF mRNA [63]. Thus, this supports a negative regulatory role for NO.

Angiopoietins and Tie-2

A second class of receptor tyrosine kinases, in addition to receptors for VEGF, termed Tie receptors (Tie-1 and Tie-2) were found to be critically involved in the formation and maturation of vessels [64–66]. Mice deficient in Tie-1 die between embryonic day 13.5 (E13.5) and birth, and display oedema and haemorrhage resulting from poor structural integrity of the endothelial cells [65,66]. In contrast, mice deficient in Tie-2 have an earlier lethal phenotype and die by E10.5 [64,66]. Recent identification of ligands for the tie-2 receptor, termed angiopoietins, provide new opportunities to study the role of Tie-2 receptor in placental angiogenesis. We have demonstrated the expression of mRNA for angiopoietin-1 and Tie-2 in the human placenta. In first trimester tissues angiopoietin-1 localises to the syncytiotrophoblast/cytotrophoblast bilayer (Fig. 8.5). The expression decreases at term and is restricted to the surrounding media of the primary blood vessels (data not shown). The Tie-2 receptor is expressed in he trophoblast layer of first trimester tissues and again becomes expressed throughout the stroma and perivascular tissues of term placental villi (Fig. 8.6). Our preliminary data demonstrate expression of these novel factors in both trophoblast and endothelium. To date, the functional role of angiopoietin in placental development is largely unknown. Angiopoietin-1-deficient mice have a phenotype similar to Tie-2 –/– mice [67], and addition of angiopoietin-1 alone to endothelial cell culture does not stimulate in vitro responses, such as proliferation or tube formation [68], previously observed with VEGF. It is thought that the angiopoetins act downstream of VEGF, mediating vessel maturation and recruitment of pericytes to the vessel walls, and as such may be of particular interest in the placenta during the formation of the paravascular capillary net throughout the second trimester.

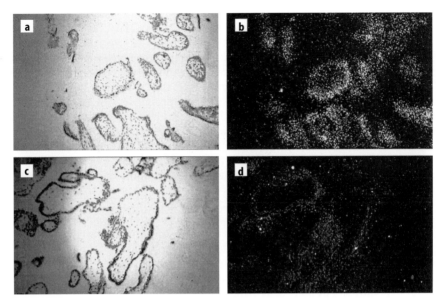

Fig. 8.5 Localization of angiopoeitin-1 mRNA in early placental villi. Photomicrograph shows hybridisation signal in early placental villi (9 weeks); intense hybridisation signal with [35S]-labelled riboprobe was localised in the syncytiotrophoblast and cytotrophoblast of the villi in: **a** brightfield and **b** darkfield optics. The specificity of the signal was confirmed by incubating a serial section with [35S]-labelled sense strand **c** and **d** (objective × 40).

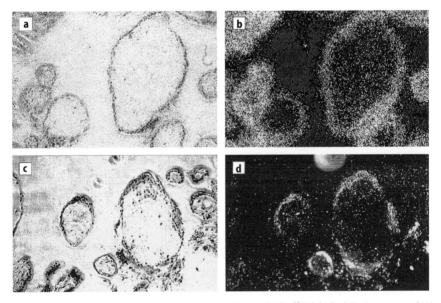

Fig. 8.6 Localisation of Tie-2 receptor mRNA in early placental villi: [35S]-labelled Tie-2 receptor cRNA probes were used for hybridisation of sections from first trimester (10 weeks' gestation) placentas. The photomicrograph shows hybridisation signal in the syncytiotrophoblast and cytotrophoblast bilayer of first trimester villi (10 weeks' gestation) under: **a** brightfield and **b** darkfield optics. The specificity of the signal was confirmed by incubating a serial section with [35S]-labelled sense strand (**c** and **d**) (objective × 40).

Effects of Oxygen on Placental Development

One other factor that should be considered during the development of the placental vasculature is the effect of the local oxygen environment during gestation. Oxygen is thought to be a major regulator of the balance between VEGF and PlGF function; hypoxia has been demonstrated to upregulate VEGF expression in tumours [69–73] and VSMC [74]; the VEGF receptor mRNA is also upregulated by hypoxia in lung tissue [75]. In placental and related chorioallantoic tissues VEGF is also upregulated by hypoxia [15,16,49,50] and downregulated by hyperoxia, while PlGF is downregulated by hypoxia but upregulated by hyperoxia [16]. Hypoxia also promotes trophoblast proliferation and limits invasion. After about the first 12 weeks of gestation the intervillous space switches from a relatively hypoxic to an enhanced oxygen environment and thus may contribute to a switch to the invasive EVT responsible for the second wave of invasion. In addition, intraplacental oxygen partial pressures have been demonstrated to increase throughout pregnancy [76], which suggests a possible mechanism for the switch from dominating VEGF effects in early pregnancy to PlGF effects in the last trimester of placental vascular development (Fig. 8.7).

Until recently the pathological complications of pregnancy, pre-eclampsia and IUGR were thought to arise simply as a result of inadequate vascular transformation of the maternal blood vessels leading to a fall in the rate of delivery of oxygenated blood to the fetus, or uteroplacental insufficiency. However, detailed ultrastructural studies in a cohort of pathological placentas complicated by absent umbilical end-diastolic flow have described three distinct types of hypoxia that may occur in the fetoplacental unit and influence fetoplacental angiogenesis [77].

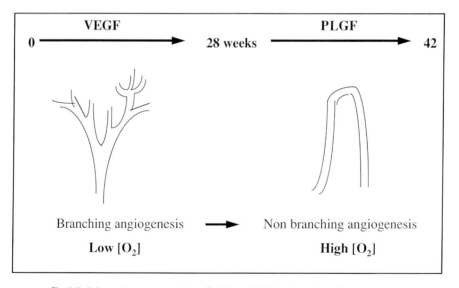

Fig. 8.7 Schematic representation of VEGF and PlGF actions throughout gestation.

Preplacental Hypoxia

The mother, the placenta and the fetus are hypoxic, as in pregnancy at high altitude, maternal anaemia and cyanotic maternal cardiac diseases. In this condition the peripheral placental villi show increased branching angiogenesis with formation of richly branched but shorter terminal capillary loops [78].

Uteroplacental Hypoxia

Maternal oxygenation is normal but, owing to impaired uteroplacental circulation, the placenta and fetus are hypoxic, as in pre-eclampsia with preserved end-diastolic flow. In this situation the peripheral placental villi similarly show formation of richly branching nets, and fetal blood flow is largely normal [79,80].

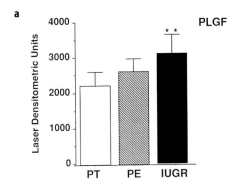

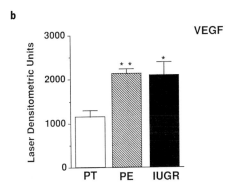

Fig. 8.8 Semiquantitative Western blot analysis of the expression of PlGF and VEGF in abnormal placenta. Immunoblot analysis of PlGF and VEGF in protein extracts from placentas. Major bands for PlGF (50 kD) and VEGF (46 kD) were detected in protein extracts from all placentas. Data are presented as laser densitometric (LD) units from Western blots of placental protein from preterm deliveries (PT, $n = 4$), pre-eclampsia (PE, $n = 6$) and IUGR (IUGR, $n = 7$). **a** Laser densitometric analysis of PlGF protein demonstrates a significant increase in IUGR placentas as compared with preterm placentas. **b** Laser densitometric analysis of VEGF protein demonstrates a significant increase in both pre-eclampsia and IUGR compared with preterm placentas. Statistical analysis on the intensity of bands was performed using Student unpaired t-test (*$P < 0.05$, **$P < 0.01$). Reproduced from: Khaliq et al. Lab Invest 1999; 79:151–70.

Semiquantitative Western blotting analysis in placentas of this type, compared with gestationally matched normal placentas, demonstrates an increased expression of VEGF (Fig. 8.8) [81], which suggests that placental hypoxia upregulates VEGF in vivo and causes the changes in angiogenesis.

Postplacental Hypoxia

The fetus is hypoxic, whereas the mother is normaxic and the placenta, owing to reduced oxygen extraction by the fetus, may show higher PO_2 levels than normal, a situation described as "placental hyperoxia" [77,82], (for commentary see [83]). In this situation the terminal capillaries are poorly developed and capillary branching is virtually absent with the resultant increase in fetoplacental flow impedance. The risk of perinatal mortality in these circumstances is over 40 per cent and survivors of neonatal intensive care are at risk of neurodevelopmental handicap. In these cases our data show a different pattern of VEGF and PlGF expression; here PlGF is significantly increased (Fig. 8.8) [81] suggesting that early onset placental hyperoxia leads to dominating PlGF effects too early in gestation, resulting in the decrease of branching angiogenesis and failure of terminal villi formation.

Conclusions

In conclusion, these data suggest that in the development of the placental vasculature the intraplacental oxygen partial pressure, the balance between VEGF and PlGF, and the balance between branching and non-branching angiogenesis all depend on each other. To date the functional studies of angiogenic factors in placental development are preliminary and would be assisted by better in vitro and in vivo cell models of placental angiogenesis and specific placental microvascular endothelial and trophoblast cell lines. Research is going on to determine the molecular mechanisms behind the hypotheses discussed in this chapter that result in normal and abnormal placental angiogenesis.

References

1. Demir R, Kaufmann P, Castelucci M, Erbengi T, Kotowski A. Fetal vasculogenesis and angiogenesis in human placental villi. Acta Anat (Basel) 1989:136:190–203.
2. Ahmed AS, Li XF, Dunk CE, Whittle MJ, Rollason T. Colocalisation of vascular endothelial growth factor and its flt-1 receptor in human placenta. Growth Factors 1995;12:235–43.
3. Davidoff M, Scheibler TH. Uber den Feinbau der Meerscwheinchenplacenta wahrend der Entwicklung. Anat Embryol (Berlin) 1970;130:234–54.
4. King, BF. Ultrastructural differentiation of stromal and vascular components in early macaque placental villi. American Journal of Anatomy 1987;178:30–44.
5. Benirschke K, Kaufmann P. Pathology of the human placenta, 3rd ennd. New York:Springer, 1995.
6. Kadyrov M, et al. Lancet 1999; in press [to add-JK]
7. Kohnen G, Kertschanska S, Demir R, Kaufmann P. Placental villous stroma as a model system for myofibroblast differentiation. Histochemistry and Cell Biology, 1996;105,415–429.
8. Demir R, Kosanke G, Kohen G, Kertschanka S, Kaufmann P. Classification of human placental stem villi: review of structural and functional aspects. Micros Res Tech 1997;38:29–41.

9. Kaufmann P, Bruns U, Leiser R, Luckhardt M, Winterhager E. The fetal vascularisation of term human placental villi. II. Intermediate and terminal villi. Anat Embryol (Berlin) 1985;173:203–14.

10. Ferriani RA, Ahmed A, Sharkey AM, Smith SK. Colocalisation of acidic and basix fibrobast growth factor (FGF) in human placenta and the cellular effects of bFGF in trophoblast cell line JEG-3. Growth Factors 1994;10:259.

11. Shams M, Ahmed A. Localisation of mRNA for basic fibroblast growth factor in human placenta. Growth Factors 1994;11:105–11.

12. Crescimanno C, Marzioni D, Persico MG, Vuckovic M, Muhauser J, Castelucci M. Expression of bFGF, PlGF and their receptors in the human placenta. Placenta 1995;16:A13.

13. Sharkey AM, Charnock-Jones DS, Boocock CA, Brown KD, Smith SK. Expression of mRNA for vascular endothelial growth factor in human placenta. J Reprod Fertil 1993;99:609–15.

14. Ahmed AS, Dunk CE, Kniss D, Wilkes M. Role of VEGF Receptor (Flt-1) in mediating calcium dependant nitric oxide release and limiting DNA synthesis in human trophoblast cells. Lab Invest 1997;76:779–91.

15. Wheeler T, Elcock CL, Anthony FW. Angiogenesis in the placental environment. Placenta 1995;16:289–96.

16. Shore VH, et al. Vascular endothelial growth factor, placenta growth factor and their receptors in isolated human trophoblast. Placenta 1997;18:657–65.

17. Vuorela P, et al. Expression of vascular endothelial growth factor and placenta growth factor in human placenta. Biol Reprod 1997;56:489–94.

18. Khaliq A, Li XF, Shams M, Sisi P, Acevedo CA, Whittle MJ. Localisation of placenta growth factor (PlGF) in human term placenta. Growth Factors 1996;13:243.

19. Rosen EM, Meromsky L, Setter E, Vinter DW, Goldberg ID. Smooth muscle derived factor stimulates mobility of human tumour cells. Invasion Metastasis 1990;10:49–64.

20. Uehara Y, et al. Placental defect and embryonic lethality in mice lacking hepatocyte growth factor/scatter factor. Nature 1995;373:702–5.

21. Kilby MD, et al. Localisation of hepatocyte growth factor (HGF) and its receptor (c-met) protein and mRNA in human term placenta. Growth Factors 1996;13:133–9.

22. Clarke DE, Smith SK, Sharkey AM, Charnock Jones DS. Localisation of VEGF and expression of its receptors flt-1 and KDR in human placenta throughout pregnancy. Hum Reprod 1996;11:1080–98.

23. Conolly DT, et al. Human vascular permeability factor: Isolation from U937 cells. J Biol Chem 1989;264:20017–24.

24. Senger Dr, Peruzzi CA, Feder J, Dvorak HF. Tumour cells secrete a vascular permeability factor that promoted accumalation of ascites fluid. Science 1983;219:983–5.

25. Dvorak HF, Brown LF, Detmar M, Dvorak AM. Vascular permeability factor/vascular endothelial growth factor, microvascular hyperpermeability, and angiogenesis. Am J Pathol 1995;146:1029–39.

26. de Vries C, et al. The fms like tyrosine kinase: a receptor for vascular endothelial growth factor. Science 1992;255:989–91.

27. Terman BI, et al. Identification of KDR tyrosine kinase as a receptor for vascular endothelial growth factor. Biochem Biophys Res Commun 1992;187:1579–86.

28. Millauer B, et al. High affinity vascular endothelial growth factor binding and developmental expression suggest Flk-1 as a major eregulator of vasculogenesis and angiogenesis. Cell 1993;72:835–46.

29. Carmieliet P, et al. Abnormal blood vessel development and lethality in embryos lacking a single VEGF allele. Nature 1996;380:435–9.

30. Shalaby F, et al. Failure of blood island formation and vasculogenesis in flk-1 deficient mice. Nature 1995;376:62–6.

31. Fong GH, Rossant J, Gersenstein M, Breitman ML. Role of the Flt-1 receptor tyrosine kinase in regulating the assembly of vascular endothelium. Nature 1995;376:66–70.

32. Maglione D, et al. Isolation of a human placental cDNA coding for a protein related to the vascular permeability factor. Proc Natl Acad Sci USA 1988;88:9267–71.

33. Dunk CE, Khaliq A, Ahmed AS. Oxygen modulates vascular endothelial growth factor (VEGF) secretion, trophoblast proliferation and VEGF receptor activation. Vigso, Denmark: European Placenta Group 1997.

34. Vuckovic M, et al. Expression of the vascular endothelial growth factor receptor, KDR, in human placenta. J Anat 1996;188:361–6.

35. Charnock-Jones DS, et al. Vascular endothelial growth factor localisation and activation in human trophoblast and choriocarcinoma cells. Biol Reprod 1994;51:524–30.

36. Athanassiades A, Hamilton GS, Lala PK. Role of vascular endothelial growth factor (VEGF) in human extravillous trophoblast proliferation, migration and invasiveness. Placenta 1998;19: 465–73.

37. Clauss M, et al. The vascular endothelial growth factor Flt-1 mediates biological activities: Implications for a functional role of placental growth factor in monocyte activation and chemotaxis. J Biol Chem. 1996;271(30):17629–34.
38. Holt VJ, et al. Normal human trophoblast express and respond to angiogenic growth factors. Placenta 1999;in press.
39. Conolly DT, et al. Tumour vascular permeability factor stimulates endothelial cell growth and angiogenesis. J Clin Invest 1989;84:1470–8.
40. Ferrara N, Henzel WJ. Pituitary endothelial cells secrete a novel heparin binding growth factor for vasculat endothelial cells. Biochem Biophys Res Commun 1989;161:851–8.
41. Plouet J, Schilling J, Gospodarowicz D. Isolation and characterisation of a newly identified endothelial cell mitogen produced by AtT-20 cells. EMBO J 1989;8:3801–6.
42. Yamane A, et al. A new communication system between hepatocytes and sinusoidal endothelial cells in liver through vascular endothelial growth factor and Flt-1 tyrosine kinase receptor family (Flt-1 and KDR). Oncogene 1994;9:2683–90.
43. Rousseau S, Huole F, Landry J, Huot J. p38 MAP kinase activation by vascular endothelial growth factor mediates actin reorganisation and cell migration in human endothelial cells. Oncogene 1997;15:2169–77.
44. Mandriota SJ, et al. Vascular endothelial frowth factor increases urokinase receptor expression of vascular endothelial cells. J Biol Chem 1995;270(17):9709–16.
45. Hauser S, Weich HA. A heparin-binding form of placenta growth factor (PlGF-2) is expressed in human umbilical vein endothelial cells and in placenta. Growth Factors 1993;9:259–68.
46. Birkenhager R, et al. Synthesis and physiological activity of heterodimers comprising different splice forms of vascular endothelial growth factor and placenta growth factor. Biochem J 1996;3126:703–7.
47. Keck PJ, et al. Vascular permeability factor, an endothelial mitogen related to PDGF. Science 1989;246:1309–12.
48. Park JE, Chen HH, Winer J, Houck KA, Ferrara N. Placenta growth factor: potentiation of vascular endothelial growth factor bioactivity, in vitro and in vivo, and high affinity binding to Flt-1 but not to Flk-1/KDR. J Biol Chem 1994;269:25646–54.
49. Wilting J, et al. Vascular endothelial growth factor (VEGF) and placenta growth factor (PlGF): homologous factors specifically affecting endothelial ells. Ann Anat 1995;178:331A.
50. Wilting J, et al. VEGF(121) induces proliferation of vascular endothelial cells and expression of Flk-1 without affecting lymphatic vessels of the chorioallantoic membrane. Dev Biol 1996;176:76–85.
51. Jackson MR, Carney EW, Lye SJ, Ritchie JW. Localisation of two angiogenic growth factors (PDECGF and VEGF) in human placentae throughout gestation. Placenta 1994;15:341–53.
52. Shiraishi S, Nakagawa K, Kinukawa N, Nakano H, Sueishi K. Immunohistochemical localisation of vascular endothelial growth factor in the human placenta. Placenta 1996;17:111–21.
53. Leiser R, Luckhardt M, Kaufmann P, Winterhager E, Bruns U. The fetal vascularisation of term human placental villi. I. Peripheral stem villi. Ana Embryol (Berlin) 1985;173:71–80.
54. Watanabe Y, Dvorak HF. Vascular permeability factor/vascular endothelial growth factor inhibits anchorage dependent apopotosis in microvessel endothelial cells by inducing scaffold formation. Exp Cell Res 1997;233:340–9.
55. Waltenberger J, et al. Different signal transduction properties of KDR and Flt-1, two receptors for vascular endothelial growth factor. J Biol Chem 1994;269:26988–95.
56. Dunk C, Ahmed A. Expression of VEGF-C and activation of its receptors VEGR-2 and VEGFR-3 in placenta: decreased expression in IUGR. Lab Invest 1999;in press.
57. Brock TA, Dvorak HF, Senger DR. Tumour secreted vascular permeability factor increases cytosolic Ca2+ and von Willebrand factor in human endothelial cells. Am J Pathol 1991;138:213–21.
58. Seymour LW, et al. Vascular endothelial growth factor stimulates protein kinase C dependant pospholipase D activity in endothelial cells. Lab Invest 1996;75:427–37.
59. van der Zee R, et al. Vascular endothelial growth factor (VEGF)/vascular permeability factor (VPF) augments nitric oxide release from quiescent rabbit and human vascular endothelium. Circulation 1997;95:1030–7.
60. Nanaev A, Chwalisz K, Frank H, Kohnen G, Hegele-Hartung C, and Kaufmann P. Physiological dilation of uteroplacental arteries in the guinea pig depends on nitric oxide synthase activity of extra villous trophoblast. Cell Tissue Res 1995;282:407–21.
61. Garg UC, Hassid A. Nitric oxide generating vasodilators and 8-bromo-cyclic guanosine monophosphate inhibit mitogenesis and proliferation of cultured rat vascular smooth muscle cells. J Clin Invest 1989;83:1774–7.

62. Gooch KJ, Dangler CA, Frangos JA. Exogenous, basal, and flow induced nitric oxide production and endothelial cell proliferation. J Cell Physiol 1997;171:252–8.
63. Tsurumi Y, et al. Reciprocal regulation between VEGF and NO in the regulation of endothelial integrity. Nat Med 1997;3(8):879–86.
64. Dumont DJ, et al. Dominant-negative and targeted null mutations in the endothelial receptor tyrosine kinase, tek, reveal and critical role in vasculogenesis of the embryo. Genes Dev 1994;8:1897–909.
65. Puri MC, Rossant J, Alitalo K, Bernstein A, Partanen J. The receptor tyrosine kinase TIE is required for integrity and survival of vascular endothelial cells. EMBO J 1995;14:5884–91.
66. Sato TN, et al. Distinct roles of the receptor tyrosine kinases Tie-1 and Tie-2 in blood vessel formation. Nature 1995;376:70–4.
67. Suri C, et al. Requisite role of angiopoietin-1, a ligand for the Tie-2 receptor, during embryonic angiogenesis. Cell 1996;87:1171–80.
68. Davis S, et al. Isolation of angiopoietin-1, a ligand for the TIE2 receptor, by secretion-trap expression cloning. Cell 1996;87:1161–69.
69. Schweiki D, Itin A, Neufeld G, Gitay-Goren H, Keshet E. Vascular endothelial growth factor induced by hypoxia may mediate hypoxia initiated angiogenesis. Nature 1992;359:843–5.
70. Plate KH, Brier G, Weich HA, Risau W. Vascular endothelial growth factor is a potential tumour angiogenesis factor in human gliomas in vivo. Nature 1992;359:845–8.
71. Brown LF, et al. Increased expression of vascular permeability factor (vascular endothelial growth factor) and receptors in kidney and bladder carcinomas. Cancer Res. 1993;59:4727–35.
72. Brown LF, et al. Increased expression of vascular permeability factor (vascular endothelial growth factor) and receptors in adenocarcinomas and gastrointestinal carcinomas. Am J Pathol 1993;143:1255–62.
73. Takaihashi Y, et al. Markedly increased amounts of mRNA for vascular endothelial growth factor and placenta growth factor in renal cell carcinomas associated with angiogenesis. Oncogene 1994;9:273–9.
74. Stavri G, Zachary I, Baskerville P, Martin J, Erusalimsky J. Basic fibroblast growth factor up-regulates the expression of vascular endothelial growth factor in vascular smooth muscle cells. Synergistic interaction with hypoxia. Circulation 1995;92:5–8.
75. Tuder RM, Flook BE, Voelkel NF. Increased gene expression for VEGF and the VEGF receptors KDR/Flk-1 and Flt-1 in lungs exposed to chronic hypoxia: modulation of gene expression by nitric oxide. J Clin Invest 1995;95:1798–1807.
76. Rodesch F, Simon P, Donna C, Jauniaux E. Oxygen measurements in endometrial and trophoblastic tissues during early pregnancy. Obstet Gynecol 1992;80:283–5.
77. Kingdom JCP, Kaufmann P. Oxygen and placental villous development: origins of fetal hypoxia. Placenta 1997;18:613–21.
78. Krebs C, Longo LD, Leiser D. Term ovine placental vasculature: comparison of sea level and high altitude conditions by corrosion cast and histomorphometry. Placenta 1997;18:43–51.
79. Kiserud T, Hellevik LR, Eik-Nes SH, Angelsen BA, Blaas HG. Estimation of the pressure gradient across the fetal ductus venosus based on Doplar velocimetry. Ultrasound Med Biol 1994;20:225–32.
80. Hitschold T, Mutefering H, Ulrich S, Berle P. Does extremely low fetoplacental impedance is estimated by umbilical artery Doppler velocimetry also indicate fetuses at risk? Ultrasound Gynecol 1996;8:39A.
81. Khaliq A, Dunk C, Jiang J. et al. Hypoxia downregulates placenta growth factor, whereas fetal growth restriction unregulates placenta growth factor expression. Molecular evidence for placental hyperoxia in intrauterine growth restriction. Lab Invest 1999; 79:151–70.
82. Macara LM, et al. Structural analysis of placental terminal villi from growth-restricted pregnancies with abnormal umbilical artery Doppler waveforms. Placenta 1996;17:37–48.
83. Ahmed A, Kilby M. Hypoxia or hyperoxia in placental insufficiency. Lancet 1997;350:70–1.

9 Placental Transfer and Intrauterine Growth Restriction

Paul Ayuk, John Hughes and Colin Sibley

Introduction

During intrauterine life, the placenta undertakes some of the functions performed postnatally by the lungs, gut and kidneys – the absorption and transfer of oxygen and nutrients to the fetus, and the elimination of carbon dioxide and other metabolic wastes. These functions are self-evidently vital to normal intrauterine development. In postnatal life, disease processes that impair the absorptive and transport functions of the gut and lungs, or the ability of the kidneys to eliminate metabolic wastes, are important causes of failure to attain the genetic growth potential (failure to thrive). The hypothesis that a failure to attain the genetic growth potential in utero is associated with an impairment of the transport functions of the placenta is therefore a logical extension. This hypothesis is strengthened by the observations that the growth-restricted fetus is at increased risk of hypoxia [1,2], hypercapnia [1], acidaemia [1], hypoglycaemia [1–23] and hypoaminoacidaemia [1,3,4].

The maternofetal exchange of nutrients and the waste products of fetal metabolism is dependent on: (1) the delivery of maternal and fetal blood to the placenta by adequate uteroplacental and fetoplacental circulations respectively, (2) the maternal and fetal plasma concentrations, and (3) the permeability and transport characteristics of the placental exchange barrier itself. Defects in any of these processes may impair net transfer in either maternofetal or fetomaternal directions with consequent effects on fetal growth. Solute metabolism by the placenta will also influence net transfer. Here, we outline the basic mechanisms of placental transfer and examine the evidence for specific defects in placental transport mechanisms in IUGR. We will focus on the solutes for which there is evidence of perturbations in the plasma concentrations of the IUGR fetus (i.e. oxygen, carbon dioxide, proton, glucose and amino acids).

The SGA infant is distinct from the growth-restricted infant [5]. The clinical literature of fetal growth tends to conflate these related concepts [6]. The definition of growth restriction differs widely among research groups and includes faltering growth both antenatally, as defined by failure to develop along ultrasound biometry percentiles [7], and postnatally, as defined by neonatal biometry [8]. To these definitions may be added antenatal abnormal umbilical vessel Doppler studies or reduced liquor volume assessed by ultrasound.

Studies examining the relationship between fetal plasma solute concentrations, placental solute transfer and fetal growth have traditionally studied "appropriate for gestational age – AGA" fetuses (usually defined as birthweight between the 10th and 90th percentiles for gestation age)[9] and "SGA" fetuses (variously defined as birthweight below the 3rd [9] or 10th [10] percentile for gestational age). More recently, however, the recognition of the value of ultrasound in the assessment of fetal well-being, in particular the use of the biophysical profile and Doppler ultrasonographic assessment of both fetal and the fetoplacental circulations [11,12], has led to more stringent subgrouping of infants in studies of placental transfer in IUGR/SGA. We will refer to studies that have used additional methods beyond birthweight alone to identify affected fetuses. We will highlight the differences in data that result from this more selective approach.

Basic Concepts of Placental Transfer

Anatomical and Morphological Considerations

The human placenta is classified as villous, and haemomonochorial [13]. The umbilical arteries and vein ramify after entering the chorionic plate at the insertion of the umbilical cord. These vessels remain paired and pierce the chorionic plate to form the blood supply to stem villi. The main stem villus forms the core of the cotyledon. These villi divide and ramify toward the basal plate of the placenta. The distal branches form either anchoring villi, which fix the placenta to the maternal decidua, or form freely suspended branches: the terminal villi. The terminal villi are the predominant villus type in the second half of gestation [14]. They are therefore considered to be the functional units of the placenta across which the majority of transfer takes place. In the terminal villi there are only two complete cell layers separating maternal and fetal blood: the syncytiotrophoblast and the fetal capillary endothelium (Fig. 9.1). The latter is a typical continuous capillary endothelium with relatively wide spaces separating the cells, through which solutes up to the size of albumen can diffuse [15]. The syncytiotrophoblast, on the other hand, forms a true syncytium, unique in the human body, and is the transporting epithelium of the placenta. Maternal blood directly bathes the maternal-facing plasma membrane of the syncytiotrophoblast. This membrane is covered with microvilli that significantly increase its surface area and give rise to the term "microvillous plasma membrane". The basal, fetal-facing, plasma membrane of the syncytiotrophoblast is apposed to the trophoblast basement membrane and villus core (Fig. 9.1).

Mechanisms of Solute Transfer across the Syncytiotrophoblast

In general terms there are three mechanisms by which solutes may be transferred across the syncytiotrophoblast: diffusion, transporter protein-mediated transcellular (traversing the plasma membranes and cytosol of the cell) transfer and endocytosis/exocytosis.

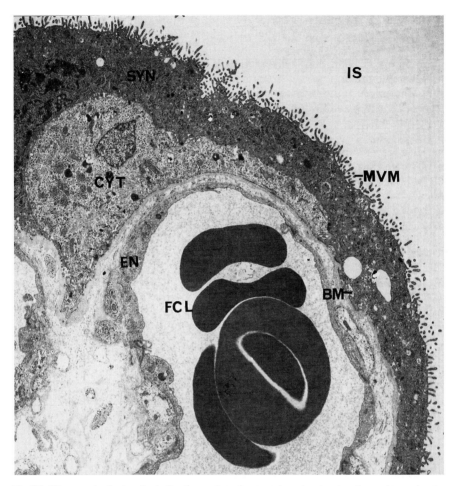

Fig. 9.1 Micrograph of a terminal villus from a term human placenta, showing the exchange barrier (SYN = syncytiotrophoblast, MVM = microvillous plasma membrane, BM = basal plasma membrane, CYT = cytotrophoblast, EN = endothelium, FCL = fetal capillary lumen, IS = intracellular space). Micrograph courtesy of Dr C.J.P. Jones

Diffusion

Diffusional transfer across the placenta, or, to use the more physiologically correct term, flux, has two components: maternofetal and fetomaternal. The net flux is the sum of these two components. For some metabolites the net flux may be magnitudes smaller than either the maternofetal or the fetomaternal flux [16].

For a given uncharged solute, the rate of transfer by diffusion is given by Fick's equation:

$$J_{net} = P[C_{maternal} - C_{fetal}]$$

where J_{net} is the rate of net flux, P is the placental permeability coefficient for a particular molecule (equivalent to the surface area of exchange barrier available for diffusion, times the diffusion coefficient in water of the solute, divided by the mean thickness of the barrier) and C represents the average concentrations or partial pressures on the maternal and fetal sides of the exchange barrier in the placenta. The relative importance of the "$[C_{maternal} - C_{fetal}]$" and "$P$" terms in the above equation is broadly dependent on the nature of the solute in question. Lipid-soluble molecules (e.g. ethanol, the respiratory gases) can dissolve in the lipid bilayer of the syncytiotrophoblast plasma membranes and so the entire surface area is available for diffusion. This process of transcellular lipophilic diffusion is rapid, and the limiting step is thus the concentration gradient ($[C_{maternal} - C_{fetal}]$), which is itself dependent on the rate of delivery of the substance to and clearance away from the exchange barrier: the blood flow. The diffusive transfer of these solutes is therefore said to be flow limited.

The lipid bilayer is relatively impermeable to densely charged and hydrophilic molecules, limiting the surface area available for exchange. Therefore, the rate of diffusive transfer of these is much slower than for the lipophilic molecules and is more dependent on the permeability (P) than on the concentration gradient or blood flow; they are said to be membrane limited.

Paracellular Diffusion: Data obtained in vivo showing a direct relationship between the rate of transfer of inert hydrophilic solutes from mother to fetus and their coefficients of diffusion in water (a measure of the size of a molecule) (Fig. 9.2), suggest that molecules are able to traverse the syncytiotrophoblast by

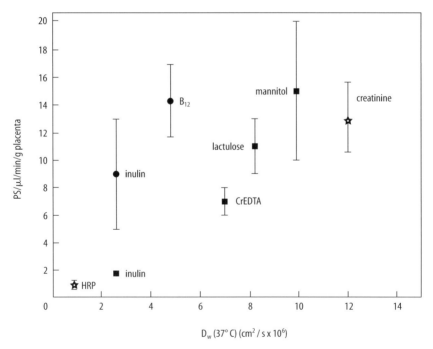

Fig. 9.2 Permeability surface area product (PS) plotted against diffusion coefficient in water at 37 °C for a variety of tracers from four studies on the human placenta (● = in vivo data [18,19], ■ = in vivo data [17], ☆ = in vitro data [20]; mean ± $s_{\bar{x}}$ is shown; reproduced from [20] with permission of Placenta).

moving through extracellular water-filled pores or channels, thus bypassing plasma membranes [17–19], that is, going through a paracellular route. The syncytiotrophoblast of the human placenta is, of course, a syncytium and therefore it is difficult to conceive of the morphological correlates of the paracellular channels. However, recent data suggest that small areas of denudation of the syncytiotrophoblast [20,21] and trophoblast channels not normally visible [22] might provide the paracellular route. Evidence derived from the in vitro dual perfusion of term placental cotyledons suggests that paracellular transfer accounts for about 80 per cent of unidirectional flux of small hydrophilic solutes such as Ca^{2+} and Cl^- [23,24].

Electrical Gradients: Diffusion of charged hydrophilic solutes will be affected by the presence of a transplacental potential difference (p.d.), an electrical gradient across the placental exchange barrier. Although there is evidence of a maternal–fetal p.d. in some species (i.e. an electrical gradient between maternal and fetal extracellular fluid), this may not be equivalent to the actual transplacental p.d. [16]. In studies in vitro of the human isolated mature intermediate villi, the transplacental p.d. is small, of the order of 3 mV, and fetus negative [25]. Measurements in vivo of the maternofetal p.d. across the first trimester and midgestational human placenta support the in vitro finding and confirm the magnitude and direction of the p.d. [26,27]. Mellor et al. [28] reported that the mean maternofetal p.d. was zero at term but these measurements may have been flawed as they followed delivery of the baby. Everything else being equal, a small fetal-side-negative transplacental p.d. will increase the net diffusion of cations towards the fetus and retard that of anions.

Transporter Protein-mediated Transfer

This mechanism involves a membrane-bound protein molecule that is specific for a restricted population of molecules that are sterically very similar (although each molecule of such a population will bind to the carrier with different affinity depending on its chemical structure). There are broadly two types of transport protein-mediated transfer: facilitated diffusion and carrier-mediated active transport.

Facilitated Diffusion: In this form of transfer diffusion across the plasma membrane is assisted by a transporter protein, but the transport is not *active* as the solute travels only down an electrochemical gradient that is already established.

Carrier-mediated Active Transport: This transport occurs against an electrical or chemical gradient and as such consumes energy: it is *active*. Active transport can be divided into two types: in primary active transport the carrier itself hydrolyses adenosine triphosphate (ATP) to provide the energy for the transport (these are termed the ATPases and are responsible for the extrusion of ions from the cell to create electrochemical gradients); in secondary active transport the carrier uses a gradient generated by an ATP-consuming system elsewhere in the cell, usually an inwardly directed gradient for sodium that is established by the action of Na^+-K^+-ATPase, thus coupling the active transport with the passive transport of a sodium ion down its chemical or electrical gradient. If this coupling is with the gradient the carrier is termed a symport or cotransporter, if against, it is an antiport or exchanger.

Endocytosis and Exocytosis

Fluid phase endocytosis is the process by which molecules are taken into the cell when an area of plasma membrane invaginates, engulfs a volume of extracellular water and subsequently pinches away from the rest of the cell surface to form an intracellular vesicle. This process may be more specific when particular molecules are additionally bound by cell surface receptors: receptor-mediated endocytosis. The intracellular vesicle, if it avoids fusion with lysosomes and other intracellular organelles, will eventually fuse with the opposite plasma membrane and extrude its contents into the extracellular space, a process called exocytosis. It is thought that immunoglobulin G crosses the placenta by this mechanism. It has not been studied in relation to IUGR and will not be considered further here.

Fetal Asphyxia

The SGA fetus is at greater risk of hypoxia, hypercapnia and acidosis than the appropriately grown fetus [1]. The severity of this metabolic and respiratory acidosis increases with worsening fetoplacental perfusion, as evidenced by umbilical arterial Doppler studies [29], and with worsening maternoplacental perfusion, as evidenced by uterine artery Doppler studies [30]. The origins of this increased incidences of asphyxia in the growth-restricted infant arise from a failure of oxygen delivery or removal of carbon dioxide and proton from the fetal circulation.

Placental Oxygen Transfer and Hypoxaemia in IUGR

Oxygen is a small lipophilic molecule that is relatively soluble in water and diffuses easily across plasma membranes. It traverses the placenta by transcellular diffusion and does not rely on a carrier molecule [31]. Because the permeability of the placenta to oxygen is so high the rate of transfer is also high and maternal and fetal circulations equilibrate rapidly (see Fick's equation above). Thus the diffusional transfer of oxygen from the maternal to the fetal circulations is flow limited. Maternal PO_2 remains constant over gestation at approximately 100 mmHg [32]. The umbilical vein PO_2 falls from 55 mmHg at 20 weeks gestation to 35 mmHg at term presenting a substantial maternofetal gradient [33]. Since oxygen transfer is flow limited, the relationship between the maternal and fetal blood flow determines the maximal amount of oxygen available for transfer to the fetus. In the mathematically ideal counter-current exchange mechanism (where blood in the uteroplacental circulation travels in the opposite direction to that in the fetoplacental circulation) the umbilical vein PO_2 should be equivalent to the uterine vein PO_2. In the human placenta this theoretical ideal is not achieved. The available data for the human best fit a multivillous pool model of the geometric arrangement of the two blood flows, which is less efficient than the countercurrent scheme [34]. Furthermore there is probably mismatching of maternal and fetal placental blood flows leading to shunting together with oxygen consumption by the placenta itself.

Despite the dependence of oxygen diffusion across the placenta on blood flow, animal data suggest that there has to be quite a marked reduction in uterine blood flow before fetal uptake of oxygen is reduced. For example, in the sheep, fetal oxygen delivery only falls when uterine blood flow is reduced by greater than 50 per cent with the placement of a balloon catheter in the uterine artery [35].

Uterine contractions reduce uteroplacental blood flow by 16 per cent in the sheep and can cause reductions in PO_2 and oxygen saturation in the fetus [36]. These reductions in fetal oxygenation are of short duration and in the healthy fetus will not lead to a profound metabolic acidosis. Using near-infrared spectroscopy of the human fetus in labour Aldrich et al. [37] demonstrated that, during a uterine contraction, cerebral oxygenation falls in the human fetus and that it recovers quickly afterward. If, however, this reduction in maternoplacental blood flow is compounded with a fetus already at the limits of compensation then hypoxia may become severe; this is the probable mechanism of the increased incidence of cardiotocographic abnormalities seen in SGA fetuses in labour [38, 39].

As on the maternal side of the placenta, data suggest that reductions in blood flow in the umbilical (fetoplacental) circulation have to be quite severe to affect fetal oxygenation in animal models. Bilateral occlusion of the ovine umbilical artery has no effect on fetal oxygen uptake until umbilical flow rates are reduced below 50 per cent of the control rates [40]. Wilkening and Meschia [41] ligated one umbilical artery and thus immediately prevented perfusion of approximately one half of the placenta. Umbilical arterial blood pressure rose by 38 per cent. Fetal oxygen consumption fell but was accompanied by an increase in the umbilical vein oxygen saturation and increased transfer of oxygen from the mother.

Clearly there are important physiological variables, in addition to blood flow, that determine oxygen delivery to the fetus in vivo that to some extent prevent reductions in oxygen transfer until large perturbations in blood flow occur. These include the oxygen affinity of haemoglobin and the haematocrit. Haemoglobin acts as the oxygen carrier molecule in both maternal and fetal circulations. In the human, the very low affinity of haemoglobin F for 2,3 diphosphoglycerate (DPG) increases oxygen affinity. As a result the dissociation curve for fetal oxyhaemo-globin is shifted to the left in most species [31] resulting in the oxygen content of fetal blood being higher than that of maternal blood for a given partial pressure. This has the result that more oxygen is extracted at the placenta but the oxygen content of fetal tissues is lower than in adult tissues.

Alteration in fetal haemoglobin type may thus affect fetal oxygen delivery. Exchange transfusion of fetal blood for adult blood causes a fall in the fetal oxygen consumption in the sheep when sampled within an hour of transfusion [42]. This fall was accentuated by a concomitant reduction in umbilical blood flow. Edelstone et al. [43] did not find a fall in fetal oxygen consumption when they transfused lambs with maternal blood unless the fetal haematocrit was also reduced. In their experiments there was no corresponding fall in umbilical flow. This may reflect the time course of the sampling in their experiments, which was more chronic than Itskovitz et al. [42], allowing adaptation by the fetus. In the human fetus, intrauterine transfusion for Rhesus disease does not lead to a fall in the umbilical PO_2, which may be explained by the narrower gap in fetal and maternal haemoglobin oxygen affinities in the human. Soothill et al. [44] found an increased umbilical PO_2 in association with an acidosis and base excess immediately after transfusion.

The fetal haematocrit is also an important determinant of oxygen uptake [45]. Oxygen uptake increases with increasing haematocrit until the blood becomes too viscous and flow is impeded. It is of note that SGA fetuses have higher haematocrits than do those of an appropriate weight. It is thought this polycythaemia is secondary to fetal erythropoietin release as a response to hypoxia [46]. Edelstone et al. [45] were able to improve fetal oxygen uptake in two SGA fetuses by isovolaemic intrauterine transfusion, which returned their haematocrit to normal suggesting that the fetal haematocrit in these SGA fetuses was too high and impeded O_2 transfer, and may have represented a maladaptive response.

Placental Carbon Dioxide Transfer and Hypercapnia in IUGR

Carbon dioxide is, like oxygen, a small lipophilic molecule that is transferred by flow-limited transcellular diffusion across the human placenta [31]. In the human fetus the PCO_2 in the umbilical vein rises marginally over gestation from 32 mmHg to 38 mmHg [33]. In humans, the uterine artery PCO_2 remains between 26 and 34 mmHg, which is lower than in the non-pregnant state because of maternal hyperventilation, and so establishes a concentration gradient [32].

The transport of CO_2 is complicated by its interconversion, catalysed by carbonic anhydrase to carbonic acid and hence proton and HCO_3^-, which is in equilibrium as expressed by the Henderson–Hasselbach equation:

$$pH = pK + \log \frac{[HCO_3]}{[CO_2]}$$

In addition to dissolved gas, CO_2 is transported in the fetal and the maternal circulation as carbaminohaemoglobin, as deoxyhaemoglobin and, after conversion in the erythrocytes, as HCO_3^-. There are low concentrations of carbonic acid (H_2CO_3) and carbonate ion (CO_3^-) in fetal plasma, although the amount of these forms is estimated to be in the order of 0.1 per cent of dissolved CO_2 [31]. Binding of CO_2 to haemoglobin in the fetal tissues facilitates oxygen release by right-shifting the haemoglobin/oxygen dissociation curve and vice versa at the placenta: the Haldane effect [32]. It is presumably of similar importance in fetal CO_2 excretion as it is in the adult in the lung. As the fetal arterial blood enters the placenta CO_2 rapidly begins to diffuse across, thus distributing the equilibrium between fetal plasma and fetal red cells so that CO_2 begins to diffuse from the red cells into the plasma. This initiates a chain of reactions that subsequently allow the transfer of CO_2 down the concentration gradient between the fetal and maternal circulation.

CO_2 may be transferred across the placenta in all of its different forms but the relative contribution of each form is not clear. In addition, HCO_3^- may be created and dissipated in both fetus and placenta. In experiments in the sheep, inhibiting fetal carbonic anhydrase, and hence fetal interconversion of CO_2 and HCO_3^-, with acetazolomide resulted in a large rise in total fetal arterial CO_2 concentrations but little change in HCO_3^- concentration [47]. It was concluded that the acetazolomide prevented catalysis of the reconversion of HCO_3^- to CO_2 in the fetal red cell at the placenta, so that the only form of CO_2 available for excretion at the placenta was the small amount of CO_2 dissolved in the plasma itself. Immediately after administration of acetazolomide, fetal excretion of CO_2 via the placenta was much less than the total fetal production of CO_2; this caused the fetal arterial PCO_2 to rise to very high levels. Subsequent administration of the strong base tris(hydroxymethyl)aminomethane (THAM) to the sheep fetus drove the CO_2/HCO_3^- equilibrium of the Henderson–Hasselbach equation in favour of HCO_3^-. This produced a rapid rise in fetal arterial HCO_3^- concentrations and a concomitant fall in the umbilical arterial PCO_2 [47]. Even in the presence of these high concentrations of HCO_3^- there appeared to be little transplacental transfer of HCO_3^- in this study. Hatano et al. [48] found that [^{14}C]-labelled HCO_3^- transfer across the guinea pig placenta was inhibited by a transport blocker, diisothio-cyano-2, 2-disulphonic stilbene (DIDS), which suggested involvement of a transporter protein on both the maternal- and fetal-facing membranes. However, 70 per cent of the total fetomaternal HCO_3^- flux was not inhibitable with DIDS. The transfer of HCO_3^- was also augmented by the presence of lactate on the fetal side, which suggested the presence of a lactate/HCO_3^- cotransporter. Thus, although there is evidence for transcellular transporter protein-mediated transfer of HCO_3^- ion in the placenta, it seems to play only a quantitatively minor role in the total fetomaternal flux.

The DIDS inhibitable transporter referred to above is probably a Cl^-/HCO_3^- exchanger. This exchanger, otherwise known as the erythrocyte anion exchanger, or band 3 protein, is one of the best-characterised transport proteins. It constitutes 25 per cent of the protein weight of the human red cell membrane [49]. In the erythrocyte it exchanges Cl^- for HCO_3^- across the cell membrane increasing the capacity of blood to transport CO_2. The exchanger is inhibited by stilbene disulphonates, such as DIDS [50]. There are at least three isoforms of the anion exchanger family identified. AE1 (anion exchanger) is the band 3 erythrocyte isoform. AE2 was originally isolated from renal tissue. AE3 seems to be of particular importance in the formation of cerebrospinal fluid (CSF) in the choroid plexus of the brain [49].

The presence of the Cl^-/HCO_3^- exchanger in the placenta was inferred from the presence of DIDS inhibitable, Na^+-independent, electroneutral Cl^- exchange in human placental microvillous membrane vesicles by Shennan et al. [51] and then confirmed by several other groups [52,53]. The expression of the anion exchanger has now been demonstrated in both the microvillous and basal plasma membranes of the syncytiotrophoblast using Western blotting [54]. The basal plasma membrane expresses a third of the level of the anion exchanger found in the microvillous plasma membrane [54]. In the SGA fetus there is no evidence of altered activity or expression of the anion exchanger [55]. This implies that any reduction in transplacental transfer of CO_2 leading to fetal hypercapnia may be due to reduced clearance of the flow limited gas as confirmed by cordocentesis studies on fetuses with abnormal umbilical arterial Doppler values [29].

To summarise the above sections on the respiratory gases, it is likely that gross reduction in fetoplacental perfusion due to abnormal umbilical arterial blood flow is the most significant contributor to the increased incidence of hypoxia in SGA fetuses. The fetus none the less possesses mechanisms that allow adequate oxygen transfer until reductions in blood flow are severe, mirroring the findings from cordocentesis studies. This reduction in oxygen transfer will of itself lead to hypercapnia that cannot be cleared because of reduced placental perfusion. The origin of the reduction in blood flow may lie in abnormal placental vascular development [56] as a consequence of poor trophoblast invasion in early pregnancy.

Placental Proton Transfer and Acidosis in IUGR

There has been little or no experimental work on the mechanisms of proton exchange across the placenta. Protons are densely charged and hydrophilic and do not cross plasma membranes easily, although the permeability of protons across lipid bilayers is anomalously high, probably owing to movement down transient "water wires" [57,58]. However, the transcellular diffusion of proton, although greater than that of sodium, is likely to be small. Several transporter proteins have now been identified that mediate proton transfer across the plasma membrane. So far, only the Na$^+$/H$^+$ exchanger has been unequivocally demonstrated to be present in the syncytiotrophoblast [54].

The Na$^+$/H$^+$ exchanger may have a role in extruding proton from the syncytiotrophoblast, and three studies have investigated the activity of the Na$^+$/H$^+$ exchanger in the microvillous plasma membrane in relation to fetal growth [9,59,60]. These studies taken in total suggest a positive correlation between birthweight and activity of this transporter, which might explain the antepartum acidosis seen in some IUGR fetuses [61]. However, only one of the studies showed a significant difference in placental Na$^+$/H$^+$ exchanger activity in relation to birthweight; activity was lower in membranes from placentas of IUGR babies compared with that in membranes from placentas of AGA babies [60].

If the syncytiotrophoblast of the IUGR fetus does lack sufficient Na$^+$/H$^+$ exchanger to deal adequately with an acid load then proton could accumulate. The resulting intracellular acidosis would have effects on the metabolism of the cell and may affect, for example, the transfer of amino acids [62]. Additionally, the placenta could have consequent difficulty excreting protons resulting in fetal acidosis and the attendant morbidities. However, it is not yet clear whether the exchanger does have a role in the transplacental transfer of protons as well as in the pH homeostasis of the syncytiotrophoblast; Hughes et al. [55] failed to find any correlation between acid–base status of the baby at delivery and placental Na$^+$/H$^+$ exchanger activity.

Placental Glucose Transfer and Hypoglycaemia in IUGR

Glucose is an important primary energy source for the fetus and its transfer from the maternal circulation by the placenta constitutes the main supply. Although the fetal plasma concentration of glucose is always lower than that in maternal plasma, paracellular diffusion alone is unable to supply sufficient glucose to meet fetal demands [63] and there is additional transporter protein-mediated transfer. Glucose transport across the placenta is by facilitated diffusion [64,65]. The mRNA encoding for two isoforms (GLUT 1 and GLUT 3) of the facilitative glucose transporter (GLUT) family of proteins has been identified in the placenta [66,67], although immunohistochemical studies and immunoblotting [68,69] have identified only GLUT 1 protein expression in the human placenta. Studies using purified microvillous [70] and basal [71] plasma membrane vesicles have identified a high capacity glucose transport system in both membranes, with similar properties. The amount of GLUT 1 transporter, per milligram membrane protein, is higher in the microvillous than in the basal plasma membrane [69].

Umbilical cord blood sampling at delivery and by cordocentesis has shown that plasma glucose concentration in SGA [1] and IUGR [3] fetuses is significantly lower than in AGA controls. Economides and Nicolaides [72] reported significantly lower umbilical artery and umbilical vein glucose concentrations at cordocentesis from SGA fetuses, compared with AGA controls. They also observed that maternal venous glucose concentrations were significantly lower in SGA pregnancies than in AGA controls. In fetuses with abnormal umbilical artery Doppler wave forms, Karsdorp et al. [3] found significantly lower glucose concentrations only in cases with absent end-diastolic velocities. Although both maternal and fetal glucose concentrations are significantly lower in SGA pregnancies, the maternofetal concentration difference is significantly higher than in AGA pregnancies [73] and there is a positive correlation between the maternofetal glucose concentration gradient and both uterine and umbilical artery impedance [73]. These findings suggest that: (1) uteroplacental and fetoplacental blood flow play an important role in determining the net maternofetal transfer of glucose, and (2) fetal hypoglycaemia in SGA pregnancies is not a direct consequence of maternal hypoglycaemia as the maternofetal glucose concentration gradient is maintained, if not augmented. Hypoglycaemia in SGA/IUGR fetuses could result from impaired placental glucose transport or abnormal placental/fetal glucose metabolism. Placental glucose transporter activity in relation to gestation and fetal growth has been examined by Jansson et al. [69] using vesicles prepared from the microvillous and basal plasma membranes. They reported a significant increase in glucose transporter (GLUT 1) expression in the basal plasma membrane between 16–22 weeks' and 27–30 weeks' gestation and a significant increase in glucose transporter activity between 16–22 weeks' gestation and term, but no change in expression or activity in the microvillous plasma membrane. They found no significant difference in GLUT 1 expression in term SGA fetuses (birthweight > 2 *sd* below mean for gestation age and sex) compared with term AGA controls. Finally, there was no significant difference in glucose uptake by microvillous or basal plasma membrane vesicles from SGA placentas compared with AGA controls. This study concluded that hypoglycaemia associated with SGA fetuses is not due to a reduction in placental glucose transporter activity. However, the finding of lower umbilical glucose concentrations in human fetuses with absent umbilical end-diastolic velocities, but not in those with reduced end-diastolic velocities [3], suggests that the net maternofetal glucose transfer may be specifically reduced in the former group of fetuses. An examination of placental glucose transporter expression and activity in such IUGR fetuses therefore remains necessary, especially in fetuses with proven hypoglycaemia.

Placental Amino Acid Transfer and Hypoaminoacidaemia in IUGR

Amino acids are essential building blocks for structural and metabolic proteins, and constitute an important primary energy source for the fetus. In addition, essential amino acids are the starting materials for the synthesis of non-essential amino acids. They may also be substrates for other metabolic processes; for example, L-arginine is the substrate for the synthesis of NO [74], a potent vasodilator and an important regulator of vascular tone in the fetoplacental circulation [75].

The concentration of amino acids is higher in fetal than in maternal plasma [76]. Furthermore, although the molar concentration of amino acids in the syncytiotrophoblast cytosol is not known, it is likely to be higher than in maternal and fetal plasma [77]. Therefore amino acid transfer across the placenta takes place against an electrochemical gradient and is an active, transporter protein-mediated process. It occurs in at least two steps: transport against the electrochemical gradient into the syncytiotrophoblast across the microvillous plasma membrane followed by "leak" down the electrochemical gradient across the basal plasma membrane into the fetal-side extracellular space.

Table 9.1 shows the various amino acid transport systems that have been identified in the human placenta, and their localisation to either microvillous or basal plasma membrane. One of the mechanisms by which transport against the electrochemical gradient across the microvillous plasma membrane is accomplished is by coupling the transport of amino acids (against a concentration gradient) to the transport of sodium (down a concentration gradient). The sodium concentration gradient is generated by Na^+-K^+-ATPase. Thus some amino acid transporters are dependent on the presence of sodium ions for their activity. By convention, sodium-dependent transporters are denoted by upper case letters (such as the system A transporter) while sodium-independent transporters are denoted by lower case letters (e.g. system 1 transporter).

Umbilical cord sampling at delivery and by cordocentesis has shown that the SGA and IUGR fetus has a hypoaminoacidaemia with an increased glycine : valine ratio typical of kwashiorkor in the infant [3,88,9]. This is mainly, but by no means exclusively, due to a reduction in the concentration of branched chain essential amino acids valine, leucine and isoleucine. By contrast, maternal plasma concentrations of essential amino acids in IUGR pregnancies are significantly higher than in AGA controls [88, 89]. The placental supply of amino acids, at least in the term fetus, may only marginally exceed fetal demands for protein synthesis. Studies using stable isotopes on term normal human pregnancies have shown that the placental supply of leucine and phenylalanine

Table 9.1 Amino acid transport systems in the human placental syncythiotrophoblast modified from Moe [78]

Transport system	Substrate	Membrane*	References
A	neutral amino acids	MVM/BM	[79]
ASC	alanine, serine, cystine, anionic amino acids	BM	[79]
N	histidine, glutamine	MVM	[80]
β	taurine	MVM	[81]
X^-_{AG}	aspartate, glutamate	MVM/BM	[82][83]
1	leucine	MVM/BM	[84]
y^+	cationic amino acids	MVM/BM	[85]
y^+L	cationic amino acids, neutral amino acids	MVM/BM	[85] [86]
b^{0+}	cationic amino acids, neutral amino acids	BM	[87]

*MVM = localised to microvillous, BM = localised to the basal plasma membrane of the syncytiotrophoblast.

exceeds fetal demands for protein synthesis by 31 per cent and 22 per cent respectively [90]. Small reductions in the supply of amino acids to the fetus may, therefore, impair protein synthesis and limit fetal growth.

The first direct study of placental amino acid transport in relation to fetal growth was that of Dicke and Henderson [10]. Using placental microvillous plasma membrane vesicles, they found that AIB (amino-isobutyric acid, a non-metabolisable amino acid analogue) uptake was significantly lower in SGA than in AGA fetuses at term. AIB is most likely to be transported by the sodium-dependent system A transporter, which is specific for neutral amino acids with short unbranched side chains such as alanine and glycine. Mahendran et al. [9] subsequently showed that both sodium-dependent (system A) and sodium-independent methylaminoisobutyric acid (MeAIB; a non-metabolisable amino acid analogue specifically transported by system A) uptake were significantly lower in microvillous plasma membrane vesicles from term SGA fetuses, compared with AGA controls. With respect to system A transporter activity, this study showed that the V_{max}, (maximum velocity, a measure of the number of trans-porters present per milligram membrane protein) but not the K_m (affinity) of this transporter was significantly lower in microvillous plasma membrane vesicles from SGA fetuses than in AGA fetuses, which suggests that the total number of system A transporters per milligram membrane protein is reduced. A diminished system A transporter activity has also been reported in preterm SGA fetuses [91]. In this latter study, when SGA fetuses were subdivided into those with normal and abnormal umbilical artery pulsitility indices (PI), system A transporter activity was found to be significantly lower only in the microvillous plasma membrane vesicles from fetuses with abnormal PI (Fig. 9.3). It should, however, be pointed out that the number of SGA pregnancies with normal umbilical artery PI in this study was small.

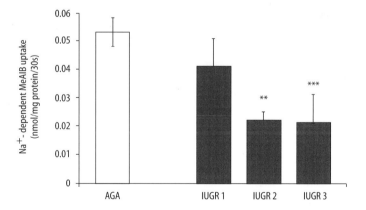

Fig. 9.3 Placental microvillous plasma membrane system A activity (measured as Na^+-dependent [^{14}C]-MeAIB uptake) in placentas from pregnancies with AGA and IUGR fetuses. IUGR-1 is a group of fetuses with birthweight below the 10th percentile but normal umbilical artery pulsatility index and fetal heart rate (FHR). IUGR-2 is a group of fetuses with birthweight below the 5th percentile and abnormal umbilical artery pulsatility index but normal FHR. IUGR-3 is a group of fetuses with birth-weight below the 5th percentile and both abnormal umbilical artery pulsatility index and abnormal FHR (mean ± se is shown; **$p < 0.01$, *** $p < 0.001$ versus AGA (ANOVA followed by Bonferroni t-test; reproduced from [91] with permission of Pediatric Research).

In a more extensive study, Dicke and Verges [92] examined alanine, leucine and glycine uptake in paired microvillous plasma membrane and basal plasma membrane vesicles from SGA and AGA pregnancies. Although the SGA fetuses in this study were born preterm (mean gestation age 36.5 weeks compared with 40.1 weeks for AGA fetuses), no difference in alanine uptake (system A and non-system A) and leucine uptake (system 1) was observed in either microvillous plasma membrane or basal plasma membrane vesicles between the two groups. Glycine uptake (system A and non-system A), was, however, significantly lower in microvillous plasma membrane and basal plasma membrane vesicles from SGA fetuses. The discrepancy between glycine and alanine uptake (both system A substrates) suggest that other transport systems may contribute significantly to the transplacental flux of these amino acids. The finding of lower microvillous plasma membrane system A amino acid transporter activity in placentas of SGA fetuses prompted the hypothesis that fetal macrosomia would be associated with increased system A activity. Surprisingly, however, system A activity was found to be significantly lower in microvillous plasma membrane vesicles from placentas of macrosomic fetuses (birthweight > 97th percentile for gestation age) born to diabetic mothers compared with AGA controls born to normal mothers; V_{max} but not K_m was reduced. There was no significant difference between system A activity in placentas of AGA fetuses born to diabetic and non-diabetic mothers [59]. Leucine uptake (system 1) was not different between any groups [59].

Data showing reduced placental microvillous plasma membrane system A transporter activity in both SGA and macrosomic fetuses present us with a paradox but a recent study (93) has provided some clarification. This study examined the relationship between placental microvillous plasma membrane system A activity and size at birth in 62 AGA fetuses born to women having normal pregnancies. A negative correlation was found between system A activity, per milligram membrane protein, and various measures of size at birth including weight and abdominal circumference. This is therefore the same trend as that seen for system A activity in placentas of macrosomic fetuses. In interpreting these data it has to be remembered that the system A activity is measured per milligram protein and that a bigger baby will have a bigger placenta and therefore more microvillous plasma membrane. Therefore the total system A activity in the whole placenta would remain constant, independently of fetal size, over the range of normal and larger birth sizes. Teleologically this might be an adaptive response, evolved to limit fetal growth, or it may be the result of a design evolved to ensure that there is always sufficient system A activity to meet the demands of the normally growing fetus, irrespective of size. Consequently the IUGR fetus may be thought of as being abnormal with respect to microvillous plasma membrane system A activity. These fetuses have suffered a double hit – reduced placental transporter activity per milligram membrane protein in conjunction with a small placenta. This could lead directly to the lower circulating plasma amino acid concentrations measured in these babies and limitation of fetal growth.

Further evidence is now emerging that the activity of other amino acid transporters is reduced in SGA/IUGR [94,95] which suggests that this deficit is a major facet of the placental pathophysiology of growth restriction in utero.

Drug Abuse, Placental Transfer and IUGR

The misuse of recreational drugs is a major medical and social problem. The association between cigarette smoking, alcohol abuse and adverse pregnancy outcome has long been recognised [96,97]. More recently, the obstetric consequences of cocaine and marijuana have been reported [98]. Less is known about the obstetric consequences of designer drugs such as ecstasy. The epidemiological association between drug abuse and intrauterine growth impairment may be confounded by several factors, not least the effects of socioeconomic deprivation.

There is, however, biological evidence that nicotine, ethanol and cocaine may interfere with placental transport mechanisms. The exposure of placental villous slices to high levels of nicotine has been reported to result in a significant reduction in AIB uptake [99] although "physiological levels" of nicotine resulted in a non-significant reduction. The addition of ethanol to nicotine-treated villous slices did not alter AIB uptake. Acetaldehyde, a metabolite of ethanol, however, had an additive effect with nicotine on AIB uptake [99] and resulted in a significant reduction in AIB uptake in villous fragments exposed to "physiological levels" of nicotine. In microvillous plasma membrane vesicles, acute exposure to "physiological levels" of nicotine and ethanol did not significantly alter alanine or cycloleucine uptake [100].

Cocaine has been demonstrated to bind to placental microvillous plasma membrane and basal plasma membrane vesicles at one and two high affinity binding sites respectively [101,102]. In both membrane fractions, cocaine (at concentrations similar to those found in recreational users) has been shown to impair system A-mediated uptake of alanine [101,102]. Sodium-independent alanine uptake and leucine uptake were unaffected by cocaine exposure in basal plasma membrane vesicles [102]. At much higher concentrations, cocaine has been shown to reduce AIB, isoleucine, lysine and aspartic acid uptake in placental villous fragments [103], AIB uptake being most sensitive.

Overall these data seem to present a picture, correlating effects of drugs on the placental amino acid transporters with reduced fetal growth, which is consistent with that described above for reduced microvillous plasma membrane system A transporter activity in non-drug-induced IUGR.

Conclusions

Classically, IUGR due to "placental insufficiency" has been thought of in relation to abnormal trophoblast invasion of the spiral arteries in early pregnancy, and consequently reduced uteroplacental blood flow, resulting in limitation of transfer of solutes across the placenta [104]. The evidence described above suggests that the fetal hypoxaemia, hypercapnia, acidosis and lower umbilical plasma concentrations of glucose and amino acids associated with IUGR can be explained only incompletely by a reduction in uteroplacental perfusion. The data on amino acid transport, in particular, suggest that syncytiotrophoblast exchange function is impaired in IUGR, although it is very difficult to know what is cause and what is effect. Clearly, the pathology known as placental insufficiency has now to be redefined in the light of modern understanding of placental morphology and transport function. Ideally morphological, biochemical and physiological methods need to be combined in studies on individual placentas from clinically well-defined pregnancies. Future efforts also need to concentrate on elucidating the fetoplacental, maternoplacental and intrinsic placental-signalling mechanisms involved in the regulation of maternofetal exchange across the placenta in normal pregnancies and those associated with growth restriction.

References

1. Soothil PW, Ajayi RA, Nicolaides KH. Fetal biochemistry in growth retardation. Early Hum Dev 1992;29:91–7.
2. Economides DL, Nicolaides KH. Blood glucose and oxygen tension levels in small-for-gestational-age fetuses. Am J Obstet Gynecol 1989;160:385–9.
3. Karsdorp VHM, van Vugt JMG, Jakobs C, Dekker GA, van Geing HP. Amino acids, glucose and lactate concentrations in umbilical cord blood in relation to umbilical artery flow patterns. Eur J Obstet Gynecol Reprod Biol 1994;57:117–22.
4. Economides DL, Nicolaides KH, Gahl WA, Bernardini I, Evans MI. Plasma amino acids in appropriate- and small-for-gestational-age fetuses. Am J Obstet Gynecol 1989;161:1219–27.
5. Altman DG, Hytten FE. Intrauterine growth retardation: Let's be clear about it. Br J Obstet Gynaecol 1989;96:1127–32.
6. Pryor J. The identification and long term effects of growth retardation. Br J Obstet Gynaecol 1997;104:1116–22.
7. Fancourt R, Campbell S, Harvey D, Norman AP. Follow-up study of small-for-dates babies. BMJ 1976;1:1435–7.
8. Beattie RB, Johnson P. Practical assessment of neonatal nutrition status beyond birthweight: an imperative for the 1990's. Br J Obstet Gynaecol 1994;101:842–6.
9. Mahendran D, Donnai P, Glazier J, D'Souza S, Boyd RDH, Sibley C. Amino acid (System A) transporter activity in microvillous membrane vesicles from the placentas of appropriate and small for gestational age babies. Pediatr Res 1993;34:661–5.
10. Dicke JM, Henderson GI. Placental amino acid uptake in normal and complicated pregnancies. Am J Med Sci 1988;295:223–7.
11. Maning FA, Bondaji N, Harman CR, Casiro O, Menticoglou S, Morrison I, Berck DJ. Fetal assessment based on fetal biopysical scoring. Am J Obstet Gynecol 1998;178:696–706.
12. Alfirevic Z, Neilson JP. Doppler ultrasonography in high-risk pregnancies: a systematic review with meta-analysis. Am J Obstet Gynecol 1995;172:1379–87.
13. Steven, editor. Comparative placentation. Essays in structure and function. London:Academic Press, 1975.
14. Kaufmann P, Scheffen I. Placental development. Section III. The placenta. In: Polin RA, Fox WW, editors. Fetal and neonatal physiology, 2nd ed vol. 1. Philadelphia USA: WB Saunders, 1998;59–66.
15. Eaton BM, Leach L, Firth JA. Permeability of the fetal villous microvasculature in the isolated perfused term human placenta. J Physiol 1993;463:141–55.
16. Sibley CPS, Boyd RDH. Control of transfer across the mature placenta. In: Clarke JR, editor. Oxford reviews of reproductive biology, vol 10. Oxford:Oxford University Press, 1988;382–485.
17. Bain MD, Copas DK, Taylor A, Landon MJ, Stacey TE. Permeability of the human placenta to four non-metabolized hydrophilic molecules. J Physiol 1990;431:505–14.
18. Willis DM, O'Grady JP, Faber JJ, Thornburg KL. Diffusion permeability of cyanocobalamin in human placenta. Am J Physiol 1986;250:R459–64.
19. Thornburg KL, Burry KJ, Adams AK, Kirk EP, Faber JJ. Permeability of placenta to inulin. Am J Obstet Gynecol 1988;158:1165–9.
20. Edwards D, Jones CJP, Sibley CP, Nelson DM. Paracellular permeability pathways in the human placenta. A qualitative and morphological study of maternal-fetal transfer of horseradish peroxidase. Placenta 1993;14:63–73.
21. Brownbill P, Edwards D, Jones C, Mahendran D, Owen D, Sibley C, Johnson R, Swanson P, Nelson DM. Mechanisms of alphafetoprotein transfer in the perfused human placental cotyledon from uncomplicated pregnancy. J Clin Invest 1995;96:2220–6.

22. Kertschanska S, Kosanke G, Kaufmann P. Is there morphological evidence for the existence of transtrophoblastic channels in human placental villi? Troph Research 1994;8:581-96.
23. Stulc J, Stulcova B, Smid M. Sach I. Parallel mechanisms of Ca transfer across the perfused human placental cotyledon. Am J Obstet Gynecol 1994;170:162-7.
24. Doughty IM, Glazier JD, Greenwood SL, Boyd RDH, Sibley CP. Mechanisms of materno-fetal chloride transfer across the in vitro perfused human placenta cotyledon. Am J Physiol 1996;271:R1701-6.
25. Greenwood SL, Boyd RDH, Sibley CP. Transtrophoblast and microvillous membrane potential difference in mature intermediate human placental villi. Am J Physiol 1993;265:C460-6.
26. Stulc J, Svihovec J, Drabkova J, Stribrny J, Kobilkova J, Vido I, et al. Electrical potential difference across the mid-term human placenta. Acta Obstet Gynecol Scand 1978;57:125-6.
27. Ward S, Jauniaux e, Shannon C, Rodeck C, Boyd R, Sibley C. Electrical potential difference between exocelomic fluid and maternal blood in early pregnancy. Am J Physiol 1998;274:R1492-5.
28. Mellor DJ, Cockburn F, Lees MM, Blagden A. Distribution of ions and electrical potential differences between mother and fetus in the human at term. J Obstet Gynaecol Br Commonw 1969;76:993-8.
29. Steiner H, Staudach A, Spitzer D, Schaffer KH, Gregg A, Weiner CP. Growth deficient fetuses with absent or reversed umbilical artery end-diastolic flow are metabolically compromised. Early Hum Dev 1995;41:1-9.
30. Aristidou A, Van der Hof M, Nicolaides KH, Campbell S. Uterine artery Doppler in the investigation of pregnancies associated with raised maternal serum alpha-fetoprotein. Br J Obstet Gynaecol 1990;97:431-5.
31. Faber JJ, Thornburg KL. Placental physiology. New York: Raven Press, 1983.
32. Meschia G. Placental respiratory gas exchange and fetal oxygenation. In: Creasy RK, Resnick R, editors. Maternal fetal medicine: principles and practice. London: WB Saunders, 1984;ch.7, 274-85.
33. Soothill PW, Nicolaides KH, Rodeck CH, Campbell S. Effect of gestational age on fetal and intervillous blood gas and acid-base values in human pregnancy. Fetal Ther 1986;1:168-75.
34. Carter AM. Factors affecting gas transfer across the placenta and the oxygen supply to the fetus. J Dev Physiol 1989;12:305-22.
35. Clapp JF. The relationship between blood flow and oxygen uptake in the uterine and the umbilical circulations. Am J Obstet Gynacol 1978;132:410-13.
36. Harding R, Sigger JN, Wickham PJD. Fetal and maternal influences on arterial oxygen levels in the sheep fetus. J Dev Physiol 1983;5:267-76.
37. Aldrich CJ, D'Antona D, Spencer JAD, Wyatt JS, Peebles DM, Delpy DT, et al. Late fetal heart decelerations and changes in cerebral oxygenation during the first stage of labour. Br J Obstet Gynaecol 1995;102:9-13.
38. Low JA, Pancham SR, Worthington D. Fetal heart deceleration patterns patterns in relation to asphyxia and weight-gestational age percentile of the fetus. Obstet Gynecol 1976;47:14-20.
39. Wennergren M, Wennergren G, Vilbergsson GSO. Obstetric characteristics and neonatal performance in a four-year small for gestational age population. Obstet Gynecol 1988;72:615-20.
40. Itskovitz J, LaGamma EF, Rudolph AM. The effect of reducing umbilical blood flow on fetal oxygenation. Am J Obstet Gynecol 1983;145:813-18.
41. Wilkening RB, Meschia G. Effect of occluding one umbilical artery on placental oxygen transport. Am J Physiol 1991;260:H1319-25.
42. Itskovitz J, Goetzman BW, Roman C, Rudolph AM. Effects of fetal-maternal exchange transfusion on fetal oxygenation and blood flow distribution. Am J Physiol 1984;247:H655-60.
43. Edelstone DI, Darby MJ, Bass K, Miller K. Effects of reductions in haemoglobin – oxygen affinity and haematocrit level on oxygen consumption and acid – base state in fetal lambs. Am J Obstet Gynecol 1989;160:820-8.
44. Soothill PW, Nicolaides KH, Rodeck CH, Bellingham AJ. The effect of replacing fetal hemoglobin with adult hemoglobin on blood gas and acid – base parameters in human fetuses. Am J Obstet Gynecol 1988;158:66-9.
45. Edelstone DI, Caine ME, Fumia FD. Relationship of fetal oxygen consumption and acid-base balance to fetal hematocrit. Am J Obstet Gynecol 1985;151:855-1.
46. Snijders RJM, Abbas A, Melby O, Ireland RM, Nicolaides KH. Fetal plasma erythropoietin concentration in severely growth retarded fetuses. Am J Obstet Gynecol 1993;168:615-23.
47. Longo LD, Delivorai-Papadopoulos M, Forster Re. Fetal CO_2 transfer after fetal carbonic anhydrase inhibition. Am J Physiol 1974;226:703-10.

48. Hatano H, Leichtweiss HP, Schroeder H. Uptake of bicarbonate/CO_2 in the isolated guinea pig placenta. Placenta 1989;10:213–21.

49. Kopito RR. Molecular biology of the anion exchanger gene family. Int Rev Cyto 1990;123:177–99.

50. Reithmeier RA. The erythrocyte anion transporter. Curr Opin Cell Biol 1994;6:583–94.

51. Shennan DB, Davis B, Boyd CAR. Chloride transport in human placental microvillous membrane vesicles. Pflügers Arch 1986;406:60–4.

52. Illsley NP, Glaubensklee C, Davis B, Verkman AS. Chloride transport across placental microvillous membranes measured by fluorescence. Am J Physiol 1988;255:789–97.

53. Byrne S, Glazier JD, Greenwood SL, Mahendran D, Sibley CPS. Chloride transport by human placental microvillous membrane vesicles. Biochim Biophys Acta 1993;1153:122–6.

54. Powell TL, Dehlin DO, Westergren K, Ingvarsson K, Jansson T. Identification of ion transporter isoforms in human placenta. Placenta 1995;16:A58.

55. Hughes JL, Glazier JD, Doughty IM, D'Souza S, Sibley CP. Cl^-/HCO_3^- Exchanger and Na^+/H^+ Exchanger activity in microvillous membrane vesicles derived from placentas of appropriate for gestational age (AGA) and small for gestational age (SGA) infants. Placenta 1997;18:A28.

56. Kingdom JCP, Kaufman P. Oxygen and placental villous development: origins of fetal hypoxia. Placenta 1997;18:613–22.

57. Illsley HE, Verkman AS. Proton permeability in microvillous membrane vesicles. J Membr Biol 1987;94:267–78.

58. Deamer DW, Nichols JW. Proton flux mechanisms in model and biological membranes. J Membr Biol 1989;107:91–103.

59. Kuruvilla A, D'Souza S, Glazier J, Mahendran D, Maresh M, Sibley C. Altered activity of the system A amino acid transporter in microvillous membrane vesicles from placentas of macrosomic babies born to diabetic women. J Clin Invest 1994;94:689–95.

60. Glazier JD, Cetin I, Perugion G, Ronzoni S, Grey AM, Mahendran D, et al. Association between the activity of the system A amino acid transporter in the microvillous plasma membrane of the human placenta and severity of fetal compromise in intrauterine growth restriction. Pediatr Res 1997;42:514–19.

61. Sibley C, D'Souza S, Doughty I, Boyd R, Glazier J, Kuruvilla A, et al. Birthweight and sodium/ proton exchanger activity in the term human placenta [letter]. Placenta 1995;16:469–70.

62. Glazier JD, O'Donnell A, Sibley CP. The effect of pH on the placental microvillous membrane system A amino acid transporter. Placenta 1996;17:A16.

63. Bain MD, Copas DK, Landon MJ, Stacey TE. In vivo permeability of the human placenta to inulin and mannitol. J Physiol 1988;399:313–19.

64. Carstensen M, Leichtweiss HP, Molsen G, Schroder H. Evidence of a specific transport of D-hexose across the human term placenta in vitro. Arch Gynaeko 1977;222:187–96.

65. Schneider H, Challier J-C, Dancis J. Transfer and metabolism of glucose and lactate in the human placenta studied by a perfusion system in vitro. Placenta 1981;2(suppl):129–38.

66. Bell GI, Kayano T, Buse JB. Molecular biology of mammalian glucose transporters. Diabetes Care 1990;13:198–208.

67. Devaskar SU, Mueckler MM. The mammalian glucose transporters. Pediatr Res 1992;31:1–13.

68. Takata K, Kasahara T, Kasahara M, Ezaki O, Hirano H. Localisation of erythrocyte/Hep G2-type glucose transporter (GLUT1) in human placental villi. Cell Tissue Res 1992;267:407–12.

69. Jansson T, Wennergren M, Illsley NP. Glucose transporter protein expression in human placenta throughout gestation and in intra-uterine growth retardation. J Clin Endocrinol Metab 1993;77:1554–62.

70. Johnson LW, Smith CH. Monosaccharide transport across microvillous membrane of human placenta. Am J Physiol 1980;238:C160–8.

71. Johnson LW, Smith CH. Glucose transport across the basal plasma membrane of human placental syncytiotrophoblast. Biochim Biophysi Acta 1985;815:44–50.

72. Economides DL, Nicolaides KH. Blood glucose and oxygen tension levels in small-for-gestational-age fetuses. Am J Obstet Gynecol 1989;160:385–9.

73. Economides DL, Nicolaides KH, Campbell S. Relation between maternal-to-fetal blood glucose gradient and uterine and umbilical doppler blood flow measurements. Br J Obstet Gynecol 1990;97:543–4.

74. Palmer RMJ, Ashton DS, Moncada S. Vascular endothelial cells synthesise nitric oxide from L-arginine. Nature 1988;333:664–6.

75. Chaudhuri G, Cuevas J, Buga GM, Ignarro LJ. NO is more important than PGI_2 in maintaining low vascular tone in feto-placental vessels. Am J Physiol 1993;265:H2036–43.

76. Matsuda T, Nakano Y, Nishikawa Y, Yamaguchi R. Feto-maternal amino acid patterns and cyclic AMP in the human placenta with abnormal pregnancies, particularly with SFD. Tohoku J Exp Med 1977;121:253–62.
77. Philipps AF, Holzman IR, Teng C, Battaglia F. Tissue concentrations of free amino acids in term human placentas. Am J Obstet Gynecol 1978;131:881–7.
78. Moe A. Placental amino acid transport. Am J Physiol 1995;268:C1321–31.
79. Hoeltzli SD, Smith CH. Alanine transport systems in isolated basal plasma membrane of the human placenta. Am J Physiol 1989;256:C630–7.
80. Karl PI, Tkaczevski H, Fisher SE. Characteristics of histidine uptake by human placental microvillous membrane vesicles. Pediatr Res 1989;25:19–26.
81. Karl PI, Fisher SE. Taurine transport by microvillous membrane vesicles and the perfused cotyledon of the human placenta. Am J Physiol 1990;258:C443–51.
82. Iioka H, Moriyama J, Itoh K, Hino K, Ichija M. Studies on the mechanisms of L-glutamate transport the effect of potassium ions in microvillous vesicles on L-glutamate uptake). J Obstet Gynecol Jpn 1985;37:2005–9.
83. Hoeltzli SD, Kelley LK, Moe AJ, Smith CH. Anionic amino acid transport systems in isolated basal plasma membrane of the human placenta. Am J Physiol 1990;259:C47–55.
84. Johnson LW, Smith CH. Neutral amino acid transport systems of microvillous membrane of the human placenta. Am J Physiol 1988;254:C773–80.
85. Furesz T, Moe AJ, Smith CH. Lysine uptake by human placental microvillous membrane: comparison of system y+ with basal membrane. Am J Physiol 1995;37:C755–61.
86. Furesz T, Smith CH. Identification of two leucine sensitive lysine transport activities in human placental basal membrane. Placenta 1997;18:649–55.
87. Furesz T, Moe A, Smith CH. Two cationic amino acid transport systems in human placental basal membrane. Am J Physiol 1991;261:C246–52.
88. Economides DL, Nicolaides KH, Gahl WA, Bernardini I, Evans MI. Plasma amino acids in appropriate- and small-for-gestational-age fetuses. Am J Obstet Gynecol 1989;161:1219–27.
89. Cetin I, Marconi A, Corbetta C, Baggiani A, Battaglia FC, Pardi G. Fetal – maternal amino acid relationships in normal and intrauterine growth retarded (IUGR) pregnancies. Troph Res 1993;7:11–23.
90. Chien PF, Smith K, Watt PW, Scrimgeour CM, Taylor DJ, Rennie MJ. Protein turnover in the human fetus studied at term using stable isotope tracer amino acids. Am J Physiol 1993;265:E31–5.
91. Glazier J, Cetin I, Perugino G, Ronzoni S, Grey A, Mahendran D, et al. Association between the activity of the system A amino acid transporter in the microvillous plasma membrane of the human placenta and severity of fetal compromise in intrauterine growth restriction. Pediatr Res 1997;42:514–19.
92. Dicke JM, Verges DK. Neutral amino acid uptake by microvillous and basal membrane vesicles from appropriate and small-for-gestational age human pregnancies. J Matern Fetal Med 1994;3:246–50.
93. Godfrey KM, Matthews N, Glazier JD, Jackson A, Wilman C, Sibley CP. Neutral amino acid uptake by the microvillous plasma membrane of the human placenta is inversely related to fetal size at birth in normal pregnancy. J Clin Endocrinol Metab 1998;83:3320–6.
94. Norberg S, Powell T, Jansson T. Intrauterine growth restriction is associated with a reduced activity of placental taurine transporters. Pediatr Res 1998;44:233–8.
95. Jansson T, Scholtbach V, Powell T. Placental transport of leucine and lysine is reduced in intrauterine growth restriction. Pediatr Res 1998;44:532–7.
96. Tuchmann-Duplessis H. Drugs acting on the central nervous system. In: Acton MA, editor. Drug effects on the fetus. Publishing Sciences Group, 1975;142–9.
97. Hasselmeyer EG, Meyer MB, Catz C, Longo LD. Pregnancy and infant health. In: Pinney JM, editor. Smoking and health: a report of the Surgeon General. Washington DC:United States Department of Health, Education and Welfare Publication No. (PHS) 79–5006, 1979;8-1–8-93.
98. Frank AD, Bauchner H, Parker S, Huber AM, Kyei-Aboagye K, Cabral H, et al. Neonatal body proportionality and body composition after in utero exposure to cocaine and marijuana. J Pediatr 1990;117:622–6.
99. Fisher SE, Atkinson M, Van Thiel DH. Selective fetal malnutrition: the effect of nicotine, ethanol and acetaldehyde upon in vitro uptake of alpha-aminoisobutyric acid by human term placental villous slices. Dev Pharmacol Ther 1984;7:229–38.
100. Schenker S, Johnson RF, Hays SE, Ganeshappa R, Henderson GI. Effects of nicotine and nicotine/ethanol on human placental amino acid transfer. Alcohol 1989;6:289–96.

101. Dicke JM, Verges DK, Polakoski KL. Cocaine inhibits alanine uptake by human placental microvillous membrane vesicles. Am J Obstet Gynecol 1993;169:515-21.
102. Dicke JM, Verges DK, Polakoski KL. The effect of cocaine on neutral amino acid uptake by human placental basal membrane vesicles. Am J Obstet Gynecol 1994;171:485-91.
103. Barnwell SL, Sastry BVR. Depression of amino acid uptake in human placental villus by cocaine, morphine and nicotine. Troph Res 1983;1:101-20.
104. Sheppard BL, Bonnar J. The maternal blood supply to the placenta in pregnancy complicated by intrauterine fetal growth retardation. Troph Res 1988;3:69-81.

10 Placental Pathology

Harold Fox

The Small for Gestational Age Infant

A baby may be small for a variety of reasons, but there are certain overt maternal and fetal factors which may lead to, or are associated with, a poor fetal growth rate. Maternal factors include severe pre-eclampsia, cigarette smoking, drug abuse and certain infections, such as malaria, whilst the most obvious fetal factors associated with a low birthweight are congenital malformations and chromosomal abnormalities. If cases such as these are removed from consideration there remains an important residue of unduly small infants who are delivered after an apparently uncomplicated pregnancy, are free from congenital malformations and have a normal karotype; it is this group that is considered here.

The placenta of the SGA infant has been the subject of many pathological studies that have utilised light microscopy [1–28], electron microscopy [29–35] and stereology [36–42]. It cannot be said, however, that the efforts of these many workers have been crowned with success in terms of any characteristic or consistent pathological picture having emerged. This lack of agreement has been due to many factors, amongst which can be included differing definitions of fetal growth retardation, selective bias, the inclusion of cases due to pre-eclampsia, a common disregard of maternal smoking habits, a failure to exclude cases in which the neonate has a low birthweight but is not SGA, a neglect of possible maternal drug abuse and a failure to distinguish between those cases of growth retardation in which the neonate has a normal ponderal index and those in which the ponderal index is abnormal. Quite apart from these methodological defects there have been two conceptual deficiencies. The first of these is the partially recognised but commonly ignored fact that idiopathic fetal growth retardation is almost certainly, even after exclusion of all known predisposing fetal and maternal factors, a heterogenous condition that is unlikely to yield a stereotyped pattern of placental findings. Secondly, in many of these studies there has been a background assumption, either stated or implied, that placental abnormalities, lesions or damage result in a state of "placental insufficiency", which is responsible for the defective fetal growth. This view ignores the fact that the placenta has a very considerable physiological reserve capacity and in only very rare cases does it suffer damage of such an extent that it becomes functionally inadequate [43].

Because there has been no agreement abut many aspects of placental pathology in cases of fetal growth restriction the description given here is largely based upon personal observations.

Placental Size

Most, though not all, small babies have small placentas and this commonplace observation has been quantitated by morphometric studies [38,39,41]; it is therefore often assumed that the baby is small *because* the placenta is small, a point of view that implies that fetal size is rigidly limited by placental mass. If, however, fetal growth were narrowly limited by placental mass this would, of necessity, imply that the placenta has little or no functional reserve capacity. Simple pathological studies of lesions such as extensive perivillous fibrin deposition indicate, however, that the placenta can withstand functional inactivation of 30–40 per cent of its villous population without any discernible effect on fetal growth or development [43]: thus the placenta does have a considerable functional reserve capacity, a finding confirmed by experiments involving surgical reduction of placental mass [44] artificially increased fetal oxygen consumption [45] or microsphere embolisation of maternal uteroplacental vessels [46]. Furthermore, the placenta has a normally unrealised potential for increased compensatory growth when in an unfavourable maternal milieu from the start of pregnancy, as is shown by the unduly large placentas seen in pregnancy at high altitude [47], in cases of severe maternal anaemia [48–50], in pregnancies in women with congestive cardiac failure [51] and in many experimental studies that have subjected the placenta to chronic hypoxia [52].

The fact that the placenta does have a very considerable reserve capacity together with a potential for compensatory growth makes it unlikely that placental mass restricts fetal growth and the point made by Gruenwald [53] appears a valid one, namely that the placenta is a fetal organ and therefore shares in any depression of fetal growth, the small fetus not only having a small liver and a small heart but also a small placenta. Thus, the placenta is small because the fetus is small, rather than the reverse. This is, perhaps, an oversimplification but a small placenta will have the capacity to transfer to the fetus all the maternal oxygen and nutrients reaching it in the maternal blood.

Gross Abnormalities

Circumvallate placentation is associated with an increased incidence of low birthweight [27, 54, 55] but most of the neonates so classified only just fall within the defined category of SGA [43]. It is unknown whether this relatively minor deficit in fetal growth is due to this form of placentation being inadequate, possibly because of distortion or constriction of the intervillous space, or whether both the abnormal placental form and the fetal growth deficiency are mutually dependent on a common causal factor.

The overall incidence of infarction tends to be increased in placentas from growth-restricted infants [28,56,57] and Laurini et al. [58] have claimed that infarction is the only placental lesion that correlates with growth retardation; the infarcts in placentas from growth-retarded infants are, however, usually small and most placentas from these infants show no infarction at all. Maternal floor infarction, very extensive perivillous fibrin deposition, widespread thrombosis of fetal arteries and unusually large, or multiple, placental haemangiomas may all be associated with diminished fetal growth [43] but such lesions are found in only a small minority of placentas from SGA infants, the vast majority of such placentas showing no significant gross lesions.

Histological Abnormalities

Histological examination of placentas from SGA infants reveals no constant or diagnostic pathological picture. Many, probably about 25 per cent, are histologically normal in all respects for the length of the gestational period. The remainder either show the features of poor fetal perfusion, evidence of having been subjected to ischaemia or, most commonly, an admixture of both ischaemic and diminished perfusion patterns [43]: the nature of these changes and their pathogenesis are discussed in later sections of this review.

A few placentas from growth-retarded infants show a delay in villous maturation, the villous tissue of a term placenta having, for example, appearances more characteristic of those in a placenta from a 30–32 weeks' gestation. It is not clear whether in these cases the process of maturation is defective from the outset of pregnancy or whether there is an "arrest" of the development of a previously normally maturing villous tree, but villous immaturity of this type is associated with a high incidence of intrauterine fetal growth restriction [59,60]. It should be stressed, however, that villous immaturity is rather a rare finding in placentas from growth-restricted neonates, the villi in most such placentas appearing fully mature for the length of the gestational period.

A villous abnormality which has consistently been shown to be associated with a high incidence of IUGR is villitis [22,28,61–66]. This term is applied to a villous lesion characterised by a chronic inflammatory cell infiltrate, and either single villi or groups of villi may be involved; although occasional instances of a very extensive villitis are encountered it is more common for the affected villi to be few in number and widely scattered. The detection of this lesion depends, to some extent, on the number of sections examined and is subject to considerable interobserver variance [67] but within these restraints the incidence of villitis in placentas from unselected Western populations is between 6 and l4 per cent [62,63]. Villitis of unknown aetiology is seen with undue frequency in placentas from SGA infants, though the reported proportion of such placentas in which this lesion has been found has been very variable, ranging from 7.5 per cent to 86 per cent [22,25,28,64–66,68–70]; most authors have found an incidence in the region of 30 per cent. The significance of this finding is, however, open to debate. A villitis is characteristic of infections reaching the placenta by a haematogenous route [22,43,62] and it has therefore been assumed that this lesion is invariably a hallmark of such infection. Nevertheless a definite infective cause can be established in only a small minority of cases and most instances of villitis are classed as being of unknown aetiology. If villitis is due to infection then its association with fetal growth restriction cannot be explained in terms of placental damage, for the extent of the villous lesions is insufficient to dissipate the functional reserve of the organ; it has therefore been suggested that villitis is indicative of an intrauterine fetal infection, acquired by transplacental passage, and that the inhibitory effect of infection on fetal DNA synthesis could be held responsible for the inadequate fetal growth [43,71].

It must undoubtedly be true that some cases of villitis of unknown aetiology are due to unrecognised infections, possibly viral in nature; indeed, molecular studies have revealed the presence of CMV DNA in a significant proportion of such cases [72,73]. In recent years it has, however, been suggested that in those cases in which a specific infective agent has not been identified the villous lesions are the morphological expression of an immunological reaction within the placental tissues, possibly a host versus graft or a graft versus host reaction [69,70,74–76]. If this is indeed the case, and it remains to be proven, then it would indicate that immunological factors of a currently unidentified nature may be implicated in fetal growth retardation.

Maternal Perfusion

The villi in placentas from growth-restricted fetuses frequently, though far from invariably, show changes that are considered to be a response to uteroplacental ischaemia [33,43]. Thus at the light-microscopic level there is an increased number of villous cytotrophoblastic cells and a degree of thickening of the trophoblastic basement membrane; the villous syncytiotrophoblast appears normal. Electron microscopy confirms the presence of an excess of prominent villous cytotrophoblastic cells; many of these are of the undifferentiated type but a significant proportion are of the intermediate type and contain many cytoplasmic organelles. At the ultrastructural level the villous syncytiotrophoblast shows focal areas of microvillous abnormality, diminished rough endoplasmic reticulum, occasionally decreased but commonly normal pinocytic activity, a reduced number of secretory droplets and small, very localised, areas of syncytial necrosis.

These changes are very similar to those seen in the placenta in pregnancy-induced hypertension [77] and are identical to those noted in placental villous tissue cultured in vitro under conditions of low oxygen tension [78,79]. They are thus very suggestive of placental ischaemia and are explicable in terms of ischaemic syncytiotrophoblastic damage with a secondary repair-hyperplasia change in the villous cytotrophoblastic cells, the stem cells of the villous trophoblast, and resulting repair of the ischaemically damaged syncytiotrophoblast.

That there is, in many cases of idiopathic IUGR, a diminished maternal blood flow to the placenta is now well established, both by the use of older techniques [79–81] and by Doppler studies of the uteroplacental circulation [82–88]; Ferrazzi et al. [89] further showed that there was a clear correlation between an abnormal uteroplacental waveform and the presence of ischaemic changes in the placenta. The pathological basis for a diminished maternal blood supply to the placenta in many cases of intrauterine fetal growth restriction is now reasonably well established. During the early stages of placentation cells from the cytotrophoblastic columns break through the trophoblastic shell and infiltrate into both the underlying decidua and the lumens of the intradecidual portion of the spiral arteries in the placental bed. Those cells entering the vessels, known as the "intravascular extravillous cytotrophoblast", replace the maternal endothelial cells, infiltrate the vessel wall, destroy the medial elastic and muscular tissue and induce deposition of fibrinoid material [90–94]. This process is complete by about the 12th week of gestation but at a later stage, between the 16th and 20th weeks of pregnancy, there is a further retrograde movement of intravascular cytotrophoblastic cells into the intramyometrial portion of the spiral arteries of the placental bed where the same process of endothelial replacement, medial destruction and fibrinoid deposition occur. These changes extend virtually to the point of origin of the spiral arteries from the arcuate vessels and their net result is to convert the thick-walled, muscular spiral arteries into thin-walled, flaccid, sac-like uteroplacental vessels that can easily dilate to accommodate the vastly increased uteroplacental blood flow, which is necessary for fetal nutrition and oxygenation as pregnancy progresses.

Although more recent studies suggest that trophoblastic invasion of the placental bed vessels may not be as temporally rigidly restricted as was originally thought to be the case [95], it nevertheless remains clear that the physiological process of conversion of the spiral arteries into uteroplacental vessels is essentially a two-stage process. It has been known for many years that, in women destined to develop pregnancy-induced hypertension, the second phase of cytotrophoblastic invasion does not occur and there is no migration of extravillous cytotrophoblast into the intramyometrial portions of the spiral arteries [96–98]; there is thus inadequate conversion of the spiral arteries into uteroplacental vessels with subsequent restriction of maternal blood flow to the placenta and a decreased ability of the mother to supply oxygen and nutrients to the fetus. It was originally thought that this defect of placentation was limited to patients with pregnancy-induced hypertension but it has since been established that an identical abnormality is found, though less consistently, in cases of normotensive idiopathic intrauterine fetal growth restriction [99–107]. It should be noted that the defective placentation is quantitative as well as qualitative. In a normal pregnancy all the approximately 150 spiral arteries of the placental bed undergo full physiological change but in cases of abnormal placentation some arteries show no physiological change at all in either their intradecidual or intramyometrial segments; others show normal changes in their intradecidual portions but an absence of change in their intramyometrial segments which, whilst often complete, may be only partial both in the sense that only some vessels are abnormal and in that some vessels may show only a partial abnormality.

The defect in placentation in many cases of idiopathic IUGR does not differ in any way from that found in patients with pregnancy-induced hypertension and is specifically associated with abnormal uterine flow velocity waveforms [108]. There must be strong grounds for presuming that the resultant restriction of maternal blood flow is a crucially important factor in the failure of fetal growth, for in animal studies experimentally induced limitation of placental blood flow will result in an unduly small fetus [52,109]. A further vascular lesion, acute atherosis, may, however, also be present in the maternal vessels in cases of idiopathic fetal growth restriction. This arteriopathy is characterised by fibrinoid necrosis of the vessel wall, an accumulation of lipophages in the damaged wall and a perivascular lymphocytic infiltrate and was originally thought to be restricted to women with pregnancy-induced hypertension [100,103]; in these patients atherosis is seen only in those vessels that have not undergone physiological change, namely the basal arteries and the intramyometrial segments of the spiral arteries of the placental bed. It is now accepted, however, that acute atherosis also occurs in the maternal uterine vasculature in some cases of normotensive IUGR [99,l01,104,107,110–113], and in two studies birthweight has been most markedly reduced in those cases in which atherosis complicated inadequate physiological change [113,114]. The pathogenesis of acute atherosis is unknown, though a strong case has been made for its having an immunological basis [115,116].

Fetal Perfusion

Histological examination of placentas from SGA infants often shows evidence of diminished fetal perfusion of the villous vessels (e.g. small or sclerosed fetal vessels, stromal fibrosis, or an increased number of syncytial knots). It was, however, only with the introduction of Doppler studies of umbilical artery blood flow velocity waveforms and umbilical vein blood flow that serious attention was paid to the possible role played by abnormalities of the placental fetal vasculature in idiopathic IUGR. Trudinger et al. [83,117] showed that in many pregnancies complicated by IUGR there were abnormal waveforms in the fetal umbilical arteries that were indicative of an increased resistance in the placental vascular bed, the inference being that fetal perfusion of the placenta was decreased in such cases. This finding was subsequently confirmed in other studies [118–123] and Doppler studies of umbilical vein blood flow have confirmed the diminished fetal perfusion of the placenta of many growth-restricted fetuses [124].

The morphological basis for the increased resistance in the placental fetal vasculature of growth-restricted fetuses is a matter for dispute. Giles et al. [125] found widespread obliteration of small muscular arteries in the tertiary stem villi in such cases and others have reported similar findings [118,120,126]. Hitschold et al. [123] thought, however, that the basic abnormality was a reduction in the vascularity of the terminal villi, whereas Macara et al. [34,127] did not think that there was any selective loss of small stem villous vessels and also suggested that the increased vascular impedance was at the level of the capillaries in the terminal villi. Because placental vascular resistance increased progressively in serial studies of growth-restricted fetuses in the cases studied by Giles et al. [125] it was thought that the vascular lesion was a progressive one and probably secondary to utero-placental ischaemia. Bracero et al. [120] noted, however, that in some cases placental vascular resistance, although still remaining abnormal, decreased as pregnancy progressed and thought that in such cases there may have been a primary defect, or arrested development, of placental angiogenesis. Jackson et al. [128] agreed, on the basis of a morphometric study, with this view and suggested that the increased vascular resistance was due to reduced villous tree elaboration with a global reduction in placental vascularity. In a not dissimilar study, Kreczy et al. [129] concluded that the high resistance in the fetal vasculature was due to a decreased number of arteries in the tertiary stem villi, a deficiency they also attributed to an early developmental arrest of placental angiogenes.

In personally studied cases a characteristic feature of many placentas from SGA fetuses is an "endarteritis obliterans" in the large stem arteries [33], a finding also noted by others [20,130,131]. This lesion, which is also often present in placentas from pre-eclamptic women [43], has been interpreted on light microscopy as a proliferation and swelling of the endothelial cells; on electron microscopy, however, the apparently swollen endothelial cells are seen to be herniations of medial smooth muscle cytoplasm into the vascular lumen [33], a phenomenon that is known to be the hallmark of a prolonged vasoconstriction. This will, if sustained, lead to a progressive sclerosis and eventual obliteration of the more distal vasculature with diminished vascularisation of the terminal villi. This dynamic vascular change is probably a response to uteroplacental ischaemia; experimental studies have clearly shown that a reduction in maternal blood flow to the placenta is followed by an increased vascular resistance within the fetal placental vasculature and decreased fetal perfusion of the villi [109,132], whereas in dually perfused human placental coyledons "maternal" hypoxia causes vaso-constriction of the fetoplacental vessels [133,134]. In teleological terms this response to placental ischaemia is part of a attempt by the deprived fetus to divert blood to the cerebral and coronary circulations, and though it may seem paradoxical to reduce placental blood flow, the placental tissue can increase oxygen extraction from the maternal blood when the fetal blood flow is decreased and can sustain a flow reduction of 50 per cent without impairing fetal oxygenation [135]. This haemodynamic view of the basis for increased fetal vascular resistance in the placenta of low birthweight infants is conceptually more appealing than the alternative concept of arrested angiogenesis, for it is difficult both to reconcile this latter view with the proven inadequate placentation in many such cases and to suggest an aetiological factor for arrested vascular development. Furthermore the concept of a fixed vascular deficiency accords ill with the observation that in many, though not all, cases of fetal growth restriction maternal hyperoxygenation decreases fetal intraplacental vascular resistance [136,137].

Cytogenetic Abnormalities

Fetal cytogenetic abnormalities are, of course, well known to be associated with diminished fetal growth, but only within recent years has it been recognised that the chromosomal constitution of the placenta is not necessarily the same as that of the fetus, discrepancies between fetus and placenta being usually due to a mosaicism that is not present in the fetus. The abnormal cell line in the placenta is usually a trisomy of chromosome 7, 16 or 18 and in such cases the zygote is often trisomic with postzygotic loss of the extrachromosomal material in the embryonic, but not the trophoblastic, precursor cells. It is a majority view that this condition of confined placental mosaicism is associated with a high incidence of intrauterine fetal growth restriction [138–144], though this has admittedly not been everyone's experience [l45–l47]; paradoxically, confined placental mosaicism also appears to be associated with an increased incidence of unusually high birthweight [141]. The quantitative contribution of confined placental mosaicism to the overall incidence of intrauterine fetal growth restriction remains to be established, though it is unlikely to be high, and it has not yet been shown that this chromosomal abnormality is associated with any histological changes in the placenta.

Conclusions

There must be a strong suspicion that the most important factor in many cases of intrauterine fetal growth restriction is faulty placentation, with inadequate conversion of spiral arteries into uteroplacental blood vessels and a consequent restraint upon the ability of the mother to supply the fetus with nutrients and oxygen, this eventually resulting in a secondary reduction in fetal villous perfusion. Histological evidence of ischaemia is frequently encountered in placentas from growth-restricted infants, whereas attempts to induce experimental fetal growth restriction rely heavily on techniques that reduce maternal placental blood flow [52,109,148].

The cause of the inadequate placentation is just as obscure in cases of idiopathic fetal growth restriction as it is in pre-eclampsia but during placentation there must be some immunological interaction between trophoblastic and maternal tissues, which probably limits the migratory capacity of the trophoblast. It could therefore be postulated that inadequate placentation is often due to an abnormal maternal–trophoblastic immune reaction [149] and that the frequently seen villitis of unknown aetiology in placentas from growth-restricted fetuses is a further hallmark of this abnormal immunological interaction. Furthermore, there is evidence that in many cases of first trimester abortion there is inadequate placentation and it has been suggested that defective trophoblastic migration and invasion may be secondary to a fetal chromosomal abnormality [150]. It is therefore possible that there is a similar defect in cases of restricted placental mosaicism, though the inadequacy of placentation may be less marked than that due to a non-mosaic chromosomally abnormal trophoblast and result in fetal growth restriction rather than first trimester loss.

Inadequate placentation, restricted placental mosaicism and villitis of unknown aetiology can therefore be linked into a unitary hypothesis, one that is admittedly speculative but nevertheless serves to emphasise the dominant role played by a reduced maternal uteroplacental blood flow in many, but certainly not all, pregnancies that result in a child which is small for its gestational age.

This view of the major importance of a restricted maternal uteroplacental flow, with consequent placental and fetal hypoxia, in intrauterine fetal growth restriction has recently been challenged, especially for those cases in which Doppler studies show absent end-diastolic flow velocity [34,35,151–153]. Whilst accepting the evidence, derived from fetal umbilical venous blood studies, that there is fetal hypoxia in such cases [154,155] it has nevertheless been maintained that there is no placental hypoxia, this claim being based on the finding of an unusually high oxygen content in uteroplacental venous blood in cases of intrauterine fetal growth restriction [156]. This apparent discrepancy between "placental hyperoxia" and fetal hypoxia has led to the view that under such circumstances there may be a primary defect in placental nutrient and gas transfer, a defect due to inhibition of the angiogenic drive to form terminal villi by the high oxygen levels in the intervillous space. This interesting and original hypothesis suffers from two major defects, both of which have been pointed out by Burton [157]. First, the theory is heavily dependent upon a single study that demonstrated that the oxygen content and saturation of the uterine venous blood was higher in cases of intrauterine growth restriction than in normal controls [156]; this study has been neither confirmed nor refuted whilst the significance and interpretation of its findings have been questioned [157]. Secondly, the theory invokes a circular argument: abnormal villous development reduces fetal uptake of oxygen with resultant placental hyperoxia, which causes abnormal villous development.

There is clearly a diversity of opinion about the placental features in intrauterine fetal growth restriction with two opposing views that are difficult to reconcile. The difference is basically between those who believe that the causal factors lie outside the placenta and those who consider that intrinsic placental abnormality is of basic importance. Which of these views will eventually prevail is currently open to question though several approaches are reasonably clear:

1. Future studies of placental pathology in intrauterine growth restriction should be closely correlated with Doppler studies and, as has been recently pointed out, a clear distinction has to be drawn between those cases associated with a normal umbilical artery Doppler flow and those in which there is absent or reversed end-diastolic flow velocity (158).

2. Investigations of the placental vasculature in fetal growth restriction should be based on the study of placentas that have been perfusion fixed rather than immersion fixed.

3. Uteroplacental venous blood oxygen levels need to be more fully studied.

4. Most controversies about placental pathology are concerned with the mechanisms by which growth restriction is produced. Less attention has been paid to the basic causes. There is a need to delineate more clearly the quantitative roles played by both villitis and confined placental mosaicism and to determine whether these factors are causally linked to growth restriction.

References

1. Botella-Llusia J Uber das Syndrom der Plazentarinsuffizienz und seine Bedeutung für die praktische Geburtshilfe. Deutsch Med 1961;12:543–6.
2. Gershon R, Strauss L. Structural changes in human placentas associated with fetal inanition or growth arrest ("placental insufficiency syndrome"). Am J Dis Child 1961;102:645–6.
3. Gruenwald P. Abnormalities of placental vascularity in relation to intrauterine deprivation and retardation of fetal growth: significance of avascular chorionic villi. N Y State J Med 1961;61:1508–13.
4. Gruenwald P. Chronic fetal distress and placental insufficiency. Biol Neonat 1963;5:215–65.
5. Rumbolz WL, Edwards MC, McGoogan LS. The small full term infant and placental insufficiency. Western J Surg 1961;69:53–61.
6. Kubli F, Budliger H. Beitrag zur Morphologie der insuffizienten Placenta. Geburts Frauenheil 1963;23:37–43.
7. Wigglesworth JS. Morphological variations in the insufficient placenta. J Obstet Gynaecol Br Cwlth 1964;71:871–84.
8. Bazso J, Gaal J. Histologische Untersuchungen der Plazenta bei im intrauterinen Wachstum zuruckgebliebenen Neugeborenen. Zentralb Gynak 1965;87:1356–66.
9. Tremblay PC, Sybuiski S, Maughan GB. Role of the placenta in fetal malnutrition. Am J Obstet Gynecol 1965;91:597–605.
10. Wilkin P. Pathologie du placenta. Paris: Masson et Cie, 1965.
11. Wong TC, Latour JPA. Microscopic measurement of the placental components in an attempt to assess malnourished newborn infant. Am J Obstet Gynecol 1966;94:942–50.
12. Schuhmann R. Hypotrophes reifes Kind am Termin aus placentarer Ursache (sogenannter placentarer Zwerg). Beitr Pathol Anat Allg Pathol 1969;138:426–35.
13. Younoszai MK, Haworth JC. Placental dimensions and relations in preterm, term and growth retarded infants. Am J Obstet Gynecol 1969;103:265–71.
14. Schrodt U. Morphometrische Untersuchungen der Placenta bei dystrophen Neuegeborenen. Zentralb Gynak 1970;92:671–3.
15. Emmrich P, Lassker G. Morphologische Plazentabefunde in Abhangigkeit vom Grad der intrauterinen Wachstumsretardierung bei Mangelgeburten. Kind Praxis 1970;38:537–9.
16. Emmrich P, Lassker G. Morphologische Plazentabefunde bei Neugeborenen mit intrauteriner Mangelentwicklung. Pathol Microbiol 1971;37:57–72.
17. Busch W. Die Placenta bei der fetalen Mangelentwicklung. Makroskopie und Mikroskopie von 150 Placenten fetaler Mangelentwicklungen. Arch Gynakol 1972;212:333-57.

18. Schuhmann R, Lehmann WD, Geier G. Beziehungen zwischen Plazentamorphologie und Ostrogenwerten im letzten Schwangerschaftsmonen: ein Beitrag zur Morphologie der insuffizienten Plazenta. Z Geburt Perinatol 1972;176:379–90.

19. Scott JM, Jordan JM. Placental insufficiency and the small-for-dates baby. Am J Obstet Gynecol 1972;113:823–32.

20. Bender HG, Werner C, Kortmann HR, Becker V. Zue Endangitisobliterans der Plazentagefasse. Arch Gynakol 1974;221:145–59.

21. Koenig UD, Paulussen F, Hansmann MA. Placentamorphologie und intrauterine Wachstummretardierung. Arch Gynakol 1975;219:377–8.

22. Altshuler G, Russell P, Ermocilla R. The placental pathology of small-for-gestational age infants. Am J Obstet Gynecol 1975;121:351–9.

23. Spaczynski M, Pisarki T, Glyda A. Zmiany morfologiczne w plytach podstawowych lozysk od plodow z niska waga urodzeniowa. (Morphological changes in the basal plates of placenta in deliveries of low weight fetuses.) Ginekol Pol 1976;41:721–6.

24. Driscoll SG. Placental lesions. Clin Perinatol 1979;6:397-402.

25. Garcia AGP. Placental morphology of low-birth-weight infants born at term: gross and microscopic study of 50 cases. Contrib Gynecol Obstet 1982;9:100–12.

26. Rayburn W, Sander C, Compton A. Histologic examination of the placenta in the growth-retarded fetus. Am J Perinatol 1989;6:58–61.

27. Liu QX. Pathology of the placenta from small for gestational age infants. Chin J Obstet Gynecol 1990;25:331–4.

28. Salafia CM, Vintzileos AN, Silberman L, Bantham KF, Vogel CA. Placental pathology of idiopathic intrauterine growth retardation at term. Am J Perinatol 1992;9:179–84.

29. Lister UM. Placental ultrastructure in dysmaturity. In: Pecile A, Finzi C, editors. The foeto-placental unit. Amsterdam: Excerpta Medica, 1969;8–17.

30. Theuring F, Kemnitz P. Electronenmikroskopische Plazentabefunde bei fetaler Wachstumretardierung. Zentralb allg Pathol 1974;118:82–9.

31. Sandstedt B. The placenta and low birthweight. Curr Top Pathol 1979;66:1–55.

32. Sheppard B, Bonnar J. Ultrastructural abnormalities of placental villi in placentae from pregnancies complicated by intrauterine fetal growth retardation: their relationship to decidual spiral arterial lesions. Placenta 1980;1:145–56.

33. Van der Veen F, Fox H. The human placenta in idiopathic intrauterine growth retardation: a light and electron microscopic study. Placenta 1983;4:65–78.

34. Macara L, Kingdom JCP, Kaufmann P, Kohnen G, Hair J, More IAR, et al. Structural analysis of placental terminal villi from growth-restricted pregnancies with abnormal umbilical artery Doppler waveforms. Placenta 1996;17:37–48.

35. Kingdom JCP, Macara L, Krebs C, Leiser R, Kaufmann P. Pathological basis for abnormal umbilical artery doppler waveforms in pregnancies complicated by intrauterine growth restriction: a review. Troph Res 1997;10:291–309.

36. Aherne W, Dunnill MS. Quantitative aspects of placental structure. J Pathol Bacteriol 1966;91:123–39.

37. Clavero-Nunez JA, Negueruela J, Botella-Llusia J. Placental morphometry and placental ciculometry. J Reprod Med 1971;6:23–31.

38. Teasdale F. Idiopathic intrauterine growth retardation: histomorphometry of the human placenta. Placenta 1984;5:83–92.

39. Boyd PA, Scott A. Quantitative structural studies on human placentae associated with pre-eclampsia, essential hypertension and intrauterine growth retardation. Br J Obstet Gynaecol 1985;92:714–21.

40. Li BZ. The stereological study on normal and intrauterine growth retardation (IUGR) placentae. Chin J Pathol 1992;21:227-8.

41. Shen Y. Stereological study of the placentae in intrauterine growth retardation with different ponderal index. Chin J Obstet Gynecol 1992;27:35l–4.

42. Karsdorp VHM, Dirks BK, van der Linden JC, van Vugt JMG, Baak JPA, van Geijn HP. Placenta morphology and absent or reversed end diastolic flow velocities in the umbilical artery: a clinical and morphological study. Placenta 1996;17:393–9.

43. Fox H. Pathology of the placenta, 2nd edn. Philadelphia: WB Saunders, 1997.

44. Robinson JS, Kingston EJ, Jones CT, Thornburn GD. Studies on experimental growth retardation in sheep: the effect of removal of endometrial caruncles on fetal size and metabolism. J Dev Physiol 1979;1:379–98.

45. Lorijn RHW, Longo LD. Clinical and physiologic implications of increased fetal oxygen consumption. Am J Obstet Gynecol 1980;136:451–7.

46. Charlton V, Johengen M. Fetal intravenous nutritional supplementation ameliorates the development of embolized induced growth retardation in sheep. Ped Res 1988;22:55-61.
47. Kruger H, Arias-Stella J. The placenta and the new born infant at high altitudes. Am J Obstet Gynecol 1970;106:586-91.
48. Beischer NA, Sivasamboo R, Vohra S, Silpisornkosal S, Reid S. Placental hypertrophy in severe pregnancy anaemia. J Obstet Gynaecol Br Commonwlth 1970;77:398-409.
49. Agboola A. Placental changes in patients with a low haematocrit. Br J Obstet Gynaecol 1975;82:225-7.
50. Godfrey KM, Redman OWO, Barker DJP, Osmond C. The effect of maternal anaemia and iron deficiency on the ratio of fetal weight to placental weight. Br J Obstet Gynaecol 1991;98:886-91.
51. Clavero-Nunez JA. La placenta de las cardiacas. Rev Esp Obstet Ginecol 1963;22:129-34.
52. Robinson JS, Owens J. The placenta and intrauterine growth retardation. In: Redman CWG, Sargent IL, Starkey PM, editors. The human placenta. Oxford: Blackwell Scientific 1993;558-78.
53. Gruenwald P. The supply line of the fetus: definitions relating to fetal growth. In: Gruenwald P, editor. The placenta and its maternal supply line. Lancaster: Medical and Technical Publishing, 1975;1-17.
54. Fox H, Sen DK. Placenta extrachorialis: a clinico-pathological study. J Obstet Gynaecol Br Commonwlth 1972;79:32-5.
55. Rolschau J. Circumvallate placenta and intrauterine growth retardation. Acta Obstet Gynecol Scand 1978;(Suppl)72:11-14.
56. Bjoro KJ. Gross pathology of the placenta in intrauterine growth retardation. Ann Chir Gynecol Fenn 1981;70:316-22.
57. Suska P, Vierik J, Handzo I, Krizko M. Vyskyt makroskopickych zmien placent u intrauterinne rastovo retardovanych novorodencov (Incidence of macroscopic changes in the placenta in intrauterine growth retardation in neonates) Brat Lek Listy 1989;90:604-7.
58. Laurini R, Laurin J, Marsal K. Placental histology and fetal blood flow in intrauterine growth retardation. Acta Obstet Gynecol Scand 1994;73:529-34.
59. Becker V. Pathologie des Ausreifung der Plazenta. In: Becker V, Shiebler T, Kubli F, editors. Die Plazenta der Menschen. Stuttgart: Thieme, 1981;266-81.
60. Schweikhart G, Kaufmann P. Endzottenmangel und klinische Relevanz. Gynakol Rundsch 1987;27:147-8.
61. Altshuler G, Russell P. The human placental villitides: a review of chronic intrauterine infection. Curr Top Pathol 1975;60:63-112.
62. Russell P. Inflammatory lesions of the human placenta. II Villitis of unknown etiology in perspective. Am J Diag Gynecol Obstet 1979;1:339-46.
63. Knox WF, Fox H. Villitis of unknown aetiology: its incidence and significance in placentae from a British population. Placenta 1984;5:395-402.
64. Bjoro KJ, Myhre E. The role of chronic non-specific inflammatory lesions of the placenta in intrauterine growth retardation. Acta Pathol Microbiol Immunol Scand 1984;92:133-7.
65. Mortimer G, MacDonald DJ, Smeeth A. A pilot study of the incidence and significance of placental villitis. Br J Obstet Gynaecol 1985;92:629-33.
66. Nordenvall M, Sandstedt B. Placental villitis and intrauterine growth retardation in a Swedish population. Acta Pathol Microbiol Immunol Scand 1990;98:19-24.
67. Khong TY, Staples A, Moore L, Byard RW. Observer reliability in assessing villitis of unknown aetiology. J Clin Pathol 1993;46:208-10.
68. Labarrere C, Althabe O, Telenta M. Chronic villitis of unknown aetiology in placentae of idiopathic small for gestational age infants. Placenta 1982;3:309-18.
69. Labarrere C, Althabe 0, Calenti E, Musculo D. Deficiency of blocking factors in intrauterine growth retardation and its relationship with chronic villitis. Am J Reprod Immunol Microbiol 1986;10:14-19.
70. Althabe O, Labarrere C. Chronic villitis of unknown aetiology and intrauterine growth-retarded infants of normal and low ponderal index. Placenta 1985;6:369-73.
71. Fox H. The placenta and infection. In: Redman CWG, Sargent IL, Starkey PM, editors. The human placenta. London: Blackwell, 1993;313-33.
72. Sachdev R, Nuovo GJ, Kaplan C, Greco MA. In situ hybridization analysis for cytomegalovirus in chronic villitis. Pediatr Pathol 1990;10:909-17.
73. Nakamura Y, Sakuma S, Ohta Y, Kawano K, Hashimoto T. Detection of the human cytomegalovirus gene in placental chronic villitis by polymerase chain reaction. Hum Pathol 1994;25:815-8.
74. Redline RW, Abramowsky CR. Clinical and pathologic aspects of recurrent placental villitis. Hum Pathol 1986;16:727-31.

75. Labarrere CA, McIntyre JA, Faulk WP. Immunohistologic evidence that villitis in human normal term placentas is an immunologic lesion. Am J Obstet Gynecol 1990;162:515–22.

76. Redline RW. Placental pathology: a neglected link between basic disease mechanisms and untoward pregnancy outcome. Curr Opin Obstet Gynecol 1995;7:10–15.

77. Jones CJP, Fox H. An ultrastructural and ultrahistochemical study of the human placenta in maternal pre-eclampsia. Placenta 1980;1:61–76.

78. Fox H. Effects of hypoxia on trophoblast in organ culture. Am J Obstet Gynecol 1970;107:1058–4.

79. MacLennon AH, Sharp F, Shaw-Dunn J. The ultrastructure of human trophoblast in spontaneous and induced hypoxia using a system of organ culture. J Obstet Gynaecol Commonwlth 1972;79:113–21.

80. Chatfield WR, Rogers TGH, Brownlee BEW, Ripon PE. Placental scanning with computer-linked gamma camera to detect impaired placental blood flow and intrauterine growth retardation. Br Med J 1975;2:120–2.

81. Lunell NO, Sarby B, Lewander R et al. Comparison of uteroplacental blood flow in normal and in intrauterine growth-retarded pregnancy. Gynecol Obstet Invest 1979;10:106–18.

82. Trudinger BJ, Giles WB, Cook CM. Uteroplacental blood flow velocity – time waveforms in normal and complicated pregnanqy. Br J Obstet Gynaecol 1985;92:39–45.

83. Trudinger BJ, Giles, WB, Cook CM. Flow velocity waveforms in the maternal uteroplacental and fetal umbilical placental circulations. Am J Obstet Gynecol 1985;152:155-63.

84. McCowan LM, Ritchie K, Mo LY, Bascom PA, Sherret H. Uterine artery flow velocity waveforms in normal and growth retarded pregnancies. Am J Obstet Gynecol 1988;158:499–504.

85. Jacobson S-L, Imhof R, Manning M, Mannion V, Little D, Rey E, et al. The value of Doppler assessment of the uteroplacental circulation in predicting preeclampsia or intrauterine growth retardation. Am J Obstet Gynecol 1990;162:110–14.

86. Bewley SM, Cooper D, Campbell S. Doppler investigation of uteroplacental blood flow resistance in the second trimester: a screening study for pre-eclampsia and intrauterine growth retardation. Br J Obstet Gynaecol 1991;98:871–9.

87. Schulman H. Uteroplacental flow velocity. In: Chervenak FA, Isaacson GC, Campbell S, editors. Ultrasound in obstetrics and gynecology. Boston: Little Brown, 1993;569–77.

88. Iwata M, Matsuzaki N, Shimizu I, Mitsuda N, Nakayama M, Suehara N. Prenatal detection of ischemic changes in the placenta of the growth-retarded fetus by Doppler flow velocimetry of the maternal uterine artery. Obstet Gynecol 1993;82:494–9.

89. Ferrazzi E, Antonio B, Gaetano B, Laura M, Alessandra P. Ischemic haemorragic placental damage and vascular lesions is associated with abnormal uteroplacental Doppler waveform in growth retarded fetuses. J Perinat Med 1994;22(suppl 1):73–8.

90. Brosens I, Robertson WB, Dixon HG. The physiological response of the vessels of the placental bed to normal pregnancy. J Pathol Microbiol 1967;93:569–79.

91. De Wolf F, De Wolf-Peeters C, Brosens I, Robertson WB. The human placental bed: electron microscopic study of trophoblastic invasion of spiral arteries. Am J Obstet Gynecol 1980;137:58–70.

92. Gerretsen G, Huisjes HJ, Hardouk MJ, Elema JD. Trophoblast alterations in the placental bed in relation to physiological changes in spiral arteries. Br J Obstet Gynaecol 1983;90:34–9.

93. Pijnenborg R, Dixon HG, Robertson WB, Brosens I. Trophoblastic invasion of human decidua from 8 to 18 weeks of pregnancy. Placenta 1980;1:3–19.

94. Pijnenborg R, Bland JM, Robertson WB, Brosens I. Uteroplacental arterial changes related to interstitial trophoblast migration in early human pregnancy. Placenta 1983;4:397–414.

95. Pijnenborg R, Anthony J, Davey DA, Rees A, Tiltman A, Vercruysse L, et al. Placental bed spiral arteries in the hypertensive disorders of pregnancy. Br J Obstet Gynaecol 1991;98:649–5.

96. Brosens I, Robertson WB, Dixon HG. The role of the spiral arteries in the pathogenesis of preeclampsia. In: Wynn RM, editor. Obstetrics and gynecology annual, 1. New York: Appleton-Century-Crofts, 1972;177–91.

97. Robertson WB, Brosens I, Dixon HG. Uteroplacental vascular pathology. Eur J Obstet Gynecol Reprod Biol 1975;5:47–65.

98. Robertson WB. Uteroplacental vasculature. J Clin Pathol 1976;(Suppl 10):9–17.

99. Sheppard BL, Bonnar J. The ultrastructure of the arterial supply of the human placenta in pregnancy complicated by fetal growth retardation. Br J Obstet Gynaecol 1976;83:948–59.

100. Brosens I, Dixon HG, Robertson WB. Fetal growth retardation and the vasculature of the placental bed. Br J Obstet Gynaecol 1977;84:656–64.

101. Sheppard B, Bonnar J. An ultrastructural study of uteroplacental spiral arteries in hypertensive and normotensive pregnancy and fetal growth retardation. Br J Obstet Gynaecol 1981;88:695–705.

102. Robertson WB, Brosens I, Dixon HG. Maternal blood supply in fetal growth retardation. In: Van Assche A, Robertson WB, editors. Fetal growth retardation. Edinburgh: Churchill Livingstone, 1981;126–38.

103. Gerretsen G, Huisjes HJ, Elema JD. Morphological changes of the spiral arteries in the placental bed in relation to preeclampsia and fetal growth retardation. Br J Obstet Gynaecol 1981;88:876–81.

104. Hustin J, Foidart JM, Lambotte R. Maternal vascular lesions in pre-eclampsia and intrauterine growth retardation: light microscopy and immunofluorescence. Placenta 1983;4:489–98.

105. Khong TY, DeWolf F, Robertson WB, Brosens I. Inadequate maternal vascular response to placentation in pregnancies complicated by pre-eclampsia and by small-forgestational-age infants. Br J Obstet Gynaecol 1986;93:1049–59.

106. Robertson WB, Khong TY, Brosens I, DeWolf F, Sheppard BL, Bonnar J. The placental bed biopsy: review from three European centers. Am J Obstet Gynecol 1986;155:401–12.

107. Khong TY, Robertson WB. Spiral artery disease. In Coulam CB, Faulk WP, McIntyre JA, editors. Immunological obstetrics. New York: Norton, 1992;492–501.

108. Lin S, Shimizu I, Suehara N, Nakayama M, Aono T. Uterine artery Doppler velocimetry in relation to trophoblast migration into the myometrium of the placental bed. Obstet Gynecol 1995;85:760–5.

108. Clapp JF. Physiological adaptation to intrauterine growth retardation. In: Ward RHT, Smith SK, Donnai D, editors. Early fetal growth and development. London: RCOG Press, 1994;371–83.

110. DeWolf F, Brosens I, Renaer M. Fetal growth retardation and the maternal arterial supply of the human placenta in the absence of sustained hypertension. Br J Obstet Gynaecol 1980;87:678–85.

111. Althabe O, Laberrere C, Telenta M. Maternal vascular lesions in placentae of small-for-gestational-age infants. Placenta 1985;6:369–73.

112. Khong TY. Acute atherosis in pregnancies complicated by hypertension, small-for-gestational-age infants and diabetes mellitus. Arch Pathol Lab Med 1991;115:722-5.

113. McFadyen IR, Price AB, Geirsson RT. The relation of birth weight to histological appearances in vessels of the placental bed. Br J Obstet Gynaecol 1986;93:47–51.

114. Frusca T, Morassi L, Pecorelli S, Grigolata P, Gastaldi A. Histological features of uteroplacental vessels in normal and hypertensive patients in relation to birthweight. Br J Obstet Gynaecol 1989;96:835–9.

115. Labarrere C, Alonso J, Manni J, Domenichini E, Althabe O. Immunohistochemical findings in acute atherosis associated with intrauterine growth retardation. Am J Reprod Immunol Microbiol 1985;7:149–55.

116. Labarrere C. Acute atherosis: a histopathological hallmark of immune aggression? Placenta 1988;9:95–108.

117. Trudinger BJ, Giles WB, Cook CM, Bombardieri J, Collins L. Fetal umbilical artery flow velocity waveforms and placental resistance: clinical significance. Br J Obstet Gynaecol 1985;92:23–30.

118. McCowan LM, Mullen BM, Ritchie K. Umbilical artery flow velocity waveforms and the placental vascular bed. Am J Obstet Gynecol 1987;157:900–2.

119. Gudmundsson S, Marsal K. Umbilical and uteroplacental blood flow velocity waveforms in pregnancies with fetal growth retardation. Eur J Obstet Gynecol Reprod Biol 1988;27:187–96.

120. Bracero LA, Beneck D, Kirshenbaum, N, Peiffer M, Stalter P, Schulman H. Doppler velocimetry and placental disease. Am J Obstet Gynecol 1989;161:388–93.

121. Ritchie JW. Use of Doppler technology in assessing fetal health. J Develop Physiol 1991;15:121–3.

122. Zacutti A, Borruto F, Bottacci G, Giannoni ML, Manzin A, Pallini M. Umbilical blood flow and placental pathology. Clin Exp Obstet Gynecol 1992;19:63–9.

123. Hitschold T, Weiss E, Beck T, Hunterfering H, Berle P. Low target birthweight or growth retardation? Umbilical Doppler flow velocity waveforms and histometric analysis of the fetoplacental vascular tree. Am J Obstet Gynecol 1993;168:1260–4.

124. Gill RW, Warren PS, Garrett WJ, Kossoff G, Stewart A. Umbilical vein blood flow. In: Chervenak FA, Isaacson GC, Campbell S, editors. Ultrasound in obstetrics and gynecology. Boston: Little, Brown, 1993;587–95.

125. Giles WB, Trudinger BJ, Baird PJ. Fetal umbilical artery flow velocity wavelengths and placental resistance: pathologic correlation. Br J Obstet Gynaecol 1985;92:31–8.

126. Fok RY, Pavlova Z, Benirschke K, Paul RH, Platt TD. The correlation of arterial lesions with umbilical artery Doppler velocimetry in the placentas of small-for-dates pregnancies. Obstet Gynecol 1990;75:578–83.

127. Macara L, Kingdom JCP, Kohnen G, Bowman AW, Greer IA, Kaufman P. Elaboration of stem villous vessels in growth restricted pregnancies with abnormal umbilical artery Doppler waveforms. Br J Obstet Gynaecol 1995;102:807–12.

128. Jackson MR, Walsh AJ, Morrow RJ, Mullen JB, Lye SJ, Ritchie JWK. Reduced placental villous tree elaboration in small-for-gestational-age newborn pregnancies: relationship with umbilical artery Doppler waveforms. Am J Obstet Gynecol 1995;172:518–25.

129. Kreczy A, Fusi L, Wigglesworth JS. Correlation between umbilical arterial flow and placental morphology. Int J Gynecol Pathol 1995;14:306–9.

130. Koenig UD. Proliferative Gefassveranderungen der kindlichen Plazentargefasse und ihre Beziehung zur Plazentarinsuffizienz und Fruhgeburt. Zeitschr Geburtsh Perinatol 1972;176: 356–64.

131. Koenig UD, Mersmann B, Haupt H. Proliferative plazentare Gefassveranderungen: Schwangerschaft und perinateler Verlauf beim Kind. Zeitschr Geburtsh Perinatol 1973;177: 58–64.

132. Stock MK, Anderson DF, Phernetton TM, McLaughlin MK, Rankin JHG. Vascular response of the fetal placenta to local occlusion of the maternal placental vasculature. J Dev Physiol 1980;2:339–46.

133. Howard RB, Hosokawa T, Maguire MH. Hypoxia-induced fetoplacental vasoconstriction in perfused human placental coyledons. Am J Obstet Gynecol 1987;157:1261–6.

134. Byrne BM, Howard RB, Morrow RJ, Whiteley KJ, Adamson SL. Role of the l-arginine nitric oxide pathway in hypoxic fetoplacental vasoconstriction. Placenta 1997;18:627–34.

135. Istkovitz J, LaGamma EF, Rudolph AM. The effect of reducing umbilical blood flow on fetal oxygenation. Am J Obstet Gynecol 1983;145:813–18.

136. Bilardo CM, Snijders RN, Campbell S, Nicolaides K. Doppler study of the fetal circulation during long-term maternal hyperoxygenation for severe early onset intrauterine growth retardation. Ultrasound Obstet Gynecol 1991;1:250–7.

137. de Rochembeau B, Poix D, Mellier G. Maternal hyperoxygenation: a fetal blood flow velocity prognosis test in small-for-gestational-age fetuses. Ultrasound Obstet Gynecol 1992;2:279–82.

138. Kalousek DK, Dill FJ, Pantzar D, McGillivray BC, Yong SL, Wilson RD. Confined chorionic mosaicism in prenatal diagnosis. Hum Genet 1987;77:163–7.

139. Kalousek DK. Confined placental mosaicism and intrauterine development. Ped Pathol 1990;10:69–77.

140. Post JG, Nijhuis JG. Trisomy 16 confined to the placenta. Prenat Diagn 1992;12:1001–7.

141. Wolstenholme J, Rooney DE, Davison EV. Confined placental mosaicism, IUGR, and adverse pregnancy outcome: a controlled retrospective U.K. collaborative study. Prenat Diagn 1994;14:345–61.

142. Kalousek DK, Langlois S. The effects of placental and somatic chromosomal mosaicism on fetal growth. In: Ward RHT, Smith SK, Donnai D, editors. Early fetal growth and development. London: RCOG Press, 1994;246–56.

143. Kalousek DK. Current topic: confined placental mosaicism and intrauterine fetal development. Placenta 1994;15:219–30.

144. Wilkins-Haug L, Roberts DJ, Morton CC. Confined placental mosaicism and intrauterine growth retardation: a case control analysis of placentas at delivery. Am J Obstet Gynecol 1995;172:44–50.

145. Schwinger E, Seidl E, Klink F, Rehder H. Chromosome mosaicism of the placenta – a cause of developmental failure of the fetus? Prenat Diagn 1989;9:639–47.

146. Kennerknecht I, Kramer S, Grab D, Terinde R, Vogel W. A prospective cytogenetic study of third-trimester placentae in small-for-date but otherwise normal newborns. Prenat Diagn 1993;13:257–69.

147. Roland B, Lynch L, Berkowitz G, Zinberg R. Confined placental mosaicism in CVS and pregnancy outcome. Prenat Diagn 1994;14:589–93.

148. Carter AM. Current topic: restriction of placental and fetal growth in the guinea-pig. Placenta 1993;14:125–35.

149. King A, Loke YW. Unexplained fetal growth retardation: what is the cause? Arch Dis Child 1994;70:F225–7.

150. Hustin J, Jauniaux E. Morphology and mechanisms of abortion. In: Barnea ER, Hustin J, Jauniaux E, editors. The first twelve weeks of gestation. Berlin: Springer-Verlag, 1992;280–96.

151. Krebs C, Macara L, Leiser R, Bowman AW, Greer IA, Kingdom JCP. Intrauterine growth restriction with absent end-diastolic flow velocity in the umbilical artery is associated with maldevelopment of the terminal placental villous tree. Am J Obstet Gynecol 1996;175: 1534–42.

152. Lyall K, Kingdom JCP, Greer IA. VEGF expression in placentas from pregnancies complicated by pre-eclampsia and/or intrauterine growth restriction. Placenta 1997;18:269–76.

153. Kingdom JCP, Kaufmann P. Current topic: oxygen and placental villous development: origins of fetal hypoxia. Placenta 1997;18:613–21.

154. Nicolaides KH, Bilardo CM, Soothill PW, Campbell S. Absence of end-diastolic frequencies in the umbilical artery: a sign of fetal hypoxia and acidosis. BMJ 1988;297:1026–7.

155. Nicolini U, Nicolaidis P, Fisk NM, Vaughan JI, Fusi I, Gleeson R, et al. Limited role of fetal blood sampling in prediction of outcome in intrauterine growth retardation. Lancet 1991;336:768–72.

156. Pardi G, Cetin L, Marconi AM, Bozzetti P, Buscaglia M, Makowski EL, et al. Venous drainage of the human uterus: respiratory gas studies in normal and fetal growth retarded pregnancies. Am J Obstet Gynecol 1992;166:699–706.

157. Burton GJ. Invited commentary: on "oxygen and placental villous development: origins of fetal hypoxia". Placenta 1997;18:625–6.

158. Kingdom J. Current topic: Adriana and Luisa Castellucci Award Lecture 1997: placental pathology in obstetrics: adaptation or failure of the villous tree. Placenta 1998;19:347–51.

Section 2
Clinical Management

11 Ultrasound Assessment

Torvid Kiserud and Karel Maršál

Introduction

The introduction of ultrasound technology in obstetrics has totally changed the antenatal scenario. In the early days, the term "screening" was used when the ultrasound examination was offered to the pregnant population and used for assessing number of fetuses, gestational age, placental localisation, fetal anatomy, and fetal size. The procedure has later been termed "routine ultrasound examination", but the ethical controversies and the discussion of its benefits have not ceased. In industrialised countries the majority of the pregnant population undergoes at least one ultrasound examination, and in some countries the ultrasound examination has become a firmly integrated part of antenatal care, involving two, three, or more examinations for screening or surveillance. The obvious advantages of ultrasound technology have favoured a rapidly increasing use of the technology in the developing world as well. The rationale for ultrasound practice, however, varies greatly because of differing standards of the equipment, skills, allocated time and resources, purpose of the examination, population characteristics, socio-economic conditions, nutritional status and morbidity pattern. This should be kept in mind when applying current knowledge in the daily clinic or when studies are planned, interpreted and evaluated. Particularly so, since much of the systematic information on ultrasound examination is collected with the best equipment in a small, privileged part of the world's population.

There is always a temptation to contrast big and healthy with small and sick. We do not want to introduce such simplistic assumptions into diagnostic ultrasound during pregnancy, but until today, this has been very difficult to escape. By our ultrasound examination we consistently stigmatise 10, 5, 3 or 2.5 per cent of the fetuses as IUGR owing to insufficient definition and diagnostic discrimination. However, a small baby may turn out to have a more favourable outcome than the well grown, for example by incurring a lower risk of obstructed labour [1]. The variation in perinatal statistics seen around the world makes it advisable to be cautious when using technology and statistics in the evaluation of individual pregnancies.

Ultrasound biometry is the key for assessing fetal age, size and growth. In the following, we shall discuss this as well as additional ultrasound examinations used to identify risk and morbidity.

The Normal Length of Pregnancy

Assessment of the duration of a normal pregnancy is a prerequisite for practically all obstetrics. However obvious it may seem, the length of the pregnancy is not unequivocally defined. For years, the LMP was used when calculating the date of confinement according to Nägele's rule with the pregnancy length set to 280 days (40 weeks). This is still commonly used in clinical work and, indeed, is the definition used by the World Health Organisation. However, a different pregnancy length has been found in a number of studies. In a study of 427,581 singleton births entered into the Swedish Medical Birth Registry during the period 1976–80, Bergsjø et al. found that, in those with reliable information about the LMP, the average duration of pregnancy from LMP to vaginal delivery was 281 days (mean), 282 days (median) and 283 days (mode) [2]. The study was criticised for including induced vaginal deliveries. Others have found the period between a certain LMP and spontaneous delivery to be slightly longer: mean and median 284 days [3,4]. When including preterm deliveries, malformations and stillbirths in a group of 865 women with certain 28 days' cycle, Kieler et al. found a mean pregnancy length of 282.5 and median 284 days for LMP dating, and, correspondingly 279.6 and 280 when using dates based on BPD measurements [4]. In a study of 9,402 singleton pregnancies and certain LMP dates, Tunón et al. found the mean to be 281.8 and median to be 283 days for LMP dating, and correspondingly 279.1 and 281 days for ultrasound [5]. Malformations, but not preterm labour, were excluded. Low maternal age, increased parity, and male fetuses favour a slightly shorter duration of pregnancy [2]. However, when using ultrasound dating, there is a tendency towards a shorter pregnancy for female fetuses [4]. This is probably due to the larger BPD found in male fetuses at the time of the ultrasound examination used for dating [6,7].

Artificially induced ovulation and in vitro fertilisation represent pregnancies with known dates of conception. The studies conducted on such groups show that the ultrasound measurements are not at great variance with previous studies of the normal population [8–10]. The problem encountered by such studies is that the number included in the statistics is small and that the group of women with subfertility problems does not reflect the general population.

There are statistical arguments for including premature deliveries and using the mode, which is less influenced by extreme values, when establishing the standard of length of pregnancy [11]. When using the mode and including the prematurely born in the statistics, there is still a difference of 3 days between the two methods [5]. As both ways of assessing gestational age are based on certain assumptions and determination by ultrasound is done some time in the second trimester, it is reasonable to assume that there is a "built-in" correction factor in the ultrasound dating charts that makes the pregnancies appear to conform with the 280 day rule, while LMP dating appears to give a shift to the right. In any case, it is wise to keep in mind that the length of a pregnancy determined by different methods may differ by 1–4 days.

Assessment of Gestational Age: LMP, Ultrasound, or Conception?

In order to assess fetal size and growth, the pregnancy has to be accurately dated. In fact, determining the gestational age was considered to be the main purpose of ultrasound screening in the early days of obstetric ultrasound development. Although ultrasound provides a reliable date of confinement in the many pregnancies with uncertain or unknown LMP, the LMP-based calculation is still a very useful and often indispensable method. It is easy, inexpensive, sufficiently accurate for the level of care otherwise achievable for the pregnant woman, and the perinatal charts still in use in many areas are actually based on LMP-data alone.

However, the assessment of gestational age based on LMP is liable to be inaccurate in quite a high proportion of the pregnant women. In some populations in the industrialised world, as many as half of the pregnancies are reported to have unreliable information on LMP, and in other cultures and traditions this number may be higher [12]. Particularly in order to cope with such problems, ultrasound biometry represents an improvement in the precision of gestational age assessment that cannot be challenged. It is quite common, however, to prefer the LMP-date if the discrepancy between the two dates is ≤ 7 days (others use ≤ 10 or ≤ 14 days). There is now growing evidence that the ultrasound method predicts spontaneous delivery more precisely than the "certain LMP" method does [4,5,13,14]. In most centres where ultrasound is extensively used, the recommendation to use ultrasound exclusively for all pregnancies dated before 21–24 postmenstrual weeks is probably a reasonable dating routine [12,15].

There are, however, some problems connected with such an approach. Even the most appropriate charts for assessing gestational age by means of ultrasound are constructed on LMP-based gestational age. For their new charts for dating, Altman and Chitty used LMP based gestational age, but excluded those with uncertain LMP, irregular cycles or a difference of > 10 days between ultrasound and LMP dating [16]. How can ultrasound then be a better predictor of spontaneous birth than a certain LMP for a woman with regular cycles? There are several possible explanations:

There are indications that certain LMP information is liable to be uncertain (how LMP was actually determined) and variation (natural fluctuation of the time of ovulation) [12]. Such uncertainties represent a higher variation. If this variation is reasonably evenly distributed around the mean, the constructed mean will not be affected. When assessing gestational age by ultrasound, the measured BPD is compared with the mean value in the chart and the corresponding age used as the new gestational age for the pregnancy, disregarding variation. If the variation of BPD measurements and biological variation of fetal size in early pregnancy are less than the variation caused by the method of certain LMP, the BPD assessment will, statistically, be a more precise predictor of date of birth. This corresponds to the findings of Kieler, Mongelli and Tonón that ultrasound predicts spontaneous birth better than accurate LMP information does [4,5,14].

Another explanation can be sought in the natural variation of fetal size and duration of pregnancy. Given that fetal size at 17–20 weeks of gestation is a stronger determinant for date of birth than actual fetal age, if age is uniformly set according to the size found by ultrasound at this stage, this will predict birth better. This will disregard a possible normal variation of actual pregnancy length expressed before the ultrasound assessment. In the majority of pregnancies, this will probably do no harm.

For the 50 per cent of fetuses smaller than the mean, however, the ultrasound assessment at 17–20 weeks consistently underestimates their gestational age. The smaller they are, the greater the underestimation. Thus the ultrasound dating shifts this group to an artificially lower gestational age at spontaneous birth – and lower preterm delivery rates [17]. In addition, the difference in size of BPD between boys and girls at 18 weeks gestation will systematically assess the female population to be younger than the male. The difference, which is reflected in growth charts, gestational age at birth, and birthweight, is small (0.7 day) and is not believed to influence clinical judgement [18].

However these issues are important for the management of the smallest fetuses in whom IUGR is not appreciated, or its detection is delayed until a later stage in pregnancy. This may become particularly relevant if valid treatment options emerge for IUGR (see Ch. 16).

Since antenatal care is especially aimed at identifying such risk pregnancies, many obstetricians offer a first trimester ultrasound examination to minimise this type of error in ultrasound dating. Indeed the role of first trimester scanning is now expanding to include aneuploidy assessment by nuchal translucency and screening for major structural abnormalities. In the absence of a reliable crown–rump length measurement, the obstetrician will have to combine all the available information to assess the pregnancy as accurately as possible.

Since ovulation induction, fertilisation and embryo transfer represent certain records for calculating gestational age, the women in such a programme will have their gestational age set at 14 days at the time of oocyte retrieval [8]. An early first trimester ultrasound examination should be performed to confirm this age and rule out a misinterpretation due to an early abortion and a later naturally conceived pregnancy.

Commonly Used Ultrasound Measurements

Crown–Rump Length (CRL)

CRL is defined as the distance between the top of the head and the rump of the embryo or fetus (Fig. 11.1). Through the years, Robinson and Fleming's charts of the embryonic and fetal CRL have proved to provide reproducible measures for first trimester assessment of gestational age [8,19–21]. With modern transvaginal equipment, this method has 95 per cent prediction intervals of ± 4.7 days when the fetal size is 1–80 mm, which corresponds to 6–11 weeks [9]. The improved resolution provided by high frequency ultrasound shows that, strictly speaking, the commonly measured greatest embryonic length is different from the true anatomical CRL [9]. As long as the difference is small, and most charts are probably based on the greatest length of the embryo anyway, the method remains the most reliable predictor of gestational age, particularly since this method is less affected by altered growth compared with the assessment at 17–20 weeks. This is a preferred method in patients with a history of previous fetal growth restriction.

Size of Head (BPD, HC)

Measurement of the fetal biparietal diameter has proved to be a very robust and practical method in the busy antenatal clinic. The normal value of the outer–inner measurement introduced by Campbell 30 years ago is probably the most widely used ultrasound standard for assessing gestational age and is reproduced today with the same 95 per cent CI, ± 8.3 days [10,16,22] (Fig. 11.2). The uncertainty increases to ± 13 days after 18 weeks and exceeds ± 19 days after

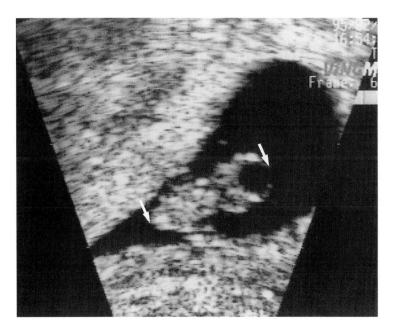

Fig. 11. 1 Measuring the CRL (12 mm between arrows) of an embryo of 7 weeks 4 days during a transvaginal coronar ultrasound scan exposing the ventricular cavity of the developing posterior portion of the brain.

24 weeks when calculated as the 90 per cent prediction range [16] (Table 11.1). In some countries (such as France, Germany, Norway) the outer-to-outer diameter is used, which also gives good results. The shape of the head has a slight influence on the prediction of gestational age. When the occipitofrontal diameter is included in the calculation, the accuracy improves [16]. However, HC gives the best precision at 18 weeks (Table 11.1). Measurement of HC by the perimeter method, by derivation from the BPD (outer–outer diameter), the outer-to-outer occipitofrontal diameter, or the head area, are equally reliable. Well-established charts exist for each method [16] and apply to the assessment of gestational age in the second trimester, usually before 21 weeks. The new charts constructed by Altman and Chitty permit the assessment of fetal age based on the fetal head bio-metry as early as 12 weeks [16]. Although not taken as a sample from a normal population, reference ranges for BPD and HC exist for gestational weeks 7–14 based on transvaginal ultrasound [23]. Correspondingly, there are new charts for head size by gestational age based on carefully conducted statistical analysis [24].

Abdominal Size (MAD, AC)

These measurements are routinely taken during pregnancy, but rarely used for assessing gestational age, as they have wider 95 per cent CI than other measure-ments, even in the first trimester [23,25]. The new charts constructed by Chitty et al. are based on a prospective cross–sectional study of 663 fetuses and seem to be an improved tool for assessing fetal size [26].

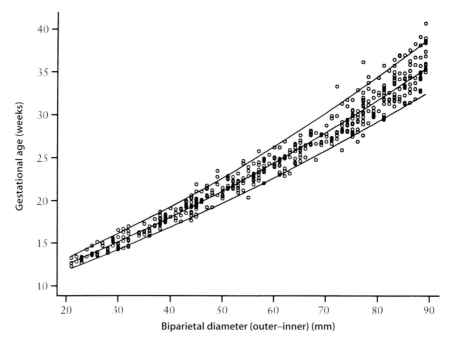

Fig. 11.2 Percentiles intended for the prediction of gestational age (5th, 50th and 95th) by outer–inner BPD measurement were constructed based on a population sample of 663 fetuses (from Altman and Chitty [16] Ultrasound Obstet Gynecol, Parthenon Publishing, London, with permission from the International Society of Ultrasound in Obstetrics and Gynecology).

Table 11.1 Prediction error (in days) for gestational age assessment by ultrasound. The numbers represent the averaged half of the 90 per cent prediction range for each interval of six weeks. HC was measured by perimetry (measured), or derived from outer–outer BPD and occipitofrontal diameter (calculated) (from Altman and Chitty [16], Ultrasound Obstet Gynecol, The Parthenon Publishing, London, with permission from International Society of Ultrasound in Obstetrics and Gynecology)

Measurement	Weeks of gestation			
	12–18	18–24	24–30	30–36
BPD (outer–outer)	8.4	13.1	18.7	24.6
BPD (outer–inner)	8.2	12.7	18.1	23.9
HC (measured)	6.7	10.5	15	19.9
HC (calculated)	8.5	9.5	14.2	23.8
Head area	8.3	9.6	14.7	24.1
Transverse cerebellar diameter	10.9	12.3	20.3	
FL	7.9	12.1	17	22.2

Femur Length (FL)

The length of the diaphysis of the fetal femur can be used to assess gestational age with an accuracy as good as that of the BPD (Table 11.1) [16,27]. When incorporated in formulas together with BPD to calculate gestational age, the prediction of gestational age is only marginally better than BPD alone [28]. FL is especially useful when malformation of the fetal head makes the BPD an unreliable predictor of gestational age. The measurement is frequently included in formulas for calculating EFW.

Precision of Ultrasound Measurements

Assessment of gestational age, fetal size and growth depends on the accuracy of the morphometric method. A single measurement of the CRL, BPD, HC etc. is quite common when assessing individual fetuses or establishing reference ranges. In Scandinavia, the convention of averaging three measurements is usually applied both in clinical routine and incorporated in the established reference ranges [4,29]. Quite a few reference standards presented in the literature do not state how the measurements were established. This is a disadvantage since such standards will only apply to the population from which they are drawn when the same measuring technique is applied. The random error of the individual diameter assessment can be reduced by averaging an increased number (n) of measurements. This is expressed in the equation $SE = sd/\sqrt{n}$, or the 95 per cent limits of the mean, 1.96·SE (Fig. 11.3). In population-based studies, a high number of participants in the sample ensures robust values of the reference standard. In the clinical routine, however, the size of random error considerably limits

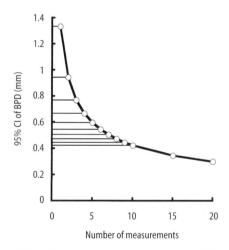

Fig. 11.3 The precision of the ultrasound measurement improves if it is calculated as a mean of repeated measurements. The graph shows how the error of BPD measurement decreases as the number of measurements included in the mean increases; sd = 0.68 mm from Chang et al. [31] is used for calculating the upper limit for the 95 per cent CI for one measurement by 1.96 sd, and for 2–20 measurements by 1.96 $sd/\sqrt{n}$

the ability to discriminate measurements in the assessment of individual patients and to compare serial measurements.

For the BPD, HC, AC and FL taken during gestational weeks 24–40, Sarmandal et al. found the 95 per cent limits of agreement (in cm) for the inter-observer variation to be {–0.8; +0.7}, {–2.4; +2.4}, {–2.2; +2.0} and {–0.7; +0.5}, respectively [30]. The consequence of these limits for a BPD measurement of 8.2 cm (10th percentile), for example, is that the discrimination is very poor. The 95 per cent limits of agreement are 7.4; 8.9 cm, which correspond to the 2nd to the 70th percentiles! Chang et al. used the average of three measurements to calculate the BPD in their interobserver variation study and found 95 per cent limits of agreement {–0.41; +0.29 mm} at a mean gestational age of 34 weeks [31]. For the BPD measurement of 8.2 cm, this corresponds to 95 per cent limits of 7.8; 8.5 cm and the 2nd to the 30th percentiles. This is an improvement of the precision compared with the results of a single measurement, but still a considerable variation. A further improvement in precision is achievable by further repeating the measurement but at an exponentially increased number of measurements (Fig. 11.3). It is obvious that the identification of the small fetus and the subsequent surveillance are uncertain undertakings, a finding that is, in fact, reflected in the literature [32–35]. For the AC, which is an important measurement when assessing fetal weight, Chang et al. found 95 per cent limits of agreement {–1.7; +1.3 cm} for the interobserver variation in small fetuses averaging three measurements [31]. The corresponding limits for their weight estimation were {–160; +124 g}. The limits were expected to be wider if the method were used in late gestation and in a busy clinical routine applying single measurements [36].

The accuracy of ultrasound measurements depends on the emitted ultrasound frequency, depth of the object, focusing of the array, resolution of the measuring callipers and the ability to catch the best image (memory function of the machine). Modern equipment offers improvement in all those aspects and probably deserves renewed evaluation. As seen from Fig. 11.3, repeated measurements improve the precision of ultrasound measurements. This important concept should be integrated into the guidelines of all obstetric ultrasound departments.

Appropriate Reference Ranges

During recent years, concern has been expressed about the way reference ranges are constructed and applied in perinatal research and clinical evaluation [16,37–39].

Generally speaking, charts for assessing gestational age are based on cross-sectional studies analysing gestational age as a function of size, i.e. CRL, BPD, HC, FL etc., with gestational age along the ordinate (y axis). Improved equipment, more appropriate recruitment of participants and optimised statistical analysis have produced better charts for ultrasound dating of the pregnancy [8,16]. Although the new standards are different at the extremes of the chart, it is reassuring that these studies conform to a large extent with the previous charts for the period of pregnancy when the gestational age usually is assessed, by the CRL at 8–11 weeks [8,9,13,19] and by the size of the fetal head at ≤ 20 weeks [8,9,13,16,19,22,40].

Charts for fetal size, EFW and various morphometric measurements according to gestational age are also commonly based on cross-sectional data. These reference ranges, specifically constructed for assessing size, cannot be used to determine gestational age.

Cross-sectional data are appropriate for assessing fetal age and size. They are also, however, commonly used for surveillance in conjunction with serial measurements, but may not reflect the growth rate correctly [41,42]. The correct approach is based on longitudinal data, particularly when assessing growth rate by EFW and growth velocity [18,29,41–44]. Constructing charts from longitudinal data is a laborious task with a high number of observations per participant. For practical reasons, this tends to limit the number of participants. However, the relatively low number of pregnancies included in such studies, makes them susceptible to exclusion bias (see below). A well-designed longitudinal study with a sufficient number of participants and frequency of observations may be used for assessing both size and growth rate, provided the ranges are correctly calculated [39,45].

Excluding certain "complications" from the statistics, such as extremely small or large fetuses, preterm deliveries, twins, malformations, smoking women, patients with medication or diabetes, restricts the applicability of a chart. Many charts in obstetric use are actually skewed due to exclusions and represent "super-normal" populations. Strictly speaking, those charts are not applicable in pregnancies with such complications, but these are the very type of condition that matters most in clinical medicine.

Different populations in different parts of the world show considerable morphometric variations. This also applies to weight and ponderal index at birth. However obvious this sounds, there are currently a number of charts that are based on populations in one part of the world, and then used in different populations, thus introducing a systematic error. This skewness hits the developing world particularly hard, which often depends on reference standards established elsewhere. Recently developed new charts show that fetal weight and growth standards, as well as birthweight charts, need to be customised for populations of different origin even in densely woven communities with mixed cultural setting [46–49]. The Nottingham obstetric database identified six non-pathological determinants that affected birthweight independently [46]. When making use of such information, customised antenatal charts for fetal weight could be applied in individual pregnancies, and false positive rates could be reduced when diagnosing IUGR (Fig. 11.4) [50]. This may prove useful for health care systems where computer resources are available. Many antenatal programmes around the world will have to cope without, but can still manage to work out a suitable chart for their populations, or make modifications for subpopulations.

Birthweight standards used as the norm for fetal weight assessment introduce two possible problems. Firstly, many of the birthweight registries were, and still are [51], based on LMP-assessed gestational age, and their data represent the skewness and variation that an uncertain LMP may cause, and they are not suitable for a comparison with data based on ultrasound measurements. Secondly, birthweight standards for gestational weeks 24–36 are based on prematurely born neonates who, on average, are smaller than their counterparts who remain in utero. An appropriate solution to these problems has been to construct new charts for EFW [42] and fetal growth (Figs 11.5 and 11.6) [18,44] and birthweight [48] based on ultrasound assessed gestational age and size during pregnancy.

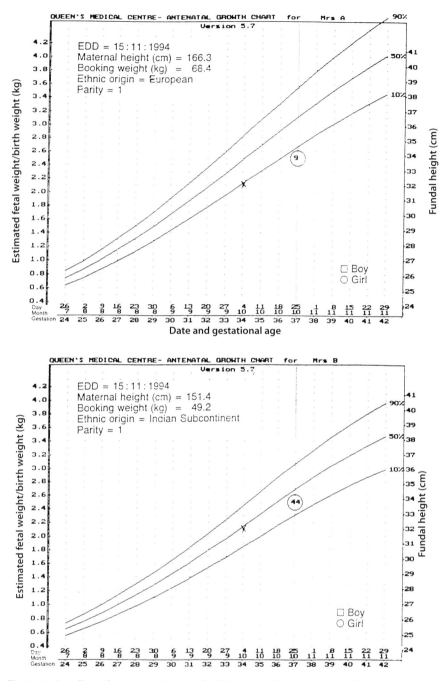

Fig. 11.4 The effect of customised charts for EFW and birthweight. A set of ultrasound meas-urements at 34 weeks gestation which corresponds to EFW < 10th percentile for a woman of European origin (upper panel) represents the average value for a woman of Indian origin (lower panel) when non-pathological determinants for fetal growth are considered (reproduced with per-mission from Gardosi J. Prediction of birth weight and fetal weight gain. Contemp Rev Obstet Gynaecol 1994;6:122–8, Parthenon Publishing Group, Carnforth).

New birthweight charts according to gestational age, largely based on ultrasound dating for 480,000 Swedish singleton deliveries, have recently been constructed [52]. When comparing these charts with the new standards for intrauterine growth (Fig. 11.5), the difference between the prematurely born population and the premature intrauterine population is apparent.

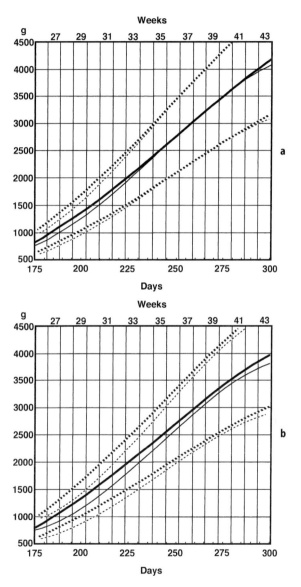

Fig. 11.5 Intrauterine growth (thick rule) compared with birthweight standards (thin rule) for boys (a) and girls (b). The difference in the curves is believed to reflect a true lower average birthweight of the prematurely born neonates compared with their intrauterine counterparts. The intrauterine growth ranges were established on a longitudinal study of EFW, and the birthweight standards were based on 480,000 pregnancies with ultrasound confirmed or corrected dates [52]. Mean ± 2 *sd* (reproduced with permission from Maršál et al. [18] Acta Pædiatr, Scandinavian University Press).

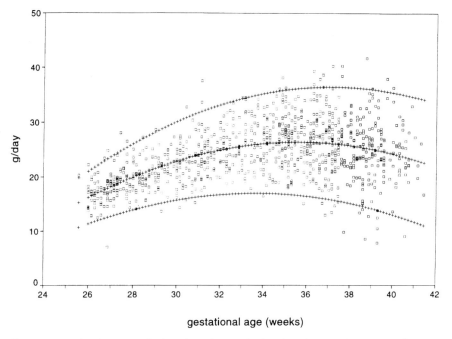

Fig. 11. 6 Growth velocity in g/day based on a longitudinal study with 2,062 observations of EFW in 274 fetuses (reproduced with permission from Owen et al. [44] Br J Obstet Gynaecol, Blackwell Science, Oxford).

Longitudinal data by themselves are not necessarily appropriate for the reference ranges. Some reference ranges presented in the literature have been criticised for being too narrow, and a more suitable method of analysis has been suggested, multilevel modelling, to establish satisfactory ranges [39,45].

Once a new chart has been constructed, it should be tested on the population it is intended for, to ensure validity [18,32,53].

Today a variety of standards are on hand for the clinician, who has to select what fits her/his population and the ultrasound technique in use, and who should also be aware of the limitations of such charts. The low predictive ability and high false positive rates of ultrasound biometry to predict fetal growth restriction is a prominent problem for the obstetrician, and, not to be ignored, a common cause of anxiety for the patients. Selection of appropriate charts for dating and growth assessment is a good start towards minimising such errors. Consistency of charts entered into machines of different companies in the same department, together with consistency between these references and manual charts used in the antenatal clinic, are likewise essential.

Assessment of Fetal Size

The single most important method of identifying a fetus with growth restriction is to measure its size by ultrasound or to use ultrasound biometry after other measures, such as the symphysis–fundus measurement, in the antenatal clinic. As mentioned previously, charts for the assessment of gestational age and size cannot be used interchangeably. Care should be taken that the charts intended to be used are specifically constructed for size assessment. Since the truncal diameter, MAD, AC, or the abdominal area all reflect the nutritional state of the fetus (subcutaneous, intra-abdominal and extraperitoneal fat, and liver size) [25,54], the nutritional state of the fetus is commonly assessed either by means of percentage deviation from the mean or by percentile [26,55]. Obviously, abdominal size alone does not reflect individual variations of body size and proportions, and a number of additional measurements have been added to refine the assessment. BPD and FL are commonly used. A ratio of head to abdominal size is particularly intended to detect asymmetrical growth of fetuses. This is based on the assumption that assymmetrical fetal size reflects the "brain-sparing" distribution of fetal cardiac output and leads to a low ponderal index at birth. Reference ranges have been constructed to facilitate the identification of such fetuses [56].

In clinical practice, the expected birthweight is a useful information for those planning antenatal care, delivery, and the level of neonatal care. Much effort has been put into establishing reliable methods of predicting birthweight and estimated fetal EFW by means of ultrasound. Fig. 11.5 emphasises the importance of appropriately constructed charts. In pregnancies before 37 weeks, the charts for EFW are intended to represent a higher and more correct weight for the unborn fetus than the charts based on birthweight (see arguments in previous sections). It is important to be aware of such distinctions and to apply EFW charts and birthweight charts based on ultrasound assessments.

In 1982, Shepard et al. presented a formula based on two measurements that came to be widely used: $\log 10(EFW) = -1.7492 + 0.166(BPD) + 0.046(AC) - 2.646 (AC \times BPD)/1000$ [57]. A refinement was introduced by Hadlock, who used four measurements [58]. Prospective evaluation studies showed that such methods had an $sd \approx 10$–12 per cent and predicted actual birthweights within 10 per cent in 60 per cent of cases [59]. The method established by Persson and Weldner [53] is an example of a formula for calculating EFW that has been in use for many years in a Scandinavian population: $EFW = BPD^{0.972} \times MAD^{1.743} \times FL^{0.367} \times 10^{-2.646}$. BPD is measured as outer–inner diameter, MAD is the mean of the anteroposterior and transverse abdominal diameters, and FL the length of the femur diaphysis. The method implies that each diameter is averaged from three measurements. The formula was shown to have an estimation error of 7.1 per cent (sd) when tested on 135 pregnancies within 48 hours of delivery [28].

An attempt to improve further the precision in predicting birthweight was made by Sabagha et al. when they established specific formulas targeted for large, appropriate and SGA groups [60]. In a subsequent evaluation, Robson et al. found no significant improvement in prediction error using targeted compared with non-targeted formulas [61].

From a theoretical point of view, there are limitations to such methods. Apart from the random error of ultrasound biometry mentioned previously, the biological variation of form and proportion implies that even the most composite formula can only be an approximation of the actual fetal volume. Interestingly, Shinozuka et al. describe differences in specific gravity of the trunk and head, and refined the formula, which then predicted EFW for the small fetuses only marginally better [62].

Assessment of Fetal Growth

Although assessing fetal growth implies assessing fetal size, the distinction is important. Growth is a dynamic process and at least two serial measurements are required to assess growth rate. The charts of fetal biometry based on cross-sectional data are commonly used for assessing growth. However, it is charts derived from longitudinal growth studies that reflect growth rate correctly [38,42,63] and, when based on a sufficiently big population sample and frequency of measurements, they can be used for size assessment as well [38,39].

Assessing fetal weight increment based on the AC measurement alone is a simple and quick method and popular in busy routine work. New charts were established by Gallivan et al. using longitudinal data from 67 low risk pregnancies, and without other exclusion criteria than premature delivery [43]. These charts represent an improvement in methodology compared to previous charts, but may have wider and more appropriate ranges when processed by multilevel modelling [45].

Maršál et al. [18] established EFW standards for a Scandinavian population applying Persson and Weldner's formula (see previous section and Fig. 11.5). They used BPD, MAD and FL from 86 pregnancies (757 observations). Ten participants had been withdrawn because of premature delivery, pre-eclampsia or birthweight below mean −2 sd. A difference of 2–3% between means for boys and girls was less than expected and assumed to be due to the difference in growth of BPD between the sexes at the time of dating. The female fetuses were smaller and believed to be systematically underestimated by 0.7 days. When the birthweights of 8,663 live singleton neonates were matched with the EFW curves, 32 per cent of the neonates born in gestational weeks 25–29 were below mean −2 sd, the corresponding figures being 11.1 per cent for 30–36 weeks, and 2.6 per cent for the term period. The high frequency of low birthweight among the prematurely born was expected and is believed to reflect the true distribution of weight classes between born and unborn at these stages of the pregnancy.

To refine the method and accommodate normal individual variation of growth, Deter and Rossavik suggested that individual growth standards should be constructed by means of a growth projection established on serial measurements in early pregnancy [64,65]. Calculation of individual growth projections has been criticised on the basis that the error of the projection is substantial towards the end of the pregnancy, and that it increases the earlier in pregnancy the growth projection is established. Another argument is the uncertainty of the nature and timing of the insult on growth. Today we expect determinants for growth restriction to occur at very early stages of pregnancy, and their impact on development might not be a short insult in time but a developmental disease or alteration that persists through a long period of the pregnancy with no sudden or obvious change in growth velocity. A longitudinal study of 134 SGA fetuses supports the assumption that a low growth pattern starts early in the second trimester or before [66]. A more recent study from Scotland has demonstrated an increased OR for IUGR in pregnancies with certain LMP where embryonic length was 2–6 days less than expected [67]. The study underscores the need to integrate LMP and ultrasound information in all patients, especially in those at risk for IUGR based on their past obstetric or medical history. Pregnancies at risk for IUGR are at risk for elevated hCG levels at 15–18 weeks, giving them false positive screen results for trisomy 21 (see Ch. 12).

A related approach to individual growth projections is found in the concept of customised growth charts. These take into account normal variations in fetal growth due to maternal height, maternal weight in early pregnancy, parity, ethnic group and fetal gender (Fig. 11.4). In a longitudinal study of 226 pregnancies, Mongelli and Gardosi showed how each factor influenced growth and suggested an adjustment of growth charts and expected birthweight on the basis of this information in order to improve diagnostic precision of the IUGR fetus [47,50,68].

Another modification designed to improve prediction and surveillance of individual growth rates is found in the conditional percentiles based on a multilevel modelling of longitudinal data [38,44,69]. Owen and Ogston used 274 low risk pregnancies dated by CRL to construct conditional percentiles for BPD, FL, abdominal area and EFW [69]. Based on the measurement done at one stage, e.g. 24 weeks, the authors have made percentile charts for the expected growth assessed by a later measurements, e.g. 28 weeks. However, Royston suggests a simpler form of documentation: to plot all measurement results and their corresponding "conditional" ranges on a common growth chart [38]. The method probably gives a more appropriate assessment of growth, but at the moment it seems better suited for computationally assisted surveillance of growth than for the direct use in charts.

Divon suggested a method specifically designed to assess growth velocity, and proposed 10 mm/14 days as the lower limit of normal AC growth [70]. In a well-designed longitudinal study, Owen et al. calculated reference ranges for growth velocity of BPD, FL, abdominal area, and EFW in per cent, mm, cm^2, and g per day (Fig. 11.6) [44]. Compared with the conventional growth charts, these types of reference ranges have not come into general use.

Predicting the Small Infant by Biometry

The routine ultrasound examination carried out in the first trimester or early second trimester was not primarily designed to identify the IUGR fetus, but rather to be the basic assessment of gestational age, and in addition, to identify risk factors such as abnormalities, placenta previa and multifetal pregnancies. These were the prerequisites for the surveillance in the second part of the pregnancy. An ultrasound assessment later in pregnancy should then be able to identify a group consisting of small fetuses. In addition to the appropriateness of the reference values and the precision of measurements, the efficacy of ultrasound biometry to predict a small fetus or infant depends on the definition of smallness, the cut-off values used in the screening, and the prevalence of SGA. The test performs better in a high risk population with high prevalence of SGA. The detection rate increases with a liberal definition of a positive test. Based on the assumption that missing IUGR can be devastating, Sarmandal and Grant used < 25th percentile as the cut-off to screen a low risk population in order to predict a ponderal index < 10th percentile at birth [34]. Their detection rate was 86 per cent (sensitivity), but the positive predictive value was 31 per cent, i.e. the vast majority of those with a positive test had a normal ponderal index at birth. In 13 studies reviewed by Secher et al. [33], the use of various morphometric ultrasound criteria and neonatal measurements led to substantial differences in sensitivity (11–94%) and positive predictive value (17–92%) in very different

Table 11.2 The ability of ultrasound screening in third trimester to predict weight deviation at birth. Secher et al. used a ratio, actual birthweight/predicted birthweight, to define their groups. Birthweight ≤80% corresponds to the lower 4% of the population, and birthweight ≤85% to the lower 10% (from Secher et al. [33], Acta Obstet Gynecol Scand, Munkgaard International Publishers, Copenhagen)

Ultrasound criterion: predicted birthweight	SGA definition: actual birthweight	Time of examination (weeks)	N SGA	N Total	Sensitivity	Specificity	Pos. predict. value	Neg. predict. value	Risk group % of total
≤80% of expected birthweight	≤80% of expected birthweight	32	37	684	0.03	0.997	0.33	0.947	0.4
		37	33	621	0.33	0.995	0.79	0.963	2.3
≤90% of expected birthweight	≤80% of expected birthweight	32	37	684	0.51	0.946	0.35	0.971	7.9
		37	33	621	0.79	0.9	0.3	0.986	14
≤85% of expected birthweight	≤85% of expected birthweight	32	75	684	0.08	0.995	0.67	0.9	1.3
		37	67	621	0.34	0.969	0.58	0.92	6.4
≤95% of expected birthweight	≤80% of expected birthweight	32	37	684	0.76	0.77	0.16	0.982	26.2
		37	33	621	0.91	0.72	0.15	0.993	14
≤95% of expected birthweight	≤85% of expected birthweight	32	75	684	0.63	0.78	0.26	0.945	26.2
		37	67	621	0.84	0.75	0.28	0.0974	14
≤95% of expected birthweight	≤80% of expected birthweight	32 and 37	24	522	0.63	0.86	0.17	0.979	16.5

populations. The risk group was 4–75% of the total population. In their own study of an unselected population, Secher et al. demonstrated how an attempt to identify SGA resulted either in low sensitivity or low positive predictive value (Table 11.2). They also showed that the ability to identify small fetuses was better at 37 than at 32 weeks. In a review of 36 studies, Chang et al. found that AC was capable of predicting small neonates (< 10th percentile) both in low and high risk populations with a common OR (95% CI) 13.5 (11.5, 15.9) and 18.4 (9.8, 34.3), respectively [71]. EFW had an even higher common OR, 39.1 (28.9, 52.8), in high risk populations. Not unexpectedly, they found in the same analysis that morphometry was superior to Doppler waveform changes as a predictor of low birthweight.

Is a growth-restricted fetus always small? It is a common view that there are newborns with a birthweight within accepted ranges who did not reach their growth potential. Low ponderal index in babies of normal weight is often taken as an indication of intrauterine redistribution of blood to the brain as a response to restricted placental function in such pregnancies. Stratton et al. made an interesting observation in a group of 75 fetuses whose birthweights dropped by more than 20 percentiles in growth during the third trimester, but maintained birthweights between the 10th and 90th percentiles [72]. These fetuses were not at a higher risk of adverse outcome than their normally growing counterparts. However, there was no information on ponderal index, and the group may not have been sufficiently large to show small differences or rare complications. In a recent cohort study of 61,000 births entered into the Swedish Medical Birth Registry during 1982–4 a comparison was made between those who underwent routine ultrasound examination during pregnancy and those who did not [73]. Apart from several beneficial effects in post-term pregnancies, there were fewer newborns with a low ponderal index at term in the ultrasound group. The study does not have the qualities of a randomised trial, but as it is based on a large population sample, the indications ought to be taken seriously in future studies.

Predicting Adverse Outcome by Biometry

There seems to be an increased perinatal morbidity and a higher risk of health impairment in later childhood and adult life for both term and preterm SGA infants [74–76]. It is therefore understandable that the identification of fetuses with low EFW does identify a group with increased morbidity and adverse outcome. As shown in Table 11.3, the frequency of low Apgar score, low pH in the umbilical vein and artery and operative delivery due to fetal distress increases with decreasing birthweight. The sensitivity and specificity of birthweight for identifying these parameters clearly depend on the cut-off level. If ultrasound biometry during pregnancy were to predict these outcomes, there would be a further reduction in precision because of the error of the method in predicting birthweight. As reviewed by Robson and Chang [36], the ponderal index or a related morphometric measurement is more suitable for identifying a group in which growth is affected during pregnancy and which is susceptible to perinatal morbidity and impaired health in later life.

Whether ultrasound biometry applied as a screening test actually improves management and outcome is a pertinent question that has been the subject of randomised trials [32,77–80]. These studies showed that the identification of a

Table 11.3 Cumulative frequency (%) of abnormal blood flow classes (BFC 1–3) in the fetal aorta, operative delivery for fetal distress (ODFD), Apgar score ≤7, umbilical arterial pH ≤7.10 and venous pH ≤7.20, related to birthweight, grouped according to the deviation from the mean. BFC is defined in Fig. 11.9. From Laurin [109] with permission

Birthweight group (sd)	BFC 1–3	ODFD	Apgar 1'	Apgar 5'	Arterial pH	Venous pH
0 – >−0.5	2	0	0	0	8	0
−0.5 – >−1.0	4	0	3	0	31	12
−1.0 – >−1.5	16	10	6	0	62	31
−1.5 – >−2.0	18	20	21	30	77	50
−2.0 – >−2.5	31	35	41	60	77	54
−2.5 – >−3.0	57	55	65	60	85	77
−3.0 – >−3.5	82	83	85	100	92	88
−3.5 – >−4.0	92	93	88	100	100	100
≤−4.0	100	100	100	100	100	100
Prevalence	51/159	40/216	34/213	10/212	13/138	26/166

group of small fetuses led to changes in management, but they failed to show improvement in perinatal death or adverse outcome measures [81].

Screening for Malformations

Malformations and chromosomal aberrations are often associated with IUGR (see Ch. 2). Ultrasound plays a major role when searching for such causes of impaired growth. Indeed assessment of fetal anatomy has become an important part of the routine ultrasound examination (screening programme) in many countries. The screening programme applied to a low risk population has failed to improve the outcome of live births, but it reduces the overall perinatal mortality by detecting abnormalities that lead to induced abortion [81]. The detection rate for major malformations may vary from setting to setting, even in well-developed countries [80,82] and is typically 36–77% depending on the particular organ system [82].

Placental Morphology

Grannum and Hobbins [83] described the changes of the placental cross-section visualised by ultrasound during the course of pregnancy. Increased echogenicity and cotyledonary segmentation was used to grade placental maturity 0–3. Obstetricians used signs of early maturation (for example grade 3 found at 28 weeks or earlier) as an indicator of placental pathology connected with IUGR and pre-eclampsia. The method never gained momentum, probably due to difficulties in distinguishing the grades and in the wide normal variation of placental ultrasound appearance. However, recent reports suggest that careful ultrasound examination of the placenta can identify changes that can be verified by microscopy (haematomas, ischaemic areas, thrombosis etc.) [84,85]. When evaluating a case of suspected IUGR, the finding of a small placenta and variations in the thickness and echogenicity should make the obstetrician more alert to this diagnosis. One interesting study, conducted in a community hospital setting, suggested a reduction in perinatal mortality where Grannum's grade 3 placentas were reported to the obstetrician [86]. However, to date this method has not been adequately investigated as a potential screening tool for IUGR.

Amniotic Fluid

Water metabolism and transport are affected during the process of fetal growth restriction and oligohydramnios is reported in such pregnancies [87]. Normally, the amniotic fluid volume increases until 22 weeks of gestation and the mean volume remains between 500 and 1,000 ml for the rest of the pregnancy [88]. For practical reasons, the ultrasound assessment of the amniotic fluid volume has been restricted to measuring the deepest pool [87] or, probably more reliably, by calculating the amniotic fluid index (AFI) [89].

The deepest pool is identified by the vertical and transverse diameters [87]. According to Manning et al., a vertical diameter of < 1 cm is classified as reduced amniotic fluid, 1–2 cm as marginal, 2–8 cm as normal, and > 8 cm as increased amniotic fluid [87,90]. In the high risk population examined by Chamberlain et al., normal amniotic volume was associated with 4.9 per cent of newborns with a birthweight < 10th percentile, and, correspondingly, marginal amniotic fluid volume was found in 20 per cent, and reduced volume in 38.6 per cent [87]. When the amniotic fluid volume was reduced, the sensitivity for picking up growth-restricted fetuses (< 10th percentile) was 5.5 per cent. The sensitivity increased to 13.2 per cent when both marginal and decreased fluid volumes were applied.

A more robust assessment would be to measure the depth of the largest amniotic pocket in four quadrants and to calculate the AFI as the sum of the four measurements [91–93]. Moore and Cayle constructed charts for normal AFI based on pregnancies with birthweights between the 10th and 90th percentiles. The 5th percentile increased from 8 cm at 16 weeks to 9.5 cm at 22 weeks, remained at that level until 30 weeks, and gradually decreased to 7 cm during the third trimester [91]. The normal ranges established by this cross-sectional study are at variance with the ranges established by the longitudinal study reported by Nwosu et al. (Fig. 11.7) [94]. Particularly for serial measurements and studies of the individual growth of the amniotic fluid volume, the chart established using longitudinal observations is recommended. Once the AFI is assessed, reference ranges for amniotic fluid growth are constructed in order to assess the development in terms of percentile at a later stage in the pregnancy [95]. The intraobserver variation has an overall *sd* of 1.6–1.9 cm, which was lowest when measuring small volumes and highest when measuring large volumes [96,97]. Correspondingly, for the interobserver variation, the overall *sd* is 2.6–2.7 cm.

Although measurement of amniotic fluid pockets has been shown to be of some value when included in the biophysical score, more prospective studies are required to assess the precision of the AFI method for predicting SGA fetuses and adverse outcomes. The method is expected to be imprecise, but could prove to be a valuable supplement to ultrasound fetometry and Doppler measurements.

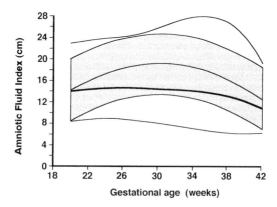

Fig.11.7 Reference ranges (3, 50 and 97th percentile) for AFI established on longitudinal observations (grey area) by Nwosu et al. [94], compared with the ranges inferred from a cross-sectional study by Moore and Cayle [91] (reproduced with permission from Nwosu et al. Br J Obstet Gynaecol, Blackwell Science, Oxford, and from Moore and Cayle. The amniotic fluid index in normal human pregnancy. Am J Obstet Gynecol 1990;162:1168–73. Mosby, St Louis).

Doppler Ultrasound Velocimetry of the Fetal Circulation

The development of pulsed and colour Doppler ultrasound techniques has helped us to envisage a composite haemodynamic assessment of the intrauterine environment. Assessment of flow characteristics in both the fetal and uteroplacental circulations gives important insights into fetal health. These techniques may therefore contribute to surveillance of the small fetus in which IUGR is suspected. Many small fetuses have developed a different haemodynamic pattern compared to their bigger counterparts. These changes include: reduced umbilical venous blood flow; reduced aortic flow; increased aortic and umbilical arterial blood flow pulsatility due to increased impedance in the fetal body and placenta; altered pressure wave propagation in the aorta; reduced pulsatility in the cerebral arteries due to reduced impedance; biphasic or reversed flow across the isthmus of the aorta; increased pulsatility in the pulmonary artery branches; reduced pulsatility in the adrenal arteries; increased pulsatility in the renal arteries; relative enlargement of the fetal heart with altered ejection force and changes in the valvular flow patterns; increased pulsatility in the precordial veins and ductus venosus; and pulsatile deflections in the umbilical venous flow. Many of these observations are incompletely explored at the present time but a selection is incorporated into a plan for intensive monitoring of the IUGR fetus. The utility of each depends to a large extent upon the severity of IUGR and gestational age – this subject is explored in detail in Ch. 13.

The concept that IUGR is an effect of chronic hypoxia is commonly held. This is based on the assumption that reduced cord blood oxygen content represents reduced oxygen availability to vital organs. Soothill et al. found that cord blood PO_2 in SGA fetuses was within the normal range in more than half of the cases [98]. The reason may be that the group studied was heterogeneous, consisting of small normally developed fetuses in addition to fetuses with compromised placental function. From animal studies we know that, if an acute reduction in oxygen delivery is maintained for a longer period in fetuses with otherwise normal circulation, the acute fetal endocrine, neural, and haemodynamic responses within the first days are transformed into metabolic adaptation with a downregulation of anabolic activity and consumption. As a consequence, the changes seen during acute hypoxaemia fade and the values gradually approach more normal levels. However, in many IUGR fetuses the condition is dominated by substantial circulatory responses and adaptation rather than changes in blood gases. Such fetuses may primarily have a compromised placental circulation and be adapted to restricted resources of oxygen and nutrients, but may never have experienced frank hypoxaemia or hypoxia. What actually induces the vascular maldevelopment in the placenta is still a controversial issue [99].

Measurement of Blood Volume Flow

Blood flow is calculated by combining the diameter measurement of the vessel with the Doppler velocimetry. This has provided valuable physiological information on the aortic and umbilical circulation in normal and growth-restricted fetus [100–104]. However, the substantial random error in estimating diameter of small fetal vessels precludes accurate assessment of volume flow [105,106], such

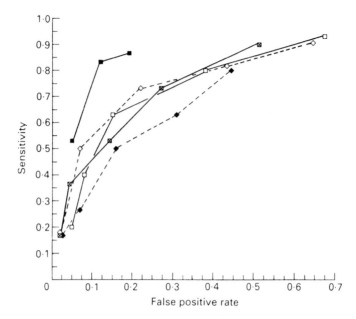

Fig. 11. 8 Receiver operating characteristic (ROC) curves showing the sensitivity and false positive rate for various parameters of blood flow in the fetal thoracic aorta predicting operative delivery for fetal distress. The waveform analysis by BFC 1–3 (closed box) is a better predictor than pulsatility index (open box), rising systolic slope (crossed box), volume flow (closed diamond), or volume flow of the umbilical vein (open diamond). BFC 1–3 are explained in Fig. 11.9 (reproduced with permission from Laurin et al. [108] Br J Obstet Gynaecol, Blackwell Science, Oxford).

that this method is inferior to waveform analysis (of blood velocity recorded in the aorta and umbilical artery) for predicting SGA fetuses and adverse outcomes (Fig. 11.8) [107–109]. The methodological problems above have restricted volume flow studies from general obstetric use in the past 10–20 years. However, a careful application of today's improved ultrasound technology may reintroduce volume flow measurement as a real option – not only for describing flow patterns in smaller vessels such as the ductus venosus [110,111], but to provide clinically relevant information for management of IUGR. Automatic phase-locked echo tracking of the pulsating vessel wall seems to be a particularly promising method of controlling diameter measurement errors [112,113].

Measurement of Blood Flow Velocity

Lower blood flow velocity in the intra-abdominal portion of the umbilical vein was found in growth-restricted fetuses and was associated with poorer outcome than that of normal-sized fetuses [101,108]. However, neither the umbilical venous nor any arterial absolute velocity measurement could compete with the more robust, dimensionless waveform analysis in clinical work (Fig. 11.8).

Doppler Waveform Analysis

By far the commonest method in clinical practice is the analysis of the waveform of pulsatile flow (Fig. 11.9). The semiquantitative assessment of waveforms in

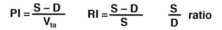

$$PI = \frac{S-D}{V_{ta}} \qquad RI = \frac{S-D}{S} \qquad \frac{S}{D} \text{ ratio}$$

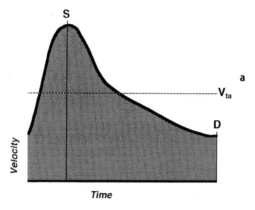

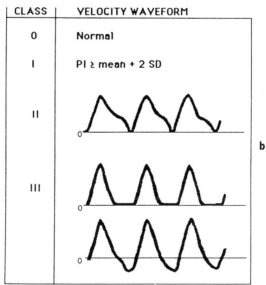

Fig. 11.9 Waveform analysis of pulsatile flow velocity is carried out by a ratio that combines the systolic maximum velocity (S), diastolic minimum velocity (D) or the time-averaged maximum velocity (V_{ta}) to form the pulsatility index, PI, according to Gosling [115], resistance index, RI, according to Pourcelot [116], or S/D ratio, according to Stuart [114] (panel **a**). A convenient alternative is the visual assessment classifying the waveforms in blood flow classes (BFC), Laurin et al. [104] (panel **b**) (panel **b** is reprinted with permission from the American College of Obstetricians and Gynecologists; Obstet Gynecol 1987;69:895–902).

four blood flow classes (BFC) is a rapid and useful method of classifying descending aorta and umbilical artery recordings (Fig. 11.9) [104]. For arteries, the pulsatile waveform can be described numerically in one of three ways; the *S/D* ratio is a simple and easy way of describing the waveform [114]. However, the PI [115] and the RI [116] are the most robust measurements and therefore commendable. Of the latter, PI is preferred on theoretical grounds.

Descending Aorta

The velocity measurement in the aorta is usually taken above the diaphragm with pulsed Doppler equipment. The Doppler shift represents a strong signal for analysis and is almost as accessible for examination as the umbilical arteries of the cord. The descending aorta and umbilical arteries have similar patterns of flow velocity in IUGR fetuses [117,118]. However, the umbilical artery waveform reflects only the fetoplacental vasculature while that of the descending aorta includes changes in the circuit of the lower fetal body – a vasculature that is more responsive to stimulation during stress. Such theoretical differences are not reflected in the diagnostic abilities as they perform equally well in screening tests. Umbilical artery velocimetry is easier to perform [119,120] and can be obtained using cheaper continuous wave Doppler equipment. Thus it has more potential as a screening test for IUGR than aortic, or other fetal Doppler waveforms that require pulsed Doppler capabilities.

Change in the descending aorta velocity waveform is capable of identifying IUGR fetuses in a high risk population during third trimester (EFW$\leq$ –2 *sd*) (prevalence 47–52%) with a sensitivity of 40–87% and a specificity of 61–87% [108,119]. When using the ratio between aortic and middle cerebral artery PI in a population at risk of IUGR (prevalence 66 per cent), Chang et al. predicted an

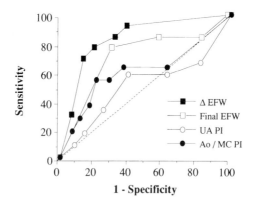

Fig.11.10 Receiver operating characteristic (ROC) curves showing the sensitivity and false positive rate in the prediction of abnormal neonatal ponderal index by EFW, EFW (growth of EFW/*sd*), umbilical artery (UA) PI and the ratio of aortal PI vs. middle cerebral artery PI (Ao/MC PI). Biometry is better than Doppler in predicting abnormal ponderal index (Chang et al. [121], reprinted with permission from the American College of Obstetricians and Gynecologists; Obstet Gynecol 1993;82:230–6).

abnormal ponderal index in the neonate with 55 per cent sensitivity and 79 per cent specificity, which was inferior to prediction by EFW (Fig. 11.10) [121].

These studies showed that it is better to use aortic velocimetry as a predictor of suboptimal perinatal outcome: sensitivity 58–91% and specificity 77–90% [108,119,120]. Follow-up studies show that fetuses demonstrating abnormal flow velocity waveforms in the descending aorta (BFC 2–3, Fig. 11.9) have an increased incidence of minor neurological dysfunction at the age of 7 years compared with their counterparts with normal aortic blood velocity [122]. Similarly, verbal and global intelligence quotients are more frequently impaired in the group with abnormal fetal blood flow velocity [123].

Umbilical Artery

Doppler measurements in the umbilical artery vary slightly according to the site of recording (placental end, free loop, or abdominal portion) though these differences are unimportant clinically. Usually, the free loop is the standard sampling site, particularly since this portion is readily accessible in all pregnancies, and the likely site of sampling with continuous wave equipment. The relationship between the PI in the umbilical artery and the impedance and resistance in the placental bed is not a direct one, but the PI gives some indication of the size of the placenta, resistance, impedance, and probably compliance of the vasculature [124–127]. Efforts are now being made to link the morphological findings of the placental microvasculature to the blood flow velocity changes found with IUGR [99]. Umbilical artery velocimetry is similar to the descending aorta velocity waveform as regards ability to predict IUGR, but both are inferior to ultrasound morphometry [121].

It is common to find an elevated PI in IUGR fetuses, and an increased PI is associated with low birthweight, low Apgar score, low pH at birth, and increased morbidity [128–132]. Interestingly, more pronounced haemodynamic changes seem to be present in IUGR diagnosed before 34 weeks than in IUGR diagnosed near term [133]. Kingdom and Smith, and Kohnen and Kingdom develop this concept further in Chs 13 and 6 respectively. ARED (BFC 3, Fig. 11.9) carries a 36 per cent risk of perinatal death [134] and, according to Tyrrell et al., predicts a venous umbilical oxygen concentration below the 2.5th percentile with a sensitivity of 78 per cent, specificity of 98 per cent, positive predictive value of 88 per cent, and negative predictive value of 100 per cent in a group of women admitted to an antenatal ward [135]. Acidaemia was predicted similarly but with a positive predictive value of 53 per cent.

Screening a low risk population by umbilical artery Doppler velocimetry is not justified. In a meta-analysis of randomised controlled trials including 11,375 low risk pregnancies, Goffinet et al. found no effect on perinatal mortality or stillbirths, nor on any other perinatal end points [136].

In contrast, the benefit from screening a high risk population is well documented [137,138]. A meta-analysis of 12 randomised trials showed that by including the information on the umbilical artery velocimetry (± uterine artery) there is a 29 per cent reduction in perinatal mortality, and fewer hospital admissions, elective deliveries, and inductions of labour [134]. Umbilical artery velocimetry is a swift method that does not require sophisticated ultrasound equipment, and is thus well suited for general use.

Cerebral Circulation

The fetal cerebral circulation is autoregulated such that blood flow remains stable within wide ranges of blood pressure, and is influenced by blood gas and acid–base values [139]. Doppler velocimetry attempts to detect changes in the cerebral circulation by describing the blood velocity waveform. There is a natural development of increased diastolic blood flow in the middle cerebral artery as the pregnancy progresses through the third trimester [140,141]. Thus, increased diastolic velocity (reduced PI) may be a more useful test in the preterm than term fetus. SGA fetuses with reduced PI in the cerebral artery seem more often to have a reduced fetal heart rate variability and an increased risk of admission to the intensive care unit [141]. Neonatal hypoxic–ischaemic encephalopathy was predicted with 77 per cent sensitivity, 75 per cent specificity and 58 per cent positive predictive value with a Cohen's kappa index of 0.58 when applying a cut-off value of mean −2 *sd* for the fetal internal carotid artery PI in IUGR fetuses [142]. However, the prevalence of encephalopathy in the group was high (33 per cent). By combining the PI of the middle cerebral and umbilical artery in a ratio, Gramellini et al. improved the prediction of SGA newborns to 70 per cent accuracy, and 90 per cent accuracy for adverse perinatal outcome [143]. A similar ratio applying the RI for the two arteries yielded 58 per cent sensitivity in predicting birthweight < 10th percentile and neonatal morbidity when the cut-off value was set to 1.0 [144]. So far, the Doppler velocimetry of the cerebral arterial circulation seems to be a promising supplement for evaluating fetuses at risk, particularly when combined with other Doppler measurements [145]. Further studies, however, are needed to give a clearer picture of the value of such measurements.

Screening by Uterine Artery Velocimetry

Based on the assumption that abnormal placentation and placental function begin with poor extravillous trophoblast invasion, "insufficiency" in this organ may in theory be detectable by Doppler abnormalities in the uterine arteries. This might be prior to the establishment of IUGR and perhaps at a stage in pregnancy where useful therapeutic interventions might be applied

Doppler studies have focused on the waveform analysis of the uterine arterial circulation during the entire pregnancy applying PI (or RI), and recently the presence or absence of an early diastolic notch (Fig. 11.11). Standardising the Doppler-sampling site in the uterine artery at the level where it crosses the external iliac artery was made possible with the advent of colour Doppler. This advance made the method reproducible and applicable as an easy screening Doppler examination. Studies thus far have focused on identifying pregnancies at risk of pre-eclampsia and fetal growth restriction. In 1983, Campbell et al. showed an association between waveform alteration (RI) in the uterine artery and pre-eclampsia [146]. Subsequent studies showed that early examination (7–16 weeks) was a poor predictor of complications or later development of pre-eclampsia and fetal growth restriction [147]. Studies at the time of routine booking of a population scanned in the second trimester confirmed the association between increased pulsatility in the uterine artery and perinatal death, fetal growth restriction, placental abruption, and pre-eclampsia [148,149]. High positive pre-

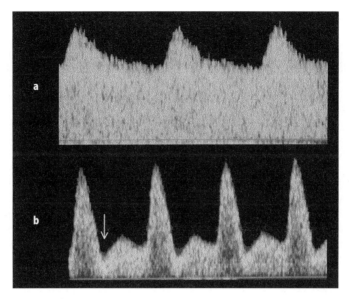

Fig. 11.11 Doppler velocimetry of the uterine artery with a normal pattern with high diastolic flow velocity (a), compared to an abnormal velocity wave (b) with increased pulsatile pattern and early diastolic notch (arrow). Both recordings are done at 28 weeks of gestation.

dictive values for these adverse outcomes were not achieved in all studies [150], reflecting variation in prevalence of obstetric complications in the underlying populations.

Attention to the presence or absence of an early diastolic notch in the test was thought to improve the test characteristics. When recording the presence or absence of a notch in one or both uterine artery velocity tracings, or RI values > 95th percentile at 24 weeks, a sensitivity of 77 per cent was achieved for predicting pre-eclampsia (proteinuric pregnancy-induced hypertension) [151]. Bilateral notching, or RI > 95th percentile for both arteries, achieved a sensitivity of 58 per cent for predicting birthweight < 10th percentile with a positive predictive value of 31 per cent in a population that developed proteinuric pregnancy-induced hypertension in 3.6 per cent and delivered 10.6 per cent of the neonates with birthweight < 10th percentile. Based on a study of 1,311 primigravida, Irion concludes that screening by Doppler of the uterine artery is not justified in a low risk population [152]. Persistent problems with the use of Doppler of the uterine artery as a screening tool include the interpretation of small notches, reliability of the method and definition of clinical endpoints [153–155]. Some centres use Doppler of the uterine artery as a screening tool at 24 weeks of pregnancy, particularly in high risk pregnancies, in order to identify a population at risk that can be assigned to a closer surveillance regimen. The benefit of such an approach still has to be proven.

Conclusions

Ultrasound examination has proven useful in assessing gestational age, fetal size and growth, and in detecting twins and malformations. Measuring fetal size and growth does identify the small fetus with adverse perinatal outcome and increased morbidity in later life. There is, however, room for improvement before these methods become good tests, especially in low risk women. Screening a population with low prevalence is likely to suffer from low sensitivity or a low positive predictive value. When applied to high risk groups, however, the diagnostic abilities are acceptable and the approach is to be commended. This is particularly true of the Doppler technology, which is recommended as a secondary screening and assessment tool. Today clinicians know that the fetus with ARED flow in the umbilical artery or aorta is at 36 per cent risk of perinatal death. They also know that including umbilical Doppler velocimetry ($\pm$ velocimetry of the uterine artery) in the assessment of high risk pregnancies improves management and outcome. These examinations are easy to perform and can be recommended. The merging pattern of the various circulatory sections of the IUGR fetus is made increasingly accessible by modern ultrasound equipment, and promises more detailed knowledge, and possibly a sounder basis for future treatment. The recently established new reference ranges for intrauterine size and growth and birthweight are expected to provide an improved basis for this development.

References

1. Garner P, Kramer MS, Chalmers I. Might efforts to increase birthweight in undernourished women do more harm than good. Lancet 1992;340:1021–3.
2. Bergsjö P, Denman DW, Hoffman HJ, Meirik O. Duration of human sigleton pregnancy. Acta Obstet Gynecol Scand 1990;69:197–207.
3. Mittendorf R, Williams MA, Berkley CS, Cotter PF. The length of uncomplicated human gestation. Obstet Gynecol 1990;75:929–32.
4. Kieler H, Axelsson O, Nilsson S, Waldenström U. The length of human pregnancy as calculated by ultrasonographic measurement of the fetal biparietal diameter. Ultrasound Obstet Gynecol 1995;6:353–7.
5. Tunón K, Eik-Nes SH, Grøttum P. A comparison between ultrasound and a reliable last menstrual period as predictor of the day of delivery in 15 000 examinations. Ultrasound Obstet Gynecol 1996;8:178–85.
6. Persson P-H, Grennert L, Gennser G. Impact of fetal and maternal factors on normal growth of biparietal diameter. Acta Obstet Gynecol Scand 1978;78(Suppl.):21–7.
7. Moore WMO, Ward BS, Jones VP, Bamford FN. Sex differences in fetal head growth. Br J Obstet Gynaecol 1988;95:238–42.
8. Daya S. Accuracy of gestational age estimation by means of fetal crown-rump length measurement. Am J Obstet Gynecol 1993;168:903–8.
9. Wisser J, Dirschedl P, Krone S. Estimation of gestational age by transvaginal sonographic measurement of embryonic length in dated human embryos. Ultrasound Obstet Gynecol 1994;4:457–62.
10. Mul T, Mongelli M, Gardosi J. A comparative analysis of second-trimester ultrasound dating formulae in pregnancies conceived with artificial reproductive techniques. Ultrasound Obstet Gynecol 1996;8:397–402.
11. Olsen O, Clausen JA. Routine ultrasound dating has not been shown to be more accurate than the calendar method. Br J Obstet Gynaecol 1997;104:1221–2.
12. Geirsson RT. Ultrasound instead of last menstrual period as the basis of gestational age assignment. Ultrasound Obstet Gynecol 1991;1:212–19.
13. Campbell S, Warsof SL, Little D, Cooper DJ. Routine ultrasound screening for the prediction of gestational age. Obstet Gynecol 1985;65:613–20.
14. Mongelli M, Wilcox M, Gardosi J. Estimating the date of confinement: ultrasonographic biometry versus certain menstrual dates. Am J Obstet Gynecol 1996;174:278–81.
15. Gardosi J. Dating of pregnancy; time to forget the last menstrual period. Ultrasound Obstet Gynecol 1997;9:367–8.

16. Altman DG, Chitty LS. New charts for ultrasound dating of pregnancy. Ultrasound Obstet Gynecol 1997;10:174–91.

17. Bakketeig LS. Ultrasound dating of pregnancies changes dramatically the observed rates of pre-term, post-term, and small-for-gestational-age births: a commentary. Iatrogenics 1991;1:174–5.

18. Maršál K, Persson P-H, Larsen T, Lilja H, Selbing A, Sultan B. Intrauterine growth curves based on ultrasound estimated foetal weights. Acta Pædiatr 1996;85:843–8.

19. Robinson HP, Fleming JEE. A critical evaluation of sonar "crown-rump length" measurements. Br J Obstet Gynaecol 1975;82:702–10.

20. Drumm JE, Clinch J, Mackenzie G. The ultrasonic measurement of fetal crown-rump length as a method of assessing gestational age. Br J Obstet Gynaecol 1976;83:417–21.

21. Pedersen JF. Fetal crown-rump length measurement by ultrasound in normal pregnancy. Br J Obstet Gynaecol 1982;89:926–30.

22. Campbell S. The prediction of fetal maturity by ultrasonic measurements of the biparietal diameter. J Obstet Gynaecol Br Commonwealth 1969;76:603–9.

23. Lasser DM, Peisner DB, Vollebergh J, Timor-Tritsch I. First-trimester fetal biometry using transvaginal sonography. Ultrasound Obstet Gynecol 1993;3:104–8.

24. Chitty L, Altman D, G., Henderson A, Campbell S. Charts of fetal size: 2. Head measurements. Br J Obstet Gynaecol 1994;101:35–43.

25. Campbell S, Wilkin D. Ultrasonic measurement of fetal abdomen circumference in the estimation of fetal weight. Br J Obstet Gynaecol 1975;82:689–97.

26. Chitty LS, Altman DG, Henderson A, Campbell S. Charts of fetal size: 3. Abdominal measurements. Br J Obstet Gynaecol 1994;101:125–31.

27. Warda AH, Deter RL, Rossavik IK, Carpenter RJ, Hadlock FP. Fetal femur length: a critical reevaluation of the relationship with menstrual age. Obstet Gynecol 1985;66:69–75.

28. Persson P-H, Weldner B-M. Reliability of ultrasound fetometry in estimating gestational age in second trimester. Acta Obstet Gynecol Scand 1986;65:481–3.

29. Persson P-H, Weldner B-M. Normal range growth curves for fetal biparietal diameter, occipito-frontal diameter, mean abdominal diameters and femur length. Acta Obstet Gynecol Scand 1986;65:759–61.

30. Sarmandal P, Bailey S, Grant JM. A comparison of three methods of assessing inter-observer variation applied to ultrasonic fetal measurement in the third trimester. Br J Obstet Gynaecol 1989;96:1261–5.

31. Chang TC, Robson SC, Spencer JAD, Gallivan S. Ultrasonic fetal weight estimation: analysis of inter- and intra-observer variability. J Clin Ultrasound 1993;21:515–19.

32. Secher NJ, Kern Hansen P, Lenstrup C, Sindberg Eriksen P, Morsing G. A randomized study of fetal abdominal diameter and fetal weight estimation for detection of light-for-gestation infants in low-risk pregnancies. Br J Obstet Gynaecol 1987;94:105–9.

33. Secher NJ, Kern Hansen P, Lenstrup C, Sindberg Eriksen P, Lykke Thomsen B, Keiding N. On the evaluation of routine ultrasound screening in the third trimester for detection of light for gestational age (LGA) infants. Acta Obstet Gynecol Scand 1987;66:463–71.

34. Sarmandal P, Grant JM. Effectiveness of ultrasound determination of fetal abdominal circumference and fetal ponderal index in the diagnosis of asymetrical growth retardation. Br J Obstet Gynaecol 1990;97:118–23.

35. Backe B, Nakling J. Effectiveness of antenatal care: a population based study. Br J Obstet Gynaecol 1993;100:727–32.

36. Robson SC, Chang TC. Measurement of human fetal growth. In: Hanson MA, Spencer JAD, Rodeck CH, editors. Fetus and neonate. Physiology and clinical application, vol 3: Growth. Cambridge: Cambridge University Press, 1995:297–325.

37. Altman D, Chitty LS. Charts of fetal size: 1. Methodology. Br J Obstet Gynaecol 1994;101:29–34.

38. Royston P, Altman DG. Design and analysis of longitudinal studies of fetal size. Ultrasound Obstet Gynecol 1995;6:307–12.

39. Royston P, Wright EM. How to construct "normal ranges" for fetal variables. Ultrasound Obstet Gynecol 1998;11:30–8.

40. Hadlock FP, Deter RL, Harrist RB, Park SK. Fetal biparietal diameter: a critical re-evaluation of the relation to menstrual age by means of real-time ultrasound. J Ultrasound Med 1982;1:97–104.

41. Deter RL, Harrist RB, Hadlock FP, Carpenter RJ. Fetal head and abdominal circumferences: II. A critical reevaluation of relationship to menstrual age. J Clin Ultrasound 1982;10:365–72.

42. Deter RL, Harrist RB, Hadlock FP, Poindexter AN. Longitudinal studies of fetal growth with the use of dynamic image ultrasonography. Am J Obstet Gynecol 1982;143:545–54.

43. Gallivan S, Robson SC, Chang TC, Vaughan J, Spencer JAD. An investigation of fetal growth using serial ultrasound data. Ultrasound Obstet Gynecol 1993;3:109–14.
44. Owen P, Donnet L, Ogston S, Christie AD, Patel N, Howie PW. Standards for ultrasound fetal growth velocity. Br J Obstet Gynaecol 1996;103:60–9.
45. Royston P. Calculation of unconditional reference intervals for foetal size and growth from longitudinal measurements. Stats Med 1995;14:1417–36.
46. Gardosi J, Chang A, Kalyan B, Sahota D, Symonds EM. Customised antenatal growth charts. Lancet 1992;339:283–7.
47. Gardosi J. Ethnic differences in fetal growth. Ultrasound Obstet Gynecol 1995;6:73–4.
48. Wilcox M, Gardosi J, Mongelli M, Ray C, Johnson I. Birth weight from pregnancies dated by ultrasonography in a multicultural British population. BMJ 1993;307:588–91.
49. Spencer JAD, Chang TC, Robson SC, Gallivan S. Fetal size and growth in Bangladeshi pregnancies. Ultrasound Obstet Gynecol 1995;5:313–17.
50. Mongelli M, Gardosi J. Reduction of fals-positive diagnosis of fetal growth restriction by application of customized fetal growth standards. Obstet Gynecol 1996;88:844–8.
51. Alexander GR, Himes JH, Kaufman RB, Mor J, Kogan M. A United States National Reference for fetal growth. Obstet Gynecol 1996;87:163–8.
52. Källén BA. A birthweight for gestational age standard based on data in the Swedish Medical Birth Registry 1985–1989. Eur J Epidemiology 1995;11:601–6.
53. Persson P-H, Weldner B-M. Intra-uterine weight curves obtained by ultrasound. Acta Obstet Gynecol Scand 1986;65:169–73.
54. Thompson HE, Holmes JH, Gottesfeld KR, Taylor ES. Fetal development as determined by ultrasonic pulse echo techniques. Am J Obstet Gynecol 1965;146:942–7.
55. Jeanty P, Cousaert E, Cantraine F. Normal growth of the abdominal perimeter. Am J Perinatol 1984;1:127–35.
56. Campbell S, Thoms A. Ultrasound measurement of the fetal head and abdominal circumference ratio in the assessment of fetal growth retardation. Br J Obstet Gynaecol 1977;84:165–74.
57. Shepard MJ, Richards VA, Berkowitz RL, Warsof SL, Hobbins JC. An evaluation of two equations for predicting fetal weight by ultrasound. Am J Obstet Gynecol 1982;142:47–54.
58. Hadlock FP, Harrist RB, Sharman RS, Deter RL, Park SK. Estimation of fetal weight with the use of head, body, and femur measurements – A prospective study. AM J Obstet Gynecol 1985;151:333–7.
59. Simon NV, Levinsky JS, Shearer DM, O'Leear MS, Flood JT. Influence of fetal growth patterns on sonographic estimation of fetal weight. J Clin Ultrasound 1987;15:376–83.
60. Sabbagha RE, Minogue J, Tamura RK, Hungerford SA. Estimation of birth weight by use of ultrasonographic formulas targeted to large-, appropriate-, and small-for-gestanional age fetuses. Am J Obstet Gynecol 1989;160:854–62.
61. Robson SC, Gallivan S, Walkinshaw SA, Vaughan J, Rodeck CH. Ultrasonic estimation of fetal weight: use of targeted formulas in small for gestational age fetuses. Obstet Gynecol 1993;82:359–64.
62. Shinozuka N, Okai T, Kohzuma S, et al. Formulas for fetal weight estimation by ultrasound measurements based on neonatal specific gravity and volumes. Am J Obstet Gynecol 1987;157:1140–5.
63. Deter RL, Harrist RB. Growth standards for anatomic measurements and growth rates derived from longitudinal studies of normal fetal growth. J Clin Ultrasound 1992;20:381–8.
64. Rossavik IK, Deter RL. Mathematical modeling of fetal growth. I. Basic principles. J Clin Ultrasound 1984;12:529–33.
65. Deter RL, Rossavik IK. A simplified method for determining indivudual growth curve standards. Obstet Gynecol 1987;70:801–5.
66. Bakketeig LS, Hoffman HJ, Jacobsen G, Hagen JA, Storvik BE. Intrauterine growth pattern by the tendency to repeat small-for-gestational-age births in successive pregnancies. Acta Obstet Gynecol 1997;76(Suppl 165):3–7.
67. Smith GCS, Smith MFS, McNay MB, Fleming JEE. First-trimester growth and risk of low birth weight. N Eng J Med 1998;339:1817–22.
68. Mongelli M, Gardosi J. Longitudinal study of fetal growth in subgroups of a low-risk population. Ultrsound Obstet Gynecol 1995;6:340–4.
69. Owen P, Ogston S. Conditional centiles for the quantification of fetal growth. Ultrasound Obstet Gynecol 1998;11:110–17.
70. Divon MY, Chamberlain PF, Sipos L, Manning FA, Platt LD. Identification of the small for gestational age fetus with the use of gestational-age dependent indices of fetal growth. Am J Obstet Gynecol 1986;155:1197–201.

71. Chang TC, Robson SC, Boys RJ, Spencer JAD. Prediction of small for gestational age infant: which ultrasonic measurement is best. Obstet Gynecol 1992;80:1030–8.
72. Stratton JF, Ni Scanaill S, Stuart B, Turner MJ. Are babies of normal birth weight who fail to reach their growth potential as diagnosed by ultrasound at increased risk? Ultrasound Obstet Gynecol 1995;5:114–18.
73. Høgberg U, Larsson N. Early dating by ultrasound and perinatal outcome. Acta Obstet Gynecol Scand 1997;76:907–12.
74. Roth S. Small-for-gestational-age infants and antenatal prediction of outcome. Ultrasound Obstet Gynecol 1996;8:149–51.
75. Piper JM, Xenakis EM-J, McFarland M, Elliott BD, Berkus MD, Langer O. Do growth-retarded premature infants have different rates of perinatal morbidity and mortality than appropriately grown premature infants. Obstet Gynecol 1996;87:169–74.
76. Barker DJP, Bull AR, Osmond C, Simmonds SJ. Fetal and placental size and risk of hypertension in adult life. BMJ 1990;301:259–62.
77. Bakketeig LS, Jacobsen G, Brodtkorb C, et al. Randomized controlled trial of ultrasonographic screening in pregnancy. Lancet 1984;ii:207–10.
78. Neilson JP, Munjaja SP, Whitfield CR. Screening for small-for-date fetuses: a controlled trial. BMJ 1984;289:1179–82.
79. Larsen T, Larsen JF, Petersen S, Greisen G. Detection of small-for-gestational age fetuses by ultrasound screening in a high risk population: a randomized controlled study. Br J Obstet Gynecol 1992;99:469–74.
80. Ewigman BG, Crane JP, Frigoletto FD, LeFevre ML, Bain RP, McNellis DA. Effect of ultrasound screening on perinatal outcome. N Eng J Med 1993;329:821–7.
81. Pearson V. Antenatal ultrasound scanning. 1997 Cochrane Library; Issue 4.
82. Saari-Kemppainen A, Karjalainen O, Ylöstalo P, Heinonen OP. Ultrasound screening and perinatal mortality: controlled trial of systematic one-stage screening in pregnancy. Lancet 1990;336:387–91.
83. Grannum PA, Hobbins JC. The ultrasound changes in the maturing placenta and their relationship to fetal pulmonic maturity. Am J Obstet Gynecol 1979;133:915–22.
84. Jauniaux E, Jurkovic D, Campbell S. In vivo investigations of the anatomy and the physiology of early human placental circulation. Ultrasound Obstet Gynecol 1991;1:435–45.
85. Jauniaux E, Ramsay B, Campbell S. Ultrasonographic investigation of placental morphometric characteristics and size during the second trimester of pregnancy. Am J Obstet Gynecol 1994;170:130–7.
86. Proud J, Grant AM. Third trimester placental grading by ultrasonography as a test of fetal wellbeing. BMJ 1987;294:1641–4.
87. Chamberlain PF, Manning FA, Morrison I, Harman CR, Lange IR. Ultrasound evaluation of amniotic fluid volume. I. The relationsship of marginal and decreased amniotic fluid volumes to perinatal outcome. Am J Obstet Gynecol 1984;150:245–9.
88. Brace RA, Wolf EJ. Normal amniotic fluid volume changes throughout pregnancy. Am J Obstet Gynecol 1989;161:382–8.
89. Phelan JP, Ahn MO, Smith CV, Rutherford SE, Anderson E. Amniotic fluid index measurements during pregnancy. J Reprod Med 1987;32:601–4.
90. Manning FA, Platt LD. Qualitative assessment of amniotic fluid volume – A rapid screen for detecting the small for gestational age fetus. Twenty-sixth Annual Meeting of the Society of Gynecologic Investigation. San Diego: Elsevier, 1979:126.
91. Moore TR, Cayle JE. The amniotic fluid index in normal human pregnancy. Am J Obstet Gynecol 1990;162:1168–73.
92. Moore T. Superiority of four-quadrant sum over the single deepest-pocket technique in ultrasonographic identification of abnormal amniotic fluid volumes. Am J Obstet Gynecol 1990;163:762–7.
93. Youssef AA, Abdulla SA, Sayed EH, Salem HT, Abdelalim AM, Devoe LD. Superiority of amniotic fluid index over amniotic fluid pocket measurement for predictig bad fetal outcome. South Med J 1993;86:426–9.
94. Nwosu EC, Welch CR, Manasse PR, Walkinshaw SA. Longitudinal assessment of amniotic fluid index. Br J Obstet Gynaecol 1993;100:816–9.
95. Owen P, Ogston S. Standards for the quantification of serial changes in the amniotic fluid index. Ultrasound Obstet Gynecol 1996;8:403–7.
96. Rutherford SE, Smith CV, Phelan JP, Kawakami K, Ahn MO. Four-quadrant assessment of amniotic fluid volume: interobserver and intraobserver variation. J Reprod Med 1987;32:587–9.

97. Bruner JP, Reed GW, Sarno AP, Harrington RA, Goodman MA. Intraobserver and interobserver variability of the amniotic fluid index. Am J Obstet Gynecol 1993;168:1309–13.

98. Soothill PW, Nicolaides KH, Campbell S. Prenatal asphyxia, hyperlactaemia and erythroblastosis in growth retarded fetuses. BMJ 1987;i:1051–3.

99. Kingdom JCP, Burrell SJ, Kaufmann P. Pathology and clinical implications of abnormal umbilical artery Doppler waveforms. Ultrasound Obstet Gynecol 1997;9:271–86.

100. Gill RW. Pulsed Doppler with B-mode imaging for quantitative blood flow measurement. Ultrasound Med Biol 1979;5:223–35.

101. Gill RW, Kossoff G, Warren PS, Garrett WJ. Umbilical venous flow in normal and complicated pregnancies. Ultrasound Med Biol 1984;10:349–63.

102. Eik-Nes SH, Brubakk AO, Ulstein MK. Measurement of human fetal blood flow. BMJ 1980;280:283–4.

103. Lingman G, Maršál K. Fetal central blood circulation in the third trimester of normal pregnancy. Longitudinal study. I. Aortic and umbilical flow. Early Hum Dev 1986;13:137–50.

104. Laurin J, Lingman G, Maršál K, Persson P-H. Fetal blood flow in pregnancies complicated by intrauterine growth retardation. Obstet Gynecol 1987;69:895–902.

105. Gill RW, Trudinger BJ, Garrett WJ, Kossoff G, Warren PS. Fetal umbilical venous flow measured in utero by pulsed Doppler and B-mode ultrasound. Am J Obstet Gynecol 1981;139:720–5.

106. Eik-Nes SH, Maršál K, Brubakk AO, Kristoffersen K, Ulstein M. Ultrasonic measurement of human fetal blood flow. J Biomed Engng 1982;4:28–36.

107. Giles WB, Lingman G, Maršál K, Trudinger BJ. Fetal volume blood flow and umbilical artery flow velocity waveform analysis; a comparison. Br J Obstet Gynaecol 1986;93:461–5.

108. Laurin J, Maršál K, Persson P-H, Lingman G. Ultrasound measurement of fetal blood flow in predicting fetal outcome. Br J Obstet Gynaecol 1987;94:940–8.

109. Laurin J. Intra-uterine growth retardation. Thesis. University of Lund, Sweden, 1987.

110. Kiserud T, Rasmussen S. How repeat measurements affect mean diameter of the umbilical vein and the ductus venosus. Ultrasound Obstet Gynecol 1998;11:419–25.

111. Kiserud T, Rasmussen S, Skulstad SM. Distribution of umbilical blood through the ductus venosus. J Soc Gynecol Invest 1998;5(Suppl 1):156–7A.

112. Sindberg Eriksen P, Gennser G, Lindström K. Physiological characteristics of diameter pulses in the fetal descending aorta. Acta Obstet Gynecol Scand 1984;63:355–63.

113. Stale H, Gennser G, Maršál K. Blood flow velocity and pulsatile diameter changes in the fetal descending aorta: A longitudinal study. Am J Obstet Gynecol 1990;163:26–9.

114. Stuart B, Drumm J, FitzGerald D, Duignan N. Fetal blood velocity waveforms in normal pregnancies. Br J Obstet Gynaecol 1980;87:780–5.

115. Gosling RG, King DH. Ultrasonic angiology. In: Harcus AW, Adamson L, editor. Arteries and veins. Edinburgh: Churchill-Livingstone, 1975:61–98.

116. Pourcelot L. Aplications cliniques de l'examen Doppler transcutane. In: Peronneau P, editor. Velocimetric ultrasonore Doppler. Paris: INSERM, 1974:213–40.

117. Jouppila P, Kirkinen P. Increased vascular resistance in the descending aorta of the human fetus in hypoxia. Br J Obstet Gynaecol 1984;91:853–6.

118. Lingman G, Laurin J, Maršál K, Persson P-H. Circulatory changes in fetuses with imminent asphyxia. Biol Neonate 1986;49:66–73.

119. Gudmundsson S, Maršál K. Blood flow velocity waveforms in the fetal aorta and umbilical artery as predictors of fetal outcome – a comparison. Am J Perinatology 1991;8:1–6.

120. Chang TC, Robson SC, Spencer JAD, Gallivan S. Prediction of perinatal morbidity at term in small fetuses: comparison of fetal growth and Doppler ultrasound. Br J Obstet Gynaecol 1994;101:422–7.

121. Chang TC, Robson SC, Spencer JAD, Gallivan S. Identification of fetal growth retardation: comparison of Doppler waveform indices and serial ultrasound measurements of abdominal circumference and fetal weight. Obstet Gynecol 1993;82:230–6.

122. Ley D, Laurin J, Bjerre I, Maršál K. Abnormal fetal aortic velocity waveform and minor neurological dysfunction at 7 years of age. Ultrasound Obstet Gynecol 1996;8:152–9.

123. Ley D, Tideman E, Laurin J, Bjerre I, Maršál K. Abnormal fetal aortic velocity waveform and intellectual function at 7 years of age. Ultrasound Obstet Gynecol 1996;8:160–5.

124. Trudinger BJ, Stevens D, Connelly A, Hales JRS, Alexander G. Umbilical artery flow velocity waveforms and placental resistance: The effects of embolization of the umbilical circulation. Am J Obstet Gynecol 1987;157:1443–9.

125. Nimrod C, Clapp JI, Larrow R, D'Alton M, Persaud D. Simultaneous use of Doppler ultrasound and electromagnetic flow probes in fetal flow assessment. J Ultrasound Med 1989;8:201–5.

126. Adamson SL, Langille BL. Factors determining aortic and umbilical blood flow pulsatility in fetal sheep. Ultrasound Med Biol 1992;18:255–66.
127. Giussani DA, Moore PJ, Spencer JAD, Hanson MA. Changes in frequency and in compliance affect the Pulsatility Index in an in vitro pulsatile flow model. J Maternal Fetal Invest 1995;5:78–82.
128. Hackett GA, Campbell S, Gamsu H, Cohen-Overbeek T, Pearce JMF. Doppler studies in the growth retarded fetus and prediction of neonatal necrotising enterocolitis, intracranial haemorrhage and neonatal morbidity. BMJ 1987;294:13–16.
129. Gudmundsson S, Maršál K. Umbilical and uteroplacental blood flow velocity waveforms in pregnancies with fetal growth retardation. Eur J Obstet Gynecol Reprod Biol 1988;27:187–96.
130. Hawton JM, Platt MPW, McPhail S, Cameron H, Walkinshaw SA. Prediction of impaired metabolic adaptation by antenatal Doppler studies in small for gestational age fetuses. Arch Dis Child 1992;67:789–92.
131. Wilson DC, Harper A, McLure G, Halliday HL, Reid M. Long term predictive value of Doppler studies in high risk fetuses. Br J Obstet Gynaecol 1992;99:575–8.
132. Arabin B, Becker R, Mohnhaupt A, Entezami M, Weitzel HK. Prediction of fetal distress and poor outcome in intrauterine growth retardation – A comparison of fetal heart rate monitoring combined with stress tests and doppler ultrasound. Fetal Diagn Ther 1993;8:234–40.
133. Kiserud T, Eik-Nes SH, Blaas H-G, Hellevik LR, Simensen B. Ductus venosus blood velocity and the umbilical circulation in the seriously growth retarded fetus. Ultrasound Obstet Gynecol 1994;4:109–14.
134. Neilson JP, Alfirevic Z. Doppler ultrasound in high risk pregnancies. 1997 Cochrane Library; Issue 4.
135. Tyrrell S, Obaid AH, Lilford RJ. Umbilical artery Doppler velocimetry as a predictor of fetal hypoxia and acidosis at birth. Obstet Gynecol 1989;74:332–6.
136. Goffinet F, Paris-Llado J, Nisand I, Bréart G. Umbilical artery Doppler velocimetry in unselected and low risk pregnancies: a review of randomised trials. Br J Obstet Gynaecol 1997;104:425–30.
137. Alfirevic Z, Neilson JP. Doppler ultrasonography in high-risk pregnancies: Systematic review with meta-analysis. Am J Obstet Gynecol 1995;172:1379–87.
138. Divon MY. Randomized controlled trials of umbilical artery Doppler velocimetry: how many are too many. Ultrasound Obstet Gynecol 1995;6:377–9.
139. Wood CE. Local and endocrine factors in the control of the circulation. In: Hanson MA, Spencer JAD, Rodeck CH, editors. Fetus and neonate. Physiology and clinical application, vol 1 Circulation. Cambridge: Cambridge University Press, 1993;100–15.
140. Wladimiroff JW, Tongue HM, Stewart PA. Doppler ultrasound assessment of cerebral blood flow in the human. Br J Obstet 1986;93:471–5.
141. Mari G, Deter RL. Middle cerebral artery flow velocity waveforms in normal and small-for gestational-age fetuses. Am J Obstet Gynecol 1992;166:1262–70.
142. Rizzo G, Arduini D, Luciano R, et al. Prenatal cerebral Doppler ultrasonography and neonatal neurologic outcome. J Ultrasound Med 1989;8:237–40.
143. Gramellini D, Folli MC, Raboni S, Vadora E, Merialdi A. Cerebral-umbilical Doppler ratio as a predictor of adverse perinatal outcome. Obstet Gynecol 1992;79:416–20.
144. Arias F. Accuracy of the middle-cerebral-to-umbilical-artery resistance index ratio in the prediction of neonatal outcome in patients at high risk for fetal and neonatal complications. Am J Obstet Gynecol 1994;171:1541–5.
145. Arbeille P, Leguyader P, Fignon A, Carles G, Locatelli H, Maulik D. Doppler ultrasonographic investigation of fetal cerebral circulation. In: Maulik D, editor. Doppler ultrasound in obstetrics and gynecology. New York: Springer-Verlag, 1996:161–80.
146. Campbell S, Diaz-Racasens J, Griffin D, Cohen-Overbeek RE, Pearce JM, Wilson K. New Doppler technique for assessing uteroplacental blood flow. Lancet 1983;1:675–9.
147. Arduini D, Rizzo G, Romanini C. Doppler ultrasonography in early pregnancy does not predict adverse pregnancy outcome. Ultrasound Obstet Gynecol 1991;1:180–5.
148. Jacobson S-L, Imhof R, Manning N, et al. The value of Doppler assessment of the uteroplacental circulation in predicting preeclampsia or intrauterine growth retardation. Am J Obstet Gynecol 1990;162:110–14.
149. Bewley S, Cooper D, Campbell S. Doppler investigation of uteroplacental blood flow resistance in the second trimester: a screening study for pre-eclampsia and intrauterine growth retardation. Br J Obstet Gynaecol 1991;98:871–9.
150. Hanretty KP, Primrose MH, Neilson JP, Whittle MJ. Pregnancy screening by Doppler uteroplacental and umbilical artery waveforms. Br J Obstet Gynaecol 1989;96:1163–7.

151. Harrington K, Cooper DCL, Hecher K, Campbell S. Doppler ultrasound of the uterine arteries: the importance of bilateral notching in the prediction of pre-eclampsia, placental abruption or delivery of a small-for-gestational-age baby. Ultrasound Obstet Gynecol 1996;7:182–8.

152. Irion O, Massé J, Forest JC, Moutquin JM. Prediction of pre-eclampsia, low birthweight for gestation and prematurity by uterine artery velocity waveforms analysis in low risk nulliparous women. Br J Obstet Gynaecol 1998;105:422–9.

153. Bower S, Kingdom J, Campbell S. Objective and subjective assessment of abnormal uterine artery Doppler flow velocity waveforms. Ultrasound Obstet Gynecol 1998;12:260–4.

154. Chappell L, Bewley S. Pre-eclamptic toxaemia: the role of uterine artery Doppler. Br J Obstet Gynaecol 1998;105:379–82.

155. Valensise H. Uterine artery Doppler velocimetry as a screening test: where we are and where we go. Ultrasound Obstet Gynecol 1998;12:81–3.

12 Biochemical Markers of Fetoplacental Growth Restriction

Gurmit Singh Pahal, Ganesh Acharya and Eric Jauniaux

Introduction

During the last 20 years maternal serum biochemical screening for neural tube defects and trisomy-21 affected fetuses has become well established and widely practised in developed countries. More recently these maternal serum biochemical markers have been found to be associated with a diverse range of pregnancy complications other than aneuploidy [1]. The single most common cause of intrauterine fetal growth restriction in developed (well-nourished) countries is pre-eclampsia, which is secondary to a defect in placentation and subsequent uteroplacental insufficiency. In this chapter we shall examine some of the evidence linking biochemical markers to fetoplacental growth restriction and its causes.

Alpha Fetoprotein

Biology

Alpha Fetoprotein (AFP), an oncofetal glycoprotein, was first identified in 1956 [2]. It is a single chain α globulin produced by the secondary yolk sac from the 2nd month of pregnancy and, from the 3rd month, by the fetal liver and gastrointestinal tract [3]. AFP is coded for by a single gene on chromosome 4, has a 65 kDa relative molecular mass, and expresses microheterogenicity in its glycan component.

Although AFP production initially increases in pregnancy, this increase is not proportional to fetal growth and so fetal serum levels of AFP decrease from 14 weeks of gestation. At 32 weeks of gestation AFP synthesis declines rapidly, to virtually cease at birth, although small quantities of AFP are detectable in adults. AFP has a half-life of 4–5 days and is thought to be the fetal form of albumin; AFP and albumin have similar physical properties and occur in inverse concentrations [4]. Male fetuses have been reported to have higher concentrations of AFP than female fetuses [5].

At an early gestational age AFP diffuses across the poorly keratinised fetal skin, and is excreted in fetal urine after 10 weeks of gestation. From that stage AFP can be detected in the amniotic fluid and subsequent levels of AFP in the amniotic fluid show a similar pattern to that seen in the fetal serum, although the concentration in the amniotic fluid is 150-fold lower. Maternal serum alpha feto-protein (MSAFP) levels slowly rise to a peak at 32 weeks of gestation but are approximately 50,000-fold lower than in the fetal serum.

High Maternal Serum Alpha Fetoprotein and Fetal Anomalies

Elevated levels of MSAFP ($\geq$ 2.5 multiples of the median (MoM)) are associated with neural tube defects [6] and initially amniocentesis was performed on preg-nancies with elevated MSAFP to measure amniotic fluid levels of AFP and confirm the diagnosis of neural tube defects. It was reported in 1978, after exam-ination of the fetal loss rate resulting from such an AFP-screening programme, that in ongoing pregnancies with elevated second trimester MSAFP (> 95th per-centile) there was a statistically significant increased risk of developing pre-eclampsia (3.8 per cent versus 0.4 per cent, $P < 0.05$) [7]. A year earlier the association between low birthweight (<2,500 g) and elevated MSAFP ($\geq$ 2.3 MoM) had also been reported (10.7 per cent versus 4.2 per cent) [8].

Other fetal abnormalities, such as abdominal wall defects and obstruction of the gastrointestinal tract, as well as placental abnormalities such as angioma, pla-cental lakes, thrombosis and infarction, have been shown to be associated with high MSAFP levels [9,10]. Maternal ethnicity, weight, diabetes mellitus and a history of early pregnancy bleeding can alter the MSAFP level. After the exclusion of these factors, and exclusion of incorrect gestational dating, multiple preg-nancy, chromosomal anomalies and structural abnormalities of the fetus, elevated MSAFP levels can be defined as unexplained.

Unexplained Elevated MSAFP and Diseases of Pregnancy

Unexplained elevated MSAFP levels have been associated with a significantly increased risk of a wide variety of pregnancy complications [1] and Table 12.1 illustrates a range of studies that have examined the relationship between unexplained elevated MSAFP and markers of fetoplacental growth restriction. Unexplained elevated MSAFP levels are statistically significantly associated with low birthweight, SGA neonates, IUGR, a higher incidence of fetal and neonatal death, preterm labour and pre-eclampsia [7,8,11–20]. However, these results cannot be considered in isolation as they may be interrelated. For example, it is important to identify clearly to what extent prematurity affects the reported increased risk of low birthweight. Even in a published retrospective study, a third of the preterm deliveries in the elevated MSAFP group were induced and not spontaneous [11].

Unexplained elevated MSAFP levels may be more closely associated with severe forms of pregnancy complications such as pre-eclampsia, haemolysis, ele-vated liver enzymes and low platelets syndrome (HELLP) and intrauterine fetal death. For example, pre-eclampsia is reported to be significantly more likely to develop than other gestational hypertensive disorders, in pregnancies with unexplained elevated MSAFP [11]. In a retrospective study of early IUGR, the presence of unexplained elevated MSAFP in the second trimester was found in five pregnancies; all five women subsequently developed severe pre-eclampsia, requiring early delivery (mean gestation 33.5 weeks). Furthermore, three developed HELLP [21].

Table 12.1 Relationship between unexplained elevated MSAFP levels and markers of fetoplacental growth restriction

Reference	Total pregnancies screened	MSAFP >/MoM	Number of cases	LBW	SGA	IUGR	IUD	PE	Preterm labour
Brock et al 1977 [8]		2.3		10.7 vs. 4.2%					
Gordon et al 1978 [7]		95th centile	102				5 vs.0%	3.8 vs. 0.4%	7.5 vs. 2%
Walters et al 1985 [11]		3.0	60	28 vs.4%				13 vs.1%	27 vs.3%
Milunsky et al 1989 [12]	13,486	2.0	530	4.0 (3.0–5.3)			8.1 (4.8–13.4)	2.3 (1.5–3.6)	
Waller et al 1991 [13]	3,113	2.0					3.2 (2.3–4.2)	8.7 (11.4–17.0)	
		2.0–2.4					2.5 (1.6–3.7)		
		2.5–2.9					2.4 (1.3–4.5)		
		≥3.0					10.4 (4.9–22.0)		
Bernstein et al 1992 [14]		2.0	95			20 vs. 4.3%	4.2 vs.0%		20 vs. 5.8%
Williams et al 1992 [15]		2.0 + placental abnormalities	201	3.7 (1.8–7.7)	4.0 (1.6–10.2)			3.8 (1.6–9.1)	3.6 (1.8–7.4)
				6.9 (2.5–18.7)	5.3 (1.2–23.5)				5.6 (2.0–15.3)
Brazerol et al 1994 [16]	776	2.0	57		10.5 vs. 4%		7 vs 0.8%	12.3 vs. 4.3%	
Waller et al 1996 [17]	51,008	2.5			3.2 (2.4–4.1)				
Wenstrom et al 1996 [18]	5,743	2.5				2.5 (1.4–4.4)	3.5 (1.4–8.3)	2.8 (1.1–7.0)	8.7 (7.1–10.7)
Morssink et al 1997 [19]	10,459	2.5						2.8 (2.3–3.4) HELLP 11 (3–47)	2.8 (2.3–3.4)
Hsieh et al 1997 [20]	5,885	2.0	176	3.7 (2.3–5.7)	1.7 (1.0–2.9)		4.0 (1.6–9.5)		2.4 (1.5–3.8)

Figures are given as percentage in elevated MSAFP group vs. control group or as relative risk (95% CI).
LBW = low birthweight, IUD = intrauterine death.

Most studies have found a significantly increased risk of fetal death until term in pregnancies with unexplained elevated MSAFP levels [11–14,16,18,20]. However, low MSAFP levels have also been associated with an increased risk of intrauterine death [22]. After fetal demise MSAFP initially increases to very high levels. As AFP is then cleared from the maternal circulation MSAFP levels rapidly decrease. Hence, the association between low levels of MSAFP and intrauterine death may be accounted for by missed abortions, if they are not excluded from the study group.

In a study of the pregnancy outcomes and serum screening levels in approximately 30 per cent of all deliveries in California, the range of MSAFP levels were divided into ten categories and the adverse pregnancy outcomes in each group were recorded. In total, there were 3,711 preterm deliveries and 2,634 SGA neonates. When compared with pregnancies with AFP levels between the 25th and 75th percentile, those pregnancies with levels outside the interquartile range were 2.3 times more likely to result in a SGA neonate, thus demonstrating a U-shaped relationship between the MSAFP level and the risk of a SGA neonate. Furthermore, there was a significant correlation between increasing risk of preterm birth and an increasing AFP concentration. A similar trend of increased risk of pre-eclampsia independent of the risk of preterm birth and SGA neonates was reported with rising levels of AFP. This large scale study demonstrated a strong association between elevated MSAFP levels and markers of fetoplacental growth restriction and, more importantly, showed that the risk of a pregnancy complication increases in proportion to the rise in MSAFP [17]. This risk has now been quantified such that an increase in AFP of 1 MoM approximately doubles the risk of a pregnancy complication [23].

The true risk of a pregnancy complication with unexplained elevated MSAFP levels may be higher than those reported, since increased surveillance may detect non-reassuring fetal testing and result in early delivery of the fetus [16]. This may prevent further intrauterine fetal hypoxia and subsequent intrauterine deaths. Once again, this highlights the need for care in quantifying unexplained elevated MSAFP levels when predicting fetoplacental growth restriction.

Table 12.2 illustrates the sensitivity, specificity and predictive values for certain pregnancy outcomes with elevated MSAFP. Due to the relatively low prevalence of these pregnancy complications, the positive and negative predictive values are respectively low and high for all these pregnancy outcomes, including neural tube defects [12]. To increase the predictive value of unexplained elevated MSAFP as a marker of fetoplacental growth restriction, levels should be used in combination with other risk factors, as will be discussed later in this chapter.

Table 12.2 Sensitivity, specificity and predictive values for certain pregnancy complications with elevated MSAFP (> 2.0 MoM)

Pregnancy Complication	Sensitivity (%)	Specificity (%)	PPV (%)	NPV (%)
anencephaly	100	96	1.7	100
spina bifida	91	96	1.9	99.9
other NTDs	50	96	0.4	99.9
low birthweight	14	96	8.1	98.0
fetal death	26	96	2.6	99.7
pre-eclampsia	9	96	3.6	98.4

PPV = positive predictive value, NPV = negative predictive value, NTD = neural tube defects.

Pathophysiology of Unexplained Elevated MSAFP

In normal pregnancy, MSAFP levels rise ninefold and fetal serum AFP concentrations fall approximately sevenfold from 20 to 32 weeks of gestation. During this period, the placental villous surface area increases by a factor of approximately only five-and-a-half and the normal rise in MSAFP levels is thought to reflect a degree of greater placental permeability. MSAFP levels may become elevated secondarily to placental pathology, which changes placental structure and function resulting in increased permeability. Investigation of growth-restricted pregnancies with abnormal umbilical artery Doppler waveforms has shown several abnormal features of the placental terminal villi, such as increased syncytial nuclei, reduced cytotrophoblast nuclei, thickened basal lamina, and increased stromal deposition of collagens and laminin [24]. Since apoptosis has also been reported to be significantly higher in these placentas it is postulated that this process may play an underlying role in these pathophysiological findings [25]. Cytochemical staining has shown that AFP transfer occurs across fibrinoid deposits at areas of discontinuity in the villous syncytiotrophoblast [26]. Further, two populations of cotyledons, one with normal permeability to AFP and the other with raised permeability to AFP, have been reported in pregnancies with elevated second trimester MSAFP levels [27]. Hence increased placental permeability to AFP may account for unexplained elevated second trimester MSAFP levels.

Women with elevated MSAFP have a higher incidence of positive Kleihauer–Betke stains, suggesting that elevated MSAFP values are secondary to fetomaternal haemorrhage [14]. A 50 per cent incidence of fetomaternal haemorrhage (> 0.1 ml) has been found in pregnancies with elevated MSAFP [28]. This is not surprising as a small degree of fetomaternal haemorrhage would result in a very large elevation of MSAFP, since fetal AFP concentrations are 50,000-fold greater than maternal serum concentrations.

A study investigating the relative merits of unexplained elevated amniotic fluid AFP or MSAFP in predicting subsequent pregnancy complications reported that a elevated amniotic fluid AFP level did not necessarily give rise to elevated MSAFP levels [18]. Hence, increased production of AFP does not always equate with elevated MSAFP. Neonatal AFP production has been shown to be increased owing to viral hepatitis with compensatory hepatocyte proliferation [29]. During the third trimester, hypoxic fetuses have been shown to have elevated levels of gamma glutamyltransferase and lactic dehydrogenase [30]. It is postulated, therefore, that early stress (infectious, hypoxic, or other) may stimulate proliferation or even destruction of fetal hepatic cells, and thus increase production or release of AFP into the fetal circulation [18]. However, it has been demonstrated in growth-restricted fetuses with absent end-diastolic flow in the umbilical artery that serum AFP levels are within normal limits [31]. This suggests, therefore, that unexplained elevated MSAFP levels are not associated with increased fetal AFP production.

Human Chorionic Gonadotrophin

Biology

Human chorionic gonadotrophin (LCG) is a glycoprotein hetrodimer of relative molecular mass 39 kDa, composed of α and β subunits is derived from the placental trophoblast, and maintains the corpus luteum for the first 7 weeks of gestation. The α subunit is coded for by a single gene on chromosome 6 and is identical in luteinising hormone LH, follicle stimulating hormone FSH and thyroid stimulating hormone TSH. The β subunit differentiates between these hormones and is coded for by six to seven genes on chromosome 19. There is an 85 per cent similarity in the β subunits in hCG and LH. The pituitary gland and fetal kidney produce small quantities of hCG, but the majority is produced by the placenta. The α and β subunits are combined in the syncytiotrophoblast, from which hCG is rapidly released directly into the maternal circulation. The rate of production of the β subunit is the rate-limiting factor in the formation of the dimer. Seventy per cent of hCG is metabolised by the kidney and liver, with 30 per cent being excreted in the urine and bile.

Intact hCG has a half-life of 6–24 hours, whereas free β-hCG, less than 0.5 per cent of intact hCG, has a half-life of 40 minutes. Free β-hCG rises to a peak in pregnancy at 9–11 weeks of gestation. Free α-hCG is 2 per cent of intact hCG, has a half-life of 15 minutes, and slowly rises to a plateau at 36 weeks' gestation. Fetal serum levels of hCG are 3 per cent of those detected in the maternal serum.

High Maternal Serum hCG (MShCG) and Fetal Anomalies

High (> 2.0 MoM) MShCG levels are associated with Down's syndrome [32] and are also found in trophoblastic disorders, for example complete hydatidform mole. High MShCG levels are also associated with triploidy, where the extra haploid chromosomal set is of paternal origin [33], and with both hydropic and non-hydropic Turner syndrome pregnancies [34]. Similar to MSAFP, elevated MShCG levels can be defined only as being unexplained after excluding known associated causes.

Unexplained Elevated MShCG and Diseases of Pregnancy

As early as 1934 a link between elevated MShCG and severe pre-eclampsia was reported [35]. The elevated MShCG levels were reported in pregnancies with established severe pre-eclampsia during the third trimester. More recently, evidence has been emerging of a link between unexplained elevated levels of MShCG during the second trimester and the subsequent development of pregnancy complications. Table 12.3 illustrates some of the studies examining the relationship between unexplained elevated MShCG levels and markers of fetoplacental growth restriction. All the markers of fetoplacental growth restriction, such as low birthweight, SGA and IUGR, and pregnancy complications, such as preterm labour, intrauterine death and hypertensive diseases of pregnancy, are significantly increased in pregnancies with unexplained elevated levels of MShCG [19,23,36–39]. More studies looking at unexplained elevated levels of MShCG have tried to differentiate between pregnancy-induced hypertension and pre-eclampsia than have those looking at unexplained elevated levels of MSAFP.

There are important differences in the value of the optimal cut-off level of MShCG for predicting fetal or maternal complications. Different assays used to measure MShCG and its subunits may contribute to the difference in the optimal cut-off levels reported. Using a receiver–operator characteristic curve, the

Table 12.3 Relationship between unexplained elevated MShCG levels and markers of fetoplacental growth restriction

Reference	Total pregnancies screened	MShCG ≥MoM	Number of cases	LBW	SGA	IUGR	IUD	PIH	PE	Preterm labour
Gonen et al 1992 [36]	6,011	2.5 4.0	271			2.8 (1–7)		4.4 (1.9–10.0) 6.8 (2.4–19.0)		3.3 (1.3–8.2)
Tanaka et al 1993 [37]	638	2.0 2.0–2.4 2.5–2.9 > 3.0	42		4.9 6.7 3.4 12.0		28.0			
Sorensen et al 1993 [38]	7,718	2.0 2.0–2.9 ≥ 3.0	180					1.8 (1.2–2.7) 1.9 (1.2–2.8) 1.4 (0.7–3.1)	6.9 (2.0–23.2) 6.9 (1.9–25.9) 6.3 (0.7–55.6)	
Lieppman et al 1993 [39]		2.0 2.0–3.9 4.0–5.9 ≥ 6	460	4.0 (1.6–9.9) 2.9 (1.0–8.4) 8.7 (3.2–25.1) 20.3 (4.0–104.0)	1.8 (1.0–3.2) 1.3 (0.7–2.5) 3.2 (1.8–6.4) 4.6 (0.9–24.3)					2.8 (1.4–5.8) 2.1 (0.9–4.8) 4.6 (2.0–10.6) 11.8 (2.6–54.5)
Benn et al 1996 [23]	25,438	3.0	316		3.0 (1.5–6.0)		fetal/neonatal death 4.4 (1.8–10.7)		6.7(2.7–17.1)	2.6 (1.7–4.0)
Morssink et al 1997 [19]	10,459	2.5							HELLP 12.0 (4.0–32.0)	

Figures are given as relative risk (95% CI)
LBW = low birthweight, IUD = intrauterine death, PIH = pregnancy-induced hypertension.

optimal cut-off level of MShCG for predicting SGA neonates was found to lie between 1.5 MoM and 2 MoM. Unexplained elevated MShCG of > 2 MoM was found to be associated with a significantly greater risk of SGA neonates [37]. A threshold effect, rather than a linear trend, in the risk for developing pregnancy-induced hypertension was reported using cut-off levels of unexplained MShCG of between 2.0 and 2.9 MoM and > 3.0 MoM [38]. However, the reported risk ratios may have been affected by the small number of pregnancies with very high MShCG levels, as reflected by the wide 95 per cent confidence intervals. In a larger series a linear trend analysis indicated that the risk of an adverse pregnancy outcome increased with increasing levels of second trimester MShCG [39]. Unexplained elevated MShCG levels were associated with increased risks of low birthweight, preterm delivery and SGA neonates. Least-square multiple regression analysis showed that an unexplained elevated MShCG $\geq$2 MoM was associated with a mean reduction of 173 g in birthweight. These reported risks were independent of MSAFP and unconjugated oestriol levels.

Furthermore, it has been reported that the greater the unexplained elevated level of MShCG, the greater is the risk of a statistically significant adverse pregnancy outcome. The risks of fetal growth restriction and preterm delivery were also increased but logistic regression analysis showed that both these risks were dependent upon the presence of pregnancy-induced hypertension [36].

Unexplained Elevated Maternal Serum β-hCG and α-hCG and Diseases of Pregnancy

An investigation into maternal serum (MS) levels of the β subunit of hCG and pre-eclampsia reported that MSβ-hCG levels were significantly higher in established pre-eclampsia, and may have become elevated before any clinical signs of disease [40]. In addition to MShCG and MSβ-hCG, MSα-hCG levels were significantly increased in the third trimester of pregnancies complicated by severe pre-eclampsia [41].

The maternal serum levels of the subunits, α-hCG and β-hCG, have been investigated in an attempt to identify their predictive value as markers of fetoplacental growth restriction. A study of over 6,000 pregnancies found a significant association between second trimester elevated β-hCG levels and the development of hypertensive disorders [42] (see Table 12.4). A sensitivity of 15.6 per cent, specificity of 90 per cent, positive predictive value of 12.8 per cent and a negative predictive value of 91.8 per cent for pre-eclampsia were calculated using a cut-off

Table 12.4 Relationship between unexplained elevated MSβhCG levels and markers of fetoplacental growth restriction

Reference	Total pregnancies screened	MSβhCG $\geqslant$MoM	Number of cases	LBW	PIH	PE
Hsieh et al 1997 [20]		2.5	416	1.9 (1.1–3.2)		
Ashour et al 1997 [42]	6,138	2.0			1.5 (1.1–2.0)	1.8 (1.3–2.6)
		2.0–2.9			1.6 (1.1–2.2)	1.7 (1.1–2.6)
		> 3.0			1.1 (0.6–2.2)	2.2 (1.2–4.3)

Figures are given as relative risk (95% CI)
LBW = low birthweight, PIH = pregnancy-induced hypertension.

level of > 2 MoM for β-hCG. However, due to the low sensitivity and positive predictive value reported, the use of β-hCG in isolation as a screening test in low risk pregnancies may be limited.

Pathophysiology of Unexplained Elevated MShCG and its Subunits

Focal cellular necrosis in the syncytiotrophoblast and increased mitotic activity with cellular proliferation in the cytotrophoblast has been noted in pre-eclampsia [43]. The proliferating cytotrophoblasts are rapidly transformed into syncytiotrophoblast [44]. Overall, the balance between cellular loss and replacement of syncytiotrophoblast may favour replacement, and hence secretion of hCG and its subunits. Thus elevated levels of hCG and its subunits in severe pre-eclampsia may reflect a secretory reaction of the placenta [41]. Similarly, it has been suggested that reduced oxygen supply to the trophoblast may result in increased hCG production owing to an increase in both differentiating cytotrophoblasts and newly transformed syncytiotrophoblast [39]. However, hypoxia has been found to stimulate cytotrophoblast proliferation but inhibit trophoblast invasion [45]. Thus early cellular proliferation creates an effective barrier to maternal oxygen transfer, allowing the early embryo to develop in hypoxic conditions. As the uteroplacental and fetoplacental circulations develop, the local oxygen tension gradients change, allowing trophoblast invasion and the completion of normal placentation, thus meeting the rising fetal demands for oxygen as pregnancy advances. It has been shown that a threefold rise in placental PO_2 corresponds to the MShCG peak seen at 9–11 weeks of gestation [46], hence hyperoxic damage to trophoblasts may give rise to the elevated maternal serum levels of hCG [47].

Alternatively, it has been postulated that unexplained elevated MSβ-hCG levels are the result of decreased renal excretion rather than increased production by trophoblasts. This results from the finding that multiparous women, who have a higher incidence of underlying chronic renal disease, had a stronger association between elevated MSβ-hCG levels and the subsequent development of hypertension [42].

AFP, hCG and Other Risk Factors

The relative merits of AFP and hCG as biological markers of adverse pregnancy outcome have been investigated and unexplained elevated MSAFP was reported to be the better predictor overall [23]. Unexplained elevated MSAFP levels alone were found to be associated with the risk of fetal growth restriction [48]. An explanation for this is that early placental vascular damage resulted in elevated levels of MSAFP and that MShCG levels remained normal because there was no associated cytotrophoblast hyperplasia. It was postulated that, overall, these changes result in poor delivery of substrate to the fetus and subsequent growth restriction. However, hCG may be the better biochemical marker for the prediction of certain diseases of pregnancy. For example, unexplained elevated MShCG levels alone were found to be associated with the increased risk of developing pre-eclampsia [48].

As second trimester unexplained elevated maternal levels of these markers are associated with pregnancy complications, the value of serial measurements has been investigated. However, in pregnancies subsequently affected by fetoplacental growth restriction, unexplained elevated maternal serum levels do not persist. Hence, serial measurements have been shown to provide no additional predictive value [10]. One must then ask, firstly, why maternal serum levels are elevated so early in pregnancy, and, secondly, why there is subsequently no difference in maternal serum levels between those pregnancies with normal and adverse outcomes.

If fetomaternal haemorrhage accounts for the high initial MSAFP levels, it would be expected that ongoing bleeding would result in early fetal loss, as reported [16]. It would also be expected that recovery from this would be associated with declining AFP levels but still carry an increased risk of future pregnancy complications. Unexplained elevated MSAFP is postulated to be the earliest marker of placental dysfunction, with increased placental permeability allowing greater transport of AFP across the placenta. Normalisation of MSAFP in high risk pregnancies could be explained if the original placental insult were limited and compensated for by the remaining placental tissue. Finally, in the unlikely event that unexplained elevated MSAFP results from increased fetal production of AFP, it is possible that ongoing stress may further compromise fetal liver metabolism, such that AFP production is reduced.

In order to maximise the positive predictive value of unexplained elevated MSAFP or MShCG as biochemical markers for fetoplacental growth restriction, other risk factors have been examined in combination with unexplained elevated MSAFP or MShCG. For example, when compared with pregnancies with unexplained elevated MSAFP alone, a history of first trimester vaginal bleeding in combination with elevated MSAFP in the second trimester was found to have an additive effect on the rate of complications [14].

Unexplained elevated MSAFP in association with abnormal placental ultrasonographic features may be a better early indicator of subsequent pregnancy complications, including fetoplacental growth restriction [9]. Unexplained elevated MSAFP and placental ultrasonographic abnormalities, such as extrachorionic or subchorionic periplacental haemorrhage, intraplacental sonolucencies or placental lakes, and thickened placenta (see Fig. 12.1), have been found to be associated with a mean reduction in birthweight of 378 g, after controlling for confounding factors, whereas unexplained elevated MSAFP alone resulted in a mean reduction in birthweight of 243 g [15].

When a uterine artery notch or an elevated (95th percentile) uterine artery resistance index is identified on Doppler ultrasound between 17 and 22 weeks' gestation, a sensitivity of 83.3 per cent and a positive predictive value of 55.6 per cent and 45.5 per cent respectively for the subsequent development of pre-eclampsia have been reported [49]. Because of the particularly high risk of an adverse pregnancy outcome associated with a combined history of unexplained elevated MSAFP and placental abnormalities, ultrasonographic examination is recommended in pregnancies with unexplained elevated MSAFP.

When unexplained elevated MSAFP and MShCG are both present, the risk of pregnancy complications and their severity both greatly increase. For example, a combined unexplained elevation in MSAFP and MShCG was found to be associated with the highest risk of preterm delivery and stillbirth (odds ratio 7.4, 95 per cent CI 1.1-168.2) [48], and the presence of unexplained elevated AFP, or hCG, or both AFP and hCG, was found to result in an 11-, 12-, or 47-fold increase, respectively, in the risk of developing HELLP [19].

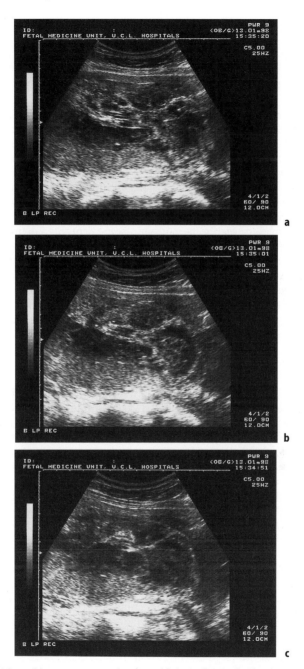

Fig. 12.1a–c A thickened heterogeneous placenta with intraplacental echo-poor sonolucencies (placental lakes) typical of a "jelly"-like placenta. A double screening test revealed unexplained elevated MSAFP and MShCG levels (6.54 MoM and 6.74 MoM, respectively). Delivery at 28 weeks of gestation was required as a result of very severe early fetoplacental growth restriction and severe maternal pre-eclampsia.

Other Biochemical Markers of Fetoplacental Growth Restriction

Unconjugated Oestriol

The precursor of oestriol is dehydroepiandrosterone sulphate, produced primarily by the fetal adrenal cortex. Dehydroepiandrosterone sulphate is hydroxylated in the fetal liver by 16 α-hydroxylase and then metabolised in the placenta to unconjugated oestriol. With advancing gestation unconjugated oestriol is excreted in increasing quantities into maternal serum. Low levels of maternal serum unconjugated oestriol are associated with reduced uteroplacental blood flow and were once used as an indicator of either fetal or placental dysfunction. Together with AFP and hCG, maternal serum levels of unconjugated oestriol comprise the triple-screening test used in some centres to determine the risk of neural tube defects and trisomy-21-affected fetuses.

Maternal serum levels of unconjugated oestriol < 0.75 MoM are reported to be statistically significantly associated with SGA, preterm delivery, pre-eclampsia and fetal death after controlling for the effects of MSAFP and MShCG (odds ratio 2.5, 95 per cent CI 1.13–5.55). Further, low maternal serum levels of unconjugated oestriol are reported to be a better predictor of subsequent adverse pregnancy outcome than either MSAFP or MShCG levels [50].

Prostacyclin

Prostacyclin is a potent vasodilator and inhibitor of platelet aggregation and its urinary metabolite levels increase during normal pregnancy. A lesser rise in prostacyclin biosynthesis has been reported in pregnancies destined to be complicated by pregnancy-induced hypertension, before any clinical manifestations of disease [51]. It is possible that this relative lack of prostacyclin may play a pathophysiological role in the subsequent development of pregnancy-induced hypertension through relative vasoconstriction and enhanced platelet activity. However, since the reported study was retrospective with regard to prostacyclin levels and pregnancy outcome, the usefulness of prostacyclin as a predictive biochemical marker of pregnancy-induced hypertension was not quantified.

Fibronectin

Fibronectin is a glycoprotein intimately associated with the vascular endothelial basement membrane and has a wide-ranging role in haemostasis and tissue repair. As pre-eclampsia results from impaired trophoblastic invasion of maternal spiral arterioles, it has been postulated that plasma fibronectin levels could act as an early biochemical marker of vascular endothelial damage, and hence of pre-eclampsia.

Early studies reported that total plasma fibronectin levels are elevated in women with pre-eclampsia and those who subsequently developed pre-eclampsia [52,53]. However, it has been shown that total serum fibronectin levels primarily reflect hepatic fibronectin and the observed rise in fibronectin may, therefore, be due not to vascular damage alone but to the hepatic dysfunction secondary to pre-eclampsia [54], thus limiting its usefulness as an early biochemical marker of pre-eclampsia.

Fetal fibronectin has been detected in maternal plasma and reported to increase with advancing gestation. However, maternal plasma fetal fibronectin levels have not been found to be associated with the subsequent development of pre-eclampsia [55].

Endothelial cell isoforms of fibronectin bearing an extra type-III domain have been identified and have been reported to be elevated before any clinical signs of pre-eclampsia [56]. Hence, they may provide an earlier and more specific marker of pre-eclampsia than total plasma fibronectin. Multivariant logistic regression analysis demonstrated that for every 1 μg/ml elevation in serum concentration of endothelial cell fibronectin the subsequent risk of developing pre-eclampsia was increased 5.4-fold.

Growth Factors

Greater mitogenic activity has been noted as early as the first trimester in the serum of women who subsequently developed pre-eclampsia [57], and the identification of this specific growth factor protein would enable the identification of the subsequent development of pre-eclampsia. IGFs were thought to be the most promising candidates and were investigated for their expressions early in pregnancy. Initially, IGFBP-3 was evaluated but no difference in this marker was noted in pre-eclamptic and normal pregnancies [58].

IGFBP-1 is an endometrial protein produced by stromal cells. In normal pregnancy a fourfold increase in serum levels of IGFBP-1 with peak levels at 22–23 weeks of gestation was demonstrated, which was concurrent with the second wave of trophoblast invasion in normal pregnancy [59]. However, no rise in maternal serum levels of IGFBP-1 at 19 weeks' gestation was observed in pregnancies with subsequent pre-eclampsia [60]. Nevertheless, the use of IGFBP-1 in screening of the general population is limited, owing to the large overlap in the maternal serum levels in normal and pre-eclamptic pregnancies.

Activin A and Inhibin A

Activin A and inhibin A are synthesised by the placenta. Activin A causes cellular proliferation in various tissues and may play a role in enhancing trophoblast proliferation during placental repair. At 30 weeks of gestation, maternal serum levels of activin A and inhibin A are reported to be elevated ninefold and eightfold respectively in pre-eclamptic pregnancies [61]. As there is no overlap of serum levels of activin A or inhibin A in normal and pre-eclamptic pregnancies, clear differentiation between pre-eclampsia and normal pregnancy is possible. However, one problem with the use of Activin A or inhibin A as a marker of the severity of pre-eclampsia is that serum levels were found not to correlate with other indices of disease severity, such as blood pressure or platelet count. Since the levels of activin A and inhibin A were measured at approximately 30 weeks' gestation in established pre-eclamptic pregnancies [61], the use of activin A and inhibin A as early biochemical markers for the prediction of pre-eclampsia cannot be commented upon at this stage.

Cytokines

The immunosuppressive cytokine IL-10 was reported to be elevated in the amniotic fluid of women who subsequently delivered SGA neonates [62]. However, a subsequent case controlled study found no difference in second trimester IL-10 levels in either the amniotic fluid or the maternal serum of women who subsequently delivered SGA neonates [63]. Hence, maternal serum IL-10 levels seem not to be predictive of the subsequent delivery of SGA neonates.

Isoferritin

A significantly reduced median level of placental isoferritin has been observed in women with diastolic notching of the uterine artery and a raised pulsatility index at 20–22 weeks and 33–34 weeks of gestation respectively, as well as in those with SGA neonates. A sensitivity of 69 per cent and specificity of 84 per cent in predicting SGA neonates, using a cut-off of 10 U placental isoferritin/ml, is reported. Due to the strong correlation between serum levels of placental isoferritin and the risk of SGA neonates, a large scale screening trial of placental isoferritin is recommended [64].

Conclusions

Evidence for biochemical markers as the predictors of pregnancies at risk of fetoplacental growth restriction has been examined in this chapter. There do appear to be biochemical markers for the prediction of fetoplacental growth restriction and the two most commonly investigated are AFP and hCG. Unexplained elevated second trimester levels of these markers have been found to be associated with fetoplacental growth restriction and there seems to be a gradient of risk, the greatest risk being associated with the highest levels of unexplained elevated MShCG or MShCG. Furthermore, when both MSAFP and MShCG are inexplicably elevated there appears to be a stronger association with pregnancy complications and, in particular, complications of a more severe nature.

A screening programme that uses both MSAFP and MShCG, in combination with other risk factors and ultrasonographic surveillance, will have a greater positive predictive value and result in the identification of high risk pregnancies from as early as 15 weeks of gestation. It has been suggested that a positive predictive value of between 20 and 40 per cent for a screening test will identify appropriate candidates for possible preventative therapies [65].

Large scale prospective studies in low risk populations need to be carried out to definitively establish and quantify the value of biochemical markers for fetoplacental growth restriction. As a result of such studies, we may be able not only to identify high risk pregnancies, but also to reassure the majority of women with normal results more strongly that their risk of developing serious pregnancy complications may actually be reduced.

Acknowledgements

We wish to acknowledge Ms Paulette Thomas, BA, of WordWorks Linguistics Services, for her invaluable assistance in the transcription and editing of the manuscript for this chapter.

References

1. Pahal GS, Jauniaux E. Maternal serum biochemical screening for pregnancy complications other than aneuploidy. Curr Opin Obstet Gynecol 1997;9:379–86.
2. Bergstrand CG, Czar B. Demonstration of a new protein fraction in serum from the human fetus. Scand J Clin Lab Invest 1956;8:174.
3. Gitlin D. Normal biology of alpha-fetoprotein. Ann NY Acad Sci 1975;259:7–16.
4. Boyd PA. Why might maternal serum AFP be high in pregnancies in which the fetus is normally formed. Br J Obstet Gynaecol 1992;99:93–5.
5. Cabellero C, Vekemaus M, Lopex del Campo JG, Robyn C. Serum alpha-fetoprotein in adults, in women during pregnancy, in children at birth, and during the first week of life: a sex difference. Am J Obstet Gynecol 1997;127:384–9.
6. Brock DJ, Sutcliffe RG. Alpha-fetoprotein in the antenatal diagnosis of anencephaly and spina bifida. Lancet 1972;2:197–9.
7. Gordon YB, Kitau MJ, Letchworth AT, Grudzinskas JG, Usherwood MMcD. Fetal wastage as a result of an alpha-fetoprotein screening programme. Lancet 1978;April:677–8.
8. Brock DJ, Barron L, Jelen P, Watt M, Scrimgeour JB. Maternal serum alpha-fetoprotein measurements as an early indicator of low birthweight. Lancet 1977;2:267–8.
9. Jauniaux E, Moscoso G, Campbell S, Gibb D, Driver M, Nicolaides KH. Correlation of ultrasound and pathologic findings of placental anomalies in pregnancies with elevated maternal serum alpha-fetoprotein. Eur J Obstet Gynecol Biol Reprod 1990;37:219–30.
10. Jauniaux E, Gulbis B, Tunkel S, Ramsay B, Campbell S, Meuris S. Maternal serum testing for alpha-fetoprotein and human chorionic gonadotropin in high-risk pregnancies. Prenat Diagn 1996;12:1129–35.
11. Walters BNJ, Lao T, Smith V, De Swiet M. α-fetoprotein elevation and proteinuric pre-eclampsia. Br J Obstet Gynaecol 1985;92:341–4.
12. Milunsky A, Juck SS, Bruell CL, MacLaughlin DS, Tsung Y-K, Jick H. Predictive values, relative risks, and overall benefits of high and low maternal serum α-fetoprotein screening in singleton pregnancies: New epidemiologic data. Am J Obstet Gynecol 1989;161:291–7.
13. Waller DK, Lustig LS, Cunningham GC, Golbus MS, Hook EB. Second-trimester maternal serum alpha-fetoprotein levels and the risk of subsequent fetal death. N Engl J Med 1991;325:6–10.
14. Bernstein IM, Barth RA, Miller R, Capeless EL. Elevated maternal serum alpha-fetoprotein: Association with placental sonolucencies, fetomaternal hemorrhage, vaginal bleeding, and pregnancy outcome in the absence of fetal anomalies. Obstet Gynecol 1992;79:71–4.
15. Williams MA, Hickok DE, Zingheimj RW, Luthy DA, Kimelman J, Nyberg DA, et al. Elevated maternal serum α-fetoprotein levels and midtrimester placental abnormalities in relation to subsequent adverse pregnancy outcomes. Am J Obstet Gynecol 1992;167:1032–7.
16. Brazerol WF, Grover S, Donnenfeld AE. Unexplained elevated maternal serum α-fetoprotein levels and perinatal outcome in an urban clinic population. Am J Obstet Gynecol 1994;171:1030–5.
17. Waller DK, Lustig LS, Cunningham GC, Feuchtbaum LB, Hook EB. The association between maternal serum alpha-fetoprotein and preterm birth, small for gestational age infants, pre-eclampsia, and placental complications. Obstet Gynecol 1996;88:816–22.
18. Wenstrom KD, Owen J, Davis RO, Brumfield CG. Prognostic significance of unexplained elevated amniotic fluid alpha-fetoprotein. Obstet Gynecol 1996;87:213–6
19. Morssink LP, Heringa MP, Beekhuis JR, De Wolf BTHM, Matingh A. The HELLP syndrome: its association with unexplained elevation of MSAFP and MShCG in the second trimester. Prenat Diagn 1997;17:601–6.
20. Hsieh TT, Hung TH, Hsu JJ, Shau WY, Su CW, Hsieh FJ. Prediction of adverse perinatal outcome by maternal serum screening for Down syndrome in an Asian population. Obstet Gynecol 1997;89:937–40.

21. Shipp TD, Wilkins-Haug L. The association of early-onset fetal growth restriction, elevated maternal serum alpha-fetoprotein, and the development of severe pre-eclampsia. Prenat Diagn 1997;17:305–9.
22. Simpson JL, Baum LD, Depp R, Elias S, Somes G, Marder R. Low maternal serum alpha-fetoprotein and perinatal outcome. Am J Obstet Gynecol 1987;156:852–62.
23. Benn PA, Horne D, Briganti S, Rodis JF, Clive JM. Elevated second-trimester maternal serum hCG alone in combination with elevated alpha-fetoprotein. Obstet Gynaecol 1996;87:217–22.
24. Macara L, Kingdom JCP, Kaufmann P, Kohnen G, Hair J, More IAR, et al. Structural analysis of placental terminal villi from growth-restricted pregnancies with abnormal umbilical artery Doppler waveforms. Placenta 1996;17:37–48.
25. Smith SC, Baker PN, Symonds EM. Increased placental apoptosis in intrauterine growth restriction. Am J Obstet Gynecol 1997;177:1395–1401.
26. Brownbill P, Edwards D, Jones C, Mahendran D, Owen D, Sibley C, et al. Mechanism of alphafetoprotein transfer in the perfused human placental cotyledon from uncomplicated pregnancy. J Clin Invest 1995;96:2220–6.
27. Brownbill P, Owen D, Mahendran D, Nelson M, Sibley C. Comparisons of the alphafetoprotein permeability of term perfused placental cotyledons from women who had above normal maternal serum alphafetoprotein levels in mid-trimester with those from women who had normal levels. Placenta 1997;18:A14.
28. Los FJ, De Wolf BTHM, Huisjes HJ. Raised maternal serum alpha-fetoprotein levels and spontaneous fetomaternal transfusion. Lancet 1979;ii:1210–12.
29. Zeltser PM, Neerhont RC, Ronkalsrud EW, Stiehm ER. Differentiation between neonatal hepatitis and biliary atresia by measuring serum alpha-fetoprotein. Lancet 1974;i:373–5.
30. Cox WL, Daffos F, Forestier F, Descomby D, Augrant C, Auger MC, et al. Physiology and management of intrauterine growth retardation: a biologic approach with fetal blood sampling. Am J Obstet Gynecol 1988;159:36–41.
31. Hubinot C, Fisk NM, Nicolini U, Rodeck CH, Johnson CH. Fetal Alpha-fetoprotein in growth retardation. Br J Obstet Gynaecol 1990;97:1233–4.
32. Bogart MH, Pandian MR, Jones OW. Abnormal maternal serum chorionic gonadotropin levels in pregnancies with fetal chromosome abnormalities. Prenat Diagn 1987;7:623–30.
33. Eiben B, Hammans W, Goebel R. Triploidy, imprinting, and hCG levels in maternal serum screening. Prenat Diagn 1996;16:377–8.
34. Laundon Ch, Spencer K, Macri JN, Anderson RW, Buchanan PD. Free Beta hCG screening of hydropic and non-hydropic Turner syndrome pregnancies. Prenat Diagn 1996;16:853–6.
35. Smith GC, Smith OW. Excessive gonad-stimulating hormone and subnormal amounts of oestrin in toxaemias of late pregnancy. Am J Obstet Gynecol 1934;107:128–45.
36. Gonen R, Perez R, David M, Dar H, Merksamer R, Sharf M. The association between unexplained second-trimester maternal serum hCG elevation and pregnancy complications. Obstet Gynecol 1992;80:83–6.
37. Tanaka M, Natori M, Kohno H, Ishimoto H, Kobayashi T, Nozawa S. Fetal growth in patients with elevated maternal serum hCG levels. Obstet Gynecol 1993;81:341–3.
38. Sorensen TK, Williams MA, Zingheim RW, Clement SJ, Hickok DE. Elevated second trimester human chorionic gonadotropin and subsequent pregnancy-induced hypertension. Am J Obstet Gynecol 1993;169:834–8.
39. Lieppman RE, Williams MA, Cheng EY, Resta R, Zingheim R, Hickok ED, et al. An association between elevated levels of human chorionic gonadotropin in the midtrimester and adverse pregnancy outcome. Am J Obstet Gynecol 1993;168:1852–7.
40. Said ME, Campbell DM, Azzam ME, MacGillivray I. Beta-human chorionic gonadotrophin levels before and after the development of pre-eclampsia. Br J Obstet Gynaecol 1984;91:772–5.
41. Hsu C-D, Chan DW, Iriye B, Johnson T, Hong S-F, Repke JT. Elevated serum human chorionic gonadotropin as evidence of secretory response in severe preeclampsia. Am J Obstet Gynecol 1994;170:1135–8.
42. Ashour AMN, Lieberman ES, Wilkins Haug LE, Repke JT. The value of elevated second-trimester β-human chorionic gonadotropin in predicting development of pre-eclampsia. Am J Obstet Gynecol 1997;176:438–42.
43. Jones CJP, Fox H. An ultrastructural and ultrahistochemical study of the human placenta in maternal pre-eclampsia. Placenta 1980;1:61–76.
44. Hoshina M, Ashitaka Y, Tojo S. Immunohistochemical interaction on antisera to hCG and its subunits with chorionic tissue of early gestation. Endocrinol Jpn 1979;26:175–84.
45. Genbacev O, Joslin R,Damsky CH, Pollitti BM, Fisher SJ. Hypoxia alters early gestation human cytotrophoblast differentiation/invasion in vitro and models the placental defects that occur in preeclampsia. J Clin Invest 1996;97:540–50.

46. Rodesh F, Simon P, Donner C, Jauniaux E. Oxygen measurements in the maternotrophoblastic border during early pregnancy. Obstet Gynecol 1992;80:283–5.

47. Kingdom JCP, Kaufmann P. Oxygen and placental villous development: Origins of fetal hypoxia. Placenta 1997;18:613–21.

48. Wenstrom KD, Owen J, Boots LR. Elevated second-trimester human chorionic gonadotrophin levels in association with poor pregnancy outcome. AM J Obstet Gynecol 1994;171:1038–41.

49. Konachak PS, Bernstein IM, Capeless L. Uterine artery Doppler velocimetry in the detection of adverse obstetric outcomes in women with unexplained elevated maternal serum α-fetoprotein levels. Am J Obstet Gynecol 1995;173:1115–19.

50. Pergament E, Stein AK, Fiddler M, Cho NH, Kupferminc MJ. Adverse pregnancy outcome after a false-positive screen for Down syndrome using multiple markers. Obstet Gynecol 1995;86:255–8.

51. Fitzgerald DJ, Entman SS, Mulloy K, Fitzgerald GA. Decreased prostacyclin biosynthesis preceding the clinic manifestation of pregnancy-induced hypertension. Pathophysiol Nat Hist 1987;75:956–63.

52. Stubbs TM, Lazarchick J, Horger EO. Plasma fibronectin levels in preeclampsia: A possible biochemical marker for vascular endothelial damage. Am J Obstet Gynecol 1984;150:885–7.

53. Lazarchick J, Stubbs TM, Romein L, Van Dorsten JP, Leadholt CB. Predictive value of fibronectin levels in normotensive gravid women destined to become preeclamptic. Am J Obstet Gynecol 1986;154:1050–2.

54. Taylor RN, Crombleholme WR, Friedman ST, Jones LA, Casal DC, Roberts JM. High plasma cellular fibronectin levels correlate with biochemical and clinical features of preeclampsia but cannot be attributed to hypertension alone. Am J Obstet Gynecol 1991;165:895–901.

55. Friedman SA, de Groot JM, Taylor RN, Roberts JM. Circulating concentrations of fetal fibronectin do not reflect reduced trophoblastic invasion in preeclamptic pregnancies. Am J Obstet Gynecol 1992;167:496–7.

56. Lockwood CJ, Peters JH. Increased plasma levels of EDI+ cellular fibronectin precede the clinical signs of preeclampsia. Am J Obstet Gynecol 1990;162:358–62.

57. Taylor RN, Heilbron DC, Roberts JM. Growth factor activity in the blood of women in whom preeclampsia develops is elevated from early pregnancy. Am J Obstet Gynecol 1990;163:1839–44.

58. Varma M, de Groot CJM, Lanyi S, Taylor RN. Evaluation of plasma insulin-like growth factor-binding protein-3 as a potential predictor of preeclampsia. Am J Obstet Gynecol 1993;169:995–9.

59. Rutanen EM, Bohn H, Seppala M. Radioimmunoassay of placental protein 12: levels in amniotic fluid, cord blood and serum of healthy adults, pregnant women, and patients with trophoblastic diseases. Am J Obstet Gynecol 1982;144:460–3.

60. de Groot CJM, O'Brien TJ, Taylor RN. Biochemical evidence of impaired trophoblastic invasion of decidual stroma in women destined to have preeclampsia. Am J Obstet Gynecol 1996;175:24–9.

61. Muttukrishna S, Knight PG, Groome NP, Redman CWG, Ledger WL. Activin A and inhibin A as possible endocrine markers for pre-eclampsia. Lancet 1997;349:1285–8.

62. Heyborne KD, McGregor JA, Henry G. Interleukin-10 in AF at midtrimester: Immune activation and suppression in relation to fetal growth. Am J Obstet Gynecol 1994;171:55–9.

63. Spong CY, Sherer DM, Ghindini A, Jenkins CB, Seydel FD, Eglinton GS. Second-trimester amniotic fluid or maternal serum interleukin-10 levels and small for gestational age neonates. Obstet Gynecol 1996;88:24–8.

64. Rosen AC, Hafner E, Auerbach L, Rosen HR, Schuchter K, Huber K, et al. Placental isoferritin in pregnancies with small for gestation age fetuses. Prenat Diagn 1996;16:641–6.

65. Schiff E, Peleg E, Goldenberg M, Rosenthal T, Ruppin E, Tamarkin M, et al. The use of aspirin to prevent pregnancy-induced hypertension and lower the ratio of thromboxane A_2 to prostacyclin in relatively high-risk pregnancies. N Engl J Med 1989;321:351–6.

13   Diagnosis and Management of IUGR

John Kingdom and Graeme Smith

Introduction

As outlined in Ch. 1, IUGR refers to a biological process in which the fetus fails to achieve its genetically programmed growth potential. Factors that interact to produce the clinical scenario of IUGR include the external environment, coexistent maternal disease, and the placental and fetal adaptive responses.

The diagnosis of IUGR is thus complex since there is neither a uniform presentation nor a standard set of diagnostic features on ultrasound. The management of this condition is compounded by variations in the gestational age at onset, the severity of coexistent maternal disease and finally by obstetrical issues such as cervical maturation, fetal presentation and previous routes of delivery.

The purpose of this chapter is to provide evidence-based diagnostic and management strategies for this condition. Unfortunately only a small proportion of contemporary decision making in IUGR is based upon the results of good quality randomised clinical trials. Recent clinicopathological information has given new insights into data from observational studies and it is hoped that this subject will be advanced by research addressing the pertinent issues.

Differential Diagnosis of SGA

The terms SGA and IUGR were defined in Ch. 1. In the absence of an underlying diagnosis for a small fetus, the term SGA is used. Thus SGA has a complex differential diagnosis [1,2] that includes a number of karyotype abnormalities (Table 13.1). Outside a tertiary referral setting, the majority of SGA fetuses will be either constitutionally small, or subject to a variable degree of uteroplacental insufficiency. [3] The more rare causes of an SGA fetus assume prominence in a tertiary setting. However, whilst seen rarely outside fetal medicine units, one has to have constant vigilance while performing ultrasound in order that these possibilities are considered. The following sequence of questions is useful to consider while performing ultrasound of the SGA fetus.

Is this a Healthy SGA Fetus?

Every small fetus should have a detailed anatomical assessment at the time of diagnosis even if a previous ultrasound has been reported as normal. During this

Table 13.1 Karyotype abnormalities in a tertiary care setting for IUGR

triploidy	36
trisomy 18	32
trisomy 21	8
trisomy 13	5
4p–	4
trisomy 22	1
rearrangements	3

Karyotype abnormalities were found in 89/458 (19 per cent) of cases in which prenatal karyotyping was performed. Triploidy was the most common abnormality presenting before 26 weeks, and trisomy 18 the most common after 26 weeks. Trisomy 21 was not a prominent cause of IUGR in this setting (adapted from [2]).

examination a biophysical profile can be undertaken and repeat measurements of BPD, HC, AC and FL can be compared with previous data. In the setting of a symmetrical fetus (normal head/abdomen circumference ratio) with a normal biophysical profile, the demonstration of normal umbilical artery Doppler confirms that this is a healthy constitutionally small fetus. The use of computerised individual percentile growth curves can improve the latter diagnosis [4] though in our opinion umbilical artery Doppler serves the same purpose. Healthy SGA fetuses by definition should be accompanied by normal uterine artery Doppler [5] and placental morphology [6].

Rare chromosomal and genetic diagnoses may have normal, or even increased amniotic fluid volume. Thus normal amniotic fluid volume per se does not exclude pathology. In this situation particular attention should be placed on examination of the face, head, heart and hands for the fetal markers of aneuploidy.

Is There a Possibility of Aneuploidy?

This should always be considered where the observations are "discordant", e.g. markedly small fetus with normal amniotic fluid volume, or where any fetal structural abnormality is detected. The risk of aneuploidy is primarily conferred by maternal age. Prior information may be helpful in refining this background risk, e.g. nuchal translucency measurement in the late first trimester (11–13 weeks) or early second trimester serum biochemistry. The latter may also support a diagnosis of IUGR due to placental insufficiency – see Ch. 12. The ultrasound finding of soft markers of aneuploidy (e.g. echogenic bowel, choroid plexus cysts, mild ventriculomegaly, intracardiac echogenic foci and pyelectasis) may have been observed at 18–20 weeks and thus this examination should be reviewed [7]. In isolation these markers may not imply a high risk for aneuploidy, since the background age-related risk may be low; however, if present at any stage, a careful examination of the more challenging parts of fetal anatomy, e.g. the heart and face, is warranted.

Intrauterine starvation itself can reproduce several soft markers of aneuploidy including short femurs and echogenic small bowel [8]. Normal placental (uterine and umbilical) Doppler studies in this setting appear to increase the risk of aneuploidy [2]. At present the quality of these data (retrospective cohort) is inadequate to accurately refine prior risk based upon either nuchal or serum screening, and the latter information ought to be used to guide the need for invasive karyotyping procedures [9].

Is this "Placental IUGR"?

A placental aetiology is usually a straightforward diagnosis before 32 weeks of gestation. It is based around the following constellation of findings:

1. Elevated PI in the umbilical arteries
2. Elevated head/abdomen circumference ratio
3. Reduced AFI
4. Coexistent pre-eclampsia
5. Elevated PI/early diastolic notches in the proximal uterine arteries
6. Abnormal appearance of the placenta.

However no single ultrasound parameter can be used to establish the diagnosis of placental IUGR. A good illustration of this is that abnormal umbilical artery Doppler has a diverse range of associated pathologies [1], in particular aneuploidy [10]. Trisomy 18 may present with a small fetus and abnormal umbilical artery Doppler, but typically the fetus is symmetrically small with normal or increased amniotic fluid. Structural abnormalities of the fetus are detectable in 80–90% of cases. Fetuses with triploidy are asymmetrically small with reduced amniotic fluid and abnormal umbilical artery Doppler. Pre-eclampsia may coexist and fetal structural abnormalities may be subtle and difficult to visualise [2,11]. Therefore, when the possibility of aneuploidy exists, karyotyping may be necessary for counselling and to avoid inappropriate delivery by CS for the compromised fetus.

In general, all SGA fetuses can be assigned to one of the three above categories – healthy small fetus, aneuploidy (or other fetal pathology), or IUGR due to placental insufficiency [3]. Comprehensive ultrasound examination, using modern equipment with color/pulsed Doppler facilities, and integration of this information with the clinical scenario, will assist the diagnostic process.

The Importance of Invasive Prenatal Diagnosis in IUGR

A comprehensive initial ultrasound assessment should be followed by appropriate investigations. Often the most important test is karyotyping. Amniocentesis, chorionic villus sampling and fetal blood sampling all carry risks of preterm delivery, premature rupture of the membranes, and/or fetal demise. Thus the test should be performed only if it will contribute to clinical management. Where late (after 24 weeks) termination of pregnancy is considered unethical or not legal (e.g. for suspected Turner syndrome or trisomy 21) invasive testing may be illogical since intervention in labour for fetal distress is generally appropriate. However, for suspected lethal abnormalities in IUGR fetuses (e.g. trisomy 18, 13, and 4p–), rapid karyotyping is essential to avoid unnecessary cesarean section. In recent years the greater availability of fluorescent in-situ hybridisation (FISH) has permitted the rapid diagnosis of the major trisomies [13, 18, 21] and triploidy from uncultured amniocytes obtained by amniocentesis [12].

Experience has taught us that early recourse to these discussions with prospective parents ensures they make the appropriate choices during the perinatal period [10]. Management of these problems is generally straightforward where termination of pregnancy after 24 weeks is not permitted for non-lethal abnormalities. However, it is clearly a complex issue for parents and health care professionals in European countries such as France [13] and the UK, which currently permit third trimester termination for non-lethal abnormalities with varying degrees of mental handicap. Indeed some authorities [14] have recently advocated deferral of invasive testing into the third trimester to avoid procedure-related losses of chromosomally normal fetuses.

Additional Tests

Ultrasound findings such as dystrophic calcification of the fetus, or asymmetrical limb deformities, should prompt investigations for congenital infections, including toxoplasmosis and varicella (see Ch. 3). Sampling for viral culture and/or antibody detection may include maternal serum and urine, amniotic fluid, or fetal blood. A recent finding has been the recognition that placental damage may be mediated by maternal [15,16] or paternal (placental) [17] pro-thrombotic disorders. These may result in placental damage and severe early-onset IUGR. Typically this scenario presents with a combined elevation in AFP and/or hCG, a small abnormal placenta and abnormal uterine and umbilical artery Doppler studies [18–20]. In a series of 16 women with early onset IUGR and absent end-diastolic flow velocity, we found thrombophilia disorders in six, including homozygous factor V Leiden (Gibson and Kingdom – submitted for publication). Thrombophilia screening should be considered, especially postpartum, where excessive (> 10 per cent) placental infarction is confirmed as the cause of IUGR and delivery at < 34 weeks' gestation.

Is the Fetus Potentially Viable?

Some IUGR fetuses are clearly non-viable at the initial ultrasound diagnosis. The typical features would be an estimated fetal weight < 500 g after 26 weeks, reversed end-diastolic flow velocity in the umbilical arteries, umbilical vein pulsations and a decelerative non-stress test (NST). Some of these features are illus-

---

Fig. 13.1 Ominous ultrasound findings in IUGR fetuses: **a** Absent end-diastolic flow velocity in the umbilical artery with a wide space between arterial signals. Florid umbilical vein pulsations are seen in the umbilical vein (lower channel). **b** Corresponding waveform for the ductus venosus showing reversed flow velocity during atrial systole. These right atrial pulsations are transmitted distally into the free portion of the umbilical vein. These gross abnormalities in venous Doppler are indicative of metabolic acidosis. **c** Markedly echogenic bowel at 20 weeks of gestation in association with absent end-diastolic flow velocity in the umbilical arteries and reduced amniotic fluid volume. This appearance is thought to be due to ischaemia since the fetus is diverting cardiac output to the brain. **d** Fetal cerebral blood flow redistribution evident at 27 weeks of gestation. Note the pulsed gate locates the middle cerebral artery along the edge of the sphenoid bone. **e** Severe waveform abnormality in the proximal uterine artery at 22 weeks of gestation characterised by diastolic notching and, in this instance, a small reversed component. **f** Normal uterine artery Doppler waveform at 22 weeks of gestation. **g** Normal umbilical artery Doppler waveform in third trimester, demonstrating positive end-diastolic flow velocity. Contrast with panel **a**. **h** Normal ductus venosus waveform at 24 weeks of gestation, demonstrating forward flow velocity throughout the cardiac cycle. Right atrial systole slows ductal flow across the right atrium – contrast with **b**.

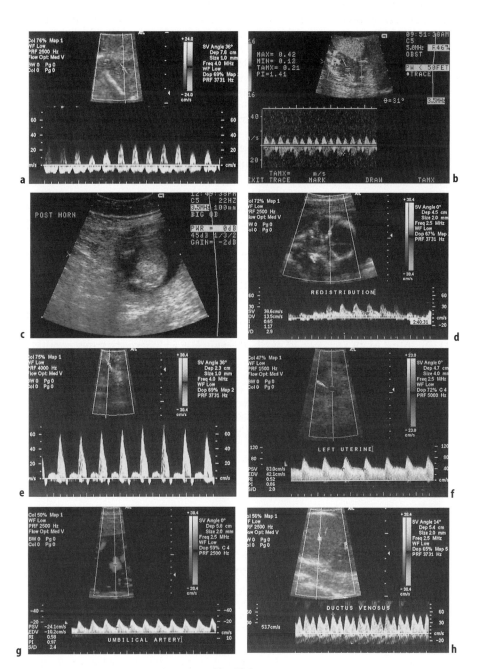

Fig. 13.1

trated in Fig. 13.1. It is important to be clear with prospective parents that such fetuses do not have the same survival statistics as appropriately grown neonates of a similar weight, yet lower gestation, that deliver spontaneously as a consequence of preterm labour. Counselling requires the coordinated input of a neonatologist closely associated with the fetal medicine unit. In our opinion, maternal administration of steroids, and a visit to the neonatal unit are not appropriate unless there is agreement on potential viability.

Outpatient screening for pre-eclampsia, via the obstetrical day unit, is essential in these instances since it occurs in 40 per cent of women with severe early onset IUGR and may include the syndrome of haemolysis, low platelets and elevated liver enzymes (HELLP) [21]. This assessment should include at least a weekly complete blood count, renal and liver biochemistry and urinalysis. Education regarding recognition of the symptoms of pre-eclampsia (headache, nausea, and upper abdominal pain) and home testing for proteinuria is worthwhile in our opinion. The development of pre-eclampsia is a valid indication for induction in these circumstances and fetal demise during labour is expected. These circumstances demand a lot of counselling time, and though difficult, is very important since a futile and possibly classical CS can be avoided [10]. Heparin therapy can be considered in future pregnancies, leading to a normal delivery at term in many cases [22].

Viable Early Onset "Placental IUGR"

This section refers to the management of pregnancies complicated by IUGR between viability and approximately 34 weeks of gestation. Pre-eclampsia co-exists in up to 40 per cent of such pregnancies, which necessitates combined maternal and fetal assessment on each occasion [21]. Pre-eclampsia may be severe and include the manifestations of HELLP syndrome. Inpatient management is generally preferable when pre-eclampsia coexists.

The woman should be encouraged to participate actively in both maternal and fetal surveillance. We use the "count-to-ten" method of fetal movement monitoring [23], discourage smoking as much as possible and reinforce knowledge of the symptoms of pre-eclampsia. We follow the therapeutic guidelines outlined Ch. 16.

Ultrasound Parameters – Which and When?

An ever-expanding list of "valuable" ultrasound observations has been reported for fetal surveillance in IUGR. Perhaps the best way to clarify their role is to view them in categories of long term (> 2 weeks), medium term (1 week) and short term (2–3 days) tests of fetal well-being based on their frequency of being repeated (Table 13.2). The inherent errors in estimating fetal weight by ultrasound (10–15%) imply that this test can only be meaningfully assessed every 2 weeks [24]. Doppler studies of the uterine arteries and placental morphological assessment likewise have only long term relevance and may be best employed as screening tools at 22–24 weeks, in order to guide the need for intensive fetal surveillance [25,26].

Medium-term tests need to be performed weekly. These include amniotic fluid index (AFI) and umbilical artery Doppler. Short term tests of fetal well-being

Table 13.2 Tests for fetal surveillance in IUGR

Long term (valid for 2 weeks)
uterine artery Doppler
placental morphology
fetal biometry

Medium term (valid for 1 week)
umbilical artery Doppler
amniotic fluid

Short term (valid for 1–3 days)
biophysical profile score
fetal arterial and venous Doppler studies
non-stress test
contraction stress test

---

focus on the assessment of fetal oxygenation. These need to be performed two or more times per week when the fetus is at risk of hypoxia and include; the ultrasound-derived BPS, middle cerebral artery (MCA) Doppler (cerebral blood flow redistribution) [27], and the non-stress test (NST)/cardiotocograph (CTG) (NST). Ideally the latter should be computerised to determine short term fetal heart rate variation [28]. An important point to emphasise is that multiple short term tests of fetal well-being are not indicated if the medium-term test are normal. Otherwise the fetus is at risk of delivery from false positive information. This may explain why the original randomised trials of NST versus no monitoring showed an increase in perinatal mortality [29]. Finally, since all three short term tests focus on fetal hypoxia, it is safe to assume the fetus is normoxic if two are normal. Thus for efficiency purposes, we omit the NST if the BPP and MCA Doppler studies are normal.

The approach to monitoring the fetus at risk for IUGR is to commence with long term assessment of growth every 2 weeks, noting amniotic fluid and asking the patient about fetal activity. If fetal growth appears to slow and/or reduced amniotic fluid is noted, medium term assessment should be added on a weekly basis, thus including umbilical artery Doppler. Reduced amniotic fluid and abnormal umbilical artery Doppler (PI values > 95th percentile) would indicate a need to step up to two per week acute tests of fetal oxygenation.

Co-existent pre-eclampsia requires two per week assessments on maternal grounds alone. Fetal health assessment at each visit is justified because the rate of deterioration in fetal health is greater when preterm IUGR is complicated by pre-eclampsia [30]. Placental pathology data [31,32] supports this view since the excessive placental thrombosis/fetal vessel occlusion in this setting may be due to an unrecognised maternal thrombophilia [33].

Whilst the literature on fetal assessment in IUGR is very substantial, it is generally of an observational nature. There are few randomised clinical trials published, some of which, for example NST versus no monitoring [29], have no applicability in contemporary practice. Undoubtedly umbilical artery Doppler should be performed in all pregnancies where IUGR is suspected before 32 weeks of gestation. Random allocation of women with IUGR pregnancies to fetal surveillance either by umbilical artery Doppler or by NST [34] demonstrates the superiority of umbilical artery Doppler. Our view is that umbilical artery assesses the cause of IUGR whereas the NST detects the consequences (i.e. fetal hypoxaemia). This rationale is supported by the current Cochrane Library meta-analysis of the impact of umbilical artery Doppler surveillance in preterm pregnancies at high risk of placental disease, on fetal and early neonatal death rates.

Timing of Delivery

At the time of publication of this book, we have no appropriate data from randomised control trials upon which to make firm recommendations about timing of delivery for early onset IUGR. A number of publications provide high quality longitudinal data from gradually "deteriorating" fetuses [30,35], though in these papers the central hypothesis was the belief that advancement of gestation will always result in improved neonatal survival and neurodevelopment. This implies that the risk of postnatal brain injury exceeds that of remaining in utero during this period of intense fetal monitoring. We have no good data to support this hypothesis. Indeed neuropathology studies of stillborn IUGR fetuses demonstrate features of chronic ischaemia [36,37]. Intensive monitoring to prolong gestation in preterm IUGR may thus confer benefit or harm depending on several factors, including gestational age, severity of IUGR, coexistent pre-eclampsia and maternal administration of steroids. The results of the GRIT study, whose primary endpoint is pediatric neurodevelopment, is due to be published in 2001 and will provide the first robust data regarding the value, or futility, of intensive fetal monitoring in preterm IUGR (see Ch. 22).

In the absence of such data, what useful conclusions can be drawn from the observational literature? The first is that abnormal umbilical artery Doppler, in particular absent end-diastolic flow velocity, is not by itself an indication for delivery. This is because the fetus may remain healthy (all short term tests of fetal oxygenation normal) for one or more several weeks [30]. Second, the fetus may tolerate mild hypoxaemia for one or more weeks (represented by cerebral blood flow redistribution) with continued movement and reassuring NSTs. While this appears to have no short term concern during infant life [38] longer term follow-up suggests that prolonged mild cerebral hypoxia may be associated with impaired cognitive function [39]. Third, most would agree it is unwise to monitor to the point of developing a metabolic acidosis before delivery [40,41], since the resultant hypotension presents additional risks to the delivered neonate (cerebral ischaemia, renal impairment, necrotising enterocolitis). Venous Doppler studies, evaluating right heart function, are useful to screen for acidosis [35,41,42], in that the failing acidotic heart transmits pulsations into the umbilical venous system (see Fig. 13.1a,b,h). Doppler studies on deteriorating non-viable fetuses indicate that this finding is associated with "loss" of cerebral blood flow redistribution [27,43], presumably due to reduced left-sided cardiac output to the brain [44]. From a mechanistic standpoint fetal cardiac failure may be the basis for "watershed" ischaemic injury to the fetal brain, leading to cerebral palsy [37]. For this reason, it may be preferable to pre-empt this degree of deterioration (usually manifest as a tachycardic decelerative NST) by consideration of delivery following maternal administration of corticosteroids.

Two additional approaches that can, in our experience, occasionally clarify timing of delivery in complex cases are: amniocentesis for assessment of lung maturation (30+ weeks' gestation) and the contraction stress test (CST).

Fetal Monitoring during Steroid Administration

IUGR is associated with advanced fetal lung maturation. The underlying reasons are not well understood, but in part comprise a stress response to hypoxaemia. In addition, the fetus may be exposed to greater amounts of maternal steroids than normal because the placental trophoblast 11β-hydroxysteroid dehydrogenase type 2 activity, which acts as an enzymatic barrier, is reduced in early onset IUGR [45]. Despite these observations, good quality follow-up data indicates improved survival and lower risks of major morbidity and handicap in preterm IUGR neonates that were exposed to corticosteroids in utero (Dr A Ohlson, Toronto – unpublished data).

Invasive monitoring of the healthy term sheep fetus demonstrates that an equivalent dose of betamethasone induces fetal hypertension, hyperglycaemia, hypoxaemia and a twofold increased in lactate levels [46]. Maternal corticosteroid administration to the fetus at risk of preterm delivery from preterm labour (not IUGR) is associated with a transient reduction in fetal heart rate variability on a computerised NST [47]. However, the ability of the human preterm IUGR fetus to tolerate these changes may be compromised by pre-existing hypoxaemia/metabolic acidosis due to reduced fetoplacental perfusion [40,48]. A recent study focusing on preterm IUGR fetuses with absent EDF in the umbilical arteries demonstrated transient reappearance of EDF for 3 days in 68 per cent following maternal betamethasone administration [49]. Acute tests of fetal oxygenation were not reported in this study, though the authors claimed the reappearance of EDF in the umbilical arteries indicated improved fetoplacental blood flow. An alternative explanation is that betamethasone induced selective vasoconstriction of the umbilical arteries and thus placed the IUGR fetus at greater risk of metabolic acidosis [50,51]. Further prospective ultrasound studies around the time of maternal corticosteroid administration for preterm IUGR are warranted in order to define potential risks of this treatment.

Late Gestation "Placental IUGR" (> 35 Weeks)

As outlined in Ch. 1, we feel it is important to consider IUGR in late gestation separately from the much smaller subgroup presenting preterm with abnormal umbilical artery Doppler. Translation of concepts regarding disease pathogenesis, and thus significance of individual tests of fetal well-being, between preterm and term IUGR may have clouded our understanding of how to manage this condition after 34–35 weeks of gestation.

Diagnosis of IUGR after 35 weeks of Gestation

Umbilical Artery Doppler?

The vast majority of fetuses with abnormal umbilical artery Doppler, especially absent EDF, will have been delivered by 35 weeks [21]. This is because the larger IUGR fetus cannot tolerate this degree of placental insufficiency. In the face of uteroplacental ischaemia, adequate transplacental gas and nutrient/waste exchange between mother and fetus depends on the balance between new placental villous growth and thrombosis – the latter taking place at three sites: spiral arteries [52], intervillous space [32] and fetoplacental vessel tree [31,53]. Continued placental villous growth is stimulated by hypoxia-sensitive growth factors such as VEGF [54]. This hypoxic drive increases peripheral villous angiogenesis (see Ch. 7) and can be demonstrated in several situations that are characterised by intraplacental hypoxia such as anaemia [55] and late gestation IUGR [56,57]. Thus fetoplacental (umbilical) vascular resistance falls (and end-diastolic flow is preserved) in the face of reduced uteroplacental blood flow. This explains why umbilical artery Doppler is typically normal in late onset IUGR [58]. In a recent series of such pregnancies evaluated at University College Hospital, London UK, we have found evidence of fetal compromise in one-third of IUGR fetuses with normal umbilical artery Doppler (Herskowitz and Kingdom – submitted for publication). Thus, contrary to earlier reports [59], "IUGR" in late pregnancy with normal umbilical artery Doppler is not a low risk situation.

Useful Additional Tests

These are shown in Table 13.3. Fetal asymmetry (increased head/abdomen circumference ratio) is a very useful guide as to the possibility of fetal starvation [60]. In our recent experience, an elevated HC/AC ratio was present in 15/16 late-gestation fetuses with cerebral blood flow redistribution (Herschkovitz and Kingdom – submitted for publication). Head measurements are typically omitted in this setting because of technical difficulty (engagement in pelvis) or because AC alone will give an adequate estimate of fetal weight [24]. From a biological perspective fetal asymmetry, rather than absolute size, should correlate with neonatal measures of IUGR. Admittedly even HC/AC ratio correlates poorly with postnatal evidence of starvation [61] and thus further research is needed to address the utility of HC measurements in late gestation.

Placental sonographic maturation, referred to as the Grannum grading system [62], may be a useful marker of placental insufficiency (see Fig. 13.2) and has been proposed as a sixth observation in the BPS [63]. Placentas with increased echogenicity (Grannum II or III) demonstrate features of adaptive villous angiogenesis, such as reduced diffusion distance for oxygen [64]. One interesting randomised control trial, performed in a community hospital setting, demonstrated a reduction in perinatal deaths where the observation of a Grannum grade III placenta was transmitted to the obstetrician [65].

Amniotic fluid volume, reported either as the 4 quadrant amniotic fluid index (AFI) or maximum vertical cord-free pool, is a widely recognised test for the recognition of fetal compromise in late pregnancy [66]. A high proportion

Table 13.3 Diagnosis of IUGR > 35 weeks of gestation

fetal asymmetry (elevated HC/AC ratio)
reduced amniotic fluid
advanced placental maturation (Grannum grade 3)
middle cerebral artery Doppler
uterine artery Doppler

Note umbilical artery Doppler is typically normal in late onset IUGR.

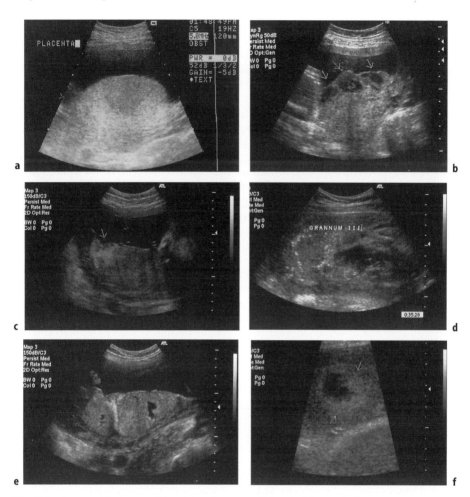

Fig. 13.2 Sonographic abnormalities of the placenta in IUGR: **a** Small "rounded" placenta projecting into the amniotic cavity. Note heterogeneous appearance, being darker in the centre. **b** These small placentas often show venous vascular malformations, with sluggish flow visible under zoom view (arrows). The placenta may be made to "wobble" with tapping, and is easily indented by fetal movement. The mobility of the placenta is thought due to the paucity of villous development and anchoring villi that would normally produce a thinner and firmer structure. Macroscopic abnormalities of the severe IUGR placenta are commonly found [70]. **c** Early infarction (arrow) is demonstrated as a segmental hyperechogenic area in an otherwise heterogeneous placenta. **d** Complete placental maturation (Grannum grade 3) characterised by bright reflective signal that delineates the lobular appearance of the placenta. **e** Infarcts in the placenta with Grannum 3 findings. This patient had pre-eclampsia and intrahepatic cholestasis with deranged liver function. **f** Magnified view of **e** demonstrating the distinction between a benign lake and an infarct. An infarct typically has a hyperechogenic ring around the cystic area, whereas a benign lake does not. Infarcts can be seen to evolve over time, whereas lakes remain static in appearance.

(> 40 per cent) of term fetuses with reduced amniotic fluid (maximum pocket < 2 cm) exhibit features of IUGR postnatally. Fetal breathing, tone (body movements) and limb movements constitute the additional components of the ultrasound-derived BPS [67] to which is added interpretation of the NST. A score of 2 for each component results in a final score of 10.

Doppler studies, other than of the umbilical arteries, may be useful in the recognition of late gestation IUGR. The middle cerebral arteries may show evidence of blood flow redistribution secondary to mild hypoxaemia. Studies in small fetuses > 35 weeks of gestation demonstrate the superiority of middle cerebral (vs. umbilical) Doppler in this setting [58] (Herschkovitz and Kingdom – submitted for publication). The proximal uterine arteries may show evidence of impaired uteroplacental blood flow in pregnancies with late gestation IUGR. Recent animal [68] and histopathological data [69] support the notion that abnormal uterine artery Doppler identifies the hypoxic-ischaemic placenta. However the principal role of uterine artery Doppler is as a screening test for IUGR (see Ch. 11). To date there is only scant information as to its potential role as a diagnostic test in this setting.

The diagnosis of IUGR in late gestation should rely on a composite of grey-scale information in addition to deriving the percentile value for the AC measurement (Table 13.3). The majority of at risk fetuses in late gestation can be recognised without the aid of Doppler. Many obstetrical day-assessment units rely on continuous-wave Doppler to determine umbilical artery Doppler, since it is a cheap test to perform. Whilst this approach may be a valid way of identifying the at-risk preterm IUGR fetus [3], the more expensive (in terms of equipment and training) colour flow techniques are needed to obtain cerebral and uterine Doppler waveforms. Given the costs of colour flow, further studies are needed to clarify the role of colour Doppler in the setting of fetal health assessment.

Management

The management of IUGR in late gestation differs in two important ways from that of early onset IUGR. First, the fetal prognosis is much better, and thus one has a lower threshold for deciding to recommend delivery. Secondly, the mode of delivery may be by induction of labour as opposed to CS.

The most mild cases of IUGR will have reduced amniotic fluid volume, an elevated HC/AC ratio, normal fetal movements and normal acute tests of fetal well-being (reactive NST, normal middle cerebral Doppler, normal biophysical profile score). Fetal BPS should be performed 2/week together with fetal movement counting. Vaginal examination should be considered from 37 weeks of gestation, to determine the suitability for induction (Bishop score) and perform membrane sweeping if the cervix is ripe. The timing of delivery represents a balance of risks for CS: failed induction due to an unripe cervix, or fetal distress during labour due to progressive placental insufficiency.

When is an Attempt at Vaginal Birth Futile?

In general a strong fetal indication for delivery at < 34 weeks would preclude a safe attempt at induction of labour. Parity, previous labour patterns and cervical ripening may influence route of delivery, especially at more advanced gestations.

The contraction stress test (CST) can be a useful adjunct to determination of route of delivery in this setting. Oxytocin is commenced intravenously at 1–2 mU/min and gradually increased until regular uterine activity is achieved. If the fetal heart rate tracing shows variable decelerations the infusion is stopped and a CS performed. If the CST is normal, labour induction can either continue with oxytocin (in parous women) or be switched to vaginal prostaglandins. This approach avoids the undesirable scenario of sever fetal distress provoked by initial use of vaginal prostaglandins in pregnancies complicated by IUGR.

What to Do at Delivery

The umbilical cord should be double-clamped to determine arterial and venous gases. This information may be useful if the newborn has unexpectedly low Apgar scores, and should be compared with the last ultrasound observations. The placenta should be weighed and inspected from both aspects (chorionic and basal plates) for evidence of infarction and gross abnormalities [70]. Placental histopathology is important, particularly in the more preterm cases [37,71]. Where the ultrasound features were "discordant" e.g. severe IUGR that is symmetrical with relatively normal amniotic fluid, the newborn should be examined carefully for external features that might indicate a genetic basis for poor growth. Screening for congenital infection (see Ch. 3) should be considered. Where the fetus is stillborn, karyotyping should be attempted if this information was not obtained prenatally, and autopsy should be considered. A full maternal thrombophilia screen should be performed following delivery < 32 weeks for severe IUGR and/or severe pre-eclampsia with HELLP syndrome [15,33].

Postnatal Role of the Obstetrician

In addition to the standard postnatal visit, the progress of the newborn should be reviewed, since this may have revealed an underlying diagnosis not appreciated during the antenatal period. Pre-eclampsia complicates up to 40 per cent of early onset/severe cases of IUGR and thus blood pressure and urinalysis are important. Persistent hypertension, especially in the presence of proteinuria and microscopic haematuria, suggests underlying renal disease and indicates the need for referral to a physician and consideration of renal biopsy. Interpretation of placental pathology and maternal thrombophilia tests is difficult at the present time owing to lack of quality prospective data. A small degree of infarction (< 5 per cent) is normal in the term placenta, but when in excess of 10 per cent, may be considered abnormal [17]. Widespread infarction is likely to impair placental function and is found in 50–75% of preterm IUGR deliveries in which ARED was observed in the umbilical arteries before delivery [32] (Gibson and Kingdom – submitted for publication. Maternal thrombophilia tests do not necessarily correlate with the degree of infarction in the placenta, which exposes our current lack of understanding of the mechanisms of placental thrombosis.

IUGR with ARED in the umbilical arteries has an overall recurrence risk of 10 per cent though no attempt was made to relate risk of recurrence to placental pathology [72]. The latter study predated the current vogue for thrombophilia testing, though the recurrence risk was lower in those women with a negative autoantibody screen. At present it is unclear whether heparin should be directed to women whose index pregnancy was complicated by excessive placental infarction or to women with thrombophilia disorders such as antiphospholipid antibody syndrome, or factor V Leiden. Longitudinal studies are in progress to assess the contribution of maternal and paternal thrombophilias to placental damage and pregnancy outcome at both University College Hospital, London and Royal Maternity Hospital, Glasgow, UK.

References

1. Wenstrom KD, Weiner CP, Williamson RA. Diverse maternal and fetal pathology associated with absent diastolic flow in the umbilical artery of high-risk fetuses. Obstet Gynecol 1991;77:374-8.
2. Snijders RJ, Sherrod C, Gosden CM, Nicolaides KH. Fetal growth retardation: associated malformations and chromosomal abnormalities. Am J Obstet Gynecol 1993;168:547-55.
3. Bobrow CS, Soothill PW. Fetal growth velocity: a cautionary tale. Lancet 1999;353:1460.
4. Mongelli M, Gardosi J. Reduction of false-positive diagnosis of fetal growth restriction by application of customized fetal growth standards. Obstet Gynecol 1996;88:844-48.
5. Chappell L, Bewley S. Pre-eclamptic toxaemia: the role of uterine artery Doppler. Br J Obstet Gynaecol 1998;105:379-82.
6. Jauniaux E, Kingdom J. Ultrasound and pathologic correlation in the placenta. In: Lewis S, Perrin E, editors. Contemporary issues in surgical pathology: the placenta. Edinburg: Churchill Livingstone, 1998.
7. Nyberg DA, Luthy DA, Resta RG, Nyberg BC, Williams MA. Age-adjusted ultrasound risk assessment for fetal Down's syndrome during the second trimester: description of the method and analysis of 142 cases. Ultrasound Obstet Gynecol 1998;12:8-14.
8. Nyberg DA, Dubinsky T, Resta RG, Mahony BS, Hickok DE, Luthy DA. Echogenic fetal bowel during the second trimester: clinical importance. Radiology 1993;188:527-31.
9. Palacio M, Jauniaux E, Kingdom J, Dell E, Sheldrake A, Rodeck CH. Perinatal outcome in pregnancies with a positive serum screening for Down's syndrome due to elevated levels of free beta-human chorionic gonadotropin. Ultrasound Obstet Gynecol 1999;13:58-62.
10. Kingdom JC, Rodeck CH, Kaufmann P. Umbilical artery Doppler–more harm than good? Br J Obstet Gynaecol 1997;104:393-6.
11. Jauniaux E, Brown R, Rodeck C, Nicolaides KH. Prenatal diagnosis of triploidy during the second trimester of pregnancy. Obstet Gynecol 1996;88:983-9.
12. Eiben B, Trawicki W, Hammans W, Goebel R, Pruggmayer M, Epplen JT. Rapid prenatal diagnosis of aneuploidies in uncultured amniocytes by fluorescence in situ Hybridization. Evaluation of > 3,000 cases. Fetal Diagn Ther. 1999;14:193-7.
13. Dommergues M, Benachi A, Benifla JL, des NR, Dumez Y. The reasons for termination of pregnancy in the third trimester. Br J Obstet Gynaecol 1999;106:297-303.
14. Fisk NM, Fordham K, Abramsky L. Elective late fetal karyotyping. Br J Obstet Gynaecol 1996;103:468-70.
15. Dekker GA, de Vries JI, Doelitzsch PM, et al. Underlying disorders associated with severe early-onset preeclampsia. Am.J Obstet Gynecol 1995;173:1042-8.
16. de Vries JI, Dekker GA, Huijgens PC, Jakobs C, Blomberg BM, van Geijn HP. Hyperhomocysteinaemia and protein S deficiency in complicated pregnancies. Br J Obstet Gynaecol 1997;104:1248-54.
17. Dizon-Townson DS, Meline L, Nelson LM, Varner M, Ward K. Fetal carriers of the factor V Leiden mutation are prone to miscarriage and placental infarction. Am J Obstet Gynecol 1997;177:402-5.
18. Hurley TJ, Miller C, O'Brien TJ, Blacklaw M, Quirk JGJ. Maternal serum human chorionic gonadotropin as a marker for the delivery of low-birth-weight infants in women with unexplained elevations in maternal serum alpha-fetoprotein. J Matern Fetal Med. 1996;5:340-4.
19. Jauniaux E, Gulbis B, Tunkel S, Ramsay B, Campbell S, Meuris S. Maternal serum testing for alpha-fetoprotein and human chorionic gonadotropin in high-risk pregnancies. Prenat Diagn 1996;16:1129-35.

20. Williams MA, Hickok DE, Zingheim RW, et al. Elevated maternal serum alpha-fetoprotein levels and midtrimester placental abnormalities in relation to subsequent adverse pregnancy outcomes. Am J Obstet Gynecol 1992;167:1032–7.

21. Karsdorp VH, van Vugt JM, van Geijn HP, et al. Clinical significance of absent or reversed end diastolic velocity waveforms in umbilical artery. Lancet 1994;344:1664–8.

22. Riyazi N, Leeda M, de Vries JI, Huijgens PC, van Geijn HP, Dekker GA. Low-molecular-weight heparin combined with aspirin in pregnant women with thrombophilia and a history of preeclampsia or fetal growth restriction: a preliminary study. Eur J Obstet Gynecol Reprod Biol 1998;80:49–54.

23. Pearson JF, Weaver JB. Fetal activity and fetal wellbeing: an evaluation. BMJ 1976;1:1305–7.

24. Smith GC, Smith MF, McNay MB, Fleming JE. The relation between fetal abdominal circumference and birthweight: findings in 3512 pregnancies. Br J Obstet Gynaecol 1997;104:186–90.

25. Bower S, Bewley S, Campbell S. Improved prediction of preeclampsia by two-stage screening of uterine arteries using the early diastolic notch and color Doppler imaging. Obstet Gynecol 1993;82:78–83.

26. Bower S, Kingdom J, Campbell S. Objective and subjective assessment of abnormal uterine artery Doppler flow velocity waveforms. Ultrasound Obstet Gynecol 1998;12:260–4.

27. Vyas S, Nicolaides KH, Bower S, Campbell S. Middle cerebral artery flow velocity waveforms in fetal hypoxaemia. Br J Obstet Gynaecol 1990;97:797–803.

28. Guzman ER, Vintzileos A, Egan JF, Benito C, Lake M, Lai YL. Antenatal prediction of fetal pH in growth restricted fetuses using computer analysis of the fetal heart rate. J Matern Fetal Med. 1998;7:43–7.

29. Kidd LC, Patel NB, Smith R. Non-stress antenatal cardiotocography – a prospective randomized clinical trial. Br J Obstet Gynaecol 1985;92:1156–59.

30. Arduini D, Rizzo G, Romanini C. The development of abnormal heart rate patterns after absent end- diastolic velocity in umbilical artery: analysis of risk factors. Am.J Obstet Gynecol 1993;168:43–50.

31. Macara L, Kingdom JC, Kaufmann P, et al. Structural analysis of placental terminal villi from growth-restricted pregnancies with abnormal umbilical artery Doppler waveforms. Placenta 1996;17:37–48.

32. Krebs C, Macara LM, Leiser R, Bowman AW, Greer IA, Kingdom JC. Intrauterine growth restriction with absent end-diastolic flow velocity in the umbilical artery is associated with maldevelopment of the placental terminal villous tree. Am J Obstet Gynecol 1996;175:1534–42.

33. Nelson-Piercy C. Inherited thrombophilia and adverse pregnancy outcome: has the time come for selective testing? Br J Obstet Gynaecol 1999;106:513–15.

34. Almstrom H, Axelsson O, Cnattingius S, et al. Comparison of umbilical-artery velocimetry and cardiotocography for surveillance of small-for-gestational-age fetuses. Lancet 1992;340:936–40.

35. Ozcan T, Sbracia M, d'Ancona RL, Copel JA, Mari G. Arterial and venous Doppler velocimetry in the severely growth- restricted fetus and associations with adverse perinatal outcome. Ultrasound Obstet Gynecol 1998;12:39–44.

36. Burke CJ, Tannenberg AE. Prenatal brain damage and placental infarction – an autopsy study. Dev Med Child Neurol 1995;37:555–62.

37. Burke CJ, Tannenberg AE, Payton DJ. Ischaemic cerebral injury, intrauterine growth retardation, and placental infarction. Dev Med Child Neurol 1997;39:726–30.

38. Scherjon SA, Smolders-DeHaas H, Kok JH, Zondervan HA. The "brain-sparing" effect: antenatal cerebral Doppler findings in relation to neurologic outcome in very preterm infants. Am J Obstet Gynecol 1993;169:169–75.

39. Scherjon SA, Oosting H, Smolders-DeHaas H, Zondervan HA, Kok JH. Neurodevelopmental outcome at three years of age after fetal "brain-sparing". Early Hum Dev 1998;52:67–79.

40. Marconi AM, Cetin I, Ferrazzi E, Ferrari MM, Pardi G, Battaglia FC. Lactate metabolism in normal and growth-retarded human fetuses. Pediatr Res 1990;28:652–6.

41. Hecher K, Snijders R, Campbell S, Nicolaides K. Fetal venous, intracardiac, and arterial blood flow measurements in intrauterine growth retardation: relationship with fetal blood gases. Am J Obstet Gynecol 1995;173:10–15.

42. Rizzo G, Capponi A, Soregaroli M, Arduini D, Romanini C. Umbilical vein pulsations and acid-base status at cordocentesis in growth-retarded fetuses with absent end-diastolic velocity in umbilical artery. Biol Neonate. 1995;68:163–8.

43. Rowlands DJ, Vyas SK. Longitudinal study of fetal middle cerebral artery flow velocity waveforms preceding fetal death. Br J Obstet Gynaecol 1995;102:888–90.

44. Ferrazzi E, Bellotti M, Marconi A, Flisi L, Barbera A, Pardi G. Peak velocity of the outflow tract of the aorta: correlations with acid base status and oxygenation of the growth-retarded fetus. Obstet Gynecol 1995;85:663–8.

45. Shams M, Kilby MD, Somerset DA, et al. 11Beta-hydroxysteroid dehydrogenase type 2 in human pregnancy and reduced expression in intrauterine growth restriction. Hum Reprod 1998;13:799–804.

46. Bennet L, Kozuma S, McGarrigle HH, Hanson MA. Temporal changes in fetal cardiovascular, behavioural, metabolic and endocrine responses to maternally administered dexamethasone in the late gestation fetal sheep. Br J Obstet Gynaecol 1999;106:331–9.

47. Henson G. Antenatal cortiscosteroids and heart rate variability. Br J Obstet Gynaecol 1997;104:1219–20.

48. Nicolaides KH, Bilardo CM, Soothill PW, Campbell S. Absence of end diastolic frequencies in umbilical artery: a sign of fetal hypoxia and acidosis. BMJ 1988;297:1026–7.

49. Wallace EM, Baker LS. Effect of antenatal betamethasone administration on placental vascular resistance. Lancet 1999;353:1404–7.

50. Adamson SL. Arterial pressure, vascular input impedance, and resistance as determinants of pulsatile blood flow in the umbilical artery. Eur J Obstet Gynecol Reprod Biol 1999;84:119–25.

51. Adamson SL, Kingdom J. Antenatal betamethasone and fetoplacental blood flow [letter]. Lancet 1999;354:255–6.

52. Sheppard BL, Bonnar J. An ultrastructural study of utero-placental spiral arteries in hypertensive and normotensive pregnancy and fetal growth retardation. Br J Obstet Gynaecol 1981;88:695–705.

53. Salafia CM, Pezzullo JC, Minior VK, Divon MY. Placental pathology of absent and reversed end-diastolic flow in growth- restricted fetuses. Obstet Gynecol 1997;90:830–6.

54. Cooper JC, Sharkey AM, Charnock-Jones DS, Palmer CR, Smith SK. VEGF mRNA levels in placentae from pregnancies complicated by pre- eclampsia. Br J Obstet Gynaecol 1996;103:1191–6.

55. Kadyrov M, Kosanke G, Kingdom J, Kaufmann P. Increased fetoplacental angiogenesis during first trimester in anaemic women. Lancet 1998;352:1747–9.

56. Olofsson P, Laurini RN, Marsal K. A high uterine artery pulsatility index reflects a defective development of placental bed spiral arteries in pregnancies complicated by hypertension and fetal growth retardation. Eur J Obstet Gynecol Reprod Biol 1993;49:161–8.

57. Todros T, Sciarrone A, Piccoli E, Guiot C, Kaufmann P, Kingdom J. Umbilical Doppler waveforms and placental villous angiogenesis in pregnancies complicated by fetal growth restriction. Obstet Gynecol 1999;93:499–503.

58. Chang TC, Robson SC, Spencer JA, Gallivan S. Prediction of perinatal morbidity at term in small fetuses: comparison of fetal growth and Doppler ultrasound. Br J Obstet Gynaecol 1994;101:422–7.

59. Burke G, Stuart B, Crowley P, Scanaill SN, Drumm J. Is intrauterine growth retardation with normal umbilical artery blood flow a benign condition? BMJ 1990;300:1044–5.

60. Crane JP, Kopta MM. Prediction of intrauterine growth retardation via ultrasonically measured head/abdominal circumference ratios. Obstet Gynecol 1979;54:597–601.

61. Colley NV, Tremble JM, Henson GL, Cole TJ. Head circumference/abdominal circumference ratio, ponderal index and fetal malnutrition. Should head circumference/abdominal circumference ratio be abandoned? Br J Obstet Gynaecol 1991;98:524–7.

62. Grannum PA, Berkowitz RL, Hobbins JC. The ultrasonic changes in the maturing placenta and their relation to fetal pulmonic maturity. Am J Obstet Gynecol 1979;133:915–22.

63. Vintzileos AM, Campbell WA, Ingardia CJ, Nochimson DJ. The fetal biophysical profile and its predictive value. Obstet Gynecol 1983;62:271–8.

64. Burton GJ, Jauniaux E. Sonographic, stereological and Doppler flow velocimetric assessments of placental maturity. Br J Obstet Gynaecol 1995;102:818–25.

65. Proud J, Grant AM. Third trimester placental grading by ultrasonography as a test of fetal wellbeing. BMJ 1987;294:1641–4.

66. Manning FA, Baskett TF, Morrison I, Lange I. Fetal biophysical profile scoring: a prospective study in 1,184 high-risk patients. Am J Obstet Gynecol 1981;140:289–94.

67. Manning FA, Snijders R, Harman CR, Nicolaides K, Menticoglou S, Morrison I. Fetal biophysical profile score. VI. Correlation with antepartum umbilical venous fetal pH. Am J Obstet Gynecol 1993;169:755–63.

68. Ochi H, Matsubara K, Kusanagi Y, Taniguchi H, Ito M. Significance of a diastolic notch in the uterine artery flow velocity waveform induced by uterine embolisation in the pregnant ewe. Br J Obstet Gynaecol 1998;105:1118–21.

69. Ferrazzi E, Bulfamante G, Mezzopane R, Barbera A, Ghidini A, Pardi G. Uterine doppler velocimetry and placental hypoxic-ischemic lesion in pregnancies with fetal intrauterine growth restriction. Placenta. 1999;20:389–94.
70. Nordenvall M, Ullberg U, Laurin J, Lingman G, Sandstedt B, Ulmsten U. Placental morphology in relation to umbilical artery blood velocity waveforms. Eur J Obstet Gynecol Reprod Biol 1991;40:179–90.
71. Salafia CM. Placental pathology of fetal growth restriction. Clin Obstet Gynecol 1997;40:740–9.
72. Farine D, Ryan G, Kelly EN, Morrow RJ, Laskin C, Ritchie JW. Absent end-diastolic flow velocity waveforms in the umbilical artery – the subsequent pregnancy. Am.J Obstet Gynecol 1993;168:637–40.

14 Management of Late Gestation IUGR: Induction or Caesarean Section?

Stephen C. Robson and Duncan W. Irons

Introduction

The principal aim of antepartum fetal monitoring is the early detection and timely delivery of fetuses with progressive acidaemia. Most fetuses with antepartum hypoxia and acidaemia will be growth restricted, secondary to placental insufficiency, and many will be SGA. In this group of fetuses, the only widely available treatment is delivery (though see Ch. 16) but the timing of this intervention remains controversial. The Growth Restriction Intervention Trial (GRIT) is currently addressing the role of early delivery in the preterm growth-restricted infant [1]. However, we are unaware of any comparable study in the term or near-term small fetus. Thus at present there are no useful data to guide clinicians as to the optimal time to deliver the SGA fetus.

Once a decision has been made to expedite delivery, the obstetrician must decide whether to induce labour or opt for a caesarean section (CS). Many factors impact on this decision. Of these, fetal condition and gestational age are the most important and will be the focus of this review. However, other factors, such as maternal disease, malpresentation and previous CS, may preclude induction of labour (IOL), independently of the fetal condition.

With respect to labour outcome, we assume that a straightforward vaginal delivery of a healthy non-acidaemic infant is the optimal outcome and that it is preferable to avoid an emergency CS for fetal distress. Thus decisions about delivery are likely to be influenced by antepartum tests that predict the development of fetal distress and acidaemia during the first stage of labour.

Outcome of Labour in the SGA Fetus

Most studies that have compared labour outcome in small and appropriately grown fetuses have defined the study populations retrospectively by birthweight, including mostly term or near-term infants. It is clear from these studies that fetal heart rate abnormalities during labour occur more frequently in SGA fetuses and their incidence increases with the degree of smallness. Low et al. [2] were the first to show a relationship between decreasing birthweight percentile and increasing frequency of total and late fetal heart rate decelerations. Subsequently Kramer et al. [3] reported an abnormal electronic fetal heart rate pattern in

25 per cent of fetuses with a fetal growth ratio (observed birthweight to mean birthweight for gestation) of 0.80–0.84 and 46 per cent of fetuses with a ratio < 0.75.

The risk of abnormal fetal heart rate patterns and emergency CS for fetal distress appears to be increased around twofold in SGA infants. Steer [4] reported that 43 per cent of SGA infants (defined as a birthweight < 5th percentile) had an abnormal heart rate pattern in labour compared with 20 per cent of AGA infants. This reflected almost double the incidence of variable and late decelerations in the SGA group. Passage of meconium- stained liquor was also more common (36 versus 17 per cent). These abnormalities were reflected in almost twice the rate of emergency CS (18.0 versus 9.8 per cent). Metabolic acidosis at delivery is also more common in SGA fetuses [4,5]; in the study of Low et al. [5] 15 per cent of AGA infants were acidotic at delivery, compared with 50 per cent of very SGA infants.

Small infants with morphometric evidence of wasting, implying fetal growth restriction rather than constitutional smallness, are at greatest risk of intrapartum complications [6]. Fay et al. [7] showed that, within a group of SGA infants over 36 weeks' gestation, the rates of fetal distress and caesarean section were higher in infants with a low ponderal index compared with those without evidence of wasting. The same relationship existed in AGA infants, although intervention rates were lower [7].

Birthweight is not known to the clinician prior to labour and therefore the outcome of SGA fetuses detected prenatally is more relevant when considering labour management. Prenatally detected small fetuses, with an AC or EFW below the 5th or 10th percentile, are also at greater risk of abnormal fetal heart rate patterns in labour. Reported rates of emergency CS for fetal distress have ranged from 6 to 45 per cent [8,9] but a figure of around 15 per cent is probably appropriate for those with an AC or EFW below the 10th percentile [10]. Serial ultrasound studies have shown that reduced fetal abdominal growth velocity is a better predictor of caesarean section for fetal distress in labour than a single measurement of fetal size prior to delivery [10,11]. These studies indicate that growth restriction is a better predictor of intrapartum complications than smallness per se.

The increased incidence of fetal distress in IUGR is due to a combination of low prelabour fetal PO_2 and pH [12,13], coupled to a higher incidence of cord compression from the associated oligohydramnios [14]. Nieto et al. [13] compared fetal pH and gases in a group of 41 SGA fetuses (birthweight <10th percentile) and 61 AGA controls. Baseline scalp PO_2 and pH, measured when the cervix was ≤ 3 cm dilated, were lower in the SGA group (mean [sd] pH 7.32 [0.05] vs. 7.34 [0.03]) as was umbilical artery pH at delivery (mean [sd] pH 7.23 [0.08] vs. 7.27 [0.08]). The calculated rate of decrease in pH during labour was greater in the SGA group (0.19 u/h vs. 0.13 u/h). The authors commented that the decline in pH was not related to fetal heart patterns. Lin et al. [15] measured umbilical artery pH, gases and lactate in 37 SGA and 108 AGA fetuses. No differences in acid–base parameters were found between the two groups when fetal heart rate patterns remained normal. However, when fetal heart rate decelerations were present, SGA fetuses had a greater fall in pH and higher lactate levels. These studies suggest that SGA fetuses enter labour with a lower PO_2 and pH than AGA fetuses. Consequently they are less able to tolerate the stress of labour, being more likely to develop metabolic acidaemia in the presence of an abnormal fetal heart rate pattern.

Thus term and near-term SGA fetuses, and particularly those with growth restriction, are at increased risk of fetal heart rate decelerations in labour and metabolic acidaemia at delivery. These infants have an increased incidence of learning deficits and minor neurological disabilities in later childhood, although most have a normal IQ [6,15]. It is unclear to what extent intrapartum complications contribute to neurodevelopmental outcome in this group of fetuses. Preterm SGA infants have higher incidences of major handicaps and learning deficits then their AGA preterm counterparts [16]. In a study of infants delivered before 32 weeks [17], SGA rather than gestational age was associated with intellectual outcome, even after allowing for the confounding effects of reading ability and social variables. Birthweight ratio, birthweight and gestational age were each independently associated with motor skills [17]. Preterm SGA infants are more likely to be growth restricted, have abnormalities on antepartum testing and be delivered by "elective" CS. Metabolic acidaemia occurring de novo in labour may therefore be less likely to contribute to long term outcome in this group.

Antepartum Tests and Outcome of Labour

Amniotic Fluid Volume

Amniotic fluid volume is assessed by ultrasound measurement of either the maximum vertical pocket (MVP) or the summation of this measurement in all four quadrants of the uterus (amniotic fluid index, or AFI). Although the majority of recent studies have used AFI, there is little evidence that this method is more predictive of perinatal complications than the MVP [18]. Antepartum oligohydramnios, however defined, increases the risk of intrapartum complications [19]. The finding of a low AFI (< 5 cm) during the third trimester is associated with around a 40 per cent risk of fetal heart rate decelerations in labour and a 20 per cent risk of meconium, resulting in a 15–20% emergency CS rate [20]. Prelabour oral maternal rehydration may restore amniotic fluid volume and improve uteroplacental perfusion, though it is not known if this approach can reduce intrapartum complications [21].

A similar association exists when oligohydramnios is detected in early labour. Sarno et al. [22] first reported that a low AFI in the latent phase of labour was associated with intrapartum fetal distress: 18 per cent of women with an AFI < 5 cm required an emergency CS for fetal distress compared with 3 per cent of women with an AFI > 5 cm. In a subsequent study we measured ultrasonic amniotic fluid volume after membrane rupture in a group of normal labouring women: the 10th percentile for AFI was 6.2 cm [14]. In a separate study population, a low AFI had a 57 per cent positive predictive value for subsequent variable decelerations in labour and operative delivery [14].

Several studies have addressed the relationship between amniotic fluid volume and fetal distress in SGA fetuses (Table 14.1). O'Brien et al. [23] performed serial AFI measurements in a group of 142 hypertensive women with SGA fetuses. Neither an initial AFI ≤ 5 cm nor a final AFI ≤ 5 cm prior to delivery were associated with abnormal fetal heart rate patterns or caesarean section. However, two

Table 14.1 Studies of oligohydramnios and fetal distress during the first stage of labour in small fetuses

Author	N	Definitions		Fetal distress (%)		Caesarean section (%)	
		SGA	Oligohydramnios	PPV	NPV	PPV	NPV
O'Brien et al. 1993 [23]	142	AC < 5th	AFI ⩽ 5 cm	14	80	43	81
			AFI ⩽ 7 cm	22	81	33	83
Tsongsong and Srisomboon 1993 [24]	242	BW < 5th	MVP < 3 cm				
Miyamura et al. 1997 [25]	69	BW < 5th	AFI < 5 cm	56	86		
Irons & Robson 2000 [UP]	130	AC < 5th	AFI < 5 cm			31	84
			AFI < 8 cm			29	87

Reference numbers shown in brackets. UP = unpublished data from Newcastle, UK.

subsequent studies have reported an association between oligohydramnios and fetal distress (defined as repetitive decelerations or bradycardia) [24,25]. Fifty-seven of the 242 small fetuses (24 per cent) reported by Tsongsong and Srisomboom [24] had a MVP < 3 cm. Ten per cent of small fetuses developed intrapartum fetal distress and in 84 per cent this was associated with oligo-hydramnios. Of the 57 subjects with a MVP < 3 cm, 20 (35 per cent) required "obstetric intervention" for fetal distress [24]. However, none of these studies reported the indications for CS and thus it is impossible to determine the predictive value of oligohydramnios for intrapartum CS due to fetal distress.

We measured AFI within 7 days of delivery in 130 singleton non-anomalous fetuses with a fetal AC < 5th percentile. Fifty-five (42 per cent) had an AFI < 5 cm. Eighty-seven fetuses subsequently experienced labour and 18 (21 per cent) developed fetal distress during the first stage of labour (confirmed by fetal scalp sampling) of which 9 (50 per cent) had oligohydramnios. The predictive values of an antepartum AFI < 5 cm and < 8 cm for CS for fetal distress during the first stage of labour are shown in Table 14.1. Taken together, these studies suggest that around one-third of small fetuses with antepartum oligohydramnios will develop fetal distress in labour necessitating CS.

Isolated oligohydramnios is not an indication for CS in an otherwise healthy small fetus. However, continuous fetal heart rate monitoring is mandatory, because of the increased risk of heart rate decelerations. Serial FBS will detect those fetuses with a progressive fall in pH that require delivery. An alternative is transcervical amnioinfusion with the aim of alleviating umbilical cord compression. Protocols for transcervical amnioinfusion vary; we infuse warmed saline to maintain an AFI > 8 cm [26]. Review of available controlled trials suggests that the procedure reduces heart rate decelerations (OR 0.54, 95 per cent CI 0.43–0.68), CS (OR 0.56, 95 per cent CI 0.42–0.75), the incidence of cord blood pH < 7.20 (OR 0.51, 95 per cent CI 0.35–0.74) and Apgar score < 7 at 1 minute (OR 0.35, 95 per cent CI 0.23–0.53) [27]. The incidence of postpartum endometritis and the length of maternal and neonatal hospital stay are also reduced [27]. Whether amnioinfusion can actually prevent a progressive decline in fetal pH in the small fetus with recurrent decelerations and oligohydramnios is unknown but is worthy of further study.

Fetal Heart Rate Monitoring

Antepartum cardiotocography (CTG), or non-stress testing (NST), remains the most widely employed test of fetal well-being, despite the lack of evidence that its use reduces perinatal mortality [28]. Fetal death rates within 1 week of a normal test are acceptably low (1–3 per 1,000 women tested) [29,30] but the positive predictive value for stillbirth and serious perinatal morbidity are very low (< 10 per cent) [29,30].

Most of the studies relating antepartum cardiotocography to fetal outcome in labour have used visual analysis and classified patterns as either reactive or non-reactive. Reactivity is very dependent upon gestational age: 7–12% of normal fetuses have a non-reactive pattern between 34 and 40 weeks' gestation, but this figure increases as gestational age declines from 18 per cent at 28–33 weeks to 45 per cent at 24–28 weeks [31,32]. Therefore the predictive value of antepartum CTG for adverse intrapartum events depends upon gestational age, the underlying indication for testing and the interval between testing and delivery. Unfortunately most studies simply report outcome by heart rate pattern.

The relationship between antepartum CTG and blood gas values obtained by percutaneous FBS has been studied in SGA fetuses (Table 14.2) [33]. A reactive CTG effectively excludes acidaemia (pH > 2 sd below mean for gestation) but around 9 per cent of small fetuses with this pattern are hypoxaemic (PO_2 > 2 s below mean for gestation). Only 2 of 13 (15 per cent) SGA fetuses with repetitive antepartum decelerations had normal gases, 9 (69 per cent) were hypoxaemic and 8 (62 per cent) were acidaemic. Of all the individual components of the CTG, an abnormal baseline variation (< 5 beats/min) had the highest positive predictive value for hypoxaemia (78 per cent), acidaemia (67 per cent) and hypoxaemia and/or acidaemia (89 per cent) [33].

The incidence of intrapartum fetal distress within 7 days of a reactive antepartum CTG is less than 2 per cent [34–36]. This figure increases to 25–30% with a non-reactive trace, whereas the overall predictive value for CS for fetal distress

Table 14.2 Relationship between the different fetal heart rate patterns and the presence or absence of hypoxaemia or acidaemia at antepartum FBS in SGA fetuses

FHR pattern	N	Normal	Hypoxaemia*	Acidaemia**	Hypoxaemia or acidaemia
reactive	45	41	4	0	4
non-reactive	5	3	1	1	2
isolated decelerations	3	2	1	0	1
repetitive decelerations	13	2	9	8	11
terminal	1	0	1	1	1
total	67	48	16	10	19

Data relate to 67 fetal heart rate traces from 67 SGA (fetal abdominal circumference >2SD below mean for gestation) fetuses.

* ΔpO_2 >2 s below mean, ** ΔpH >2 s below mean.

Definitions: Reactive; ≥ 2 accelerations (amplitude ≥ 10 beats/min and duration ≥ 15 s) in a period of ≤ 30 min at ≤ 36 weeks' gestation or ≤ 40 min after 36 weeks' with no decelerations. Non-reactive; oscillation amplitude > 5 beats/min but less than 2 accelerations in a period of ≤ 30 min at ≤ 36 weeks' gestation or ≤ 40 min after 36 weeks' with no decelerations. Decelerations were considered to be significant if they were late (U shaped after Braxton–Hicks contractions with a decrease from the baseline of ≥ 10 beats/min) or variable (V shaped, not necessarily related to contractions and with a decrease from baseline of ≥ 20 beats/min). Terminal; completely flat with late decelerations after each contraction (Reproduced from [33] with permission).

is 13–27% [24,34,35,37]. The majority of non-reactive patterns do not have decelerations [34] and these confer a greater risk of morbidity. Between 30 and 35 per cent of fetuses with a terminal heart rate pattern (defined as one with a baseline variability of < 5 beats/min and repeated late decelerations in relation to Braxton–Hicks contractions) die within 7 days of testing [36,38]. Most surviving fetuses are not exposed to the additional risks of labour and over 70 per cent will be acidaemic at "elective" CS [38]. This compares with fetuses with a non-terminal decelerative pattern, of which only 8 per cent are acidaemic after CS [38].

Induction of labour may be considered (depending on obstetrical history and favorability) in fetuses with a non-terminal decelerative heart rate pattern. However, almost 70 per cent of these fetuses are hypoxaemic prior to induction [33], and as such up to 80 per cent will require an emergency CS because of persistent or deteriorating heart rate decelerations in labour [34]. Visser and Huisjes [36] reported an umbilical artery pH ≤ 7.15 at delivery in < 10 per cent of such cases, though many were delivered by CS owing to abnormal fetal heart rate patterns early in the first stage of labour. By contrast, an isolated decelerative CTG pattern is much less likely to be associated with antenatal hypoxaemia (Table 14.2) [33]; operative delivery for fetal distress in labour is required in only 12–16% of these cases [35,39].

Computer analysis of antepartum CTG is increasingly employed since it removes the subjectivity of visual analysis [40]. Studies in which computerised measurement of fetal heart rate (FHR) variation have been used as a predictor of fetal hypoxaemia/acidaemia have shown inconsistent results in terms of predicting fetal distress. Ribbert et al. [41] found that antepartum hypoxaemia in SGA fetuses was not reliably predicted until FHR variation fell to < 20 ms. By contrast, Guzman et al. [42], in a study of SGA fetuses delivered by CS before the onset of labour, found that a short term variation < 3.5 ms predicted acidaemia (defined as an umbilical artery pH < 7.20) with a sensitivity of 100 per cent and a positive predictive value of 57 per cent.

In a longitudinal study of 13 SGA fetuses ultimately delivered because of late decelerations, Snijders et al. [43] found that heart rate variation remained within the normal range until (or even after) late decelerations occurred. Furthermore Soothill et al. [44] found that computerised measurement of FHR variability did not predict short term morbidity in either SGA or AGA fetuses. Chang [45] studied the ability of computerised measurement of FHR variation to predict CS for fetal distress in women undergoing prostaglandin IOL. Thirty per cent of the fetuses were SGA. Using a cut-off of both short term variation < 3 ms and mean variation < 30 ms, computerised analysis had a sensitivity of 33 per cent and a positive predictive value of only 9 per cent. The negative predictive value was 95 per cent. Taken together, these studies suggest that computerised FHR analysis confers no additional benefit over visual analysis in deciding the mode of delivery in SGA fetuses.

Tongsong and Srisboom [24] compared the predictive value of CTG and amniotic fluid volume for intrapartum fetal distress in a large cohort of SGA fetuses (Table 14.3). Although both tests were significantly associated with fetal distress, there were no statistically significant differences in the predictive ability of the two tests. However, decisions regarding delivery are usually made with the knowledge of both tests and the incidence of a non-reactive antepartum FHR pattern increases from 1.2 per cent with a normal AFI (5–15 cm) to 28 per cent with

Table 14.3 Comparison of the accuracy of antepartum fetal heart rate monitoring and amniotic fluid volume for determining intrapartum fetal distress

	AFHR	MVP
sensitivity (%)	88.0	84.0
specificity (%)	70.1	83.4
positive predictive value (%)	25.3	36.8
negative predictive value (%)	98.1	97.8

Prevalence of intrapartum fetal distress 50/242 (20 per cent).
AFHR = antepartum fetal heart rate monitoring (a non-reactive pattern or a reactive pattern with variable or late decelerations was interpreted as abnormal); in MVP, a maximum vertical < 3 cm was interpreted as abnormal (reproduced from [24] with permission).

oligohydramnios (AFI < 5 cm) [20]. Hoskins et al. [46] reported the incidence of operative delivery for fetal distress in a large cohort of high risk fetuses tested after 33 weeks' gestation and delivered at a mean gestation of 36.3 weeks (Fig. 14.1). One-quarter of fetuses with severe variable decelerations and oligo-hydramnios (AFI ≤ 5 cm) developed late decelerations in labour and 46 per cent required CS for fetal distress.

Biophysical Profile Score (BPS)

The most widely adopted scoring system for the fetal biophysical profile is that of Manning [47] in which the five biophysical variables (breathing, movements, tone, amniotic fluid volume and CTG) are each assigned a score of 2 (normal) or 0 (abnormal). Manning [48] provides an excellent recent overview of the BPS. Several studies have compared antepartum fetal acid–base status with the BPS. A normal BPS (10/10, 8/10 with normal amniotic fluid volume, or 8/8 in the absence of a CTG) excludes acidaemia; in a total of 609 cases reported, none had an umbilical venous $pH < 7.25$ [48]. The risk of acidaemia (umbilical venous $pH < 7.25$) increases with declining score; 10 per cent (6/10), 35 per cent (4/10), 70 per cent (2/10) and 100 per cent (0/10) [49]. Assessment of acute biophysical variables immediately prior to elective CS indicates that fetal heart rate reactivity and breathing movements are lost at a higher mean [sd] umbilical artery pH (7.21 [0.10] and 7.21 [0.12] respectively) than are fetal movements (7.08 [0.10]) and tone (7.03 [0.04]) [50].

A normal BPS provides optimum reassurance that a fetus is healthy; the risk of fetal death within 7 days of a normal BPS is 0.6/1000 [48]. The risk of developing fetal distress in labour necessitating emergency CS increases with declining BPS [47,51]. With a normal score (8–10/10) the likelihood of developing fetal distress is 2.9–9.7%. This increases to 23–25% with an equivocal score (6/10) and 67 per cent with an abnormal score (0–4/10). In the initial Manning series [47] the results of the BPS were concealed from clinicians: five of five fetuses with a score of 0/10, three of four with a score of 2/10 and four of ten with a score of 4/10 required emergency delivery because of abnormal fetal heart rate patterns in labour. In a subsequent report of 18 fetuses with a BPS of 0/10, 17 (94 per cent) developed fetal distress and 13 (72 per cent) underwent emergency CS [52].

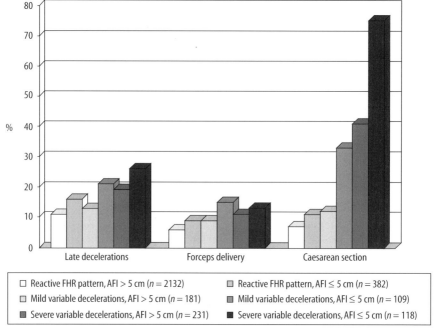

Fig. 14.1 Frequency of intrapartum late decelerations and operative delivery (forceps and CS) for fetal distress in a cohort of 3,158 pregnancies tested by antepartum FHR monitoring and measurement of AFI after 33 weeks' gestation. Mild variable decelerations (lasting ≤ 15 s with a decline ≤ 20 beats/min) and an AFI ≤ 5 cm predicted emergency CS for fetal distress with a sensitivity, specificity, PPV and NPV of 71.5, 83.3, 23.2 and 97.9 per cent respectively. Comparable figures for severe variable decelerations (lasting > 15 s with a decline > beats/min) were 84.5, 87.2, 43.6 and 91.2 per cent respectively (reproduced from [46] with permission).

Doppler Ultrasound

Doppler ultrasound allows detailed assessment of the placental and fetal haemodynamic modifications that are known to occur in IUGR. The umbilical artery is the mostly widely studied vessel. Abnormal waveforms range from a reduction in end-diastolic velocities (EDV) (elevated PI) to absent (AEDV) and ultimately reversed end-diastolic velocities (REDV). Reduced end-diastolic velocities are associated with increased vascular resistance in the fetoplacental circulation and adverse pregnancy outcome [53]. Between 40 and 45 per cent of fetuses with abnormal umbilical artery waveforms but EDV present are hypoxaemic (fetal $PO_2 > 2$ s below mean for gestation) and 20–30% are acidaemic (fetal pH > 2 sd below mean for gestation) [54,55]. In contrast, 80–90% of fetuses with AEDV are hypoxaemic and 45–80% are acidaemic [54–56].

Fetal bood flow redistribution in response to hypoxaemia is well documented in animal models and can be readily assessed in the human fetus by pulsed and colour Doppler (see Chs 5 and 13). Decreased PI values from the middle cerebral artery waveform, indicating cerebral vasodilatation, begins during mild to moderate hypoxaemia and is maximal when fetal PO_2 is 2–4 sd below the mean for gestation [57]. The incidence of redistribution, defined as a middle cerebral artery PI < 2 *sd* below the mean for gestation, ranges from 46 to 76 per cent among fetuses with abnormal umbilical artery Doppler waveforms [58]. Assessment of fetal arterial and venous Doppler waveform may be used to refine the risk of fetal hypoxia/acidaemia [59,60] and is discussed further in Ch. 13.

Umbilical artery Doppler has been subjected to more rigorous assessment by randomised trials than any other antepartum test of fetal health. Review of available trials indicates that umbilical artery Doppler reduces the odds of perinatal death in high risk pregnancies, most of which were suspected of being SGA, by 38 per cent (95 per cent CI 15–55) [53]. The rates of intrapartum fetal distress and emergency CS for fetal distress are also reduced, the latter by 52 per cent (95 per cent CI 24–69) [53], presumably because of more timely IOL. Thus delivery may be expedited because of deteriorating umbilical artery PI, but before EDV are lost and fetal compromise develops. This is supported by the trend towards increased preterm delivery in women randomised to revealing umbilical Doppler tests to clinicians (OR for delivery < 37 weeks + 36 per cent, 95 per cent CI –7, 8). There have been no trials to determine whether the use of fetal arterial or venous Doppler information improves perinatal mortality or morbidity.

The incidence of intrapartum late fetal heart rate decelerations is increased in SGA fetuses with abnormal umbilical artery Doppler waveforms. In women who labour with a small fetus, those with normal Doppler indices have a 3–8% risk of requiring an emergency CS for fetal distress [8,61]. In contrast, when the umbilical artery PI is > 2 *sd* above the mean for gestation but EDV are present, the incidence increases to 33–38% [61]. Once end-diastolic frequencies are absent or reversed the risk of intrapartum fetal heart rate decelerations necessitating CS is around 75 per cent, although this figure varies from 50 to 95 per cent in different series [62]. Most fetuses with AEDV in the umbilical artery are preterm; in the largest series from nine European centres, the mean gestational age at diagnosis of AEDV and REDV were 30 and 27.7 weeks respectively [63]. The mean gestation at delivery in these two groups was 31.5 weeks and 29.0 weeks respectively and 96 per cent of pregnancies were delivered by CS [63]. At these gestational ages the cervix is usually extremely unfavourable and induction has a high failure rate.

In SGA fetuses with abnormal umbilical artery Doppler indices the risk of intrapartum fetal distress and emergency CS is increased in those with evidence of cerebral blood flow redistribution [64] and abnormal venous waveforms [58,59,64]. If umbilical venous pulsations are present then the likelihood that the fetus will tolerate labour is less than 10 per cent [59]. The presence of an abnormal CTG also increases the risk of CS for fetal distress in fetuses with abnormal umbilical artery Doppler from 28 to 75 per cent [65]. In fetuses with AEDV in the umbilical artery, the interval between the first documentation of this finding and the development of late decelerations on a CTG ranges from 1 to 26 days (median 7 days) [66]. Gestational age less than 29 weeks and the presence of maternal hypertension and umbilical venous pulsations are associated with a reduced interval [66].

Almstrom et al. [67] compared umbilical artery Doppler with CTG as the primary method of antenatal surveillance in a group of 426 SGA fetuses (EFW > 2 *sd* below mean for gestation) ⩾ 31 weeks' gestation. Fetuses randomised to the Doppler group and found to have an abnormal PI but EDV present were examined twice a week while those with AEDV or REDV were delivered the same day. In comparison with the CTG group, the Doppler group had fewer antepartum monitoring occasions (4.1 vs. 8.2), fewer hospital admissions (31 vs. 46 per cent), fewer inductions of labour (10 vs. 22 per cent), fewer emergency CSs for fetal distress (5 vs. 14 per cent) and fewer admissions to neonatal intensive care. These results, together with those from other trials [53,44], strongly suggest that umbilical artery Doppler ultrasound should be the primary mode of antepartum fetal monitoring in the SGA fetus. This strategy, probably supplemented by selective use of the BPS, aids the clinical decision as to whether delivery should be by planned CS or by IOL – in the latter case the implication being that the fetus will likely tolerate labour.

Induction of Labour

Methods and Outcome

Clear guidelines on IOL methods and indications have recently been published by the RCOG [68]. When the cervix is favourable (Bishop score $\geq$ 4) intravenous oxytocin or intravaginal prostaglandin E_2 (either gel or tablets) [68] can be used to induce labour. Oxytocin is often ineffective in nulliparous women with an unfavourable cervix (Bishop score 0–3). Prostaglandin priming of the cervix increases cervical compliance and thus more closely mimics the physiological onset of labour; this approach has a lower incidence of operative delivery and a reduced need for epidural analgesia compared with oxytocin. However, the principal disadvantage of prostaglandin is the risk of uterine hypertonus, to which the IUGR fetus is most vulnerable [69]. An oxytocin contraction stress test (CST), using 2–4 mu/min intravenous oxytocin can be used initially to select out fetuses who will not tolerate IOL, thereby avoiding this particular risk in the IUGR fetus. Additional maternal complications associated with IOL include chorioamnionitis, uterine dehiscence, postpartum haemorrhage and hyponatraemia. One or more of these complications occur in 7 per cent of cases [70].

Parity, previous obstetrical history and the state of the cervix prior to IOL can reliably predict labour outcome. Failed induction, defined as the inability to enter the active phase of labour despite adequate exposure to cervical priming and oxytocin, is increased in women with an unfavourable cervix, particularly nulliparas [70] (Fig. 14.2). Compared with spontaneous labour, the risk of CS is increased four- to fivefold in women induced with a Bishop score of 0–3 (primiparas OR 3.7, 95 per cent CI 2.3–6.1; multiparas OR 4.7, 95 per cent CI 2.6–6.7) and two- to threefold in women with a more favourable cervix (primiparas OR 1.8, 95 per cent CI 1.1–2.9; multiparas 4.2, 95 per cent CI 2.6–6.7) [70].

Induction of Labour in the Small Fetus

There have been no published randomised trials addressing the optimum timing for, or mode of, delivery in the healthy term or near-term SGA fetus. In the absence of such data many clinicians opt for IOL between 37 and 40 weeks' gestation. Suspicion of a small fetus is the primary indication for delivery in 7–18% of labour inductions [70,71]. Not surprisingly, knowledge that a fetus is small has been shown to increase the rate of IOL for this indication. In a randomised trial of ultrasound screening in a population of low risk women [72], the rate of IOL

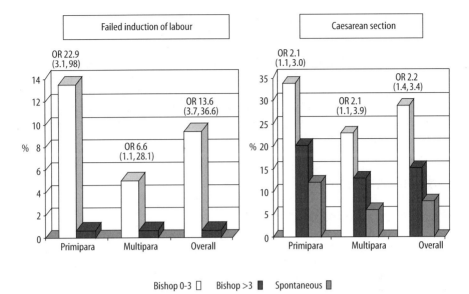

Bishop 0-3 ☐   Bishop >3 ■   Spontaneous ▨

Fig. 14.2 Rates of failed induction and CS in women undergoing induction of labour stratified by parity and Bishop's score at entry. Odds ratios (95 per cent CI) relate to comparisons between women induced with a Bishop score of 0-3 and those with a Bishop score > 3. Women with a Bishop score 0-3 (n = 202) were given PGE_2 3 mg intravaginally every 6 hours until they attained a score of > 7 or until a maximum of three PG doses had been administered. The same PG regimen was used in women with a Bishop score of 4-6 (n = 216), while those with a score > 6 were given oxytocin (n = 179). No statistically significant differences in induction outcome were demonstrated between women with a score of 4-6 and those with a score of > 6 and the data are presented together. The results are compared with a cohort of women in spontaneous labour (n = 2,204) (reproduced from [70] with permission).

for an SGA fetus was twofold higher in the revealed arm compared with the concealed arm (9 vs. 4 per cent, OR 2.37, 95 per cent CI 1.32–4.29). In those pregnancies with SGA infants, the higher rate of IOL in the revealed arm (41 vs. 11 per cent) was associated with a reduced incidence of emergency CS for "asphyxia" (14 vs. 34 per cent). Induction rates in pregnancies with an ultrasonically confirmed small fetus vary between 10 and 52 per cent [8,67], although most series report a rate in excess of 30 per cent. This figure is undoubtedly influenced by fetal condition; in the study of Burke et al. [8], the rate of IOL in small fetuses (AC < 5th percentile) with normal umbilical artery Doppler waveforms was 52 per cent compared with only 13 per cent in those with AEDV.

There is very little information published on the outcome of IOL in small fetuses. Almstrom et al. [73] reported the outcome of 80 women induced at term with an unfavourable cervix and a small fetus (ultrasonic size > 2 sd below the mean for gestation). Cervical ripening and IOL was undertaken with 0.5 mg intracervical prostaglandin E_2 gel. The cohort was divided into those confirmed to be small at birth (birthweight > 2 sd below the mean for gestation, n = 50) and those with a normal birthweight (n = 30). The cervical-ripening effect did not differ between the groups: failed induction occurred in two of 50 in the study group and one of 30 in the control group. The frequency of operative deliveries for fetal distress was higher in the study group (14 of 50, 28 per cent) compared with the control group (three of 30, 10 per cent). In a consecutive series of 30 small fetuses (AC < 5th percentile) with normal umbilical artery Doppler waveform induced between 36 and 41 weeks with vaginal prostaglandin E_2 gel, we encountered no cases of failed IOL, and the rate of emergency CS for fetal distress was 13 per cent [Irons and Robson unpublished data].

Experience of IOL in women with pre-eclampsia is relevant since up to 52 per cent of fetuses are SGA [74]. Xenakis et al. [75] studied the outcome of IOL in 183 women with pre-eclampsia (mean gestational age 38 weeks) and 461 controls. Around 70 per cent of women in each group were given 3 mg prostaglandin E_2 gel every 6 hours until a Bishop score of 7 was achieved or a maximum of three doses were administered. Failed IOL was fivefold higher (8.2 vs. 1.7 per cent) and CS twofold higher (28 vs.16 per cent) in the pre-eclamptic group. This effect persisted after controlling for parity, Bishop score and epidural anaesthesia. The increased risk of CS was not apparently related to a higher prevalence of fetal distress in this study. However, Regenstein et al. [76] have previously shown that when prostaglandin IOL is attempted remote from term in women with pre-eclampsia, nearly 50 per cent of fetuses will be delivered by CS because of fetal intolerance of labour.

Based on the very limited data available it seems reasonable to attempt IOL in the healthy term or near-term small fetus. When the cervix is favourable, amniotomy and oxytocin is the preferred method. With an unfavourable cervix, intravaginal prostaglandin E_2 (1–2 mg) should be administered 6 hourly [68]. If amniotomy is deemed unfeasible after three doses it is reasonable to undertake a CS. Fetal heart monitoring is usually undertaken for an arbitrary period (30–60 min) after administration of prostaglandin since this procedure is acting as a contraction stress test (CST). Continuous fetal heart rate monitoring of the suspected IUGR fetus is mandatory once uterine contractions become established. The small, presumably IUGR, fetus is at increased risk of developing an abnormal fetal heart rate pattern in labour. Given the increased risk of significant acidosis in this group, there should be early recourse to fetal scalp sampling; where metabolic acidosis is found, delivery by CS should be considered since metabolic acidosis is more progressive in this group compared with well-grown fetuses.

Caesarean Section

Rates and Complications

In developed countries 15–25% of all deliveries are performed by CS [77]. The CS rate has increased fourfold in USA over the last 30 years, whereas in the UK the increase has been less marked (approximately 2.5-fold). The commonest indication for CS in nulliparas is failure to progress in labour (35–42%) [78,79] followed by elective repeat CS (29 per cent) [78]. Maternal mortality associated with CS has remained relatively stable in the UK since 1985 [80]. Deaths from emergency procedures now contribute 36 out of 50 (72 per cent) direct deaths in women having CS [80]. Morbidity related to CS includes haemorrhage, urinary tract and wound infection, endomyometritis and thromboembolism. The reported incidence of urinary tract and wound infection after elective CS ranges from 2 to16 per cent [77,81] but the rate can be reduced with prophylactic antibiotics.

Caesarean Section in the SGA Fetus

The reported proportion of SGA fetuses delivered by CS varies dramatically from 15 to 92 per cent [82,83]. This is likely to reflect the type of population studied, the incidence of associated fetal compromise and the presence of pre-eclampsia. The coexistence of pre-eclampsia has been associated with up to a tenfold increase in the rate of CS [84]. Interestingly, even after adjusting for obstetric history and the presence of pre-eclampsia, the misdiagnosis of an SGA fetus has been shown to increase the rate of CS by up to fivefold relative to undiagnosed small fetuses [84].

In the majority of cases with an SGA fetus, CS can be performed through a Pfannenstiel skin incision followed by a transverse lower uterine segment incision. In the very preterm growth-restricted fetus, where there is often marked oligohydramnios and a poorly formed lower segment, consideration should be given to using a vertical uterine segment incision, termed classical CS. Misguided attempts to deliver compromised fetuses (< 750 g) through transverse incisions lead to fetal trauma, asphyxia, additional uterine incisions (J or T) and excessive blood loss. The reluctance to perform planned classical CS stems from the knowledge that any future delivery then has to be by elective CS. A modification of the vertical incision by de Lee, commencing in the lower segment and extending upwards, may permit delivery without incising the fundus – if so, a trial of labour is acceptable in future pregnancies [85].

Careful consideration should be given to the mode of anaesthesia for CS. In the great majority of appropriately monitored SGA fetuses, a planned emergency CS can be performed. Aside from acute fetal distress due to placental abruption, there should be little necessity for unplanned emergency procedures requiring general anaesthesia. Many elective CSs in the UK and North America are now performed under spinal block because of the rapid onset of reliable, high quality surgical anaesthesia. However, there are several concerns about using this form of anaesthesia in a compromised SGA fetus. Maternal hypotension is reported in up to 80 per cent of cases and neither fluid preload nor ephedrine has been shown to prevent this reliably [86]. In healthy AGA fetuses delivered by elective CS, mean umbilical arterial pH is lower and the incidence of acidaemia (pH < 7.10) is higher with spinal compared with epidural or general anaesthesia [87]. Fetal pH, and umbilical artery PI correlate poorly with changes in blood pressure after regional anaesthesia [88], reinforcing the fact that upper limb blood pressure measurement is a poor predictor of placental perfusion (which is itself compromised by poor development of the uteroplacental vessels (see Ch. 6). Thus it is possible that spinal anaesthesia may prejudice the fetal condition, which in turn is not recognised by maternal monitoring. Therefore continuous fetal heart rate monitoring is mandatory in the anaesthetic room and should be continued right up until the point that the surgeon cleanses the skin. The already compromised fetus with AEDV is likely to be the most at risk and there is an urgent need for a randomised trial of spinal versus epidural anaesthesia in this group of fetuses. Until evidence is available that spinal anaesthesia is as safe as epidural anaesthesia, we believe epidural anaesthesia should remain the technique of choice in SGA fetuses with abnormal umbilical artery Doppler waveforms or an abnormal BPS.

Conclusions

The conclusions that can be drawn from this review are limited. The absence of any randomised trial addressing the implications of mode of delivery in the SGA fetus means that it is impossible to formulate evidence-based guidelines on delivery management. Although many studies have reported the risks of intrapartum fetal distress after individual antepartum tests, few combine the results of different tests. As decisions about the mode and timing of delivery in high risk fetuses are rarely made on the basis of a single test, most of these studies are of limited relevance to the current debate. Studies relating BPS to labour outcome in fetuses with abnormal umbilical artery Doppler waveform would be particularly valuable in this respect. The following conclusions therefore reflect the author's current practice. They assume there are no other maternal or fetal factors that preclude an attempt at vaginal delivery. Emphasis is placed on the condition of the fetus and the likelihood of successful IOL.

1. Term SGA fetus: IOL should be attempted with normal umbilical artery Doppler waveform and/or a normal BPS. If the cervix is unfavourable (Bishop score 0–3), intravaginal prostaglandin E_2 should be used to prime the cervix. An attempt at IOL is also appropriate in fetuses with an elevated umbilical artery PI, but EDV present, provided the BPS is normal. If decelerations develop in pregnancies with documented oligohydramnios, amnioinfusion should be considered, provided acidaemia can be excluded by fetal scalp blood sampling. In our experience most fetuses with a very abnormal BPS (0–2) have abnormal Doppler indices and delivery is best undertaken by a planned emergency CS. The most difficult group comprises fetuses with AEDV but a normal BPS and those with an equivocal BPS but EDV present. The risk of emergency CS in such cases may be as high as 50 per cent but is likely to be very dependent on the state of the cervix. When the cervix is favourable, it may be appropriate to consider amniotomy and oxytocin with early recourse to scalp sampling to assess the fetal condition.
2. Preterm SGA fetus: The main reason for delivering a SGA fetus before 37 weeks gestation is concern about fetal well-being. The earlier in gestation this issue is considered the more likely it is that the fetus has IUGR and in turn that the umbilical artery Doppler waveform is abnormal. We would not consider delivering an SGA fetus before 34 weeks unless there was AEDV/REDV and/or an abnormal BPS. Under such circumstances a planned emergency CS is the preferred option. This reasoning would also apply nearer to term if abnormal umbilical or middle cerebral artery Doppler indices were associated with a persistently abnormal BPS. In the absence of any proven benefit, we would generally not deliver a healthy SGA fetus with EDV before 37 weeks to avoid failed IOL. However, if delivery were deemed necessary, we feel it is reasonable to consider an attempt at IOL where the cervix is favourable.

References

1. The GRIT study group. When do obstetricians recommend delivery for a high risk preterm growth retarded fetus? Eur J Obstet Gynecol Reprod Biol 1996;67:121–6.

2. Low JA, Pancham SR, Worthington D. Fetal heart deceleration patterns in relation to asphyxia and weight-gestational age percentile of the fetus. Obstet Gynecol 1976;47:14–20.
3. Kramer MS, Olivier M, McLean FH, Willis DM, Usher RH. Impact of intrauterine growth retardation and body proportionality on fetal and neonatal outcome. Pediatrics 1990;86:707–13.
4. Steer PJ. Intrapartum monitoring in IUGR. In: Sharp F, Fraser RB, Milner RDG, editors. Fetal growth. London: RCOG, 1989;381–7.
5. Low JA, Karchmar J, Broekhoven L, Leonard T, McGrath MJ, Pancham SR, et al. The probability of fetal metabolic acidosis during labor in a population at risk as determined by clinical factors. Am J Obstet Gynecol 1981;141:941–51.
6. Robson SC, Chang TC. Intrauterine growth retardation. In: Reed G, Claireaux A, Cockburn F, Connor M, editors. Diseases of the fetus and newborn, 2nd edn. London: Chapman & Hall, 1995;275–83.
7. Fay RA, Dey PL, Saadie CMJ, Buhl JA, Gebski VJ. Ponderal index: a better definition of the "at risk" group with intrauterine growth problems than birth-weight for gestational age in term infants. Aust N Z J Obstet Gynecol 1991;31:17–9.
8. Burke G, Stuart B, Crowley P, Scanaill SN, Drumm J. Is intrauterine growth retardation with normal umbilical artery Doppler blood flow a benign condition? BMJ 1990;300:1044–5.
9. Arabin B, Becker R, Mohnhaupt A, Entezami M, Weitzel HK. Prediction of fetal distress and poor outcome in intrauterine growth retardation – a comparison of fetal heart rate monitoring combined with stresss tests and Doppler ultrasound. Fetal Diagn Ther 1993;8:234–40.
10. Chang TC, Robson SC, Spencer JAD, Gallivan S. Prediction of perinatal morbidity at term in small fetuses: comparison of fetal growth and Doppler ultrasound. Br J Obstet Gynaecol 1994;101:422–7.
11. Owen P, Harrold AJ, Farrell T. Fetal size and growth velocity in the prediction of intrapartum caesarean section for fetal distress. Br J Obstet Gynaecol 1997;104:445–9.
12. Nicolaides KH, Economides DL, Soothill PW. Blood gases, pH and lactate in appropriate and small for gestational age fetuses. Am J Obstet Gynecol 1989;161:996–1001.
13. Nieto A, Villar J, Matorras R, Serra R, Valenzuela P, Kellar J. Intrauterine growth retardation: fluctuation of fetal pH measured between beginning and at completion of labour. J Perinat Med 1994;22:329–35.
14. Robson SC, Crawford RA, Spencer JAD, Lee A. Intrapartum amniotic fluid index and its relationship to fetal distress. Am J Obstet Gynecol 1992;166:78–82.
15. Lin CC, Moawad AH, Rosenow PJ, River P. Acid–base characteristics of fetuses with intrauterine growth retardation during labour and delivery. Am J Obstet Gynecol 1980;137:553–9.
16. Low JA, Handley-Derry MH, Burke SO, Peters RD, Pater EA, Killen HL, et al. Association of intrauterine growth retardation and learning deficits at age 9 to 11 years. Am J Obstet Gynecol 1992;167:1499–505.
17. Hutton JL, Pharoah POD, Cooke RWI, Stevenson RC (1997). Differential effects of preterm birth and small gestational age on cognitive and motor development. Arch Dis Child 75: F75–81.
18. Ajayi RA, Soothill PW. Ultrasound assessment of amniotic fluid volume: a comparison of the single deepest pool and amniotic fluid index to predict perinatal morbidity. Ultrasound Obstet Gynecol 1991;1:401–4.
19. Varma TR, Bateman S, Patel RH, Chamberlain GVP, Pillai U. Ultrasound evaluation of amniotic fluid: outcome of pregnancies with severe oligohydramnios. Int J Gynecol Obstet 1988;27:185–92.
20. Anandakumar C, Biswas A, Arulkumaran S, Wong YC, Malarvishy G, Ratnam SS. Should assessment of amniotic fluid volume form an integral part of antenatal fetal assessment of high risk pregnancy? Aust N Z J Obstet Gynaecol 1993;33:272–5.
21. Flack,NJ, Sepulveda,W, Bower S, Fisk, NM. Acute maternal hydration in third-trimester oligohydramnios: effects on amniotic fluid volume, uteroplacental perfusion, and fetal blood flow and urine output. Am J Obstet Gynecol 1995;173:1186–91.
22. Sarno AP, Ahm MO, Brar HS, Phelan JP, Platt LD. Intrapartum Doppler velocimetry, amniotic fluid volume and fetal heart rate as predictors of subsequent fetal distress. Am J Obstet Gynecol 1989;161:1508–14.
23. O'Brien JM, Mercer BM, Friedman SA, Sibai BM. Amniotic fluid index in hospitalised hypertensive patients managed expectantly. Obstet Gynecol 1993;82:247–50.
24. Tongsong T, Srisomboon J. Amniotic fluid as a predictor of fetal distress in intrauterine growth retardation. Int J Gynecol Obstet 1993;40:131–4.
25. Miyamura T, Masuzaki H, Miyamoto M, Ishimaru T. Comparison between the single deepest pocket and amniotic fluid index in predicting fetal distress in small for gestational age fetuses. Acta Obstet Gynecol Scand 1997;76:123–7.

26. Strong TH, Hetzler G, Sarno AP, Paul RH. Prophylactic intrapartum amnioinfusion; a randomised clinical trial. Am J Obstet Gynecol 1990;162:1370–5.
27. Hofmeyer GJ. Amnioinfusion in intrapartum umbilical cord compression (Cochrane review). In: The Cochrane Library, Update Software, 1999.
28. Neilson JP. Cardiotocography for antepartum fetal assessment (Cochrane review), In: The Cochrane Library, Updated Software, 1999.
29. Schneider EP, Hutson JM, Petrie RH. An assessment of the first decade's experience with antepartum fetal heart rate testing. Am J Perinatol 1988;5:134–41.
30. Boehm FH, Salyer S, Shah DM, Vaughn WK. Improved outcome of twice weekly nonstress testing. Obstet Gynecol 1986;67:566–8.
31. FIGO. Guidelines for the use of fetal monitoring. Int J Gynaecol Obstet 1987;25:159–67.
32. Druzin ML, Fox A, Kogut E, Carlson C. The relationship of the nonstress test to gestational age. Am J Obstet Gynecol 1985;153:386–9.
33. Visser GHA, Sadovsky G, Nicolaides KH. Antepartum heart rate patterns in small-for-gestational age third-trimester fetuses: correlation with blood gas values obtained at cordocentesis. Am J Obstet Gynecol 1990;162:698–703.
34. Flynn AM, Kelly J. Evaluation of fetal wellbeing by antepartum fetal heart monitoring. BMJ 1977;i:936–9.
35. Keegan KA, Paul RH. Antepartum fetal heart rate testing IV. The nonstress test as a primary approach. Am J Obstet Gynecol 1980;136:75–80.
36. Visser GHA, Huisjes HJ. Diagnostic value of the unstressed antepartum cardiotocogram. Br J Obstet Gynaecol 1977;84:321–6.
37. Freeman RK, Anderson G, Dorchester W. A prospective multi-institutional study of antepartum fetal heart rate monitoring I. Risk of perinatal mortality and morbidity according to antepartum fetal heart rate results. Am J Obstet Gynecol 1982;143:771–7.
38. Visser GHA, Redman CWG, Huisjes HJ, Turnbull AC. Nonstressed antepartum heart rate monitoring: implications of decelerations after spontaneous contractions. Am J Obstet Gynecol 1980;138:429–35.
39. Meis PJ, Ureda JR, Swain M, Kelly RT, Penry M, Sharp P. Variable decelerations during nonstress tests are not a sign of fetal compromise. Am J Obstet Gynecol 1986;154:586–90.
40. Guzman ER, Vintzileos AM. Computerized analysis of antepartum fetal heart rate tracings. Fetal Matern Med Rev 1997;9:19–34.
41. Ribbert LSM, Snijders RJM, Nicolaides KH, Visser GHA. Relation of fetal blood gases and data from computer-assisted analysis of fetal heart rate patterns in small for gestation fetuses. Br J Obstet Gynaecol 1991;98:820–3.
42. Guzman ER, Vintzileos AM, Martins M, Benito C, Houlihan C, Hanley M. The efficacy of individual computer heart rate indices in detecting acidemia at birth in growth-restricted fetuses. Obstet Gynecol 1996;87:969–74.
43. Snijders RJM, Ribbert LSM, Visser GHA, Mulder EJH. Numeric analysis of heart rate variation in intrauterine growth-retarded fetuses: a longitudinal study. Am J Obstet Gynecol 1992;166:22–7.
44. Soothill PW, Ajayi RA, Campbell S. (1991) Prediction of morbidity in small and normally grown fetuses by fetal heart rate variability, biophysical profile score and umbilical artery Doppler studies. Br J Obstet Gynaecol 100:742–745.
45. Chang TC. Computerised analysis of fetal heart rate variation: prediction of adverse perinatal outcome in pateints undergoing prostaglandin induction of labour at term. Ann Acad Med (Singapore) 1997;26:772–5.
46. Hoskins IA, Frieden FJ, Young BK. Variable decelerations in reactive nonstress tests with decreased amniotic fluid index predict fetal compromise. Am J Obstet Gynecol 1991;165:1094–8.
47. Manning FA, Platt LD, Sipos L. Antepartum fetal evaluation: the development of a fetal biophysical profile score. Am J Obstet Gynecol 1980;136:787–95.
48. Manning FA. Fetal biophysical profile; a critical appraisal. Fetal Matern Med Rev 1997;9:103–23.
49. Manning FA, Snijders RJM, Harman CR, Nicolaides KH, Menticoglou S, Morrison I. Fetal biophysical profile scoring. VI. Correlation with antepartum umbilical venous fetal pH. Am J Obstet Gynecol 1993;169:755–63.
50. Vintzileos AM, Fleming AD, Scorza WE, Wolf EJ, Balducci J, Campbell WA, et al. Relationship between fetal biophysical activities and umbilical cord blood gas values. Am J Obstet Gynecol 1991;165:707–13.
51. Baskett TF, Gray JH, Prewett SJ, Young LM, Allen AC. Antepartum fetal assessment using a fetal biophysical profile. Am J Obstet Gynecol 1984;148:630–3.

52. Manning FA, Harman CR, Morrison I, Menticoglou S. Fetal assessment based on fetal biophysical profile scoring. III. Positive predictive accuracy of the very abnormal test (biophysical profile score = 0). Am J Obstet Gynecol 1990;162:398–402.

53. Alfirevic Z, Neilson JP. Doppler ultrasonography in high risk pregnancies: systematic review with meta-analysis. Am J Obstet Gynecol 1995;172:1379–87.

54. Nicolini U, Nicolaidis P, Fisk NM, Vaughan JI, Fusi L, Gleeson R, et al. Limited role of fetal blood sampling in prediction of outcome in intrauterine growth retardation. Lancet 1990;336:768–72.

55. Tyrell S, Obaid AH, Lilford RJ. Umbilical artery Doppler velocimetry as a predictor of fetal hypoxia and acidosis at delivery. Obstet Gynecol 1989;74:332–7.

56. Nicolaides KH, Bilardo CM, Soothill PW, Campbell S. Absence of end diastolic frequencies in umbilical artery: a sign of fetal hypoxia and acidosis. BMJ 1988;297:1026–7.

57. Vyas S, Nicolaides KH, Bower S, Campbell S. Middle cerebral artery flow velocity waveforms in fetal hypoxaemia. Br J Obstet Gynaecol 1990;97:797–803.

58. Hornbuckle J, Thornton JG. The fetal circulatory response to chronic placental insufficiency and relation to pregnancy outcome. Fetal Matern Med Rev 1999; in press.

59. Rizzo G, Capponi A, Soregaroli M, Arduinin D, Romanini C. Umbilical vein pulsations and acid-base status at cordocentesis in growth-retarded fetuses with absent end-diastolic velocity in umbilical artery. Biol Neonate 1995;68:163–8.

60. Rizzo G, Capponi A, Arduini D, Romanini C. The value of fetal arterial, cardiac and venous flows in predicting pH and blood gases measured in umbilical blood at cordocentesis in growth retarded fetuses. Br J Obstet Gynaecol 1995;102:963–9.

61. Mires GJ, Patel NB, Dempster J. The value of fetal umbilical artery flow velocity waveforms in the prediction of adverse fetal outcome in high risk pregnancies. J Obstet Gynecol 1990;10:261–70.

62. Forouzan I. Absence of end diastolic flow velocity in the umblical artery: A review. Obstet Gynaecol Survey 1995;50:219–27.

63. Karsdrop VHM, van Vugt JMG, van Geijn HP, Kostense PJ, Arduini D, et al. Clinical significance of absent or reversed end diastolic velocity waveforms in umbilical artery. Lancet 1994;344:1664–8.

64. Gramellini D, Folli MC, Raboni S, Vadora E, Merialdi A. Cerebral–umbilical Doppler ratio as a predictor of adverse perinatal outcome. Obstet Gynecol 1992;79:416–20.

65. Farmakides G, Schulman H, Winter D, Ducey J, Guzman E, Penny B. Prenatal surveillance using nonstress testing and Doppler velocimetry. Obstet Gynecol 1988;71:184–7.

66. Arduini D, Rizzo G, Romanini C. The development of abnormal heart rate patterns after absent end-diastolic velocity in umbilical artery; analysis of risk factors. Am J Obstet Gynecol 1993;168:43–50.

67. Almstrom H, Axelsson O, Cnattingius S, Ekman G, Maesel A, Ulmsten U, et al. Comparison of umbilical-artery velocimetry and cardiotocography for surveillance of small-for-gestational age fetuses. Lancet 1992;340:936–40.

68. RCOG. Induction of labour. Guideline no 16. London: RCOG, 1998;1–10.

69. Brennand J, Greer I. Induction of labour: new horizons. Hosp Med 1998; 59: 856–60.

70. Xenakis EMJ, Piper JM, Conway DL, Langer O. Induction of labour in the nineties: Conquering the unfavourable cervix. Obstet Gynecol 1997;90:235–9.

71. Shepherd JH, Bennett MJ, Laurence D, Moore F, Sims CD. Prostaglandin vaginal suppositories; a simple and safe approach to induction of labor. Obstet Gynecol 1981;58:596–600.

72. Larsen T, Larsen JF, Petersen S, Greisen G. Detection of small-for-gestational-age fetuses by ultrasound screening in a high risk population: a randomized controlled trial. Br J Obstet Gynaecol 1992;99:469–74.

73. Almstrom H, Ekman G, Granstrom L. Preinductive cervical ripening with PGE2 gel in term pregnant women with ultrasonically diagnosed intra-uterine growth-retarded. Acta Obstet Gynecol Scand 1991;70:555–9.

74. Ferrazzani S, Caruso A, De Carolis S, Martino IV, Mancuso S. Proteinuria and outcome of 444 pregnancies complicated by hypertension. Am J Obstet Gynecol 1990;162:366–71.

75. Xenakis EMJ, Piper JM, Field N, Conway D, Langer O. Preeclampsia: Is induction of labor more successful? Obstet Gynecol 1997;89:600–3.

76. Regenstein AC, Laros RK, Wakeley A, Kitterman JA, Tooley WH. Mode of delivery in pregnancies complicated by preeclampsia with very low birth weight infants. J Perinatol 1995;15:2–6.

77. Dickinson JE. Cesarean section. In: James DK, Steer PJ, Weiner CP, Gonik B, editors. High risk pregnancy, 2nd edn. London: WB Saunders, 1999;1153–65.

78. Taffel SM, Placek PJ, Liss T. Trends in the United States caesarean section rate and reasons for the 1980–1985 rise. Am J Public Health 1985;77:955–9.

79. Leitch CR. Walker JJ. The rise in caesarean section rate: the same indications but a lower threshold. Br J Obstet Gynaecol 1998;105:621–6.

80. HMSO. Report on confidential enquiries into maternal deaths in the United Kingdom 1994–1996. London: HMSO, 1998.

81. Nielson TF, Hokegard KH. Postoperative caesarean section morbidity: A prospective study. Am J Obstet Gynecol 1983;146:911–16.

82. Farrell SJ, Anderson HF, Work BA. Caesarean section: indications and post operative morbidity. Obstet Gynecol 1980;56:696–700.

83. Langhoff Roos J, Lindmark G. Obstetric interventions and perinatal asphyxia in growth retarded term infants. Acta Obstet Gynecol Scand (Suppl 165) 1997;76:39–43.

84. Ringa V, Carrat F, Blodel B, Breart G. Consequences of misdiagnosis of intrauterine growth retardation on preterm cesarean section Fetal Diagn Ther 1993;8:325–30.

85. Depp R. Cesarian delivery in: Obstetrics: Normal and problem pregnancies, edited by Gabbe SG, Niebyl J and Simpson JL, 3rd Ed. 1996. Churchill Livingstone, New York.

86. Howell P. Spinal anaesthesia in severe preeclampsia: time for reappraisal, or time for caution? Int J Obstet Anaesth 1998;7:217–19.

87. Mueller MD, Bruhwiler H, Schupfer GK, Luscher KP. Higher rate of fetal acidemia after regional anaesthesia for elective cesarean section. Obstet Gynecol 1997;90:131–4.

88. Robson SC, Boys RJ, Rodeck C, Morgan B. Maternal and fetal haemodynamic effects of spinal and extradural anaesthesia for elective caesarean section. Br J Anaesth 1992;68:54–9.

15 Coexistent Maternal Disease and Intrauterine Growth Restriction

Janet R. Ashworth and Philip N. Baker

Introduction

A plethora of different coexistent maternal diseases has been linked to the development of IUGR; if any maternal disease is of sufficient severity, IUGR may ensue. Examples of reported associations with IUGR include maternal diabetes, cardiac disease, thyrotoxicosis, asthma, anaemia and chronic hypertension.

Maternal *diabetes* may produce alterations in red blood cell oxygen release and placental blood flow [1]. Reduced uterine blood flow is thought to contribute to the increased incidence of IUGR observed in pregnancies complicated by diabetic vasculopathy. Investigations using radioactive tracers have suggested a relationship between poor maternal metabolic control and reduced uteroplacental blood flow [2]. In diabetic ketoacidosis, hypovolaemia and hypotension caused by dehydration may further reduce blood flow through the intervillous space. Diabetic nephropathy has recently been reported to be associated with IUGR in 15 per cent of individuals [3]. The risk of IUGR is increased in pregnancies complicated by all forms of *cardiac* disease [4]. *Thyrotoxicosis* is associated with an overall decrease in the mean infant birthweight [5]; thyroid hormones are though to influence fetal growth via a complex mechanism involving IGF-I [6]. Although studies have been sparse and conflicting, there is little evidence to suggest that maternal hypothyroidism leads to an increased risk of IUGR. Although IUGR is an oft-cited complication of *asthma*, IUGR occurs in only a very few cases of maternal asthma when patients are permanently hypoxaemic [7]. In a large retrospective study, Godfrey et al. [8] reported a correlation between maternal iron deficiency *anaemia* and an increased placenta : infant birthweight ratio, suggesting that maternal iron deficiency leads to poor fetal growth. Sickle cell disease leads to a high incidence of IUGR owing to both an impaired oxygen supply and sickling infarct in the placental circulation [9]. Finally, the incidence of IUGR is directly related to the severity of *chronic hypertension* and is particularly high in the presence of superimposed pre-eclampsia.

This chapter will focus on two situations in which there are particularly strong associations with IUGR; the first of these is the pregnancy complication pre-eclampsia, and the second is an underlying maternal thrombophilic tendency.

The Association of Pre-eclampsia with Intrauterine Growth Restriction

IUGR has traditionally been difficult to diagnose accurately, studies being flawed by the erroneous inclusion of constitutionally small babies. Similarly, a major difficulty in compiling any review of pre-eclampsia is the use of variable or imprecise criteria for the diagnosis of the disease by different authors. In this chapter "pre-eclampsia" implies significant hypertension and proteinuria, although a myriad of different thresholds have been used. This important caveat must be considered when comparing even the more recent studies.

A strong association between IUGR and pre-eclampsia is well documented [10,11], and following pregnancies complicated by pre-eclampsia, restricted infant growth as late as at 2 years of age has been reported [12]. The degree of growth restriction appears to correlate with the severity of the pre-eclampsia [10], although this correlation is dependent upon which parameters are used to quantify the severity of pre-eclampsia [13]. In a prospective study of 332 hypertensive pregnant women (the hypertension being of mixed aetiology and duration), Redman et al. [13] demonstrated that fetal outcome, and particularly perinatal mortality, correlated poorly with the degree of hypertension, but was closely related to the level of maternal hyperuricaemia. This study included large numbers of women with either chronic hypertension or non-proteinuric pregnancy-induced hypertension. Many of the women studied did not have pre-eclampsia, and hence diseases with entirely different aetiologies were interpreted *en masse*. What can, however, be gleaned from this study, is that in pregnancies complicated by non-proteinuric pregnancy-induced hypertension, the fetus appears to be at an advantage when compared with pregnancies complicated by pre-eclampsia.

The pathogenesis of pre-eclampsia is thought to involve the action of the predisposing genes being mediated via trophoblast cells and immunologically active decidual cells [14]. There is evidence from a number of morphological studies that in many cases of pre-eclampsia there is inadequate trophoblastic invasion of spiral arteries, with a resultant failure of complete dilatation of the spiral arteries. In addition, not so many vessels show evidence of trophoblast invasion [15–17]. The shallow endovascular trophoblast invasion leads to an inadequate development of the uteroplacental blood supply. Pre-eclampsia is associated with a reduced uteroplacental flow index [18], and non-invasive MRI techniques have demonstrated reduced placental perfusion in pre-eclampsia and IUGR [19]. The diminished uteroplacental blood supply leads to reduced fetal perfusion as indicated by abnormal Doppler waveforms in the fetal umbilical arteries, resulting from an increased resistance in the placental vascular bed [20–22]. In pre-eclampsia, the reduced perfusion of trophoblast tissue is thought to result in the production of a circulating agent(s) that is released into the systemic circulation and induces dysfunction of endothelial cells throughout the body [14].

Rather than being a complication of pre-eclampsia, there is much evidence that IUGR shares features of the pathophysiology that causes the clinical syndrome of pre-eclampsia. IUGR is not merely a result of decreased placental perfusion due to maternal intramyometrial vasoconstriction in pre-eclampsia. Just as there are many cases of pre-eclampsia where there is no element of fetal growth restriction, there are also cases of IUGR in the absence of pre-eclampsia; in these pregnancies a similar failure of spiral artery remodelling has also been reported [15,23]. Normotensive pregnancies complicated by IUGR are consequently associated with a reduced uteroplacental blood flow. A prospective study by Nylund et al. [24] used intravenous maternal injection of indium-113m chloride and a gamma camera to measure maternal placental blood flow, and to compare normal, uncomplicated pregnancies with those complicated by IUGR. In all pregnancies complicated by IUGR, there was a reduced uteroplacental flow index, the median value being 50 per cent that in the control group. When pregnancies complicated by pre-eclampsia were removed from consideration, there remained a significantly lower value for the uteroplacental flow index in the cases with IUGR than in those with babies of normal size for gestational age and fetal sex [24]. Nylund et al. [24] attempted to subdivide pregnancies complicated by IUGR into those with fetal congenital abnormalities and those with no fetal malformation. Although the group with fetal malformations generally had smaller placentae, no difference in uteroplacental blood flow index was demonstrated between these two subgroups.

Further evidence of similarities in the pathogenesis of the two conditions is provided by studies of blood vesssel function. The first direct evidence of altered resistance artery function of women with pre-eclampsia was provided by McCarthy et al., who found impaired acetylcholine-mediated relaxation in subcutaneous arteries of women with pre-eclampsia compared with arteries from normotensive pregnant women [25]. We have established a technique for the study of myometrial and systemic (omental) arteries. Arteries of 200–500 μm were dissected from myometrial and omental biopsies obtained from non-pregnant women and from pregnant women whose pregnancies were uncomplicated or complicated by pre-eclampsia or IUGR. Cases of IUGR were identified by ultrasound scans; however, the final arbiter was an individualised birthweight ratio (IBR) below the 10th percentile. The IBR is a ratio relative to a predicted birthweight, calculated using independent coefficients for gestation at delivery, fetal sex, parity, ethnic origin, maternal height and booking weight. IBR enables a more accurate prediction of pregnancies that end in a poor outcome than birthweight for gestational age alone [26]. Vessels were mounted on Mulvany wire myographs as a ring preparation, being held by two wires passing through the lumen. This allows isometric force exerted circumferentially on the wires to be measured. For each pair of myometrial or omental arteries, one vessel had the endothelium removed with a human hair, and the endothelium of the other artery was left intact. Vessels were contracted with vasopressin and then relaxed with the endothelium-dependent vasodilator, bradykinin. We found myometrial and omental resistance arteries in humans to show endothelium-dependent relaxation, which persists in pregnancy. However, the endothelium-dependent relaxation to bradykinin was markedly reduced in vessels from patients with pre-eclampsia, the greatest difference between the groups being found when myometrial vessels were studied (Fig. 15.1) [27]. Interestingly, when vessels from pregnancies complicated by IUGR were studied, the results were similar to those found in pre-eclampsia (Fig. 15.1).

Support for the concept of a circulating factor(s) in pre-eclampsia [14] is provided by studies examining the effect of plasma or serum from pre-eclamptic women on endothelial cells in vitro. These studies have demonstrated alterations in a wide variety of parameters such as PDGF mRNA and protein production, intracellular triglycerides, cellular fibronectin release, NO release and

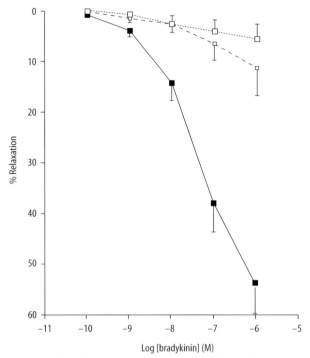

Mean % relaxation of vessels from women with normal pregnancies to bradykinin; s_x is shown for each point.

Mean % relaxation to bradykinin of vessels from women with pregnancies complicated by pre-eclampsia; s_x is shown for each point.

Mean % relaxation of vessels from women with IUGR pregnancies to bradykinin; s_x is shown for each point.

Figure 15.1 The relaxation of myometrial resistance vessels from women with uncomplicated pregnancies, and from those with pregnancies complicated by pre-eclampsia or IUGR.

prostacyclin generation [28,29]. Further evidence of a circulating factor altering endothelial-dependent function was provided by our finding that incubation of vessels from normal pregnant women with plasma from patients with pre-eclampsia resulted in the vessel response to bradykinin mimicking the diminished response of vessels from women with pre-eclampsia [30]. Preliminary studies from our laboratory indicate that plasma from women whose pregnancies are complicated by IUGR evokes similar differences in the function of vessels from those of normal pregnant women.

Several factors influence whether pregnancies complicated by pre-eclampsia will also be affected by IUGR. Maternal smoking is associated with a reduced risk of pre-eclampsia [31]. However, in pregnancies complicated by pre-eclampsia, smoking was associated with a significantly increased risk of IUGR; rates of 68 per cent have been reported [31].

Maternal parity is also factor in whether a pregnancy complicated by pre-eclampsia is also likely to exhibit fetal growth restriction. A retrospective study of

133 women with pre-eclampsia and 132 normal pregnant women compared the likelihood of primiparous and multiparous women to have a growth-restricted baby; 28 per cent of women with pre-eclampsia had growth-restricted babies, compared with just 5 per cent of normal pregnant women. However, when the groups were subdivided on the basis of parity, further differences were apparent. Primiparous women with normal pregnancies were more likely to have a growth-restricted baby than were their multiparous counterparts. In those women with pre-eclampsia, however, it was the multiparous women who were more likely to have the further complication of IUGR. In multiparous women with pre-eclampsia who had a history of pre-eclampsia in a previous pregnancy, the proportion of growth-restricted babies was higher still. The only clinical difference between the primiparous and multiparous women was that the duration of hypertension prior to delivery was longer in the multiparous women, but this difference did not correlate with likelihood of IUGR. All other biochemical, haematological and clinical measures were similar between the two groups [32]. The selection of pre-eclamptic patients appears to have been rigorous in this study. Birthweight below the 10th percentile on standard growth charts was used to define IUGR, with no individualisation of expected fetal weights. However, the trend for multiparous women to have larger babies than primiparous women was reversed in the population with pre-eclampsia, which suggests that this limitation [26] was not of significance in influencing the overall results.

The effect of parity on the development of pre-eclampsia [33], and the finding that the protective effect of multiparity may be lost after a change of partner [34], has led to investigation of the immune system. Although evidence of a widespread disturbance in pre-eclampsia is contradictory [35], serum concentrations of immunoglobulins and components of the complement system are altered in pre-eclampsia [36,37]. The role of autoimmunity in the link between the pathogenesis of pre-eclampsia and IUGR has been investigated [38]. Neither pre-eclampsia nor IUGR was associated with an alteration in total immunoglobulin levels, compared with normal pregnancy. However, levels of autoantibodies (those measured included a mixture of antiphospholipid, antihistone and antipolynucleotide autoantibodies) correlated well with various complications of pregnancy. Women with severe pre-eclampsia, but not those with chronic hypertension, had significantly higher levels of autoantibodies than did normal pregnant women. Normal pregnant women whose pregnancies were complicated by IUGR also had raised autoantibody levels. The most common autoantibodies found in association with IUGR were the antiphospholipid antibodies of the IgG isotype. In pregnancies complicated by both pre-eclampsia and IUGR, autoantibody levels were further raised [38].

The Association Between Maternal Thrombophilias and Intrauterine Growth Restriction

Patients with an underlying thrombophilic tendency can be subdivided into:

1. those in whom antiphospholipid (APA) antibodies have been detected
2. those in whom an alteration in proteins that regulate coagulation has been identified.

Antiphospholipid Autoantibodies

Two types of antiphospholipid antibodies have been identified and associated independently with adverse pregnancy outcome. These are anticardiolipin antibodies and lupus anticoagulant. Antiphospholipid antibodies (APA) may be generated in response to various infections or as a result of endogenous stimuli.

In 1941 an antibody was identified that reacted to the VDRL antigen of *Treponema pallidum*, the infective agent in syphilis [39]. This antigen consisted of a unique combination of cardiolipin, phosphatidylcholine and cholesterol, the phospholipids being arranged around a core of cholesterol. The APA identified in patients with syphilis did not bind to protein–phospholipid complexes. A similarly inactive anticardiolipin has been identified in a significant proportion of patients with HIV [40]. Other viral infections, including measles, mumps, Epstein–Barr virus, varicella, as well as bacterial infections such as pneumococcal pneumonia and parasitic episodes including malaria, have been recognised to induce transient, asymptomatic expression of anticardiolipin or lupus anticoagulant antibodies [41]. The antiphospholipids generated following infection do not appear to be associated with an increased risk of thrombosis development, and have not been independently associated with adverse pregnancy outcome, although clearly the infections giving rise to the APA may in themselves be risk factors in pregnancy.

In contrast, APA that arise from endogenous stimuli may have considerable implications for fetal growth. In 1952, two patients with systemic lupus erythematosus (SLE) were reported to have false positive serological tests for syphilis and a plasma inhibitor of *in vitro* clotting assays [42]. The inhibitor was named "lupus anticoagulant" [43], and it may be defined as an APA prolonging phospholipid-dependent clotting assays. The definitive diagnosis of lupus anticoagulant (LAC) activity requires the phospholipid-specific prolongation of a phospholipid-dependent clotting assay, in the absence of any clotting factor deficiency [41,44,45]. LAC may be associated with clotting factor depletion, and any resultant false negative tests for LAC may be ruled out with a dilute Russel viper venom test [46]. In 1983 an APA was identified that reacted against all anionic phospholipids. It was designated as anticardiolipin antibody (ACA), as it was identified while using cardiolipin as the target phospholipid. ACA is detected by sensitive ELISA [47], and a positive test should be confirmed by repeating in 6–8 weeks, because of the possibility of transient, infection-induced APA expression [46]. Assay results are expressed semiquantitatively, and APA syndrome is associated with medium or high ACA-positive results [41].

Both "lupus anticoagulant" and "anticardiolipin antibody" are misleading terms, as not all patients with LAC have lupus, or indeed any recognised autoimmune disease, and ACA are not specific to cardiolipin, recognising all anionic phospholipids when part of a protein–anionic phospholipid complex. Patients with SLE may have either LAC (34 per cent) or ACA (44 per cent) [48], but the presence of either APA carries a fourfold increased risk of thrombosis or thrombocytopenia [41]. Notably, many women with antiphospholipid syndrome are symptomatic only in association with pregnancy [46].

Patients with APA syndrome have been estimated to have a total fetal loss rate of 25 to 29 per cent [41,49]. Women with APA associated with SLE have a fetal loss rate of 59 per cent, whereas those with SLE in the absence of APA will lose approximately 20 per cent of fetuses [41]. In pregnancies of women with APA, the incidence of IUGR is increased. A prospective study of 860 pregnant women found a 7 per cent prevalence of ACA; the incidence of IUGR in pregnant women with ACA was 11.7 per cent compared with 1.9 per cent in the ACA-negative pregnant women [49]. Similarly, Polzin et al. [50] found that 24 per cent of the women delivering growth-restricted fetuses were positive for ACA, whereas ACA was found in only 2.5 per cent of the general pregnant population. It appears likely that higher levels of ACA correlate more strongly with fetal growth restriction or loss, as studies accepting lower levels of ACA frequently fail to show any association with adverse pregnancy outcome [46,51–55].

The pathophysiology linking APA and fetal demise or growth restriction has been suggested to lie in repeated thromboses leading to extensive placental infarction, with vasculopathy in the underlying uteroplacental arteries. De Wolf et al. [56] demonstrated decidual vasculopathy and extensive placental infarction in patients with APA and poor obstetric histories.

Pregnancy outcome has been shown to be improved by treatment in women with APA, and hence women with recurrent pregnancy loss or IUGR should be investigated for APA so that treatment may be considered. A study determining ACA status in 259 women with a range of adverse pregnancy outcomes, including recurrent abortion, intrauterine death, IUGR and pre-eclampsia, found ACA in 20.5 per cent of women; this proportion was significantly higher than that found in a normal pregnant control group [57].

Katano et al. [58] advocated the use of beta-2-glycoprotein I-dependent ACA (autoimmune type) as a general screening test. Sixteen hundred pregnant women were screened in the first trimester and their pregnancies were observed; 0.7 per cent of the population screened positive for the antibody. The outcome of many of these pregnancies was poor, with IUGR in 37.5 per cent of cases (2.9 per cent in antibody-negative women), and an intrauterine fetal death in 25 per cent of cases (0.5 per cent in antibody-negative women) [58]. Ketano's group suggested that this antibody should be used to screen for potential adverse outcome and to facilitate prophylactic treatment, but whether their results can be extrapolated to other pregnant populations has yet to be assessed.

Two main approaches have been taken in the active management of pregnancies in which APA have been identified. Antibody load may be targeted with therapy, usually glucocorticoid, or the procoagulant effects of APA may be reduced. The former usually involves chronic prednisolone administration, with or without low dose aspirin. Although this has been shown to increase the live delivery rate in women with APA, compared with when no treatment is given [59], morbidity and premature delivery rate are increased, and the mother is subjected to the potential of diabetogenic and osteopoenic side-effects. The alternative is to consider anti-coagulant therapy, which may constitute low dose aspirin with or without sub-cutaneous heparin. The combination of low dose aspirin and subcutaneous heparin have been shown to increase the live birth rate in women with APA, with lower rates of fetal morbidity and prematurity than when prednisolone was used [59]. The prolonged usage of heparin again predisposes to osteopoenic effects, which may be minimised by the use of low molecular weight heparin, such as Fragmin.

Proteins that Regulate Coagulation

The glycoprotein antithrombin III, manufactured by the liver, is recognised as an important physiological inhibitor of coagulation, and forms irreversible complexes with all activated factors except VIIIa. Increased formation of antithrombin III occurs in association with coagulation activation. A decrease in the antithrombin III activity level indicates increased thrombin binding secondary to increased thrombin generation and is found after thromboembolic events, in disseminated intravascular coagulopathy, and after major surgery. Antithrombin III activity levels are unchanged in normal pregnancy, although marginal decreases have been described [60,61]. Low antithrombin III concentrations have been associated with placental infarctions, perinatal morbidity and mortality and maternal morbidity [62–64]. In particular, decreased levels of antithrombin III activity have been demonstrated in the majority of women with pre-eclampsia, [62–64].

Protein C, a serine protease, is probably also synthesised by the liver and is activated by contact with thrombin and thrombomodulin on the surface of endothelial cells. It is a potent inhibitor of activated factor V and VIII, and is an activator of fibrinolysis [65,66]. Protein C is highly sensitive to consumption and reduced levels are found after surgery, thromboembolic events and in disseminated intravascular coagulation. Protein C levels appear to be unchanged in normal pregnancy compared with the non-pregnant state [67]. The prevalence of protein C deficiency in the general pregnant population is less than 0.5 per cent [68]. Protein C deficiency has also been connected with adverse pregnancy outcome, being detected in 17 per cent of pregnancies complicated by an intrauterine death [69], and in 7.5 per cent of women who deliver SGA babies [70], although only a small number of women were involved in the latter study.

Protein S serves as a cofactor for activated protein C in the degradation of the activated factors V and VIII, acting by binding to lipid and platelet surfaces [71,72]. Levels of protein S in pregnancy may decrease to those found in patients with congenital protein S deficiency [73]. Deficiency of protein S results in a thrombophilic state, and has been connected with adverse pregnancy outcome [68–70]. The prevalence of protein S deficiency in the general population has been estimated to be between 0.2 and 2 per cent [68]. In a study in the Netherlands, protein S deficiency was found in 23 per cent of 13 successively recruited women with babies delivered SGA [70].

In 1993 a hereditary limitation in anticoagulant response to activated protein C was reported. The affected families had a history of venous thromboses that was not explained by deficiencies of protein C, protein S or antithrombin III [74]. The source of the hereditary activated protein C resistance has been identified as a point mutation on the gene coding for factor V, which results in the synthesis of a factor V molecule that is not properly inactivated by protein C [75]. The resultant mutation has become known as "factor V Leiden", as the work to identify the mutation was carried out in the Dutch town of Leiden [75]. Both heterozygotes and homozygotes for the factor V Leiden mutation are affected, the defect being inherited in an autosomal dominant fashion [74,76]. The risk of developing deep-vein thrombosis in people with factor V Leiden is seven times greater than that of the general population [77]. Prevalence of the factor V Leiden mutation varies between populations, and is in the range of 2–7% [75,77–79]. When measured in patients having their first confirmed episode of deep-vein thrombosis, the prevalence of activated protein C resistance in one study was 21 per cent [77].

Activated protein C resistance is a common cause of deep-vein thrombosis associated with pregnancy. Hellgren et al. [80] reported that when women who suffered a deep-vein thrombosis in pregnancy had their activated protein C resistance measured in the non-pregnant state, the prevalence of activated protein C resistance was 59 per cent. Measurement of activated protein C resistance in pregnancy is potentially confounded, however, by physiological changes in resistance levels as pregnancy progresses [80–82]. A Canadian cross-sectional study of healthy, non-smoking, normal pregnant women with no history of thromboembolism measured activated protein C resistance in patients of varying gestation [78]. Resistance was expressed as a ratio, with a value of less than two constituting the definition of activated protein C resistance [78,83]. In non-pregnant women the mean ratio was 2.5. This figure fell throughout pregnancy, from 2.4 in the first trimester to 1.9 in the third trimester. Using a ratio of less than two to define activated protein C resistance, 5 per cent of the non-pregnant group were resistant, compared with 12 per cent in the first trimester, 46 per cent in the second and 62 per cent in the third [78]. The decreased availability of the protein S cofactor may contribute to the rising activated protein C resistance of late pregnancy [78]. In contrast, the prevalence of the factor V Leiden point mutation in the pregnant population in this study was 7.3 per cent. In a pregnant patient, DNA testing for the factor V Leiden mutation is thus a more effective method of assessing any suspected thrombophilia than the determination of the ratio for activated protein C resistance.

The discovery and characterisation of activated protein C resistance is relatively recent, and population-based studies upon which to draw an accurate picture of the increased risks of fetal loss or IUGR in the presence of the factor V Leiden mutation are awaited. One study in Israel comprised seven patients presenting by referral over an 18 month period with recurrent pregnancy loss, IUGR and pre-eclampsia who had activated protein C resistance. All had ratios of below 1.7 and had the factor V Leiden mutation identified by PCR; one women was homozygous and the remainder were heterozygous for the mutation [84]. One patient had a prior history of thromboembolism, and another three women had a family history of thromboembolic events. The described cohort of patients clearly suggest a strong link between factor V Leiden and adverse pregnancy outcome, but this study made no attempt to obtain an overview of the prevalence of this problem in the population from which these patients were referred. As the probable population prevalence of the factor V Leiden mutation is around 5 per cent, women with recurrent pregnancy loss, a history of IUGR or a personal or strong family history of thromboembolism should be tested for this mutation, and prophylactic anticoagulant treatment should be considered during the pregnancy and puerperium.

Conclusions

It is to be expected that general maternal health is likely to influence the nutrition and growth of the dependent, developing fetus. A number of clinically diagnosable disorders that may already affect the health of the mother or may arise during pregnancy have a recognised association with IUGR. Careful fetal surveillance to detect compromise in placental function and growth should be integral to the antenatal care of women with disorders such as diabetes mellitus, thyroid disorders and hypertension, including pre-eclampsia when it is diagnosed. Additionally there are a number of disorders in which a history of poor obstetric outcome, including recurrent pregnancy loss or IUGR, may be an

indicator of an underlying disorder. This is particularly true with the thrombophilias, and in such women the diagnosis of the disorder, preferably preconceptually, would permit antenatal treatment likely to benefit both mother and
fetus.

References

1. Madsen H. Fetal oxygenation in diabetic pregnancy. Dan Med Bull 1986;33:64.
2. Nyland L, Lunell NO, Lewander R et al. Uteroplacental blood flow in diabetic pregnancy:
   Measurements with indium 113m and a computer linked gamma camera. Am J Obstet Gynecol
   1982;144:298.
3. Reece EA, Leguizamon G, Homko C. Pregnancy performance and outcomes associated with
   diabetic nephropathy. Am J Perinatol 1998;15:413–21.
4. Niswander KR, Berendes H, Deutschberger J. Fetal morbidity following potentially anoxygenic
   obstetric conditions. Organic heart disease. Am J Obstet Gynecol 1967;98:871–6.
5. Vander Spruy ZM and Jacobs HS. Management of endocrine disorders in pregnancy. Thyroid and
   parathyroid disease. Postgrad Med J 1984;60:245–52.
6. Owens JA. Endocrine and substrate control of fetal growth: placental and maternal influences
   and insulin-like growth factors. Reprod Fertil Dev 1991;3:501–17.
7. Sims CD, Chamberlain GVP, de Swiet M. Lung function tests in bronchial asthma during and after
   pregnancy. Br J Obstet Gynaecol 1976;88:434–7.
8. Godfrey KM, Redman CWG, Barker DJP, Osmond C. The effect of maternal anaemia and iron
   deficiency on the ratio of fetal weight to placental weight. Br J Obstet Gynaecol 1991;98:886–91.
9. Charache S, Niebyl JR. Pregnancy in sickle cell disease. In: Letsky EA, editor. Haematological
   disorders in pregnancy. Clinics in haematology, vol 14. London: WB Saunders, 1985;720–46.
10. Sibai BM, Spinnato JA, Watson DL, Hill GA, Anderson GD. Pregnancy outcome in 303 cases with
    severe preeclampsia. Obstet Gynecol 1984;64:319–25.
11. Wildschutt HIJ, Triffers PE, Hart AAM. The effect of hypertension on fetal growth. Clin Exp
    Hypertens 1963;B2:37–43.
12. Szymonowicz W, Yu VYH. Severe pre-eclampsia and infants of very low birth weight. Arch Dis
    Child 1987;62:712–16.
13. Redman CWG, Beilin LJ, Bonnar J, Wilkinson RH. Plasma-urate measurements in predicting fetal
    death in hypertensive pregnancy. Lancet 1976;i:1370–3.
14. Cooper JC, Milton PJ, Baker PN (1995). Pre-eclampsia; current theories of. In: Asch R, Studd J,
    editors. Progress in reproductive medicine, vol 2. London: Parthenon, 1995;165–76.
15. Brosens IA, Robertson WB, Dixon HG. The role of the spiral arteries in the pathogenesis of
    preeclampsia. Obstet Gynecol Annu 1972;1:177–91.
16. Sheppard BL, Bonnar J. The ultrastructure of the arterial supply of the human placenta in
    pregnancy complicated by fetal growth retardation. Br J Obstet Gynaecol 1976;83:948–59.
17. Khong TY, DeWolf F, Robertson WB, Brosens I. Inadequate maternal vascular response to pla-
    centation in pregnancies complicated by pre-eclampsia and by small-for-gestational age
    infants.Br J Obstet Gynaecol 1986;93:1049–59.
18. Lunell N-O, Nylund L, Lewander R, Sarby B (1982). Uteroplacental blood flow in pre-eclampsia.
    Measurements with indium-113m and a computer-linked gamma camera. Clin Exp Hypertens
    B1: 105–117.
19. Francis ST, Duncan K, Moore RW, Baker PN, Johnson IR, Gowland PA. Non-invasive imaging of
    placental perfusion in normal pregnancies and in pregnancies complicated by intrauterine
    growth restriction. Lancet 1998;351:1397–400.
20. Cameron AD, Nicholson SF, Nimrod CA, Harder JR, Davies DM. Doppler waveforms in the fetal
    aorta and umbilical artery in patients with hypertension in pregnancy. Am J Obstet Gynecol
    1988;158:339–45.
21. Trudinger BJ, Cook, CM. Doppler umbilical and uterine flow waveforms in severe pregnancy
    hypertension. Br J Obstet Gynaecol 1990;97:142–8.
22. Zacutti, A., Borruto, F., & Bottacci, G. Umbilical bloodflow and placental pathology. Clin Exp
    Obstet Gynecol 1992;19:63–9.
23. Brosens I, Dixon HG, Robertson WB. Fetal growth retardation and the arteries of the placental
    bed. Br J Obstet Gynaecol 1977;84:656–63.

24. Nylund L, Lunell N-O, Lewander R, Sarby B. Uteroplacental blood flow index in intrauterine growth retardation of fetal or maternal origin. Br J Obstet Gynaecol 1983;90:16–20.
25. McCarthy A, Woolfson RG, Raju SK, Poston L. Abnormal endothelial cell function of resistance arteries from women with preeclampsia. Am J Obstet Gynecol 1993;168:1323.
26. Wilcox MA, Johnson IR, Maynard PV, Smith SJ, Chilvers CED. The individualised birthweight ratio: a more logical outcome measure of pregnancy than birthweight alone. Br J Obstet Gynaecol 1993;100:342–7.
27. Ashworth JR, Warren AY, Baker PN, Johnson IR. Loss of endothelium-dependent relaxation in myometrial resistance arteries in pre-eclampsia. Br J Obstet Gynaecol 1997;104:1152–8.
28. Roberts JM, Redman CWG. Pre-eclampsia: more than pregnancy-induced hypertension. Lancet 1993;341:1447–51.
29. Baker PN, Davidge ST, Roberts JM. Plasma from women with preeclampsia increases endothelial cell nitric oxide production. Hypertension 1995;26:244–8.
30. Ashworth JR, Warren AY, Johnson IR, Baker PN. Plasma from pre-eclamptic women induces a functional change in myometrial resistance arteries. Br J Obstet Gynaecol 1998;105:459–61.
31. Cnattingius S, Mills JL, Yuen J, Eriksson O, Salonen H. The paradoxical effect of smoking in preeclamptic pregnancies: smoking reduces the incidence but increases the rates of perinatal mortality, abruptio placentae and intrauterine growth restriction. Am J Obstet Gynecol 1997;177:156–61.
32. Eskenazi B, Fenster L, Sidney S, Elkin E. Fetal growth retardation in infants of multiparous and nulliparous women with preeclampsia. Am J Obstet Gynecol 1993;169:1112–18.
33. MacGillivray I. Some observations on the incidence of preeclampsia. J Obstet Gynaecol Br Commonwlth 1958;65:536–9.
34. Feeney JG, Scott JS. Pre-eclampsia and changed paternity. Eur J Obstet, Gynaecol Reprod Biol 1980;11:35–8.
35. Redman CWG. Immunological aspects of pre-eclampsia. Bailiere's Clin Obstet Gynaecol 1992;6:601–15.
36. Petrucco O. Aetiology of pre-eclampsia. In: Studd J, editor. Progress in obstetrics and gynaecology. Edinburgh: Churchill Livingstone, 1981;51–69.
37. Haeger M, Unander M, Bengtsson A. Complement activation in relation to development of pre-eclampsia. Obstet Gynecol 1991;78:46–9.
38. El-Roeiy A, Myers SA, Gleicher N. The relationship between autoantibodies and intrauterine growth retardation in hypertensive disorders of pregnancy. Am J Obstet Gynecol 1991;164:1253–61.
39. Pangborn MC. A new serologically active phospholipid from beef heart. Proc Soc Exp Biol Med 1941;48:484–6.
40. Johnstone FD Kilpatrick DC, Burns SM. Anticardiolipin antibodies and pregnancy outcome in women with human immunodeficiency virus infection. Obstet Gynecol 1992;80:92–6.
41. McNeil HP, Chesterman CN, Krills SA. Immunology and clinical importance of antiphospholipid antibodies. Adv Immunol 1991;49:193–280.
42. Conley CL, Hartman RC. Hemorrhagic disorder caused by circulating anticoagulant in patients with disseminated lupus erythematosus. J Clin Invest 1952;31:621–2.
43. Feinstein DI, Rapaport SI. Acquired inhibitors of blood coagulation. Proc Hemast Thromb 1972;1:75–95.
44. Triplett DA, Brandt JT, Musgrove KA, Orr CA. The relationship between lupus anticoagulants and antibodies to phospholipid. JAMA 1988;259:550–4.
45. Triplett DA, Brandt J. Laboratory identification of the lupus anticoagulant. Br J Haematol 1989;73:139–42.
46. Lockwood CJ, Rand JH. The immunology and obstetrical consequences of antiphospholipid antibodies. Obstet Gynecol 1994;49:432–41.
47. Gharavi AE, Harris EN, Asherson RA. Anticardiolipin antibodies: Isotope distribution and phospholipid specificity. Ann Rheum Dis 1987;46:1–6.
48. Love PE, Santoro SA. Antiphospholipid antibodies: Anticardiolipin and the lupus anticoagulant in systemic lupus erythematosus (SLE) and in non-SLE disorders. Ann Intern Med 1990;112:682–98.
49. Yasuda M, Takakuwa K, Tokunaga A, Tanaka K. Prospective studies of the association between anticardiolipin antibody and outcome of pregnancy. Obstet Gynecol 1995;86:555–9.
50. Polzin WJ, Kopelman JN, Robinson RD. The association of antiphospholipid antibodies with pregnancies complicated by fetal growth restriction. Obstet Gynecol 1991;78:1108–11.
51. Bendon RW, Hayden LE, Hurtubise PE. Prenatal screening for anticardiolipin antibody. Am J Perinatol 1990;7:245–50.

52. Toyoshima K, Makino T, Sugi T. Correlation between trimester of fetal wastage and anti-cardiolipin antibody titer. Int J Fertil 1991;36:89–93.

53. Infante-Rivard C, David M, Gauthier R, Rivard G-E. Lupus anticoagulants, anticardiolipin antibodies, and fetal loss. N Engl J Med 1991;325:1063–6.

54. Haddow JE, Rote NS, Dostal-Johnson D, Palomaki GE, Pulkkinen AJ, Knight GJ. Lack of an association between late fetal death and antiphospholipid antibody measurements in the second trimester. Am J Obstet Gynecol 1991;165:1308–12.

55. Lockshin MD, Sammaritano LR. Antiphospholipid antibodies and fetal loss [letter]. N Engl J Med 1992;326:951–3.

56. De Wolf F, Carreras LO, Moerman P, Vermylen J, Van Assche A, Renaer M. Decidual vasculopathy and extensive placental infarction in a patient with repeated thromboembolic accidents, recurrent fetal loss, and a lupus anticoagulant. Am J Obstet Gynecol 1982;142:829–34.

57. De Carolis S, Caruso A, Ferrazzani S, Carducci B, De Santis L, Mancuso S. Poor pregnancy outcome and anticardiolipin antibodies. Fetal Diagn Ther 1994;9:296–9.

58. Katano K, Aoki A, Sasa H, Ogasawara M, Matsuura E, Yagami Y. Beta 2-Glycoprotein I-dependent anticardiolipin antibodies as a predictor of adverse pregnancy outcomes in healthy pregnant women. Human Reprod 1996;11:509–12.

59. Cowchock FS, Reece EA, Balaban D, Branch DW, Plouffe L. Repeated fetal losses associated with antiphospholipid antibodies: a collaborative randomized trial comparing prednisolone with low-dose heparin treatment. Am J Obstet Gynecol 1992;166:1318–23.

60. Stirling Y, Woolf L, North WR, Seghatatchian MJ, Meade TW. Haemostasis in normal pregnancy. Thromb Haemost 1984;52:176–82.

61. Weiner CP. Evaluation of clotting disorders during pregnancy. In: Sciarra JJ, Eschenbach DA, Depp R, editors. Gynecology and obstetrics, vol 3. Hagerstown MD, Harper & Row, 1990;1.

62. Maki M. Coagulation, fibrinolysis, platelet and kinin-forming systems during toxaemia of pregnancy. Biol Res Preg 1983;4:152–4.

63. Weiner CP, Brant J. Plasma antithrombin III activity: an aid in the diagnosis of pre-eclampsia-eclampsia. Am J Obstet Gynecol 1982;142:275–81.

64. Saleh AA, Bottoms SF, Welch RA, Ali MA, Mariona FG, Mammen EF. Preeclampsia, delivery, and the haemostatic system. Am J Obstet Gynecol 1987;157:331–6.

65. Brant JT. Current concepts of coagulation. Clin Obstet Gynecol 1985;28:3–14.

66. Comp PC, Jacocks RM, Ferrell GL, Esmon CT. Activation of protein C in vivo. J Clin Invest 1982;70:127–34.

67. Gonzalez R, Alberca I, Vincente V. Protein C levels in late pregnancy, post partum and in women on oral contraceptives. Thromb Res 1985;39:637–41.

68. Dekker GA, de Vries JIP, Doelitzch PM, Huijgens PC, Von Blomberg BME, Jakobs C. Underlying disorders associated with severe early onset pre-eclampsia. Am J Obstet Gynecol 1995;173:1042–8.

69. Preston FE, Rosendaal FR, Walker ID, Briet E, Berntorp E, Conard J, et al. Increased fetal loss in women with heritable thrombophilia. Lancet 1996;348:913–16.

70. De Vries JIP, Dekker GA, Huijgens PC, Jakobs C, Blomberg BME, van Geijn HP. Hyperhomocysteinaemia and protein D deficiency in complicated pregnancies. Br J Obstet Gynecol 1997;104:1248–54.

71. Cunningham FG, Macdonald PC, Gant NF. Williams obstetrics, 19th edn. East Norwalk, CT: Appleton & Lange, 1993;763–817.

72. Paternoster D, Stella A, Simioni P, Trovo S, Plebani P, Girolami A. Clotting inhibitors and fibronectin as potential markers in pre-eclampsia. Int J Gynaecol Obstet 1994;47:215–21.

73. Fernandez JA, Estelles A, Gilabert J. Functional and immunologic protein S in normal pregnant women and in full term neonates. Thromb Haemost 1989;61:474–8.

74. Dahlback B, Carlsson M, Svensson PJ. Familial thrombophilia due to a previously unrecognised mechanism characterised by poor anticoagulant response to activated protein C. Proc Natl Acad Sci USA 1993;90:1004–8.

75. Bertina RM, Koeleman BPC, Koster T, Rosendaal FR, Dirven RJ, de Ronde H, et al. Mutation in blood coagulation factor V associated with resistance to activated protein C. Nature 1994;369:64–7.

76. Svensson PJ, Dahlback B. Twenty novel families with thrombophilia and inherited resistance to activated protein C. Thromb Haemost 1993;69:1252 [abst].

77. Koster T, Rosendaal FR, de Ronde H, Briet E, Vandenbroucke JP, Bertina RM. Venous thrombosis due to poor anticoagulant response to activated protein C: Leiden Thrombophilia Study. Lancet 1993;342:1503–6.

78. Walker MC, Garner PR, Keely EJ, Rock GA, Reis MD. Changes in activated protein C resistance during normal pregnancy. Am J Obstet Gynecol 1997;177:162–9.
79. Lee DH, Henderson PA, Blajchman MA. Prevalence of factor V Leiden in a Canadian blood donor population. Can Med Assoc J 1996;155:285–9.
80. Hellgren M, Svensson PJ, Dahlback B. Resistance to activated protein C as a basis for venous thromboembolism associated with pregnancy and oral contraceptives. Am J Obstet Gynecol 1995;173:210–13.
81. Cumming AM, Tait RC, Fildes S, Yoong A, Keeney S, Hay CR. Development of resistance to activated protein C during pregnancy. Br J Haematol 1995;90:725–7.
82. Mathonnet F, Demazancourt P, Bastenaire B, Morot M, Benattar N, Beufe X. Activated protein C sensitivity ratio in pregnant women at delivery. Br J Haematol 1996;92:244–6.
83. Zoller B, Svensson PJ, He X, Dahlback B. Identification of the same factor V gene mutation in 47 out of 50 thrombosis-prone families with inherited resistance to activated protein C. J Clin Invest 1994;94:2521–4.
84. Rotmensch S, Liberati M, Mittelman M, Ben-Rafael Z. Activated protein C resistance and adverse pregnancy outcome. Am J Obstet Gynecol 1997;177:170–3.

16 Prevention and Treatment of IUGR

James J. Walker, Graeme Smith, Gustaaf A. Dekker

Introduction

Birthweight is the most important determinant of perinatal outcome and as such IUGR remains a major cause of perinatal morbidity and mortality. It should be stressed when reading the literature that there is significant conflict in publications between those based exclusively upon neonatal weight percentiles to diagnose IUGR and those in which antenatal and/or neonatal clinical information is available. In the latter group, low birthweight is more likely to be secondary to pathology (e.g. uteroplacental insufficiency) than in the former group, which contains largely healthy SGA newborns (Ch. 1). From a clinical perspective the diagnosis of IUGR can be problematic and the underlying aetiology multifactorial (Table 16.1). Thus consideration of a broad range of preventive measures, applicable to the general pregnant population, may be more effective than resorting to focused therapeutic measures. It therefore follows that the management and/or

Table 16.1 Factors associated with IUGR; many of these factors are interrelated

fetal
fetal abnormality
intrauterine infection

placental
placental maladaption
reduced fetal placental blood ow
reduced maternal placental blood ow

maternal
maternal infection
chronic maternal disease
low maternal prepregnancy weight
poor maternal nutrition
poor maternal weight gain
maternal smoking
maternal caffeine intake
excessive physical activity
inadequate maternal haemodynamic adaptation

social
lower social class
single mothers
teenage pregnancy
deficient antenatal care

treatment must be individualised. This chapter critically evaluates various treatment and management regimens. It must be realised that no one therapeutic approach will be suitable for all; in the majority of cases no treatment other than close fetal surveillance and timely delivery may be available.

There are three traditional approaches to disease prevention: primary, secondary and tertiary [1]. As it pertains to IUGR, *primary prevention* is aimed at preventing growth restriction before it develops, thus reducing the incidence of the disease. An example of this would be population-based or community-based nutritional supplementation programmes or facilitating antenatal visits. *Secondary prevention* involves the early detection and treatment of the disease (IUGR) in an "asymptomatic" period before it progresses. An example of this would be close antenatal surveillance (i.e. ultrasound) of high risk groups (e.g. previous affected pregnancy) and institution of means to improve placental blood flow or maternal/fetal energy supplementation if expected fetal growth is not maintained. *Tertiary prevention* attempts to reduce complications of IUGR by treatment. An example of this would be the use of corticosteroids to improve fetal maturation or timely delivery to reduce the incidence of stillbirth. There is clearly an overlap between these "divisions" and published management/therapeutic trials for IUGR include women in all three groups. Thus very little of our current clinical practice in IUGR can be said to be "evidence based".

An infant's birthweight is primarily dependent upon two factors, gestational age at delivery and the rate of fetal growth. Fetal growth is a balance of supply, demand and utilisation. On the maternal side, adequate energy supply (e.g. nutrients, oxygen), uteroplacental perfusion, proper placentation and placental function are required to supply the fetal energy needs. On the fetal side, placental perfusion and substrate utilisation are essential. Any impairment in these processes will result in reduced fetal growth. Prevention and/or therapy for IUGR needs to be directed at one or more of these parameters.

Antenatal Care

Fetal growth is a complex, multifactorial phenomenon, influenced by the maternal and uterine environments. While placental pathology may be the primary aetiologicol factor, multiple social factors are also associated with poor fetal growth and thus presumably the quality of placentation (Table 16.1). These include being a single mother, teenage pregnancy, low maternal weight, maternal malnutrition, increased caffeine intake, smoking and chronic maternal ill health [2–4].

Primary prevention can be aimed at whole populations, or focused on perceived "high risk" groups such as those with a past history of IUGR, in an attempt to reduce the overall incidence of IUGR (Table 16.2). Such an approach was tried in Tennessee [5]. Project HUG (Helping Us Grow) included care provider referrals, visit scheduling, transportation and nutritional and health education to potentially "high risk" pregnant woman who were enrolled in the USA government Medicaid system. Those women who were HUG participants were more likely to utilise antenatal care and other benefits such as antenatal vitamin supplementation compared retrospectively with a similar cohort of pregnant Medicaid users who did not receive HUG services. However, there was no

Table 16.2 Methods of screening and diagnosis of IUGR

history
maternal past pregnancy history
maternal medical history
maternal social history

clinical assessment
maternal booking weight
maternal weight gain
fundal height measurement

ultrasound monitoring
Doppler ultrasound of the uterine arteries
fetal biometry
Doppler ultrasound of the umbilical artery
Doppler ultrasound of fetal cerebral arteries

significant reduction in the incidence of preterm births or of very low birthweight infants [5]. Other randomised controlled trials have examined different methods of intervention (e.g. dietary supplementation, smoking reduction, pharmaceutical intervention with aspirin) for "high risk" groups. Unfortunately, these interventions have, for the most part, failed to show any significant effects on overall short term perinatal outcome [6]. The impact of optimal contemporary obstetrical management upon perinatal morbidity may at best be marginal. Targeting a group of pregnancies deemed to be "high risk" will not probably have a major impact on the overall rate of preterm birth, low birthweight and IUGR because the majority of adverse pregnancy outcomes occur in women not deemed to be in "high risk" groups [7]. Therefore, a community-wide approach offers a potentially more effective way to promote healthier babies than one directed solely at improving antenatal care [7]. If obstetrical complications in general, and IUGR in particular, are to be reduced then there needs to be an increased commitment to assuring adequate individual and family support.

Dietary Supplementation

There is evidence that the IUGR fetus is malnourished in utero, based on postpartum demonstration of muscle wasting and reduced glycogen and fat stores [8]. In addition, FBS studies have demonstrated that the IUGR fetus is hypoglycaemic [9] with a reduced circulating concentration of certain essential amino acids (e.g. valine, leucine, isoleucine, threonine) and total a-aminonitrogen levels [10]. Nutrient requirements during the first trimester are quantitatively small, but deprivation during this period can adversely affect placental structure and ultimately birthweight [11]. However, later in gestation, maternal malnutrition can also have profound effects. The classic example of this was the Dutch famine (1944–5) at the end of World War II [12]. During this time, there was severe caloric restriction of significantly less than 1500 calories per day. Third trimester exposure accounted for the whole effects of the famine. There was a 9 per cent reduction in birthweight, 15 per cent reduction in placental weight and approximately a 2.5 per cent reduction in neonatal length and head circumference at birth. For infants born in the period following the famine, all these parameters had returned to normal [12]. Animal studies have confirmed that severe maternal malnutrition throughout pregnancy causes IUGR [13].

Inadequate nutrient supply to the fetus may represent a final common aetiological pathway in the IUGR fetus. IGUR, in both human and experimental animals, is characterised by fetal hypoglycaemia and hypoxaemia [9]. Experimental IUGR in pregnant sheep has demonstrated that consumption of glucose and oxygen is similar per unit weight to that of the normally grown fetus [14,15], which suggests that fetal growth rate may be limited by the supply of these substrates. Therefore prevention of, and therapy for, IUGR fetuses has been directed at improving fetal nutrient supply.

Both maternal prepregnancy weight and weight gain during pregnancy influence fetal growth. However, the effect of weight gain lessens as prepregnancy weight increases [11,16]. In women with a normal prepregnancy weight, excessive weight gain did not enhance fetal growth or length of gestation [17]. In underweight mothers, prepregnancy nutritional supplementation had a greater effect on birthweight than supplementation during the pregnancy in question [18]. Interpregnancy nutritional supplementation results in higher birthweights as well as other benefits to the mother (e.g. higher mean haemoglobin) [19]. Therefore, maternal prepregnancy weight appears to be fundamental in achieving adequate fetal growth; maternal nutritional supplementation during pregnancy may be beneficial in preventing the development of IUGR only in those women with a severely deficient diet.

Reduced intake of protein, minerals and B vitamins all correlate with birthweight [20]; birthweight progressively falls with a decrease in maternal intake but only in those women with lower birthweight fetuses. These "at risk" women are found in all social classes. It is in these women that nutritional supplementation may improve fetal growth [21]. Specific nutrient supplements (e.g. vitamin A, folic acid, iron, calcium and magnesium) have all been suggested to reduce the incidence of low birthweight. However, in studies of dietary interventions, including protein/energy, vitamin, mineral and fish oil supplementation, as well as the prevention and treatment of anaemia, only the balanced protein/energy supplementation reduced the risk of developing IUGR [22]. The effect is due, in part, to a prolongation of gestation [11]. For example, a study of zinc supplementation in pregnant women found that birthweights were significantly higher than in control pregnancies; this was related to a prolongation of gestation at delivery rather than a reduction in the incidence of IUGR per se [23].

Although oral dietary supplementation appears to be of limited value in preventing and certainly treating IUGR, parenteral treatment may have more of an effect. Furthermore, intra-amniotic infusion of amino acids may be even more effective in prevention and/or treatment of IUGR than maternal intravenous infusion, particularly those cases where placental pathology results in impaired placental transport. As much as 10 per cent of fetal protein requirements are obtained from amniotic fluid that is swallowed [24]. Experimental oesophageal ligation is associated with growth restriction [25]. Administration of nutrients either into the amniotic cavity or directly into the stomach has been tested as a therapeutic strategy. The intragastric infusion of amniotic fluid in rabbit fetuses with experimental oesophageal ligation reversed the growth restriction [25,26]. Replacement with specific components such as dextrose, amino acids and lipids could not reverse the experimental growth restriction, which suggests that impaired nutrient delivery is not the limiting factor in this model [26,27]. Direct intravascular nutrient supplementation to the chronically catheterised sheep fetus was able to prevent the growth restriction associated with placental embolisation [28]. These strategies are clearly not clinically practical at this point, given the attendant risks of invasive fetal procedures, and little evidence from data in human pregnancies that either of these feeding strategies is of benefit.

Whilst there is some evidence to support the concept that maternal nutritional supplementation improves fetal growth and pregnancy outcome [29,30], there is a lack of quality randomised controlled studies addressing the issue of nutritional supplementation to women *with* an IUGR fetus. In pregnant sheep, prolonged malnourishment results in fetal growth restriction, but once established cannot be reversed by refeeding the mother [31]. This experimental model may be analogous to the human situation since poor postnatal growth is a feature of IUGR, though the underlying mechanism remains unknown [32].

Nutritional supplementation may not be risk free for the IUGR fetus either. Maternal metabolic conditions, such as phenylketonuria (PKU), which results in high circulating levels of the amino acid phenylalanine, can significantly impair fetal growth and development. Intravenous amino acid supplementation to pregnant humans and to sheep has demonstrated elevated fetal concentrations of ammonia and urea and lower PO_2 and pH at the time of delivery [33,34]. Similarly, administration of intravenous glucose solutions to mothers of normally grown fetuses results in the development of fetal acidaemia [35] secondary to a resultant increase in fetal oxygen consumption [36]. Glucose supplementation in pregnancies complicated by IUGR has been shown to produce a fall in pH [37] and an increase in the rate of fetal demise [36]. In the face of already reduced PO_2 at delivery [9], an increase in IUGR fetal oxygen consumption, provoked by a glucose load, would clearly be detrimental.

Thus in summary prepregnancy and early prenatal nutritional counselling should be an integral component of all antenatal care, particularly in those women deemed to be at high risk for an IUGR fetus [11,38]. By contrast, intensive nutritional therapy, commenced alter IUGR has been diagnosed, does not appear to improve either fetal growth or perinatal morbidity/mortality.

Drug Abuse During Pregnancy

Smoking has been shown to decrease fetal weight by approximately 200 g per pack cigarettes smoked per day [39]. Although this is not a dramatic amount of weight reduction, it may be magnified by additional insults such as poor nutritional intake and other drug use. Presumably once the underlying placental pathology is established, maternal–fetal transfer cannot be augmented. This subject is addressed in Ch. 4. Other drugs have been associated with restricted fetal growth although, again, it is difficult to determine by what degree because of other confounding variables. As an example, women with a high caffeine intake (> 300 mg/day; equivalent to approximately three cups of coffee or seven cups of tea) also have a significantly higher proportion of growth-restricted babies. However, the effect of caffeine is not significant when confounding variables (e.g. smoking) are taken into account [40]. In human pregnancies, it is difficult to differentiate the effects of cocaine abuse from the tendency of this group of women to smoke and abuse other drugs, specifically alcohol, as well. It is certainly recommended that woman who abuse drugs in pregnancy should stop or reduce their use to improve outcome (i.e. growth, neurodevelopment, etc.) of the infants. To this end, epidemiological data have demonstrated that cessation of alcohol use in the later half of pregnancy in women who had significant consumption early on improved fetal/neonatal outcome [41,42]. Birthweights and neurodevelopmental parameters were better than those who continued to abuse alcohol but not as good as those that did not consume alcohol during pregnancy. However, there is a paucity of studies demonstrating that cessation of drug use in pregnancies *already* complicated by IUGR will improve neonatal outcome.

Physical Activity

Evidence suggests that women who undertake manual-type work during pregnancy have an increased incidence of IUGR, though significant confounding variables, (e.g. low socioeconomic class, poor working conditions, and smoking) make the association difficult to establish. There is some evidence that a reduction in physical effort in these women may be beneficial [43]. However, there is no good evidence to support empirical bed rest in women whose physical effort is not excessive. Reduced physical activity results in decreased peripheral blood flow and thus in theory an increased proportion of cardiac output will enter the uteroplacental circulation. In fact, there is no good evidence that uteroplacental blood flow increases with rest, presumably because cardiac output falls. Furthermore, bed rest increases the risk of deep venous thrombosis (DVT) and pulmonary embolus. This is an important consideration as some IUGR pregnancies result from maternal thrombophilia, and many will be delivered by CS, thus amplifying their inherent risk of DVT. In a large prospective trial of pregnancies complicated by IUGR (detected sonographically at 32 weeks' gestation), hospitalisation with bed rest for an average of 30 days had no effect on either fetal growth or pregnancy outcome compared with outpatient management and normal activity [44]. Likewise the combination of hospitalisation, bed rest and oral *b*-mimetic therapy had no effect on birthweight or perinatal outcome, compared with outpatient monitoring alone [45].

Antenatal Treatment

Low Dose Aspirin

An imbalance in the ratio of the vasoconstrictor/platelet aggregator effects of thromboxane (T_x) to the vasodilator/platelet inhibitory effects of prostacyclin (PGI_2) has been proposed as an aetiological factor in pre-eclampsia, and possibly IUGR. Aspirin, an irreversible inhibitor of the cyclo-oxygenase enzyme, has a greater effect on platelets (which preferentially produce T_x) than on endothelial cells (which preferentially produce PGI_2) because platelets lack the ability to generate new enzyme. Studies of maternal urinary excretion of prostaglandin metabolites in IUGR demonstrated a reduction in prostacyclin generation and increased thromboxane production. Aspirin was therefore proposed as a therapy for IUGR by returning the imbalance of T_x/PGI_2 to normal. Whilst initial studies suggested this hypothesis to be true, the effectiveness of aspirin for the prevention and treatment of IUGR (and/or pre-eclampsia) has not been realised in subsequent larger studies with sufficient power.

Initial small clinical series suggested that aspirin therapy produced a reduction of the recurrence of IUGR [46]. Because of these positive findings the prescription rate for low dose aspirin increased markedly from 1989 to 1991 in some countries [47]. However, subsequent larger multicentre trials did not support these findings [48,49]. The largest of these trials was the CLASP trial [49] . Although this trial corroborated other studies that found no increased risk of placental abruption or increased perinatal mortality [50], it did not find any overall benefit of low dose aspirin therapy in the prevention of IUGR. However, subgroup analysis suggested a possible benefit in women with severe early onset placental problems. A recent study, addressing this issue as a primary outcome measure, found no benefit of aspirin over placebo for women with a variety of high risk conditions for IUGR [51]. The evidence for a beneficial effect of aspirin in the prevention and/or treatment of IUGR has thus receeded to the point that individual physicians need to reconsider their prescribing practice carefully. This is an important issue as some obstetrical anaesthetists view current low dose aspirin use as a relative contraindication to regional anesthesia for caesarean section.

Oxygen Therapy

Fetal tissue oxygenation is critical to the maintenance of normal growth. The adaptive response of the fetus to chronic hypoxaemia, known as "brain sparing", involves redistribution of fetal cardiac output to vital organs such as the brain, heart and adrenal glands. Reduced renal blood flow results in oligohydramnios, a common finding in IUGR. These effects are at the expense of blood flow to certain "non-critical organs", such as the fetal liver, which grows at a slower rate producing asymmetrical IUGR. Maternal medical conditions (e.g. cyanotic heart disease) and environmental conditions (e.g. high altitude), which impair/reduce maternal oxygen delivery to the fetus by preplacental hypoxia, are also associated with reduced fetal growth.

Experimental data from pregnant sheep demonstrate that fetal PO_2 could restored to normal by maternal hyperoxygenation in moderate but not in severe growth restriction [32]. No increase in fetal oxygen consumption could be demonstrated, presumably because impaired placental transfer of basic nutrients precluded anabolic growth. Of more concern, cessation of treatment was followed by a period of impaired fetal oxygenation that was worse than that prior to supplementation. This phenomenon was worse when no initial improvement was observed in the fetal condition [52].

Data from human pregnancies are more reassuring. In a study of IUGR pregnancies in which FBS was performed for karyotyping purposes, 37 per cent (14/38) had low oxygen tension values, compared with published data for normally grown fetuses of similar gestational age [9]. As a result, it has been postulated that improving fetal oxygenation may be useful in preventing or reversing IUGR. Initial animal data supported supplemental maternal oxygen inhalation to improve survival and marginally improve growth in rat fetuses compromised by experimental uteroplacental insufficiency [53]. In a series of five human IUGR fetuses, maternal therapy with 55 per cent humidified oxygen for 15–24 hours per day until delivery (5 days to 9 weeks), resulted in improved PO_2 on FBS and normalisation of fetal redistribution [54]. No improvement in fetal growth could be demonstrated over the treatment period. In fact, all fetuses continued to fall off their individual growth curves and one intrauterine death occurred. The 80 per cent fetal survival compared well with historic control pregnancies with severe IUGR (15 per cent), suggesting that oxygen improved fetal survival in severe IUGR with abnormal umbilical artery Doppler waveforms [54]. In a more recent randomised study of fetuses with severe IUGR ($n = 36$), continuous maternal administration with humidified 55 per cent oxygen (vs. no supplemental oxygen), for approximately 10 days, resulted in improved fetal Doppler ultrasound findings and improved fetal acid–base balance [55]. No difference was seen in fetal growth velocity and no difference was observed in birthweights between the groups. This is not surprising given the short treatment time period but is of lesser importance since the treatment was associated with a significant reduction in perinatal mortality (29 vs. 68 per cent). Maternal oxygen therapy thus appears to confer benefit to the IUGR fetus. However, this treatment modality has not gained popularity outside a research setting. Possible reasons include reluctance for inpatient monitoring, lack of evidence for an effect upon fetal growth, and finally a belief that timing of delivery and quality of immediate postnatal care vastly override any potential benefit derived from oxygen. As discussed in the Ch. 22, we do not at present know whether prolongation of gestation in severe IUGR reduces the risk of major pediatric morbidity. Should the GRIT trial demonstrate a benefit from prolongation of gestation then it would logically follow that the issue of oxygen therapy be revisited.

Growth Factors

Fetal growth is influenced by various growth factors such as GH, insulin and IGF-1. One area that has recently gained a lot of interest is the involvement of IGFs in fetal growth; circulating fetal levels of IGF-l are reduced in both experimental animal models of IUGR and human IUGR [56–59]. Human genetic studies indicate that IGF-1R defects (chromosome l5q25–26) [60,61] are also associated with IUGR. A significant increase in IGFBP-1, which would decrease the bioavailability of IGF-l, has also been reported in experimental and human IUGR [59,62,63]. A balance of IGF-l and IGFBP-l appears to be involved in the regulation of fetal growth; elevated IGFBP-l, in the presence of nutritional insult, may act to reduce the fetal growth rate. In essence, the fetus is adapting to its environment by raising IGFBP-l. It is important to note that reduced IGF-l and elevated IGFBP-l were found only in growth-restricted fetuses that demonstrated evidence of placental insufficiency and not in those without placental insufficiency [63]. Infusion of IGF-l into fetal sheep significantly altered placental metabolism reducing placental lactate production and demand for amino acids allowing more to be available to the fetus [64]. Therefore, fetal IGF-l may act to coordinate fetal and placental metabolism. Maternal infusion with IGF-l did not affect fetal IGF-l levels in pregnant sheep, but did increase placental lactate production by over 50 per cent. Lactate is utilised by the fetus for oxidative metabolism [65] and thus maternal IGF-l may affect fetal growth by its effect on placental carbohydrate metabolism, facilitating transfer of nutrients to the fetus. Interestingly, in the studies mentioned earlier demonstrating intragastric amniotic fluid replacement, but not replacement with nutrients, improved fetal growth [25,26], the effect may be in part to IGF-1 in the amniotic fluid; swallowed amniotic fluid contains IGF-1 and may effect both fetal growth and gut maturation [66].

Experimentally, the maternal administration of GH and IGF-1 can affect placental function and increase fetal growth. This suggests a potential role for growth factors given maternally, intra-amniotically or postnatally in IUGR fetuses [66]. Since placental insufficiency is a feature of IUGR, it would seem more likely that direct intra-amniotic therapy or fetal therapy might be more likely to be beneficial. However, the underlying block in the transfer of maternal supply of nutrients (other than oxygen, which can be supplied via the mother) prevents the fetus from increasing its growth. By contrast, postpartum therapy might allow an increased catch-up for the affected fetus since nutritional supply is no longer an issue [66].

Attempts at Improving Fetoplacental Blood Flow

Recent histopathological data from delivered placentas of IUGR pregnancies has challenged the hypothesis that the placenta is hypoxic in the presence of utero-placental insufficiency [67,68]. Where AEDF is found in the umbilical arteries, fetal hypoxaemia is due to a block in oxygen transfer across the placenta. Intraplacental PO_2 rises towards arterial values, which in turn inhibits placental vascular development via the suppression of critical growth factors [68]. Attempts to treat fetal hypoxaemia by maternal administration of supplemental oxygen are therefore likely to inhibit villous vascularisation and development further [69]. Thus strategies that selectively promote fetaplacental blood flow in IUGR pregnancies with absent uterine artery end-diastolic flow are likely not only to attenuate the block in oxygen transfer to the fetus, but in doing so may restore the normal hypoxic drive (via VEGF) to villous placental angiogenesis (see Ch. 8). Prostaglandin synthetase (cyclo-oxygenase) inhibitors (e.g. acetyl saliclyclic acid, ASA) (see earlier discussion) and NO donor drugs, specifically nitroglycerin (glyceryl trinitrate, GTN) and sodium nitroprusside (SNP), have been proposed to reduce fetoplacental vascular resistance [70,71]. Of concern with the use of any vasoactive drug in pregnancy, antepartum or intrapartum, is the effect on utero-placental perfusion. Drugs that cause proportionately greater vasodilation in the non-uterine vasculature may decrease uterine blood flow.

NO is involved in regulation of blood flow in the placenta. In animal studies, a chronic reduction in NO production results in significant IUGR [72,73]. These changes are reversed by treatment with L-arginine, the precursor of NO [74]. Furthermore, in an hypoxia-induced fetal growth restriction model in the rat, supplementary L-arginine improves fetal growth [75]. These findings lend support to the potential for use of NO donors in the treatment and prevention of IUGR. However, studies of NO metabolite levels in human pregnancy have produced inconsistent results. Furthermore, immunohistochemical studies show that there appears to be an increase in endothelial NO synthase (eNOS) expression, and hence an increase in local NO production in the fetoplacetnal vasculature in pregnancies complicated by IUGR [76]. Therefore, IUGR does not appear to be associated with endothelial NO deficiency in human pregnancy. Indeed, this may be a compensatory response in an attempt to improve blood flow. Longer-acting nitrates, such as isosorbide mononitrate, have been shown to lower uterine artery vascular resistance in normal pregnancies [77], but as yet no data are available to assess its potential role in the management of IUGR.

Is there a Role for Improving Uteroplacental Blood Flow?

As discussed above, despite perhaps 50 per cent reductions in uteroplacental blood flow in pregnancies complicated by severe early onset IUGR, oxygen transfer to the fetus is limited by the more profound defect in fetoplacetnal blood flow represented by absent end-diastolic flow velocity in the umbilical arteries. If this argument is accepted from a scientific standpoint, it makes little sense to direct treatment at the uteroplacental circulation, for example to women with abnormal uterine artery Doppler at 22–24 weeks of gestation [78]. The placenta is intrinsically capable of making adaptive changes to reduced uteroplacental blood flow such that flow-dependent transfer of oxygen is preserved without recourse to "vasodilator" therapy [79].

Undoubtedly the uteroplacental arterial vasculature is responsive to vasoactive agents – at least in early gestation. In pregnant women at 8 to 10 weeks of gestation, prior to elective termination, intravenous administration of GTN decreased the uterine artery PI (= the systolic velocity – diastolic velocity/time average maximum velocity), and thus increased the mean velocity of uterine arterial blood flow [77]. Exposure of low risk pregnant women, at 17 to 24 weeks of gestation, to sublingual isosorbide dinitrate (ISDN) resulted in a significant reduction in Doppler impedance in the uterine arteries – and an associated drop in maternal blood pressure [80]. At 24 to 26 weeks of gestation, in women with documented abnormal uteroplacental blood flow, GTN infusion produced a similar decrease in the PI of the uterine artery [77]. No changes were observed in maternal or fetal heart rate, maternal blood pressure, or the PI for the umbilical and maternal carotid arteries. In patients with severe pre-eclampsia at 31 to 35 weeks of gestation, the use of I.V. GTN to decrease maternal diastolic blood pressure to 100 mmHg improved fetoplacental perfusion without adversely affecting uteroplacental perfusion [81]. This effect was seen primarily in fetuses with an abnormal umbilical artery PI prior to GTN infusion. There was no effect of GTN on the fetal heart rate and thus likely no effect on fetal blood pressure [81]. Sublingual GTN administration was shown to improve the umbilical artery systolic/diastolic velocity ratio in 37- to 38-week-old fetuses with abnormal umbilical artery velocity ratio associated with pregnancy-induced hypertension and IUGR [82]. Transdermal GTN has been used for women with previously noted bilateral uterine diastolic notching on Doppler waveform and either pre-eclampsia or IUGR [83]. There was a 16 per cent decrease in the uterine artery PI that was maximal by 60 hours. The PI had returned to baseline values by 36 hours following removal of the GTN patch.

In most of these studies, there was no placebo treatment, which severely limits the conclusions that can be drawn. The findings are also somewhat confusing as the apparent beneficial effect of GTN was much longer than would be predicted from the kinetics of GTN metabolism. This drug is quickly metabolised and cleared from the system following removal of the GTN patch.

In summary, NO donors represent a novel approach to the prevention or management of pregnancies complicated by IUGR. At least in theory, selective improvement of fetoplacental blood flow will probably confer perinatal benefit whilst improvements in uteroplacental blood flow are unlikely to influence flow-dependent transfer across the placenta. Good quality placebo-controlled studies are required to address these issues, using paediatric morbidity as the primary outcome measure. NO donors have potential risks and thus their continued use must be evidence based.

Abdominal Decompression

A physical method of attempting to improve uterine blood flow is intermittent abdominal decompression [84,85]. Case series suggested that early onset IUGR may be improved by abdominal decompression produced by wearing a plastic suit over a rigid frame in which pressure can be reduced with a vacuum. Twice a day, a negative pressure (70 mmHg) was applied for 30 seconds every minute for 30 minutes. Theoretically, the device is supposed to improve placental intervillous blood flow. There are no controlled studies that assess the technique. Moreover, the method requires cumbersome equipment, although newer methods using plastic shells are being investigated. There are no data to demonstrate that this device actually improves uteroplacental perfusion.

Maternal Haemodilution

Women destined to have an IUGR fetus appear to mount an inadequate haemo-dynamic response during the first trimester of pregnancy. The resultant effect is a reduced plasma volume expansion [86,87], which is counteracted by an increased sympathetic tone to preserve blood pressure [88]. Placental blood flow may be impaired because the incompletely transformed spiral arteries can constrict to endogenous catecholamines. Furthermore the relatively high maternal haemo-globin concentration increases blood viscosity. Initial studies of haemodilution, designed to counteract these potentially harmful events, demonstrated an increase in both placental perfusion and fetal cardiovascular status [89]. In the presence of pre-eclampsia, heavy proteinuria may lower plasma oncotic pressure. Colloid volume expansion is designed to counteract this process, and appears to improve amniotic fluid volume and coexistent abnormal umbilical artery Doppler waveforms [89]. Colloid volume expansion is an established method of reducing maternal blood pressure and restoring tissue perfusion in pre-eclampsia. Experimental animal studies and randomised clinical trials are necessary to investigate further the role, if any, of maternal volume expansion in normotensive IUGR.

Antenatal Corticosteroids and Timed Delivery

In 1995, the National Institute of Child Health and Human Development (NICHD) convened a consensus conference promoting the use of antenatal corticosteroids to decrease the incidence of respiratory distress syndrome, necrotising entero-colitis, periventricular haemorrhage perinatal mortality. The vast majority of the data available pertain to women in preterm delivery with normally grown fetuses. However, recent data from the Vermont–Oxford Trials Network and the NICHD Neonatal Research Network indicate a beneficial effect of antenatal cortico-steroids to reduce the morbidity and mortality associated with SGA [90,91]. The consensus is that it is reasonable to administer steroids in this situation, especially if preterm delivery is planned.

Of concern with the use of corticosteroids especially involving cases of IUGR, is the effect on fetal heart rate variability and fetal behaviour [92,94]. The effect of antenatal corticosteroids to decrease the baseline fetal heart rate, heart rate variability and fetal movements lasted for approximately 48 hours after adminis-tration. As biophysical profile scoring and heart rate monitoring are the main-stay of fetal assessment, alterations in an already compromised IUGR fetus might push one's hand towards intervention (i.e. delivery). This needs to be taken into account when administering antenatal steroids to this "high risk" group.

Conclusions

It is obvious that there should be continued efforts at reducing the incidence of IUGR and its associated morbidity and mortality. Most efforts to date have failed in part because of the many aetiologies of IUGR, the intervention(s) for which will probably vary based on the aetiology. Preconception counselling and close antenatal follow-up are perhaps the best methods currently available to improve neonatal outcome though, the evidence that it can reduce the incidence of IUGR is poor. However, we can encourage the reduction of drug use (e.g. smoking) and improve maternal nutrition and general health. The cornerstone of management during pregnancy remains close fetal surveillance, a well-planned timely delivery (+/- antenatal corticosteroids) and close collaboration with the neonatologists.

References

1. Shah CP, Shah SS, Shah RR. Concepts, determinants and promotion of health. In: Anonymous public health and preventive medicine in Canada, 3rd edn. Toronto: University of Toronto Press, 1994:1–20.
2. Sayers S, Powers J. Risk factors for aboriginal low birthweight, intrauterine growth retardation and preterm birth in the Darwin Health Region. Aust N Z J Health 1997;21:524–30.
3. Scholl TO, Hediger ML. Weight gain, nutrition, and pregnancy outcome: findings from the Camden study of teenage and minority gravidas. Sem Perinatol 1995;19:171–81.
4. Petridou E, Trichopoulos D, Revinthi K, Tong D, Papathoma E. Modulation birthweight through gestational age and fetal growth. Child Care Health Dev 1997;22:37–53.
5. Piper JM, Mitchel EF, Ray WA. Evaluation of a program for prenatal care management. Family Planning Perspectives 1996;28:65–8.
6. Gulmezoglu M, de Onis M, Villar J. Effectiveness of interventions to prevent treat impaired fetal growth. Obstet Gynecol Surv 1997;52:139–49.
7. Stewart PJ, Nimrod C. The need for a community-wide approach to promote healthy babies and prevent low birthweight. Can Med Assoc J 1993;149:281–5.
8. Naeye RL. Probable cause of fetal growth retardation. Arch Pathol 1965;79:284–91.
9. Soothill PW, Nicolaides KH, Campbell S. Prenatal asphyxia, hyperlacticaemia, hypoglycaemia, and erythroblastosis in growth retarded fetuses. BMJ 1987;294:1051–3.
10. Cetin I, Marconi AM, Bozzetti P, Sereni LP, Corbetta C, Pardi G, et al. Umbilical amino acid concentrations in appropriate and small for gestational age infants: a biochemical difference present in utero. Am J Obstet Gynecol 1988;158:120–6.
11. Luke B. Nutritional influences on fetal growth. Clin Obstet Gynecol 1994;37:538–49.
12. Stein Z, Susser M. The Dutch Famine, 1944–1945, and the reproductive process. I. Effects on six indices at birth. Pediatr Res 1975;9:70–6.
13. Woodall SM, Breier BH, Johnston BM, Gluckman PD. A model of intrauterine growth retardation caused by chronic maternal undernutrition in the rat: Effects on the somatotrophic axis and postnatal growth. J Endocrinol 1996;150:231–42.
14. Owens JA, Falconer J, Robinson JS. Effect of restriction of placental growth on oxygen delivery to and consumption by the pregnant uterus and fetus. J Dev Physiol 1987;9:137–50.
15. Owens JA, Falconer J, Robinson JS. Effect of restriction of placental growth on fetal and uteroplacental metabolism. J Dev Physiol 1987;9:225–38.
16. de Jong CL, Gardosi J, Baldwin C, Francis A, Dekker GA, van Geijn HP. Fetal weight gain in a serially scanned high-risk pop4lation. Ultrasound Obstet Gynecol 1998;11:39–43.
17. Scholl TO, Hediger ML, Schall JI, Ances IG, Smith WK. Gestational weight gain, pregnancy outcome, and postpartum weight retention. Obstet Gynecol 1995;86:423–7.
18. Viteri FE, Schumacher L, Silliman K. Maternal malnutrition and the fetus. Sem Perinatol 1989;13:236–49.
19. Caan B, Horgen DM, Margen S, King JC, Jewell NP. Benefits associated with WIC supplemental feeding during the interpregnancy interval. Am J Clin Nutr 1987;45:29–41.

20. Chabra S, Bhandari V. Some medico-socio-demographic factors and intra-uterine growth retardation. J Indian Med Assoc 1996;94:127–30.
21. Wynn SW, Wynn AH, Doyle W, Crawford MA. The association of maternal social class with maternal diet and the dimensions of babies in a population of London women. Nutr Health 1994;9:303–15.
22. de Onis M, Villar J, Gulmezoglu M. Nutritional interventions to prevent intrauterine growth retardation: evidence from randomized controlled trials. Eur J Clin Nutr 1998;52:583–93.
23. Garg HK, Singhal KC, Arshad ZA. Study of the effect of oral zinc supplementation during pregnancy on pregnancy outcome. Indian J Physiol Pharmacol 1999;37:276–84.
24. Charlton V, Rudolph AM. Digestion and absorption of carbohydrates by the fetal lamb in utero. Pediatr Res 1979;13:1018–23.
25. Mulvihill SJ, Albert A, Synn A, Fonkalsrud EW. In utero supplemental fetal feedings in an animal model: Effects on fetal growth and development. Surgery 1985;98:500–5.
26. Buchmiller TL, Kim CS, Chopourian L, Fonkalsrud EW. Transamniotic fetal feeding: Enhancement of growth in a rabbit model of intrauterine growth retardation. Surgery 1994;116:36–41.
27. Flake AW, Villa-Troyer RL, Adzick NS, Harrison MR. Transamniotic fetal feeding. II. The effect of nutrient infusion on fetal growth retardation. J Pediatr Surg 1986;21:481–4.
28. Charlton V, Johengen M. Fetal intravenous nutritional supplementation ameliorates the development of embolization-induced growth retardation in sheep. Pediatr Res 1987;22:55–61.
29. Mesaki N, Kubo T, Iwasaki H. A study of the treatment for intrauterine growth retardation. Acta Obst Gynaec Jpn 1980;32:879–85.
30. Beischer NA. Treatment of fetal growth retardation. Aust NZ J Obstet Gynaecol 1978;18:28–33.
31. Mellor DJ, Murray J. Effects on the rate of increase in fetal girth of refeeding ewes after short periods of severe undernutrition during late pregnancy. Res Vet Sci 1982;32:377–82.
32. Harding JE, Owens JA, Robinson JS. Should we try to supplement the growth retarded fetus? A cautionary tale. Br J Obstet Gynaecol 1992;99:707–10.
33. Benny PS, Legge M, Aickin DR. The biochemical effects of maternal hyperalimentation during pregnancy. NZ Med J 1978;88:283–5.
34. Charlton V, Johengen M. Intraamniotic administration of nutrients. Pediatr Res 1984;18:136A
35. Lawrence GF, Brown VA, Parsons RJ, Cooke ID. Fetomaternal consequences of high-dose glucose infusion during labour. Br J Obstet Gynaecol 1982;89:27–32.
36. Phillips AF, Porte PJ, Stabinski S, Rosenkrantz TS, Raye JR. Effects of chronic fetal hyperglycemia upon oxygen consumption in the ovine uterus and conceptus. J Clin Invest 1984;74:279–86.
37. Nicolini U, Hubinont C, Santolaya J, Fisk NM, Rodeck CH. Effects of fetal intravenous glucose challenge in normal and growth retarded fetuses. Horm Metab Res 1990;22:426–30.
38. Alexander GR, Korenbrot CC. The role of prenatal care in preventing low birth weight. Future Child 1995;5:103–20.
39. Conter V, Cortinovis I, Rogari P, Riva L. Weight growth in infants born to mothers who smoked during pregnancy. BMJ 1995;310:768–71.
40. Mills JL, Holmes LB, Aarons JH, Simpson JL, Brown ZA, Jovanovic-Peterson LG, et al. Moderate caffeine use and the risk of spontaneous abortion and intrauterine growth retardation. JAMA 1993;269:593–7.
41. Coles CD, Smith I, Fernhoff PM, Falek A. Neonatal neurobehavioral characteristics as correlates of maternal alcohol use during gestation. Alcohol Clin Exp Res 1985;9:454–60.
42. Rosett HL, Weiner L, Zuckerman B, McKinlay S, Edelin KC. Reduction of alcohol consumption during pregnancy with benefits to the newborn. Alcohol Clin Exp Res 1980;4:178–84.
43. Bergsjo P, Villar J. Scientific basis for the content of routine antenatal care II. Power to eliminate or alleviate adverse newborn outcomes; some special conditions and examinations. Acta Obstet Gynecol Scand 1997;76:15–25.
44. Laurin J, Persson P-H. The effect of bedrest in hospital on fetal outcome in pregnancies complicated by intra-uterine growth retardation. Acta Obstet Gynecol Scand 1987;66:407–11.
45. Cabero L, Cerqueira MJ, del Solar J, Bellart J, Esteban-Altirriba J. Long-term hospitalization and b-mimetic therapy in the treatment of intrauterine growth retardation of unknown etiology. J Perinat Med 1988;16:453–8.
46. Wang Z, Li W. A prospective randomized placebo-controlled trial of low-dose aspirin for prevention of intra-uterine growth retardation. Chin Med J (Engl) 1996;109:238–42.
47. Bremer HA, Wallenburg HC. Low-dose aspirin in pregnancy: changes in patterns of prescription in The Netherlands. Eur J Obstet Gynecol Reprod Biol 1993;52:29–33.

48. ECPPA (Estudo Colaborativo para Prevencao da Pre-eclampsia com Aspirina) Collaborative Group. ECPPA: randomized trial of low dose aspirin for the prevention of maternal and fetal complications in high risk pregnant women. Br J Obstet Gynaecol 1996;103:39–47.

49. CLASP Collaborative Group. CLASP: a randomized trial of low-dose aspirin for the prevention and treatment of pre-eclampsia among 9364 pregnant women. Lancet 1994;343:619–29.

50. Hauth JC, Goldenberg RL, Parker CR Jr, Cutter GR, Cliver SP. Low-dose aspirin: lack of association with an increase in abruptio placentae or perinatal mortality. Obstet Gynecol 1999;85:1055–8.

51. Caritis SN, Sibai B, Hauth JC, Lindheimer MD, Klebanoff M, Thom E, et al. Low-dose aspirin to prevent preeclampsia in women at high risk. N Engl J Med 1998;338:701–5.

52. Arduini D, Rizzo G, Romanini C, Mancuso S. Hemodynamic changes in growth retarded fetuses during maternal oxygen administration as predictors of fetal outcome. J Ultrasound Med 1989;193–6.

53. Vileisis RA. Effect of maternal oxygen inhalation on the fetus with growth retardation. Pediatr Res 1985;19:324–7.

54. Nicolaides KH, Bradley RJ, Soothill PW, Campbell S, Bilardo CM, Gibb D. Maternal oxygen therapy for intrauterine growth retardation. Lancet 1987;1:942–5.

55. Battaglia FC, Artini PG, D'Ambrogio G, Galli PA, Segre A, Genazzani AR. Maternal hyperoxygenation in the treatment of intrauterine growth retardation. Am J Obstet Gynecol 1992;167:430–5.

56. Bernstein IM, DeSouza MM, Copeland KC. Insulin-like growth factor-I in substrate deprived growth retarded fetal rats. Pediatr Res 1991;30:154–7.

57. Kind KL, Owens JA, Robinson JS. Effect of restriction of placental growth on expression of IGFs in fetal sheep: Relationship of fetal growth, circulating IGFs, and binding proteins. J Endocrinol 1995;146:23–34.

58. Nieto-Diaz A, Villar J, Matorras-Weinig R, Valenzuela-Ruiz P. Intrauterine growth retardation at term: Association between anthropomorphic and endocrine parameters. Acta Obstet Gynecol Scand 1995;75:127–31.

59. Giudice LC, de Zegher F, Gargofsky SE. Insulin-like growth factors and their binding proteins in the term and preterm human fetus and neonate with normal and extremes of intrauterine growth. J Clin Endocrinol Metab 1995; 80:1548–55.

60. Roback EW, Barakat AJ, Dev VG, Mbikay M, Chretien M, Butler MG. An infant with deletion of the distal long arm of chromosome 15 (q26.1—-qter) and loss of insulin-like growth factor 1 receptor gene. Am J Med Genet 1991;38:74–9.

61. Woods KA, Camacho-Hubner C, Savage MO, Clark AJ. Intrauterine growth retardation and post-natal growth failure associated with deletion of the insulin-like growth factor I gene. N Engl J Med 1996;335:1363–73.

62. Unterman TG, Simmons RA, Glick RP, Ogata ES. Circulating levels of insulin, insulin-like growth factor-I (IGF-1), IGF-2, and IGF-binding proteins in the small for gestational age fetal rat. Endocrinology 1993;132:327–36.

63. Langford K, Blum W, Nicolaides K, Jones J, McGregor A, Miell J. The pathophysiology of the insulin-like growth factor axis in fetal growth failure: A basis for programming by under-nutrition. Eur J Clin Invest 1994;24:851–6.

64. Harding JE, Liu L, Evans JA, Gluckman PD. IGF-1 alters feto-placental protein and carbohydrate metabolism in fetal sheep. Endocrinology 1994; 134:1509–15.

65. Liu L, Harding JE, Evans JA, Gluckman PD. Maternal insulin-like growth factor-1 infusion alters fetoplacental carbohydrate and protein metabolism in pregnant sheep. Endocrinol 1994;135:890–5.

66. Gluckman PD, Harding JE. The physiology and pathophysiology of intrauterine growth retardation. Horm Res 1997;48(suppl 1):11–16.

67. Krebs C, Macara LM, Leiser R, Bowman AW, Greer IA, Kingdom JCP. Intrauterine growth restriction with absent end-diastolic flow velocity in the umbilical artery is associated with maldevelopment of the placental terminal villous tree. Am J Obstet Gynecol 1996;175:1534–42.

68. Kingdom JCP, Kaufmann P. Oxygen and placental villous development: Origins of fetal hypoxia. Placenta 1997;18:613–21.

69. Ahmed A, Kilby MD. Hypoxia or hyperoxia in placental insufficiency? Lancet 1997;350:826–7.

70. Smith GN, Bobier HS, Brien JF. The role of nitric oxide in the maintenance of normal pregnancy and preeclampsia. In: Lee RV, Garner PR, Barron WM, Coustan DR, editors. Current Obstetric Medicine. Toronto: Mosby-Year Book, 1996;103–27.

71. Smith GN, Brien JF. The use of nitroglycerin for uterine relaxation. Obstet Gynecol Surv 1998;53:559–5.

72. Molnar M, Suto T, Toth T, Hertelendy F. Prolonged blockade of nitric oxide synthesis in gravid rats produces sustained hypertension, proteinuria, thrombocytopenia, and intrauterine growth retardation. Am J Obstet Gynecol 1994;170:1458–66.

73. Diket AL, Pierce MR, Munshi UK. Nitric oxide inhibition causes intrauterine growth retardation and hind- limb disruptions in rats. Am J Obstet Gynecol 1994;1243–50.

74. Helmbrecht GD, Farhat MY, Lochbaum L, Brown HE, Yadgarova KT, Eglinton GS, et al. L-Arginine reverses the adverse pregnancy changes induced by nitric oxide synthase inhibition in the rat. Am J Obstet Gynecol 1996;175:800–5.

75. Vosatka RJ, Hassoun PM, Harvey-Wilkes KB. Dietary L-arginine prevents fetal growth restriction in rats. Am J Obstet Gynecol 1999;178:242–6.

76. Myatt L, Eis AL, Brockman DE, Greer IA, Lyall F. Endothelial nitric oxide synthase in placental villous tissue from normal, pre-eclamptic and intrauterine growth restricted pregnancies. Human Reprod 1999;12:167–72.

77. Ramsay B, De Belder A, Campbell S, Moncada S, Martin JF. A nitric oxide donor improves uterine artery diastolic blood flow in normal early pregnancy and in women at high risk of pre-eclampsia. Eur J Clin Invest 1994;24:76–8.

78. Poston L. Nitrovasodilators – will they be useful in lowering uterine artery resistance in pre-eclampsia and intrauterine growth restriction? Ultrasound Obstet Gynecol 1998;11:92–3.

79. Kingdom J. Adriana and Luisa Castellucci Award Lecture 1997: Placental pathology in obstetrics: Adaptation or failure of the villous tree? Placenta 1998;19:1–5.

80. Thaler I, Amit A, Jakobi P, Itskovitz-Eldor J. The effect of isosorbide dinitrate on uterine artery and umbilical artery flow velocity waveforms at mid-pregnancy. Obstet Gynecol 1996;88:838–43.

81. Grunewald C, Kublickas C, Carlstrom K, Lunell N-O, Nisell H. Effects of nitroglycerin on the uterine and umbilical circulation in severe preeclampsia. Obstet Gynecol 1995;86:600–4.

82. Giles W O'Callaghan S, Boura A, Walters W. Reduction in human fetal umbilical–placental vascular resistance by glyceryl trinitrate. Lancet 1992; 340:856.

83. Cacciatore B, Halmesmaki E, Kaaja R, Teramo K, Ylikorkala 0. Transdermal nitroglycerin administration reduces uterine artery impedance in pregnancies with preeclampsia and IUGR. Hypertension in Pregnancy 1997;16:92 (abst).

84. Shimonovitz S, Yagel S, Zacut D, Ben Chetrit A, Hochner Celnikier D, Ron M. Intermittent abdominal decompression: An option for prevention of intrauterine growth retardation. Br J Obstet Gynaecol 1992;99:693–5.

85. Hofmeyr GF, Metrikin DC, Williamson I. Abdominal decompression: new data from a previous study. Br J Obstet Gynaecol 1990;97:547–8.

86. Duvekot JJ, Cheriex EC, Pieters FA, Peeters LL. Severely impaired fetal growth is preceded by maternal hemodynamic maladaptation in very early pregnancy. Acta Obstet Gynecol Scand 1995; 74:693–7.

87. Duvekot JJ, Cheriex EC, Pieters FA, Menheere PP, Schouten HJ, Peeters LL. Maternal volume homeostasis in early pregnancy in relation to fetal growth restriction. Obstet Gynecol 1995;85:361–7.

88. Schobel HP, Fischer T, Heuszer K, Geiger H, Schmieder RE. Preeclampsia – a state of sympathetic overactivity. N Engl J Med 1996;335:1480–5.

89. Karsdorp VH, van Vugt JM, Dekker GA, van Geijn HP. Reappearance of end-diastolic velocities in the umbilical artery following maternal volume expansion: a preliminary study. Obstet Gynecol 1992;80:679–83.

90. Wright LL, Verter J, Younes N, Stevenson D, Fanaroff AA, Shankaran S, et al. Antenatal corticosteroid administration and neonatal outcome in very low birth weight infants: The NICHD Neonatal Research Network. Am J Obstet Gynecol 1995;175:269–74.

91. Horbar JD, Vermont Oxford Network. Antenatal corticosteroid treatment and neonatal outcomes for infants 501 to 1500 gm in the Vermont–Oxford Trials Network. Am J Obstet Gynecol 1995;173:275–81.

92. Henson G. Antenatal corticosteroids and heart rate variability. Br J Obstet Gynaecol 1997;104:1219-20.

93. Magee LA, Dawes GS, Moulden M, Redman CWG. A randomised controlled comparison of betamethasone with dexamethasone: effects on the antenatal fetal heart rate. Br J Obstet Gynaecol 1997;104:l233–8.

94. Mulder EJH, Derks JB, Visser GHA. Antenatal corticosteroid therapy and fetal behaviour: a randomised study of the effects of betamethasone and dexamethasone. Br J Obstet Gynaecol 1997;104:1239–4.

17 Management of Antepartum Fetal Death

Jeremy Chipchase and Donald M. Peebles

Introduction

The death of a fetus in utero is a tragic event irrespective of gestation. The importance of appropriate psychological support for the parents at such a time is well recognised and has been reviewed recently [1]. This chapter will focus on the clinical management of antepartum fetal death from 20 weeks gestation with particular reference to IUGR.

Fetal death occurring in utero is a problem with which most clinicians have to deal regularly. The late fetal loss rate (number of fetal deaths between 20 and 23 weeks + 6 days' gestation or with a birthweight of less than 500g/total number births, including live births, stillbirths and late fetal losses) for the UK was 2.29 per 1,000 in 1995 [2]. The stillbirth rate (fetal loss after 24 weeks' gestation/total number of live births and stillbirths) was 5.48 per 1,000. Both late fetal loss and stillbirth rates have demonstrated a slight upward trend within the 3 years of operation of the rapid reporting system. It is however difficult to derive from these statistics either the number of fetuses that were growth restricted or the contribution of growth restriction to the cause of death, as neither the Extended Wigglesworth nor the Obstetric classification system (shown in Table 17.1) used by the Confidential enquiries into stillbirth and deaths in infancy DoH report (CESDI) includes a specific category for IUGR. Using the

Table 17.1 The Extended Wigglesworth and Obstetric Classifications

Extended Wigglesworth classification	Obstetric classification
congenital defect/malformation	congenital abnormality
unexplained antepartum fetal death	isoimmunisation
death from intrapartum asphyxia, trauma	pre-eclampsia
immaturity	antepartum haemorrhage
infection	mechanical including cord prolapse, breech, etc.
other specific causes:	maternal conditions e.g. hypertension
fetal conditions e.g. hydrops	miscellaneous:
neonatal	specific fetal conditions
paediatric	neonatal condition
due to accident or non-intrapartum trauma	unexplained < or > 2.5 kg
sudden infant death	unclassifiable
unclassifiable	

Wigglesworth classification the largest group were unexplained antepartum still-births (3.8 per 1,000) of which the majority weighed less than 2.5 kg. If postnatal weight is plotted on an ultrasound derived chart of estimated weight for gestation such as that described by Hadlock et al. [3], rather than neonatal charts, over 50 per cent of unexplained stillbirths are shown to be below the 10th per-centile [4], suggesting that a substantial number of this group may be growth restricted. However, as the majority of fetal deaths occur in unmonitored preg-nancies, many stillbirths will not meet the following definition of IUGR used by CESDI: "an ultrasound derived diagnosis of a weight < 10th percentile as esti-mated by serial measurement of the abdominal circumference, occasionally by clinical impression alone" [5].

Despite these problems with classification CESDI makes some important points about the management of fetuses with IUGR. In some cases ultrasound was not used to corroborate a clinical impression of fetal growth restriction. In other cases with clear risk factors for IUGR there was no planned protocol for regular or even single ultrasound examination measurements. Even when ultrasound was used, and a small fetus detected, appropriate action was not always taken. Reviewers also commented on the inappropriateness of isolated biparietal diameter measurement for assessment of fetal growth, the need to plot measurements based on an accurate estimate of gestation, and the use of appropriate levels of surveillance, even when results appear to return to normal in a high risk pregnancy.

Obstetric Management

Diagnosis of Antepartum Fetal Death

In a small number of cases, fetal death will have been anticipated as a result of previous monitoring and the parents counselled about this possibility. High mor-tality rates and incidence of severe neurological handicap in survivors of preg-nancies with evidence of early onset (< 32 weeks) severe IUGR and absent end-diastolic flow in the umbilical artery [6,7] mean that, in some cases, con-servative obstetric management with the expectancy of fetal demise in utero may be appropriate [8]. In this situation suitable investigations and counselling will be performed before fetal death occurs and the shock normally associated with this event diminished.

The majority of antepartum fetal deaths are unexpected, occurring in appar-ently normal pregnancies. Presentation will be in a variety of ways: maternal per-ception of a cessation of fetal movements, absence of fetal cardiac activity at a routine antenatal check or more rarely with clinical signs of placental abruption or disseminated intravascular coagulation (DIC). The mainstay of diagnosis is ultrasound. If fetal death in utero is suspected the initial ultrasound examination should be performed by a clinician experienced in ultrasonography and of sufficient seniority to inform the parents of the result. Sonographic features of fetal death are absence of fetal movements, no evidence of cardiac activity on a four-chamber view and absence of blood flow in the heart, aorta and umbilical artery using colour Doppler. Other findings include a clot or gas in the fetal heart or umbilical vessels, fetal maceration and deformity and dilated loops of fetal bowel [9]. The presence of Spalding's sign (overlapping skull sutures), originally defined radiographically but easily detected by ultrasound, suggests that fetal death was not a recent event. Documentation of oligohydramnios is useful as this cannot be demonstrated postnatally. Although, using these criteria, the diagnosis of fetal death can be made with confidence, many parents will wish to have a second ultrasound examination to confirm the findings; this is an important part of coming to terms with this traumatic event and should not be denied.

Timing of Delivery

The interval between the diagnosis of an antepartum fetal death and delivery is determined by several factors, the most important of which is parental choice. Obviously it is a period of great distress for the parents and some will decide to get the fetus delivered as quickly as possible; it is, however, important, in the absence of rare medical indications such as abruption or DIC, not to impose any element of haste. In a study of 69 women with an intrauterine fetal death [10] just over 50 per cent chose to wait for spontaneous delivery compared with immediate induction. If mifepristone is used to prime the uterus before induction of labour with prostaglandins a 48 hour delay is necessary for optimal therapeutic effect. The complications of retaining the fetus are described below.

Complications of Fetal Death

The potential medical complications of retaining a dead fetus in utero are infection and DIC. It is rare, however, for chorioamnionitis to occur in the absence of ruptured membranes. Conversely, if the membranes are ruptured delivery should be expedited.

In 1950 Weiner et al. [11] described the development of coagulation system changes in immunised Rhesus-negative women carrying a dead fetus. Subsequently the presence of the dead fetus was identified as the cause of the coagulopathy [12]. The course of DIC associated with antepartum fetal death tends to be chronic and is not normally manifest until the fetus has been dead in utero for more than 4 weeks [13,14]. At this stage the continuing presence of the fetus leads to tissue factor release, explosive production of thrombin and uncontrolled conversion of fibrinogen to fibrin. At first the mother can compensate for the fall in fibrinogen concentration, which often levels off at about 1 g/l. This steady state can persist for several days [15,16]. However, decompensation with severe coagulopathy eventually occurs unless the uterus is evacuated. Data on the incidence of this severe complication of antepartum fetal death are scanty, presumably because in the majority of cases the fetus is delivered within a 4 week period.

The diagnosis of DIC is essentially a clinical one with laboratory tests providing confirmatory evidence. Thrombocytopenia occurs with associated prolongation of the prothrombin time and activated partial thromboplastin time with low fibrinogen concentrations and elevated levels of fibrin and fibrinogen degradation product [17-20].

Treatment is by removal of the fetus and placenta, which usually results in rapid resolution of the condition. Monitoring of the haematological indices will guide management postdelivery and decisions regarding replacement of platelets and coagulation factors can be made with the haematologist. Heparin can restore fibrinogen concentrations, although the indications for giving heparin are not well established [21].

Induction of Labour

Induction of labour for fetal death in utero differs from induction for other indications in that it occurs over a wider range of gestational age and fetal well-being is not an issue. The principal aims of induction are therefore to achieve a short induction to delivery time with minimal maternal side effects. The performance of available methods is reviewed below.

The introduction of prostaglandins in the 1970s has superseded the use of intra-amniotic instillation of hypertonic solutions such as saline, glucose and urea for induction of labour. Only 20 per cent of patients will abort within 24 hours when hypertonic saline is used [22] and maternal deaths have been recorded with both hypertonic saline [23] and glucose [24]. However, some still advocate extra-amniotic saline infusion as a cost-effective method in countries where the newer prostaglandin analogues are not available [25].

Prostaglandins

Natural prostaglandins and their analogues have been administered by a variety of routes for the induction of labour including intra- and extra-amniotic infusion, intramuscular and intravenous injection and vaginally, using tablets, pessaries or gel. The extra-amniotic approach was the principal method for terminating pregnancies in the second trimester, although it has a high rate of side-effects, including vomiting in 45 per cent and diarrhoea in 17 per cent of women [26]. As a result the procedure lost popularity in favour of vaginally administered prostaglandin analogues. Sakamoto et al. [27] were the first to report the use of gemeprost, a PGE_1 analogue in pessary form, with a mean induction to abortion time of 16 hours. These findings were later confirmed in a review of over 900 second trimester abortions [28].

Mifepristone

The next major advance in the management of labour induction for fetal death was the introduction of mifepristone (RU486). Mifepristone is a 19 nor-steroid with an affinity for the human progesterone receptor three times greater than that of progesterone. Administration of mifepristone sensitises the myometrium prior to the use of prostaglandins and has been shown to reduce the induction to abortion interval and the total prostaglandin dose required to achieve abortion; 200 mg of mifepristone administered 24 hours prior to extra-amniotic administration of PGE_2 significantly reduced both the induction to abortion time and total dose of PGE_2 compared with [29]. Roger and Baird [30] randomly allocated patients to receive either 600 mg of mifepristone or placebo prior to administration of 1.0 mg of cervagem every third hour. In mifepristone-pretreated group, 94 per cent of the patients aborted within 24 hours compared with 80 per cent of the placebo group. The mean induction to abortion interval was reduced significantly, from 15.8 hours to 6.8 hours. The women pretreated with mifepristone also reported significantly less pain than the women who received placebo. Therefore the use of mifepristone in combination with a prostaglandin analogue has evolved as the method of choice to terminate the pregnancy during the second trimester.

Misoprostol

Although very effective in combination with mifepristone, several features of gemeprost, such as the need for repeated vaginal examinations, the short shelf-life if not adequately refrigerated and its cost, prompted the search for new prostaglandin analogues. Misoprostol is an orally active prostaglandin E_1 analogue that was first developed as a treatment for gastric ulcers. The first report, published in 1991, that examined the use of misoprostol in combination with mifepristone for induction of abortion showed a success rate close to 95 per cent with minimal side-effects [31].

El Refaey et al. [32] further demonstrated its practical value by randomising 60 patients at 13 to 20 weeks' gestation, pretreated with mifepristone, to either oral misoprostol with vaginal gemeprost or gemeprost alone. There were no significant differences in outcome measures. In 77 per cent of patients, use of misoprostol alone was sufficient to induce abortion. Only five out of 60 patients had a retained placenta, which compares favourably with the 53 per cent reported by Rogers and Baird with mifepristone and gemeprost. No patients had to discontinue misoprostol because of side-effects.

The combination of vaginal and oral misoprostol was assessed in 70 patients who were randomised to either vaginal misoprostol (600 μg then 400 μg 3 hourly) or one 600 μg vaginal dose followed by 3 hourly oral 400 μg doses [33]. No significant differences were found between the two groups in terms of outcome measures. The mean induction abortion time for the study population was 6.4 hours with total misoprostol doses up to 2200 μg, and 97 per cent aborted within 14 hours. These results are comparable to regimens using mifepristone and gemeprost where approximately 95 per cent of patients abort within 24 hours [30]. Retained placenta occurred in six patients, the only other side-effect being mild gastrointestinal symptoms that did not require discontinuation of the regimen. Single doses of 800 μg of misoprostol given vaginally have also been successful in 94 per cent of patients with a mean induction interval of 14 hours [34]. Table 17.2 shows a safe, effective and non-invasive regimen for induction of labour in the second trimester based on the above research.

Table 17.2 A regimen for the induction of labour with antepartum fetal death in the second trimester

1. Administer mifepristone (RU486) 600 mg orally.
2. Readmission 36–48 hours later.
3. Misoprostol 800 μg administered vaginally.
4. Three hours later give oral misoprostol 400 μg (two tablets). The oral dose should be repeated at 3 hourly intervals to a maximum of four oral doses.
5. If this course is unsuccessful give 600 μg of mifepristone with the last misoprostol dose and repeat the misoprostol regimen as above, starting the following morning beginning with 800 μg vaginal dose.
6. In cases of intrauterine death patients may not want to wait 36 hours before starting misoprostol. In these cases it is advisable to give mifepristone 600 mg and defer the misoprostol until the following day.

   A 12 hour mifepristone–misoprostol treatment interval is recommended. If a patient refuses to wait she should still receive the mifepristone with the rst misoprostol dose.

   If mifepristone is not available the misoprostol component could be followed without prior treatment with mifepristone.

While most studies have investigated the role of misoprostol in termination of pregnancy during the second trimester there is evidence that it can be used safely in doses of 50 μg, given vaginally to induce labour in the third trimester [35].

Caesarean Section

There are relatively few absolute indications for CS in the presence of a dead fetus. These include a major degree of placenta praevia, previous classical CS, two or more previous CS and uterine rupture. With CS becoming increasingly safe for the mother [36] and experience of destructive fetal procedures such as craniotomy declining, the management of impacted transverse lie is much more likely to be by CS. Perhaps cleidotomy (division of the fetal clavicles) to achieve delivery in the presence of shoulder dystocia is the only destructive procedure to retain a place in current obstetric practice.

Twin Intrauterine Death

Intrauterine death in twin pregnancies can occur at any gestation. Before 20 weeks the vanishing twin syndrome and fetal papyraceous may occur. The prevalence of fetal death in the late second and third trimester is generally quoted as 0.5–6.8 per cent of all twin pregnancies [37]. Contributing factors are an increased rate of intrauterine growth restriction of one or both twins, twin-to-twin transfusion syndrome, velamentous insertion of the cord, true cord knot, congenital anomaly and pre-eclampsia [38].

Although constituting only 20 per cent of twin pregnancies, 50–70 per cent of IUDs will occur in monochorionic twins with twin to twin transfusion syndrome being the main aetiological factor [38]. The presence of a shared circulation makes death of one monochorionic twin particularly hazardous for the survivor [39]. Acute haemodynamic imbalance around the time of death can lead to cerebral hypoperfusion and subsequent severe neurological handicap in between 15 and 36 per cent of the survivors of twin to twin transfusion syndrome [40,41]. As this is most likely to occur at the time of death, delivery of the surviving twin is unlikely to change the outcome. The survivor should, however, be monitored in utero to look for ultrasonographic markers of brain injury, such as the development of porencephalic cysts. Neonatal evaluation of the survivor should include high resolution ultrasonography, computerised tomography (CT) and renal function studies.

The main hazard following death of one dichorionic twin in utero is pre-term delivery, as labour will occur within 3 weeks of the diagnosis in approximately 90 per cent of cases [42]. Expectant management is appropriate if death occurs before 37 weeks' gestation with serial coagulation studies, ultrasound and Doppler evaluation.

Investigations

The importance of appropriate investigation of the factors that lead to fetal growth restriction and death in utero cannot be overstated, both to classify correctly the cause of death but also to give a prognosis for and plan treatment in a

Table 17.3 A list of relevant investigations after death of a growth-restricted fetus in utero

full blood count	thyroid function tests
glycosylated haemoglobin	blood group and antibodies
random blood glucose	Kleihauer test
congenital infection screen toxoplasmosis, rubella, parvovirus and CMV)	thrombophilia screen (including APA)
urea and electrolytes	karyotype of placenta and fetus
urates	postmortem
liver function tests	

future pregnancy. For instance, treatment of women in whom an hereditary thrombophilia has been identified has been shown to improve pregnancy outcome [43]. Each unit should have a checklist to ensure that all the appropriate tests are performed and one member of staff should be identified as the person responsible for arranging the investigations and checking the results. Table 17.3 lists the appropriate investigations. The rationale for and optimal timing of some of these tests is detailed below.

Many cases of fetal growth restriction will share a common pathology with and present in women with pre-eclampsia [44]. Careful investigation for clinical, haematological and biochemical evidence of a pre-eclamptic process is therefore indicated. Maternal serum can be compared with serum taken at booking to detect changing antibody titres or development of IgM antibodies suggesting recent infection with rubella, CMV, parvovirus or toxoplasmosis. It is estimated that congenital infection is the cause of between 0.3 and 3.5 per cent cases of growth restriction [45,46]. Gestational diabetes is more likely to present with macrosomia than growth restriction but should be screened for with a measurement of glycosylated haemoglobin levels. If there are clinical or pathological features suggesting glucose intolerance then a glucose tolerance test should be performed in a future pregnancy.

Thrombophilia Screening

The association between APA and the components of the antiphospholipid syndrome, thrombosis, thrombocytopenia and recurrent pregnancy loss are well known. More recently both anticardiolipin and lupus anticoagulant antibodies have been shown to be strongly related to the risk of developing both IUGR and pre-eclampsia [47,48]. There is also an increased prevalence of IgG anticardiolipin antibodies in women with a third trimester fetal death [49]. Additionally, a whole range of inherited thrombophilias have been implicated in the aetiology of severe early onset pre-eclampsia [50] and intrauterine fetal death [43]. Activated protein C resistance due to heterozygosity for the factor V Leiden mutation leads to a twofold increase in the OR for stillbirth compared with controls [51] whilst protein C, S and antithrombin-III deficiency also carry an increased risk of intrauterine fetal death [51,52]. The relationship between IUGR and thrombophilia is discussed further in Ch. X.

A full thrombophilia screen is recommended in patients where there has been early onset severe growth restriction, pre-eclampsia or unexplained fetal loss. Such a screen should include a coagulation screen (activated partial thromboplastin time, prothrombin time and thrombin time), functional assays of "natural anticoagulants" (antithrombin III, protein C and protein S), a test for lupus anticoagulant and quantification of anticardiolipin antibodies [53]. In addition the point mutation responsible for factor V Leiden can be detected [54]. It is recommended that thrombophilia screening is performed at least 6 weeks' postpartum as pregnancy alters the concentrations of haemostatic factors, with increases in many procoagulants and the anticoagulant protein C, and decreasing levels of protein S.

Cytogenetics

Chromosomal analysis is indicated if the fetus is dysmorphic or growth restricted, as approximately 2 per cent of IUGR fetuses are aneuploid [45]. If the fetus has not already been karyotyped in utero a postmortem sample will have to be sent. The "UK Collaborative Study on solid tissue culture in clinical cytogenetics" reported a culture success rate of only 16 per cent using skin samples from intrauterine deaths [55]. By contrast the success rates using placental or villous specimens were 67 and 79 per cent respectively. Interestingly, tissue from pregnancies terminated with prostaglandins in the second trimester have a successful culture rate of only 50 per cent. The mechanism for this is unknown.

To optimise the chances of successful culture the following samples should be sent: a biopsy from muscle or fascia lata, a skin sample, a placental biopsy, and cardiac or cord blood. Biopsies should be sent in transport medium and blood in a lithium–heparin tube. If the fetus is severely macerated, it can be sent to the histopathologists in saline to obtain a ribcage or ovary for cytogenetic assessment. Before 24 weeks, the whole fetus and placenta can be sent in a dry sterile container, prior to postmortem.

Postmortem

An autopsy can contribute to diagnosis of the cause of antepartum fetal death in three ways: by confirming the diagnosis made antepartum, by identifying unexpected disorders and by excluding other conditions that may have been contributory. One recent audit showed that perinatal autopsy provided new diagnostic information in 28 per cent of cases, confirmed the diagnosis in 43 per cent and provided useful negative information (excluding other possible causes of death) in 15 per cent [56]. The Wigglesworth classification of death was altered after postmortem in 20 per cent cases, mostly as the result of identification or exclusion of infection or congenital anomaly. Despite increasingly sophisticated ultrasound technology, there remains a discrepancy of about 25 per cent between the findings from antenatal fetal ultrasound and postnatal autopsy [57]. These findings are in line with those from other regional audits and provide the basis for a recommendation by a joint working party of the Royal College of Pathologists and Royal College of Obstetricians and Gynaecologists that a perinatal autopsy should be performed in at least 75 per cent of cases [58].

Postmortem assessment should therefore always be offered, even when the cause of death is known, and the benefits, particularly with regard to the prognosis for future pregnancies, explained. However, whilst all parents should have the option of an autopsy they should not feel under pressure to do so. A limited autopsy, where only specified parts of the baby are examined, or even a detailed external examination combined with radiography, may be more acceptable.

Guidelines for performing a perinatal autopsy, recommended by CESDI, have been approved by the Royal College of Pathologists [59]. Fetuses should be weighed, measured and X-rayed. Photographs and additional X-rays should be taken if there are signs of dysmorphism. An internal examination should be performed on the body cavities and all major organs should be weighed. A systematic description of all major organs, should be performed. Histological sections of at least one block of the major organs, especially lung, liver, kidney and placenta, should be undertaken. However, it is stressed that these are minimum guidelines and clinical judgement should be used to conduct specialist investigations as indicated by the case or family history.

There is an argument for postmortems to be performed by a specialist perinatal–paediatric pathologist. Rushton [60] found that 44 per cent of examinations by general histopathologists in the West Midlands region (UK) were substandard, whilst Thornton showed that 95 per cent "substandard" postmortems were performed by a general histopathologist, as compared with "good" postmortems where 60 per cent were carried out by a specialist perinatal pathologist [55]. The quality of information is improved if the pathologist is provided with a comprehensive description of the clinical scenario and specific questions are raised.

Placental Pathology

As described in previous chapters, problems at the placental maternofetal interface underlie many cases of fetal growth restriction. Placental pathology should, therefore, be sought in all cases of antepartum fetal death. Worryingly, a recent study showed that placental histology was not available in 30 per cent of stillbirths and 75 per cent of neonatal deaths [61]. This highlights the need to have clear unit policies on retaining the placenta for at least a month in all cases where the infant goes to the special care unit, and routinely studying placental histology in all stillbirths.

The four major patterns of placental abnormality described in association with fetal growth restriction by Fox [62] suggest the histological and karyotypic features that should be sought at routine examination.

1. Abnormal placentation with subsequent restriction of maternal blood flow to the placenta can occur as a result of failure of the normal transformation of maternal spiral arteries into low resistance vessels. Many of the histological sequelae, such as the presence of intraluminal EVT, atherosclerotic changes and thrombosis, are better detected in placental bed biopsies than sections of the basal plate obtained at routine histology. Information about the uteroplacental circulation is therefore restricted outside a research protocol. However, placental infarctions, which are areas of localised ischaemic villous necrosis secondary to lesions in the maternal uteroplacental blood supply, can be detected macroscopically on routine histology. As the placenta has a large functional reserve capacity, infarcts occupying less than 10 per cent of the parenchyma are probably insignificant. The only gross lesions of the placenta that are linked to defective growth are the rare large isolated or multiple placental haemangiomata [63].
2. The presence of an intravillous inflammatory infiltrate, or villitis, of unknown aetiology is significantly associated with both IUGR and pre-eclampsia [64].

3. Restricted placental mosaicism is considered by some to be associated with a high incidence of IUGR [65], although this is not always the case [66]. Sending both fetal and placental samples for cytogenetic analysis will detect this abnormality.
4. Defective villous vascularisation as a cause of abnormal Doppler waveforms in the fetal umbilical arteries was first by described by Giles et al. [67], who found widespread obliteration of small muscular arteries in the tertiary stem villi. Subsequent authors have reported a range of abnormalities of villous development associated with fetal growth restriction including a reduction in the density of gas-exchanging terminal villi [68] and abnormal villous morphology [69].

The fact that some of these features will not be detected on routine histology should not obscure the relevance of this crucial aspect of the investigation of antepartum fetal death.

After Delivery and Follow-up

Inhibition of lactation should be discussed and can be achieved with dopamine agonists. The long-acting cabergoline is now the drug of choice [70] as concern has been raised over the use of bromocriptine in women with pre-eclampsia [71]. However, many find that good breast support and analgesia suffice.

Before leaving hospital parents should be offered mementoes of their child, including photographs and hand or foot prints. If they do not wish to take them they should be stored in the patient notes. The provision of adequate support is important and a comprehensive checklist detailing the personnel to be informed is useful.

A postnatal follow-up appointment should be made with the consultant obstetrician. Traditionally this has been done at 6 weeks but most results, including the postmortem should be available in 2 weeks. It has been suggested that early discussion may help the grieving process [1]. This discussion should address the cause of death including events leading up to the death and results of investigations. Not all parents will be thinking about a future pregnancy at this stage but it is useful anyway to discuss the prognosis. Broadly speaking the prognosis will be that of the underlying aetiology, although an overall recurrence rate of 23 per cent [72] has been reported. This will obviously be partly dependent on the occurrence of aetiological factors in a subsequent pregnancy.

References

1. Fox R, Pillai M, Porter J, Gill G. The management of late fetal death: a guide to comprehensive care. Br J Obstet Gynaecol 1998;104–10.
2. Department of Health. Confidential enquiries into stillbirth and deaths in infancy; 4th Annual Report, 1 January–31 December 1995. London: DoH, 1997.
3. Hadlock FP, Harrist RB, Martinez-Poyer J. In-utero analysis of fetal growth: a sonographic weight standard. Radiology 1991;181:129–33.
4. Gardosi J, Mul T, Mongelli M, Fagan D. Analysis of birthweight and gestational age in antepartum stillbirths. Br J Obstet Gynaecol 1998;105:524–30.
5. Department of Health. Confidential enquiries into stillbirth and deaths in infancy; Annual Report, 1 January–31 December 1993. London: DoH, 1995.

6. Guzman ER, Benito CW, Vintizeleos AM, et al. Intrauterine growth restriction prior to 24 weeks of gestation associated with abnormal uterine and umbilical artery Doppler velocimetry [abstract]. J Soc Gynecol Invest 1996;3: 240A.
7. Valcamonico A, Danti L, Frusca T, et al. Absent end-diastolic velocity in umbilical artery: risk of neonatal morbidity and brain damage. Am J Obstet Gynecol 1994;170:796–801.
8. Kingdom JCP, Rodeck CH, Kaufmann P. Umbilical artery Doppler – more harm than good? Br J Obstet Gynaecol 1997;104:393–6.
9. Nolan RL. The maternal abdomen and pelvis in pregnancy. In: Sauerbrei EE, Nguyen KT, Nolan RL, editors. A practical guide to ultrasound in obstetrics and gynaecology, 2nd edn. New York: Lippincott-Raven, 1998;503–35.
10. Kellner KR, Donnelly WH, Gould SD. Parental behaviour after perinatal death: lack of predictive demographic and obstetric variables. Obstet Gynecol 1984;63:809–14.
11. Weiner AE, Reid DE, Roby CC, Diamond LK. Coagulation defects with intrauterine death from Rh isosensitization. Am J Obstet and Gynaecol 1950;60:1015–21.
12. Pritchard JA, Ratnoff OD. Studies of fibrinogen and other haemostatic factors in women with intrauterine death and delayed surgery. Surg Gynaecol Obstet 1995;10:467–77.
13. Pritchard JA. Fetal death in utero. Obstet Gynaecol 14:573–80.
14. Pritchard JA. Haematological problems associated with delivery, placental abruption, retained dead fetus, and amniotic fluid embolism. Clin Haematol 1973;2(3):563–86.
15. Baglin T. Disseminated intravascular coagulation: diagnosis and management. BMJ 1996;312: 683–7.
16. Tindall VR, Reid GD. The management of intrauterine death. In: Studd J, editor. Progress Obstet Gynaecol, vol. 7. London: Churchill Livingstone, 1987;ch 13, 199–215.
17. Colman R, Robboy S, Minna J. Disseminated intravascular coagulation (DIC): an approach. Am J Med 1972;52;679–87.
18. Seigel T, Seligsohn U, Agahi E, Modan M. Clinical and laboratory aspects of DIC; A study of 118 cases. Thromb Haemost 1978;39:122–34.
19. Spero J, Lewis J, Hasiba U. Disseminated intravascular coagulation. Findings in 346 patients. Thromb Haemost 1980;3:28–33,
20. Carr J, Mckinney M, McDonnagh J. Diagnosis of disseminated intravascular coagulation. Role of D-dimer. Am J Clin Pathol 1989;91:280–7.
21. Williams E. Disseminated intravascular coagulation. In: Loscalzo J, Schafer A, editors. Thrombosis and haemorrhage. Boston: Blackwell Science 1994;921–44.
22. Urquhart DR. Therapeutic abortion; methods used in the second trimester. Curr Obstet Gynaecol 1993;3:17–22.
23. Wagatsuma T. Intra amniotic injection of saline for therapeutic abortion. Am J Obstet Gynaecol 1993;93:743–5.
24. MacDonald D, O'Driscoll MK, Geoghegan FJ. Intra-amniotic dextrose – a maternal death. J Obstet Gynaecol Br Commonwealth 1965;72:452–5.
25. Mahomed K, Jayaguru A. Extra amniotic saline infusion for induction of labour in ante-partum fetal death: a cost effective method worthy of wider use. Br J Obstet Gynaecol 1997;104(9):1058–61.
26. Hill NCW, MacKenzie IZ. 2308 second trimester terminations using extra-amniotic or intra-amniotic prostaglandin E2: an analysis of efficacy and complications. Br J Obstet Gynaecol 1989;96:1421–31.
27. Sakamoto S, Satoh K, Nishiya I, Kunimoto K, Chimura T, Oda T. Abortifacient effect and uterine cervix-dilating action of 16,16-dimethyl-trans-delta2 PGE 1 methylester(ONO8O2) in the form of a vaginal suppository (a randomized double-blind controlled study in the second trimester of pregnancy). Prostaglandins Leukotrienes 1982;9:349–61.
28. Thong KJ, Robertson AJ, Baird DT. Retrospective study of 932 second trimester terminations using gemeprost (16,16 dimethyl-trans PGE1 methyl ester). Prostaglandins 1992;44:65–74.
29. Urquhart DR, Templeton AA. Mifepristone and second trimester pregnancy Lancet 1987;ii:1405.
30. Roger MW, Baird DT. Pretreatment with mifepristone (RU486) reduces the interval between prostaglandin administration and expulsion in second trimester abortion. Br J Obstet Gynaecol 1990;97:41–5.
31. Aubeny E, Baulieu EE. Activite contragestive de 1 association auRU486 d' une prostaglandine active par voie orale. CR Acad Sci III 1991;312:539–45.
32. El-Refaey H, Hinshaw K, Templeton A. The abortifacient effect of misoprostol in the second trimester. A randomized comparison with gemeprost in patients pre-treated with mifepristone(RU486). Hum Reprod 1993;8(10):1744–6.

33. El-Refaey H, Templeton A. Induction of abortion in the second trimester by a combination of misoprostol and mifepristone: a randomized comparison between two misoprostol regimens. Hum Reprod 1995;10(2):475–8.

34. Bugalho A, Bique C, Almeidia L, Faundes A. The effectiveness of intravaginal misoprostol (Cytotec) in inducing abortion after eleven weeks of pregnancy. Stud Fam Plann 1993;24:319–23.

35. Marguilies M, Perez MC, Vato L. Misoprostol to induce labour. Lancet 1992;339:64.

36. Report on confidential enquiries into maternal deaths in England and Wales. HMSO, 1997.

37. Enborm JA. Twin pregnancy with intrauterine death of one twin. Am J Obstet Gynaecol 1985;152:429–9.

38. D'Alton ME, Newton ER, Cetrulo A. Intrauterine fetal demise in multiple gestation. Acta Genet Med Gemellol 1984;33:43–9.

39. Murphy K. Intrauterine death in a twin: implications for the survivor. In: Ward RH, Whittle M, editors. Multiple pregnancy. London: RCOG Press, 1995.

40. Pinette MG, Pan Y, Pinette SG, Stubblefield PG. Treatment of twin-to-twin transfusion syndrome. Obstet Gynecol 1993;82:841–6.

41. Trespidi L, Boschetto C, Caravelli E, Villa L, Kustermann A, Nicolini U. Serial amniocentesis in the management of twin-to-twin transfusion syndrome: when is it valuable? Fetal Diagn Ther 1997;12:15–20.

42. Dippel AL. Bull Johns Hopkins Hosp 1934;54:24.

43. Brenner B, Blumfield Z. Thrombophilia and fetal loss. Blood Rev. 1997;11:72–9.

44. Salafia CM, Ernst LM, Pezz. The very low birthweight infant: maternal complications leading to preterm birth, placental lesions, and intrauterine growth. Am J Perinatol 1995;12(2):106–10.

45. Allen MC. Developmental outcome and follow-up of the small for gestational age infant. Semin Perinatol 1984;8:123–9.

46. Taylor DI. Low birth weight and neurodevelopmental handicap. Clin Obstet Gynecol 1984;11:525–31.

47. Katano K, Aoki A, Sasa H, Ogasawara M, Matsuura E, Yagami Y. Beta 2-glycoprotein I-independent anticardiolipin antibodies as a predictor of adverse pregnancy outcomes in healthy pregnant women. Hum Reprod 1996;11:509–12.

48. Pattison NS, Chamley LW, McKay EJ, Liggins GC, Butler WS. Antiphospholipid antibodies in pregnancy: prevalence and clinical associations. Br J Obstet Gynaecol 1993;100:909–13.

49. Draycott TJ, Kaloo P, Locke R, Fox R, Smith P, Read M. A case–control study of anticardiolipin antibodies after unexplained fetal loss from 24 weeks of gestation(abstract). Br J Obstet Gynaecol 1996;103:484.

50. Dekker GA, de Vries JIP, Doelitzsch PM, Huijgens PC, von Blomberg BME, Jakobs C, et al. Underlying disorders associated with severe early-onset preeclampsia. Am J Obstet Gynecol 1995;173:1042–8.

51. Preston FE, Rosendale FR, Walker ID. Increased fetal loss in women with heritable thrombophilia. Lancet 1996;348:913–16.

52. Sanson BJ, Friederich PW, Simioni P. The risk of abortion and stillbirth in anti-thrombic-protein C–and protein S-deficient women. Thromb Haemost 1996;75:387–8.

53. Maternal and Neonatal Haemostasis Working Party. Guidelines on the prevention, investigation and management of thrombosis associated with pregnancy. J Clin Pathol 1993;46:489–96.

54. Bertina RM, Koeleman BPC, Koster T, Rosendaal FR, Dirven RJ, de Ronde H. Mutation in blood coagulation factor V associated with resistance to activated Protein C. Nature 1994;369:64–7.

55. Waters. UK Collaborative Study: Solid tissue culture in clinical cytogenetics. Association Clinical Cytogeneticists Working Party Report.

56. Thornton CM, O'Hara MD. A regional audit of perinatal and infant autopsies in Northern Ireland. Br J Obstet Gynecol 1998;105:18–23.

57. Weston MJ, Porter HJ, Andrews HS, Berry PJ. Correlation of antenatal ultrasonography and pathological examination in 153 malformed fetuses. J Clin Ultrasound 1993;21:387–92.

58. Joint Working Party of the Royal College of Pathologists and Royal College of Obstetricians and Gynaecologists. Report on fetal and perinatal pathology. London: Royal College of Obstetricians and Gynaecologists, 1988.

59. Royal College of Pathologists. Guidelines for post mortem reports. London: Royal College of Pathologists, 1993.

60. Rushton DI. West Midlands perinatal mortality survey: an audit of 300 perinatal autopsies. Br J Obstet Gynaecol 1991;98:624–7.

61. Wright C, Cameron H, Lamb W. A study of the of perinatal autopsy in the former Northern region. Br J Obstet Gynaecol 1998;105:24–8.

62. Fox H. The placenta in intrauterine growth retardation: Ward RHT, Smith SK, Donnai D, editors. Early fetal growth and development. London: RCOG press, 1994;23–44.
63. Fox H. Non-trophoblastic tumours of the placenta. In: Fox, editor. Obstetrical and gynaecological pathology, 3rd edn. Edinburgh, Churchill Livingstone, 1030–44.
64. Salafia CM, Vintzileos AM, Silberman L. Placental pathology of idiopathic intrauterine growth retardation at term. Am J Perinatol 1992;9:179–84.
65. Stioui S, de Silvestris M, Molinari A. Trisomic 22 placenta in a case of severe intrauterine growth retardation. Prenat Diagn 1989;9:673–6.
66. Schwinger B, Seidl B, Klink F. Chromosome mosaicism of the placenta – a cause of development failure of the fetus? Prenat Diagn 1989;9:639–47.
67. Giles WB, Trudinger BJ, Baird PJ. Fetal umbilical artery flow velocity wavelengths and placental resistance: pathological correlation. Br J Obstet Gynaecol 1985;92:31–8.
68. Jackson MR, Walsh AJ, Morrow RJ, Mullen JBM, Lye SJ, Knox-Ritchie JW. Reduced placental villous tree elaboration in small-for-gestational age pregnancies: relationship with umbilical artery Doppler waveforms. Am J Obstet Gynecol 1995;172:518–25.
69. Krebs C, Macara LM, Leiser R, Bowman AWF, Greer IA, Kingdom JCP. Intrauterine growth restriction with absent end-diastolic flow velocity in the umbilical artery is associated with maldevelopment of the terminal placental villous tree. Am J Obstet Gynecol 1996;175:1534–42.
70. Rains CP, Bryson HM, Fitton A. Cabergoline. Drugs 1995;49:255-79.
71. Iffy L. Lethal cardiovascular complications in patients receiving bromocriptine for ablactation. Medical law 1995;14:99–104.
72. Kuno N, Itakura A, Kurachi O, Mizutani S, Kazeto S, Tomoda Y. Decrease in severity of intrauterine growth retardation in subsequent pregnancies. Int J Gynaecol Obstet 1995;51:219–24.

18 Paediatric Implications – Neonatal Complications

Neil Marlow

Introduction

The literature concerning neonatal aspects of babies who have failed to thrive in the intrauterine environment is intermingled with data on babies who are SGA. This latter concept, which may be defined as having a birthweight below the 10th or 3rd percentile of birthweight for gestational age, was designed for postnatal use to define an at-risk group at a time when antenatal fetal assessment was inadequate, but has value because of the ease of definition. Following improvements in our ability to define antenatal growth, it is clear that the concept of the "SGA baby" is different from the baby identified to have restricted intrauterine growth. In the former category, babies with IUGR are mixed with appropriately small babies (from primarily genetic causes) or those with congenital malformations or infections. Furthermore, some babies who have restricted growth may not be small for gestational age when defined by the 10th percentile, having been potentially large babies whose growth potential has been impaired, but not sufficiently to bring them below the arbitrarily chosen centile.

Even within the IUGR group without malformation or infection, several subgroups of infants may be identified, for example those exposed to marginal intrauterine hypoxia, those exposed to preterminal chronic hypoxia and those who have experienced acute-on-chronic hypoxia. In discussing the neonatal consequences of growth restriction, therefore, it is critical to define populations as precisely as possible – something that has really become possible only over the past few years following the development of techniques of haemodynamic, behavioural and invasive fetal assessment. Indeed this knowledge of antenatal pathophysiology offers the chance to evaluate the effects of growth restriction more accurately.

The postnatal identification of growth-restricted babies, however, is as important as their antenatal assessment. Most studies still mix babies together as an SGA group, even if labelled "IUGR". Attempts to define subsets have been made using auxological parameters such as symmetry/asymmetry of weight and HC growth, mid arm circumference (MAC) or MAC:HC ratios, a variety of skinfold thickness (SFT) measures (of which the quadriceps SFT appears the most useful), redefined birthweight charts using measures based upon estimated fetal weights using ultrasound, markers of symmetry of antenatal growth or individualised birthweight assessments allowing for genetic or racial parameters and parity [1]. Of these, individualised birthweight assessments, the least used, may be the most useful as the mean anticipated birthweight is adjusted for a range of important influences and the actual birthweight expressed as a ratio of that expected. This allows the definition of failure to achieve expected growth without the use of arbitrary points on charts based on the whole population.

Antenatal identification of babies in whom nutrient supply failure is suspected is an equally important issue. The pattern of fetal responses to mild to moderate hypoxia, initially using Doppler assessment of umbilical vessel flow velocity, has been refined since the late 1980s [2–4], culminating in a meta-analysis of trials that concluded "there is now compelling evidence that women with high risk pregnancies ... should have access to Doppler ultrasonographic study of umbilical arterial waveforms" [5]. The classical description of the fetus whose growth velocity initially begins to fall, followed by a reduction in end-diastolic velocity on ultrasound, as an indication for delivery is now commonplace. The natural history is that this may then be followed with a reduction in liquor volume, changes in fetal behaviour, a reduction in fetal movements and abnormalities of cardiotochograph trace as increasingly preterminal signs [3].

Technically it is now possible to make more detailed assessment of fetal acid–base balance and circulatory status, the latter by evaluating Doppler velocities from the aorta and several organs, including the brain. Such assessments are necessarily associated with increased intervention and adverse assessment with increasing fetal death. Intervention probably improves pregnancy outcome, although to date there have been no randomised trials of action based upon the results of such studies. Observational studies [6] have indicated that fetal hypoxia, as measured by fetal circulatory redistribution to increase flow to the fetal brain using middle cerebral artery waveform indices (or relating these to umbilical waveforms), leads to more preterm delivery, lower birthweight for gestational age, increased fetal acidosis and, in one study, increased neonatal complications. The finding of a pulsatile umbilical venous flow appears to be particularly ominous in terms of adverse outcome [7].

The early detection of fetal hypoxia, treatment with antenatal steroids and delivery of infants before preterminal hypoxia supervenes may be expected to alter the spectrum of neonatal mortality, and hence the large literature base concerning babies with suspected IUGR will have to be re-evaluated. Furthermore, studies of outcome after pregnancies where decision making using newer assessment tools must evaluate the effect of intervention based upon them. Decision making with respect to delivery and IUGR is currently the subject of a major randomised UK-based trial (GRIT) [8].

Immediate Condition at Birth and Resuscitation

Despite a threefold increased risk of obstetric intervention for "fetal distress" for babies who are SGA or have asymmetric body proportions, condition at birth is generally good. In the recently reported Scandinavian SGA Study, only 3.8 per cent of such infants had Apgar scores < 8 at 1 minute and 3 out of 1,435 infants (0.7 per cent) at 5 minutes [9].

In contrast, when infants are classified as growth restricted according to a neonatal growth assessment score performed on the results of two ultrasound scans over the middle trimester, compared with AGA predictions greater numbers were in poor immediate condition (Apgar score < 8 at 1 minute: 33.3 vs. 8.3 per cent), or had acidosis (cord pH < 7.2: 27.8 vs. 6.7 per cent) [10]. Despite these differences similar proportions were admitted to the neonatal intensive care unit (NICU) (5.6 vs. 2.5 per cent respectively) and reclassification using conventional birthweight criteria did not worsen the prediction.

In studies of FBS performed in babies with IUGR, there is a progressive hypoxaemia and acidosis [11]. In such babies a poorer condition at birth may be anticipated. Where fetal compromise has been identified by using Doppler and/or biophysical profile, there appears to be a progressive increase in the need for resuscitation and worsening of condition at birth as two or more abnormalities are identified [2–4]. Careful assessment of fetal haemodynamics, behaviour and Cardio Tochography (CTG) may therefore identify babies at risk and, in these, early delivery should alter the immediate neonatal condition of such populations. However, despite increasing the likelihood of CS because of CTG abnormality before or during labour, meta-analysis of trials of Doppler assessment have failed to shown improved early neonatal condition defined by Apgar score at 1 or 5 minutes [5].

Mortality

Logic determines that, in the unmonitored state, the growth-restricted hypoxic and acidaemic fetus must be at higher rate of perinatal death compared with a normally grown fetus with normal oxygen tensions. For example, in a 15 year hospital cohort, babies less than the 10th percentile of weight for gestation had higher mortality at each gestational age to 36 weeks, in contrast to birthweight groups where AGA children fared worse from 750 to1500 g [12].

The heterogeneity encountered by the use of SGA as a definition to identify populations at risk may often be associated with little increased risk for babies whose birthweight lies between the 3rd and 10th percentile. These form the majority in any study and therefore association with increased perinatal mortality may not be found [13]. In contrast, those babies at the extreme range of birthweight for gestational age may be more likely to have congenital abnormality, infection or hypoxia and are at greater risk. For example Lund [14], in a study of very preterm infants born with IUGR and using a birthweight chart modified using intrauterine estimated fetal weights, found mortality in the group of children considered to be SGA was higher than in AGA infants, because of excess morbidity in the severely growth-restricted group (birthweight $\geq$ 3 sd below the mean – OR for perinatal death 2.24 (95 per cent CI 1.26–3.99).

The early descriptions of progressive ultrasound signs of fetal compromise were associated with parallel increasing risk of perinatal death [3] and groups of babies described with AEDV had high mortality and rates of oligohydramnios and CTG abnormality [2]. Application of Doppler assessment of the circulation has had a major impact on perinatal mortality. In meta-analysis there was a reduction in the OR of perinatal death by 38 per cent (95 per cent CI 15–55), of stillbirth by 37 per cent (95 per cent CI 3–62) and by 38 per cent (95 per cent CI 7–59) in neonatal death, using Doppler indices to guide perinatal management [5].

It is likely that the relationship between gestational age, intrauterine growth and mortality is therefore complex, and previously observed relationships are being modified by current assessment techniques and intervention. Among extremely premature infants, the presence of growth failure is associated with a increased rate of neonatal complications and is likely to lead to neonatal death [15]. At more mature gestations (28–32 weeks), even quite marked growth failure, delivered before preterminal compromise, may result in improved neonatal survival because of accelerated pulmonary maturation due to mild hypoxia or intervention with steroids. However, the superimposition of severe hypoxia, either as an acute obstetric event or by progression of chronic hypoxia due to worsening nutrient transfer failure, may reverse this advantage at any gestation. Reversal of end-diastolic flow on Doppler assessment is associated with worsening fetal compromise and a high perinatal mortality [16]. At gestations over 32 weeks, however, even severely acidotic growth-restricted fetuses may survive [17].

The underlying pregnancy illness may also interact with mortality. Overall, mortality in normotensive SGA pregnancies is higher than in hypertensive pregnancies (OR 1.9, 95 per cent CI 1.3–2.9) but at term this may be reversed (OR hypertension > normotension 2.42, 95 per cent CI 1.7–3.4). For the preterm, therefore, hypertension may have advantage for the SGA baby [18].

In the post-term pregnancy, perinatal mortality rises significantly from 40 to over 42 weeks, mainly in terms of intrauterine fetal death [19]. There is an interaction with low birthweight for age in that the OR both of intrauterine fetal death and of neonatal death rises progressively among the SGA groups at each gestational age, with less-marked increases for intrauterine fetal death only among AGA children.

Specific Neonatal Conditions

Many studies use admission to a neonatal unit as an endpoint denoting adverse outcome. This itself may be gestation or birthweight dependent and, unless term infants are considered alone, is unlikely to be helpful. Some studies have looked at

Table 18.1 Conditions specifically associated with IUGR

Neonatal condition	Reason for association
perinatal hypoxia	poor glycogen reserves and metabolic adaptation (q.v.) result in poor tolerance of intrapartum hypoxia; at term and post-term particularly associated with meconium aspiration syndrome
necrotising enterocolitis	fetal gut ischaemia (see text)
RDS and respiratory complications	lung maturity dependent upon several factors (see text)
hypoglycaemia	metabolic adaptation (see text)
polycythaemia	bone marrow response to hypoxia; may be modified by cord-clamping practice
anaemia, leucopenia and low platelets	associated with preterminal marrow response to hypoxia; especially common when pre-eclampsia present
postnatal growth	some groups exhibit good catch-up growth (see text)

more specific neonatal morbidity, and these have tended to show higher rates of many neonatal conditions in SGA or IUGR babies, though for other neonatal conditions the association is more difficult to show. For instance, respiratory distress syndrome (RDS) may interact with growth restriction in various ways (see below) (Table 18.1).

Of more interest than these generalisations is to look within the at-risk obstetric group to which markers are associated with neonatal condition. James and colleagues [3] evaluated the outcome for 100 pregnancies referred because of suspected chronic fetal asphyxia. A sequential deterioration in ultrasonographic and cardiotochographic findings was observed, with a variable time scale. Doppler studies initially became abnormal, followed by a reduction in AC and finally BPS. Five subgroups were identified (Table 18.2) depending upon fetal characteristics. Prognosis was most impaired in the last category, in terms of both mortality and neonatal morbidity. In a further analysis, controlling for gestation, between 11 babies from each of the two highest risk groups there remained many more complications in the babies who had an abnormal BPS.

Table 18.2 Relationship between indices of compromise in fetuses thought to be at risk of chronic intrauterine hypoxia and outcome [3]

Condition	A: normal (hypertension only) $n=23$	B: low AC $n=16$	C: abn. Doppler $n=7$	D: abn. Doppler + low AC $n=29$	E: abn Doppler, low AC, low BPS $n=28$
neonatal survivors	23 (100%)	16 (100%)	7 (100%)	29 (100%)	21 (75%)
fetal death	—	—	—	—	2 (7.1%)
neonatal death	—	—	—	—	5 (18%)
gestational age at delivery weeks (r)	37 (29–40)	38 (35–41)	38 (34–40)	36 (28–40)	32.5 (26–39)
resuscitation at birth	3 (13%)	1 (6.3%)	—	8 (28%)	19 (68%)
RDS	2 (8.7%)	3 (18.8%)	—	5 (17%)	8 (29%)
ventilated	2 (8.7%)	—	—	3 (10%)	8 (29%)
patent ductus	—	—	—	2 (6.9%)	1 (3.6%)
chronic lung disease	—	—	—	—	3 (11%)
polycythaemia	1 (4.4%)	1 (6.3%)	—	4 (14%)	4 (14%)
anaemia	—	—	—	—	3 (11%)
low platelets	—	—	—	2 (6.9%)	3 (11%)
intraventricular haemorrhage	—	—	—	1 (3.5%)	3 (11%)
NEC	—	—	—	—	3 (11%)
hypoglycaemia	2 (8.7%)	—	1 (14%)	5 (17%)	5 (18%)
minor dysmorphism	—	1 (6.3%)	—	1 (3.5%)	5 (18%)
no neonatal problems	13 (57%)	11 (69%)	6 (86%)	11 (38%)	3 (11%)

The SGA Term Infant Without Risk Factors

At term the simple use of low birthweight (without other obstetric risk factors) to identify a group at risk has been challenged [20]. Indeed it is logical that, among a group of term infants, a significant proportion of this group will be genetically small and therefore not at increased risk. Part of the issue is the hypothesis that PI varies normally with decreasing birthweight and that "asymmetric growth restriction" is indeed a natural biological phenomenon. None the less, careful study is necessary before this hypothesis can be accepted. Minior and Divon [21] report a case–control study where matched AGA term infants were compared with a group of SGA babies without obstetric risk factors or anatomical abnormality. The SGA group had higher rates of perinatal morbidity over a range of outcomes, including immediate condition at birth, hypoglycaemia, respiratory symptoms, thrombocytopenia and hyperbilirubinaemia.

Metabolic Adaptation

The dominant determinant of intrauterine growth is oxygen and nutrient delivery to the fetus and this is modulated by the action of IGFs, which have been primarily studied in animal models [22]. In the human and sheep models, circulating IGF-I levels correlate with birth size [23]. Maternal starvation or undernutrition in the sheep leads to a decline in levels of IGF-I, which is mediated by glucose supply via insulin secretion by the pancreas. Changes in the concentrations of IGF-binding proteins mean that the bioavailability of IGF-I may be more affected by changes in nutrient supply antenatally than postnatally. Although GH is not a primary growth factor before birth, infusion studies have demonstrated its ability to enhance fetal growth in late gestation and the fetal somatotrophic axis appears to be active before birth. Fascinatingly, the maternal somatotrophic axis may also affect fetal growth and thus exert an external non-genetic influence over fetal growth potential [22].

In parallel with changes in IGF-I concentrations in cord blood from babies with IUGR, insulin and TSH levels may be reduced and GH levels elevated. Associated with these endocrinological changes, cord blood analysis shows reduced glucose, albumin and cholesterol concentrations [24] and elevated concentrations of lactate and non-esterified fatty acids [25]. Low cord blood glucose correlates with birthweight standard deviation score [26].

Babies with IUGR have long been recognised to be at risk for neonatal hypoglycaemia [27] and aggressively managed to maintain normoglycaemia, although the long term effects of mild to moderate brief periods of hypoglycaemia are far from clear. Children at risk for hypoglycaemia tend to be slimmer than babies without symptom, as measured using MAC or SFT [27]. The major risk for neonatal hypoglycaemia in IUGR babies occurs in the first 24 hours, although it may take longer to resolve in some children. The major difference between the term AGA and IUGR child is that the former seems able to generate and use alternative fuels for gluconeogenesis, such as ketone bodies, which may offset any significant detrimental effect of low glucose levels, whereas, in contrast, the baby who is preterm or has IUGR seems unable to do so. Total gluconeogenic substrate for babies with IUGR, determined by low MAC : HC ratio, is actually high in the first 6–12 hours after birth, representing failure of utilisation or increased release of substrate under the influence of stress hormones, but thereafter concentrations decline to values consistently lower than AGA children over the remainder of the first week [25]. The normal relationships between plasma glucose and counterregulatory hormones are not present in babies with IUGR, and gluconeogenic substrate remains low even when blood glucose is low [26]. Preterm infants behave in a similar manner to children with growth restriction. In these elegant studies by Hawdon and colleagues [26], it seems clear that current early feeding regimens that encourage increased caloric intake over the first few days are successful in avoiding biochemical hypoglycaemia. The failure to utilise gluconeogenic substrate over the first 12 hours and ketogenesis over the first week indicate that the growth-restricted infant is unable to respond appropriately to hypoglycaemic stress and that strategies to encourage metabolic adaptation are required.

The role of this impaired metabolic adaptation in IUGR term infants in pathogenesis of the well-described association with adult disease patterns remains to be elucidated (see Ch. 15).

Necrotising Enterocolitis

Progressive hypoxia during intrauterine growth results in a redistribution of blood flow to various fetal organs. This "brain-sparing" effect is associated with reductions in blood flow to muscles, kidneys and the gut. That these changes produce particular hypoxia in the bowel, which may then respond to the stress of feeding with the development of necrotising enterocolitis (NEC), has been known since the earliest description of an association by Hackett and colleagues [2]. There were seven cases of NEC (27 per cent) among a group of 26 babies < 2000 g birthweight with documented fetal AEDV, compared with none in the comparison group. Further small studies have tended to confirm these data [28–30], although these and other studies have really been too small to produce definitive results in a time frame when the incidence of NEC seems to be falling.

Kempley and colleagues [31] have studied the natural history of splanchnic blood flow following delivery. AEDV was associated with reduction in superior mesenteric and coeliac axis blood flow velocities and by an elevated PI, indicating increased resistance in the splanchnic bed. These changes were observed on the 1st day but persisted for over 1 week. Furthermore the normal rise in gut blood flow, seen when feeding is commenced, is not seen in babies with IUGR.

These and other observations have dictated caution in the commencement of feeding in an attempt to prevent NEC in babies who have known fetal AEDV. Early feeding has been associated with an increasing risk of symptoms in the face of AEDV [32] but the data from a number of studies have failed to really establish whether or not delaying feeds does prevent risk of NEC [33]. Confounding factors, such as the use of breast milk, a slow rate of feed increment or the commencement of minimal enteral feeding in an attempt to prime the gut to receive full feeds, have also shown inconsistent results when NEC is considered. The delaying of feeds and the early use of total parental nutrition (TPN) with its attendant complications are risks that have to be balanced. We currently delay feeds for up to 72 hours (48 hours if colostrum is available) and then commence cautiously for babies who are < 3rd percentile or have a history of fetal AEDV, acknowledging that the evidence for this plan is rather weak.

Respiratory Distress Syndrome

It is generally held that RDS is less frequently encountered following IUGR, although this may be modified by the superimposition of an acute hypoxic insult around delivery. The published evidence, however, is more difficult to interpret. Although publications point to a preventative effect on RDS when gestation is controlled [122], other data point to a differential effect that is dependent upon gestational age. In a study from Lund using a novel intrauterine growth curve to determine appropriateness of growth [14], SGA infants born between 29 and 32 weeks were at lower risk of RDS, in contrast to infants born before 29 weeks from pregnancies complicated by pre-eclampsia. Interestingly, in this study SGA infants appeared to benefit less from antenatal steroids in terms of mortality, RDS and perinatal brain lesions than AGA infants. In a contrasting study, evaluation of a range of birthweight grids and estimates of gestational age failed to demonstrate this difference and consistently showed an excess of RDS in SGA babies at all gestations from 27 weeks to term [34]. It is clear that the interaction of antenatal intervention with steroids and timely delivery may modify these risks considerably and that evaluations of the risk of RDS in relationship to growth restriction should be designed to account for these confounders.

Neurological Effects of Fetal Growth Restriction

The effects of growth restriction on the incidence of major intracranial injury are equally difficult to tease out. In one neuropathological study of 274 intrauterine or early neonatal deaths [35], babies with evidence of ischaemic brain injury had lower weights for gestation. Other studies evaluating the frequency of intraventricular haemorrhage (IVH) or of periventricular leucomalacia (PVL) have produced inconsistent results.

Extrapolating from studies based upon the Western Australia Cerebral Palsy Register, Blair and Stanley [36] have observed a gestational-age-dependent increase in risk of spastic cerebral palsy as appropriateness of birthweight for age falls. For babies born before 34 weeks' gestation there was no increased risk if birthweight was below the 10th percentile. At term there was a moderate increase in risk for children with birthweights both below the 3rd and between the 3rd and 10th percentiles. But between 34 and 37 weeks gestation the risk of cerebral palsy rose dramatically as birthweight for gestation fell. Data such as these give clinical credence to the observations of Gaffney and colleagues [35], even though studies looking for in vivo evidence of brain injury show conflicting results. The examination of other data for the confounding effect of gestation may also reveal such interactions.

Indeed, studies evaluating blood flow redistribution show gestational-age-dependent differences. At term there would appear to be a rapid return to normality [37], whereas in the preterm there tends to be a switch to high resistance patterns [38]. Increasing risk of cerebral injury in the preterm growth-restricted infant may therefore have a physiological basis. In the very preterm the risk of brain injury as a result of IVH, PVL or other ill-defined cortical injury may relate to many other factors, such as nutritional or systemic blood flow changes, and the resultant effect of IUGR is lost.

Alternative hypotheses as to the clinical significance of blood flow redistribution have been advanced, in that the antenatal high cerebral flow state may confer some advantage to the developing brain [6]. This would be consistent with a protective effect on major markers of brain injury (IVH, PVL). Some evidence has been advanced to support this, in that visual evoked potentials may show accelerated development over the first 6 months, an effect that has disappeared by 12 months of age and is reflected in a lack developmental advantage demonstrable at 2 years. Indeed in longer term follow-up studies of the same group the converse is true, there being an 8.8 point reduction in IQ scores for those with evidence of "sparing" defined as an umbilical:cerebral PI ratio of < 0.73 [39]. The nature of the brain injury that produces cognitive impairment remains unclear. In a detailed study of outcome for children in mainstream school following very low birthweight birth, appearances of periventricular leucomalacia on MRI at 16 years did not correlate with school or cognitive performance [40].

It is more logical that outcome may relate to fetal condition as opposed to overall size or focal white matter injury, through markers that may relate to a more global hypoxic cerebral insult. There is evidence from several studies to support this contention.

In a study of 65 children who had FBS and blood gas measurement [41], low Griffith's Developmental Scores at between 12 and 66 months were associated with low pH ($r^2 = 0.17$) and low oxygen tension ($r^2 = 0.06$) as opposed to the severity of growth restriction. Developmental measures are poor predictors of cognitive outcomes, especially when measured early in postnatal life, and there are concerns over the value of Griffith's testing applied to such a wide age range without considering other confounders; thus confirmation of these fascinating data is required.

In the same study [41], reduction in mean aortic blood flow velocity was also associated with lower developmental scores. A larger longitudinal study following 178 pregnancies has demonstrated a reduction in verbal and global IQ scores between 6 and 7 years [42] (Table 18.3), together with an excess of minor neurological signs in children with absent or reversed end-diastolic flow in fetal life. Results of Doppler waveforms independently predicted cognitive and neurological outcome.

Table 18.3 Outcome at 6–7 years related to fetal Doppler findings [42]

Fetal aortic blood flow velocity	n	Verbal IQ	Global IQ
abnormal	41	96 ± 17.7	95.9 ± 15.7
normal	105	102.1 ± 12.2	102.9 ± 13.2

Other Problems Encountered in Preterm Infants

Haematological changes have been described that relate to hypoxia, namely both anaemia and polycythaemia. Anaemia may relate to extreme hypoxic compromise or to fetal infection, whereas polycythaemia is usually considered the result of chronic marginal hypoxia. Both may be modified by placental transfusion at delivery. Thrombocytopenia is frequently observed in SGA or IUGR babies. This may be a result of chronic hypoxia, or of maternal thrombocytopenia as part of systemic or hypertensive illness or response to fetal intrauterine infection. It may also be part of the pathological process associated with NEC. Other areas of import relate to polycythaemia

Cardiorespiratory adaptation may differ between otherwise healthy SGA and AGA children after birth. In a study comparing results of sleep studies in 26 SGA and 31 AGA children at 2–6 days of age [43], despite similar respiratory rates, SGA children showed significantly more pauses lasting 2–5 seconds and 5–10 seconds respectively, with higher proportions of non-breathing time and periodic breathing. These disturbances of respiratory rhythm control are associated with a higher resting heart rate [44] and may relate to dysfunctional neurological maturation during the antenatal period of hypoxaemia, despite evidence of protection of brain growth and architecture.

Growth over the First Year

The heterogeneity of samples of SGA babies followed after birth makes generalisation with respect to IUGR difficult. The restriction in intrauterine growth is partially abolished by catch-up in postnatal growth over the 1st year, and parameters at 1 year seem to relate to genetic factors. In a recent study of term infants born in the late 1980s, SGA (< 10th percentile) infants were still lighter and shorter than AGA infants at 13 months of age, despite having had higher growth velocities in terms of length and HC and a smaller drop in PI, but not weight [45]. Where intrauterine growth had been asymmetric, PI remained lower at 13 months than in children who were symmetrically small at birth [46]. Poor prenatal and postnatal head growth is associated with poor developmental outcome and this group may be that at most risk for growth and developmental problems.

In the more selected group of premature SGA children enrolled into the Infant Health and Development Program (< 37 weeks) [47], limited catch-up in length and weight did occur over the first 4 postnatal months, with growth paralleling the centiles subsequently. In this group the symmetrically small babies were consistently smaller and shorter than "short-for-age" or "asymmetric IUGR" groups.

Nonetheless it would appear that functional measures of fetal health may provide better indicators of risk than conventional growth assessment.

Greater sophistication in the detection of intrauterine growth restriction, better quantification of fetal health and growth potential and more sophisticated assessment of developmental performance are likely to demonstrate differences.

Conclusions

Fetal growth restriction has serious implications for the newborn infant, in terms of immediate condition, neonatal adaptation and later growth and development. Older literature points to conflicting results in terms of neonatal disadvantage.

More recent studies, in which fetal well-being has been assessed, point to markers that may indicate those at most risk in both the short and long term.

The balance of risks for the growth-restricted fetus remains very difficult to assess. On the one hand, the fetus may be faced with making adaptive changes in a hypoxic intrauterine environment, with the attendant risk of perinatal death and acute compromise. This must be balanced against early delivery and the superimposition of risk from prematurity. It is this balance that at present is difficult to quantify and there is a need for randomised trials of perinatal management for this group, given the evidence that delayed delivery of the fetus may produce short term advantage but longer term cognitive and neurological impairment, which is discussed in further detail in the following chapter.

References

1. Sanderson DA, Wilcox MA, Johnson IR. The individualised birthweight ratio: a new method of identifying intrauterine growth retardation. Br J Obstet Gynaecol 1994;101:310–14.
2. Hackett GA, Campbell S, Gamsu H, Cohen-Overbeek T, Pearce JM. Doppler studies in the growth retarded fetus and prediction of neonatal necrotising enterocolitis, haemorrhage, and neonatal morbidity. BMJ 1987;294:13–16.
3. James DK, Parker MJ, Smoleniec JS. Comprehensive fetal assessment with three ultrasonographic characteristics. Am J Obstet Gynecol 1992;166:1486–95.
4. Karsdorp VH, van Vugt J, van Geijn HP, Kostense PJ, Arduini D, Montenegro N, et al. Clinical significance of absent or reversed end diastolic velocity waveforms in umbilical artery. Lancet 1994;344:1664–8.
5. Alfirevic Z, Neilson JP. Doppler ultrasonography in high-risk pregnancies: systematic review with meta-analysis. Am J Obstet Gynecol 1995;172:1379–87.
6. Hornbuckle J, Thornton JG. The fetal circulatory response to chronic placental insufficiency and relation to pregnancy outcome. Fetal Matern Med Rev 1998;10:137–52.
7. Kiserud T, Eik-Nes SH, Blaas HG, Hellevik LR, Simensen B. Ductus venosus blood flow velocity and the umbilical circulation in the seriously growrh retarded fetus. Ultrasound Obstet Gynecol 1994;4:109–14.
8. [Anonymous] When do obstetricians recommend delivery for a high-risk preterm growth-retarded fetus? The GRIT Study Group. Growth Restriction Intervention Trial. Eur J Obstet Gynecol Reprod Biol 1996;67:121–6.
9. Langhoff-Roos J, Lindmark G. Obstetric interventions and perinatal asphyxia in growth retarded term infants. Acta Obstet Gynecol Scand (suppl) 1997;165:39–43.
10. Ariyuki Y, Hata T, Kitao M. Evaluation of perinatal outcome using individualized growth assessment: comparison with conventional methods. Pediatrics 1995;96:36–42.
11. Nicolaides KH, Economides DL, Soothill PW. Blood gases, pH and lactate in appropriate and small for gestational age fetuses. Am J Obstet Gynecol 1989;161:996–1001.
12. Piper JM, Xenakis EM, McFarland M, Elliott BD, Berkus MD, Langer O. Do growth-retarded premature infants have different rates of perinatal morbidity and mortality than appropriately grown premature infants? Obstet Gynecol 1996;87:169–74.
13. Amin H, Singhal N, Sauve RS. Impact of intrauterine growth restriction on neurodevelopmental and growth outcomes in very low birthweight infants. Acta Paediatr 1997;86:306–14.
14. Ley D, Wide-Swensson D, Lindroth M, Svenningsen N, Marsal K. Respiratory distress syndrome in infants with impaired intrauterine growth. Acta Paediatr 1997;86:1090–6.
15. Batton DG, DeWitte DB, Espinosa R, Swails TL. The impact of fetal compromise on outcome at the border of viability. Am J Obstet Gynecol 1998;178:909–15.
16. Wang KG, Chen CP, Yang JM, Su TH. Impact of reverse end-diastolic flow velocity in umbilical artery on pregnancy outcome after the 28th gestational week. Acta Obstet Gynecol Scand (suppl) 1998;77:527–31.
17. Soothill PW. Diagnosis of intrauterine growth retardation and its fetal and perinatal consequencs. Acta Obstet Gynecol Scand (suppl) 1994;399:55–8.
18. Piper JM, Langer O, Xenakis EM, McFarland M, Elliott BD, Berkus MD. Perinatal outcome in growth-restricted fetuses: do hypertensive and normotensive pregnancies differ? Obstet Gynecol 1996;88:194–99.

19. Divon MY, Haglund B, Nisell H, Otterblad PO, Westgren M. Fetal and neonatal mortality in the postterm pregnancy: the impact of gestational age and fetal growth restriction. Am J Obstet Gynecol 1998;178:726–31.
20. Chard T, Costeloe K, Leaf A. Evidence of growth retardation in neonates of apparently normal weight. Eur J Obstet Gynecol Reprod Biol 1992;45:59–62.
21. Minior VK, Divon MY. Fetal growth restriction at term: myth or reality? Obstet Gynecol 1998;92:57–60.
22. Gluckman PD, Cutfield W, Harding JE, Milner D, Jensen E, Woodhall S, et al. Metabolic consequences of intrauterine growth retardation. Acta Paediatr (suppl) 199;417:3–6.
23. Soothill PW, Ajayi RA, Campbell S, Ross EM, Nicholiades K. Fetal oxygenation at cordocentesis, maternal smoking and childhood neurodevelopment. Eur J Obstet Gynecol Reprod Biol 1995;59:21–4.
24. Nieto-Diaz A, Villar J, Matorras-Weinig R, Valenzuela-Ruiz P. Intrauterine growth retardation at term: association between anthropometric and endocrine parameters. Acta Obstet Gynecol Scand 1996;75:127–31.
25. Hawdon JM, Ward PM. Metabolic adaptation in small for gestational age infants. Arch Dis Child 1993;68:262–8.
26. Hawdon JM, Weddell A, Aynsley-Green A, Ward PM. Hormonal and metabolic response to hypoglycaemia in small for gestational age infants. Arch Dis Child 1993;68:269–73.
27. Drossou V, Diamanti E, Noutsia H, Konstantinidis T, Katsougiannopoulos V. Accuracy of anthropometric measurements in predicting symptomatic SGA and LGA neonates. Acta Paediatr 1995;84:1–5.
28. McDonnell M, Serra-serra V, Gaffney G, Redman CWG, Hope PL. Neonatal outcome after pregnancy complicated by abnormal velocity waveforms in the umbilical artery. Arch Dis Child Fetal Neonatal Edn 1994;70:F84–89.
29. Eronen M, Kari A, Pesonen E, Kaaja R, Wallgren EI, Hallman M. Value of absent or retrograde end-diastolic flow in fetal aorta and umbilical artery as a prediction of perinatal outcome in pregnancy induced hypertension. Acta Paediatr 1993;82:919–24.
30. Malcolm G, Ellwood D, Devonald K, Beilby R, Henderson-Smart DJ. Absent or reversed end diastoloic flow velocity in the umbilicial artery and necrotising enterocolitis. Arch Dis Child Fetal Neonatal Edn 1991;66:805–7.
31. Gamsu HR, Kempley ST. Enteral hypoxia/ischaemia and necrotizing enterocolitis. Semin Neonatol 1997;2:245–54.
32. Yu VYH, James B, Hendry P, MacMahon RA. Total parenteral nutrition in very low birth weight infants: a controlled trial. Arch Dis Child 1979;54:653–61.
33. Williams AF. Role of feeding in the pathogenesis of necrotizing enterocolitis. Semin Neonatol 1997;2:263–72.
34. Tyson JE, Kennedy K, Broyles S, Rosenfeld CR. The small for gestational age infant: accelerated or delayed pulmonary maturation? Increased or decreased survival? Pediatrics 1995;95:534–8.
35. Gaffney G, Squier MV, Johnson A, Flavell V, Sellers S. Clinical associations of prenatal white matter injury. Arch Dis Child Fetal Neonatal Edn 1994;70:F101–6.
36. Blair E, Stanley F. Intrauterine growth and spastic cerebral palsy. I. Association with birth weight for gestational age. Am J Obstet Gynecol 1990;162:229–37.
37. Ley D, Marsal K. Doppler velocimetry in the cerebral vessels of small for gestational age infants. Early Hum Dev 1992;31:171–80.
38. Scherjon SA, Oosting H, de VB, de WT, Zondervan HA, Kok JH. Fetal brain sparing is associated with accelerated shortening of visual evoked potential latencies during early infancy. Am J Obstet Gynecol 1996;175:1569–75.
39. Sicco S, Briet J, Oosting H, Kok JH. The discrepancy between maturation of visual evoked potentials and cognitive outcome at five years in very preterm infants with and without hemodynamic signs of fetal brain sparing. Pediatrics 1999;in press.
40. Cook RWI, Abernethy LJ. Cranial magnetic resonance imaging and school performance in very low birthweight children in adolescence. Arch Dis Child Fetal Neonatal Edn 1999;81:F116–F121.
41. Soothill PW, Ajayi RA, Campbell S, Ross EM, Nicolaides KH. Fetal oxygenation at cordocentesis, maternal smoking and childhood neuro-development Eur J Obstet Gynecol Reprod Biol 1995;59:21–4.
42. Ley D, Tideman E, Laurin J, Bjerre I, Marsal K. Abnormal fetal aortic velocity waveform and intellectual function at 7 years of age. Ultrasound Obstet Gynecol 1996;8:152–65.
43. Curzi-Dascalova L, Peirano P, Christova E. Respiratory characteristics during sleep in healthy small-for-gestational age newborns. Pediatrics 1996;97:554–9.

44. Curzi-Dascalova L, Spassov L, Eiselt M. Development of cardiorespiratory control and sleep in newborns. In: Cosmi AV, Renzo GC, editors. Current progress in perinatal medicine. London: Parthenon, 1994;303–8.
45. Markestad T, Vik T, Ahlsten G, Gebre-Medhin M, Skjaerven R, Jacobsen G, et al. Small-for-gestational-age infants born at term: growth and development during the first year of life. Acta Obstetr Gynecol Scand (suppl) 1997;76:93–101.
46. Strauss RS, Dietz WH. Effects of intrauterine growth retardation in premature infants on early childhood growth. J Pediatr 1997;130:95–102.

19 Paediatric Implications of IUGR with Special Reference to Cerebral Palsy

Eve Blair

Criteria for the Inference of IUGR

Intrauterine growth restriction is a concept signifying that the fetus has not grown as fast as it ought to have grown. The growth-restricted baby would have been bigger were it not for suboptimal genetic and/or environmental factor(s) (Ch. 1). Since we do not know exactly what size the individual newborn ought to be, IUGR cannot be measured directly and its presence has been inferred from several surrogate measures, as outlined in Ch. 1.

Individual adverse paediatric outcomes such as cerebral palsy occur rarely, and cannot be reliably ascertained until the children are several years of age. The large sample size and long term follow-up required to study them prospectively frequently make the cost prohibitive. However, the functional measures from which the inference of IUGR is most valid, such as ultrasonically ascertained deviation from the antenatal growth trajectory, require data that are not routinely recorded. Therefore many studies considering paediatric outcomes of IUGR are retrospective and limited to investigating the less accurate surrogates for IUGR such as birthweight and birthweight for gestational duration because only these data are retrospectively available. The use of these surrogate measures of IUGR increases the number of epidemiological pitfalls in this field of research, outlined below.

Potential Confounders in Studies of the Association Between Paediatric Outcomes and Measures of Growth

The most common confounders of the study of outcomes of IUGR involve preterm births and result from attempting to control for maturity.

Selecting Cohorts using Birthweight Criteria

Many studies assessing the impact of SGA birth in preterm infants consider samples selected by birthweight criteria, such as < 1500 g. This means that older infants must be SGA in order to meet the birthweight criterion and the older they are the more growth restricted they must be. Size for gestation (a frequent measure of IUGR) is then inextricably correlated with duration of gestation, but duration of gestation is a stronger determinant of paediatric outcome than size for gestation [1]. For studies considering samples selected using birthweight criteria, the results pertaining either to intrauterine growth or to variables associated with intrauterine growth are misleading and should be ignored. Clues concerning the existence of this bias may be subtle. For example Commey and Fitzhardinge [2] selected cases using the gestational duration criterion of < 37 weeks and birthweight < –2 s. However, they were selected from referrals to an NICU and almost all were < 1500 g. If an unstated criterion for referral to the NICU were birthweight < 1500 g, as the authors suggest, there would be a strong correlation between gestational age and growth. Adjustment for gestational age in the analysis or by matching on gestation can be achieved only by going outside the sample selected using birthweight criteria.

Matching for Birthweight in Case-control Studies

Matching controls by birthweight, particularly to low birthweight cases, results in the same bias as above: growth in the controls will be inversely correlated with maturity [1].

Inadequate Control for Gestation of Delivery

To control for maturity, duration of gestation must be controlled very closely. It is not sufficient to observe that the *mean* gestation of two groups is not statistically significantly different to assume that the effects of gestation can be ignored. To avoid confounding, the *distribution* of gestational age at delivery in the groups with and without growth restriction must also be *as close as possible*, since a difference of even 1 week has a significant effect on outcome in infants born very preterm. Thus the presence of just a few subjects at the earliest gestations can have a profound effect on the incidence of infrequent suboptimal outcomes. If the most premature infants are concentrated in one group, which tends to be the AGA group given the high mortality of the extremely premature SGA infant, the comparison is biased.

The following three arguments compete with the interpretation that SGA is protective for infants born very preterm.

Control for Gestational Duration in Preterm Infants

Virtually all preterm infants have a pathological cause for their preterm birth; therefore comparing outcomes of SGA and AGA infants born very prematurely compares not one pathology with no pathology, but two different pathologies. In humans the effects of premature birth cannot be separated from those of the cause of premature birth because induction of premature birth at random is unethical and mistaken iatrogenic very preterm delivery fortunately very rare. No ideal comparison group is available.

Systematic Differences in Perinatal Care

The perinatal care of SGA infants born prematurely may differ systematically from that of AGA prematures, because the timing of the birth of a premature SGA infant is frequently easier to anticipate [3]. SGA premature births may then be more likely than AGA premature births to have planned deliveries in tertiary level facilities and to have received antenatal steroids.

Mortality

Only neonatal survivors can exhibit a paediatric outcome. Mortality increases with decreasing gestation of delivery, and more so for the SGA infant. If a very preterm SGA infant has to be otherwise healthier than an equally preterm AGA infant in order to survive, a better paediatric outcome might be anticipated. Death should always be included among the outcomes considered.

The above considerations apply primarily to studies of premature births. The following may also apply to term births.

The Cause of Growth Restriction

The causes of growth restriction are described in earlier chapters. They include: aneuploidy, congenital infection, environmental agents and social deprivation, multiple pregnancy, uteroplacental malfunction and placental anomalies. Paediatric outcome varies with causes of IUGR [4]. For example, disability is inevitable following trisomies, several congenital syndromes and untreated phenylketonuria. Several congenital infections and toxic exposures are associated with a significant risk of disability, whereas maternal hypertension and low social class are associated with minimal disabilities.

The severity and pattern of IUGR and gestation of onset may also be associated with cause. Trisomies are associated with early onset and proportionately small infants, congenital CMV infection (see Ch. 3) with microcephalic infants of normal length [4], while smoking reduces lean body mass [5].

The gestation of delivery, which is very strongly associated with paediatric outcome, is also associated with cause. Very preterm SGA birth has been reported [6] to be associated with maternal hypertension while multiple pregnancy was more commonly associated with moderately preterm birth. The incidence of chromosomal, toxic or infective causes among SGA births increased with increasing gestation of delivery but did not exceed 16 per cent. The cause of the majority of SGA births at term is often less well understood [6].

The distribution of cause in IUGR infants varies with the health and lifestyle of each population [4] so observations may not be generalisable between populations unless they are cause specific.

The heterogeneity of aetiology is appreciated. Several studies seek more homogeneous populations by excluding multiple birth, congenitally malformed or chromosomally abnormal children and/or those with recognised congenital infection. More rarely, specific causes such as pre-eclampsia are studied [7, 8].

Controlling for Factors on the Causal Path from IUGR to Outcome

The mechanisms whereby growth restriction is associated with poor pediatric outcomes are not well understood and may vary with the cause of restriction. If poor outcome is the direct result of an intervening factor to which growth restriction predisposes the fetus, it is not appropriate to control for this factor. Although such factors would be associated with both restriction and the poor outcome they are not confounders but steps in the causal path. Candidates for such intervening factors include intrapartum hypoxia, hypoglycaemia, hypothermia, neonatal complications such as necrotising enterocolitis and intraventricular haemorrhage and even gestation of delivery.

With these caveats in mind, the literature of the paediatric implications of IUGR is now reviewed.

Studies Investigating Associations Between Paediatric Outcomes and IUGR

Cohort studies can examine a wide range of outcomes, but seldom have the power to consider rare outcomes. Specific outcomes are best investigated with retrospective case-controlled studies.

Cohort Studies of Term or Predominantly Term Infants

IUGR Defined by Size

In her 1984 review of studies that frequently excluded congenital anomaly and multiple pregnancy, Allen [4] reported that SGA term infants were *at slightly increased risk of cerebral palsy and mental retardation* but *the vast majority of term SGA infants have no major handicap*. The numbers with major handicap observed in each study reviewed were small, in contrast to more frequent outcomes such as minimal brain dysfunction and school failure, for which an increased frequency among SGA infants was more apparent. Some studies found suboptimal outcomes more frequent for SGA boys than girls. Observed gender differences could have resulted from failure to adjust for gender in the assignment of birthweight percentile, resulting in more severe IUGR among selected boys than girls in some (e.g. [9, 10]) but not all (e.g. [11]) studies and gender differences were not observed in some studies that did not adjust for gender (e.g. [12, 13]).

IQ scores and school performance correlated poorly with degree of IUGR as measured by proportion of expected birthweight (PEBW)[9], which argues against a direct causal role for restriction. Socioeconomic circumstance may confound the investigation of neurodevelopment outcomes because it is associated with major [14] as well as minor suboptimal outcomes and with poor intrauterine growth. Since Allen's review [4] further studies have investigated the role of social class. Hawdon et al. [15] compared 10–11 year outcomes of 38 singleton boys born between 36 and 42 weeks' gestation below the 2nd percentile birthweight for gestation with those of a singleton control group of AGA infants matched for age and social class, where social class was estimated by father's social class and single parenthood. Two of the 38 SGA infants (5.3 per cent) were profoundly handicapped, a much (but not statistically significantly) higher proportion than anticipated in a term population. The other 36 SGA boys were very similar to their matched controls for IQ, verbal and reading quotients but showed more features reminiscent of attention deficit disorder. This observation was supported by another briefly reported Swedish study [16] which excluded subjects with signs of perinatal asphyxia. Two of 25 SGA infants, but none of 21 AGA controls matched for social class, showed signs of mental retardation or cerebral palsy at 18 months. The remaining SGA group showed more developmental and behavioural problems, with retarded cortical development and accelerated brainstem development suggesting uneven neural development relative to AGA infants.

Two studies of unselected 1960s birth cohorts measured paediatric outcomes by measures of size for gestational duration. First, Rantakallio [17] studied an unselected geographically defined Finnish cohort ($n = 12,058$). Only 14 children (0.12%) were lost to follow-up at 14 years of age and there were no exclusions of chromosomal or other congenital anomaly or infection. Below median birthweight, the proportion of children with IQ below 85 increased with decreasing percentile birthweight. Of children who had weighed more than 2 s below mean birthweight, 8 per cent had an IQ < 85 compared with 2.5 per cent of infants at or above median birthweight for gestation. This increase was composed of a steady increase in the proportion with IQ in the 50–85 range with decreasing birthweight percentile and a sharp increase in incidence of IQ < 50 among those with birthweights more than 2 s below the mean. Low birthweight for gestation percentiles were also strongly associated with poor school performance (with or without physical handicap), but not with physical handicap accompanying normal school performance.

Secondly, The National Collaborative Perinatal Project (NCPP) recruited approximately 54,000 births from several US centres and followed the children to 7 years of age. Analysis of the whole cohort by birthweight percentile [18] suggested an association of low birthweight percentiles with cerebral palsy, but not epilepsy in the absence of cerebral palsy. More thorough analysis of the Boston arm of the study ($n = 5,363$)[19, 20] reported that birthweight below the 10th percentile was significantly associated with neurological abnormality (P 0.03) although the relative risk was not high (14.45 per cent in the SGA group vs. 11.43 per cent in the AGA group). The association was slightly stronger for SGA with normal ponderal index than for SGA with low ponderal index. Neurological abnormality was also associated with head circumference < 10th percentile and length < 10th percentile at birth. While suboptimal neurological outcome was increased in infants with low birthweight percentiles, it is not clear what these outcomes consisted of.

IUGR Defined (at least Partially) by Size-Independent Criteria

Doppler-Measured Umbilical Blood flow.   Valcamonico et al. [21] measured end-diastolic flow in pregnancies in which IUGR was suspected. Mortality and neurological morbidity were associated with the Doppler findings, as shown in Table 19.1. Both mortality and severity of neurological impairment correlated inversely with flow. Trisomies were concentrated in infants with reversed or absent end-diastolic flow, while those with congenital anomalies had less severe reductions in flow.

Chan et al. [22] studied Doppler blood flow longitudinally through pregnancy for 74 antenatally recruited patients with severe growth restriction ($n = 47$), pre-eclampsia ($n = 19$), major congenital anomaly ($n = 5$) or abruptio placenta ($n = 3$). They followed postnatally only the 30 of 63 perinatal survivors who were either below 3rd percentile weight for gestation or had perinatal complications. Poor outcome was associated with the lowest flow rates.

Table 19.1 Mortality and outcome at 12–24 months by end diastolic flow [21]

| | Pattern of end diastolic flow | | Reduced | Normal |
	Reversed	Absent		
Mortality				
Numbers of subjects (%)	5	26	23	17
Trisomies {deaths}	1 {0}(20)	2 {2}(8)	0	0
Congenital anomaly {deaths}	0	0	1 {0}(4.3)	4 {3}(23.5)
Other perinatal death	2 (40)	6 (23)	1 (4.3)	1 (6)
Paediatric neurologic outcome in survivors of reversed or absent end diastolic flow and individually gestational age matched survivors with reduced or normal end diastolic flow.				
Number of subjects (%)	2	18	16	10
Major sequelae	1 (50)	2 (11.1)	1 (6.2)	0
Minor sequelae	0	2 (11.1)	0	0
Minimal	0	2 (11.1)	1 (6.2)	0
Normal	1 (50)	12 (46.2)	14 (87.5)	10 (100)

Marsál and Ley [23] measured developmental outcome in 149 7-year-old children stratified as AGA/SGA (birthweight more or less than 2 *s* below mean birthweight), maturity (term and preterm birth) and Doppler-measured end-diastolic flow measurement. Approximately half of 129 subjects estimated to be SGA at 33 weeks' gestation by routine ultrasound fetometry were born AGA. A further 20 AGA infants were added to the control group. Thus the majority of infants who were AGA at birth had been estimated antenatally to be SGA and were therefore not representative of all AGA births. Observed differences reflect chiefly the impact of continuing or more severe growth deficit compared with less severe restriction. End-diastolic blood flow abnormalities were more frequent among infants born SGA, particularly if born preterm. There were few preterm infants and the major difference in neurological outcome between SGA and AGA infants born at term was in coordination and balance.

More definitive assessment of the association between intrauterine blood flow and paediatric outcome awaits the results of neurological assessments at 2 years in the ongoing Growth Restriction Intervention Trial [24]. Doppler studies have tended to focus on infants with absent or reversed end-diastolic flow, which represents such an exceedingly compromised group of infants that the wisdom of their attempted salvage has been questioned [25]. Follow-up of infants exhibiting lesser reductions in umbilical end-diastolic flow may clarify outcomes of the less severely growth restricted, who are more numerous.

Fetal Blood pH at FBS. Soothill et al. [26] defined SGA as abdominal circumference below 5th percentile for gestational duration. They followed those delivered at more than 32 weeks of gestational for 1–5 years and assessed neurodevelopmental outcomes in relation to fetal blood pH at FBS. These criteria were chosen after confirming that the oxygen tension at FBS of SGA infants was below the gestation specific mean [27]. The correlation between developmental quotient and continuous measures of either gestation specific weight or pH deficit was measured. Three of the 64 infants had cerebral palsy: the one with the lowest pH, one with borderline and one with high pH at FBS, reflecting the heterogenous aetiology of cerebral palsy even among the SGA. Among subjects without cerebral palsy, developmental quotient correlated with deviation of pH from the mean at FBS ($r = 0.41$, $P = 0.0008$) but not with deviation of birthweight from the mean. The authors concluded that neurodevelopment was impaired in SGA fetuses with uteroplacental dysfunction sufficiently severe to cause chronic acidosis, but cautioned that the acidosis need not be the causal factor since placental dysfunction has many other nutritional and metabolic effects. It also suggests an association with cerebral palsy, since 4 per cent is a high frequency for infants delivered after 32 weeks' gestation.

Deviation of Intrauterine Head Growth.   Two studies categorised SGA cohorts born at term without major congenital abnormalities or congential infections by the gestation of onset of restriction in growth of head circumference as observed on serial ultrasound. In about 20 per cent of both cohorts, restriction commenced before 26 weeks of gestation. Ability to concentrate and school achievement [11] and development quotient at 4 years [28] were associated with age of onset. Onset of restriction before 26 weeks had significantly worse outcomes, which was seen exclusively in boys in the analysis stratified on gender [11]. Spinillo et al. [29] followed a cohort born after 33 weeks' gestation with idiopathic IUGR (excluding maternal disease, including pre-eclampsia and chronic hypertension, and fetal congenital or chromosomal anomaly). IUGR was defined as a ratio of head to abdominal circumference greater than 2 s above the mean or failure of head or abdominal circumference growth on two consecutive ultrasound scans 2 weeks apart. The study is unusual in both aetiology and definition of IUGR. Neurological outcome was examined at 2 years, stratified into three equal-sized groups by PEBW (not severity or onset of IUGR). The frequency of cerebral palsy and minor neurodevelopment impairment (not further described) tended to increase with decreasing PEBW. Despite small numbers, frequencies were significantly higher than in the control population, with an OR of 12.0 (3–49) for cerebral palsy.

In summary, cohort studies of term or predominantly term births suggest that IUGR is associated with: (a) cognitive deficit, which may be mediated through socioeconomic circumstance, (b) behavioural disturbances reminiscent of attention deficit disorder than may be more pronounced in boys and (c) although there is an increased frequency of major disability, particularly cerebral palsy, the majority of term IUGR births develop free of disability.

Cohort Studies of very Preterm Infants

As discussed previously, control for birthweight invalidates much of this literature and may be responsible for the variety of conclusions concerning the impact of growth restriction in infants born preterm [30]. Four studies are discussed: the first is very small but likely to produce valid results, the other three have possible sources of confounding.

Robertson et al. [31] compared 36 Canadian non-syndromic children without evidence of congenital infection, of < 1501 g birthweight and < 5th percentile birthweight for gestation with 36 AGA infants matched for gestational duration, gender, mother's educational grade level and father's social class as determined by occupation. The mean birthweight of the SGA group was 1226 g ($s = 236$ g) compared with 1818 g (569 g) for the gestation-matched control group. Six (17 per cent) of the SGA group were disabled compared with five (14 per cent) of the AGA group, with five (14 per cent) of the SGA having cerebral palsy compared with three (8 per cent) of the AGA group, giving a non-statistically significant OR of 1.77 (0.39–8.05). There were no differences in IQ or school performance at 8 years other than a non-significantly higher rating score on the Davids Scale of Hyperkinesis for the SGA group.

Wocadlo and Rieger [32] studied a cohort of 438 infants born at < 30 weeks' gestation. Perinatal mortality among SGA (< 10th percentile) was 64 per cent in contrast to 23 per cent in AGA infants, and postneonatal mortality was 5.3 per cent and 1.1 per cent respectively. Thus only 18 SGA survived to follow-up at 1 year. The authors compared their outcomes with 18 controls individually matched not only for gender and gestational duration but also for incidence of chronic lung disease (CLD) and head ultrasound at discharge and found four cases (22.2 per cent) of developmental abnormality in each group. If growth restriction predisposes to CLD and/or ultrasound observable cerebral damage the controls may have been overmatched: matched for factors on the causal path. While the frequency of abnormal head ultrasounds was the same for SGA and for all AGA survivors the frequency of CLD was 40.5 per cent in surviving AGA infants but 50 per cent surviving SGA infants, and CLD was also associated with poorer outcomes. The importance of this design error is difficult to quantify, but casts a shadow of doubt on the validity of the conclusion that SGA does not increase the risk of poor paediatric outcome relative to gestational age-matched controls.

Both the following studies selected children by gestational age from larger samples previously selected by birthweight. Morley et al. [33] investigated outcome at 18 months of 429 infant born at < 31 weeks selected from a larger cohort with birthweights < 1850 g. Hutton et al. [34] investigated outcome at 8–9 years of 182 infant born in Merseyside at < 33 weeks of gestation selected from a cohort of infants of < 2000 g birthweight. The assumption in both studies was that no infants delivered at or before the cut-off gestation would have been excluded by the birthweight criterion of the larger sample. It would be reassuring to know the percentile or PEBW value that the cut-off birthweight represented at the cut-off gestation. Scottish National norms published in 1986 [35] with birthweights above those from New South Wales [36] but below those from Denmark [37] or Western Australia [38] indicate a mean birthweight (and standard deviation) at 30 weeks of 1524 g (358 g) and at 32 weeks of 1843 g (371 g). Including only those < 1850 g would exclude 18 per cent of infants born at 30 weeks and including only those < 2000 g would exclude 33 per cent of infants born at 32 weeks of gestation. These may not be the appropriate reference values and it is reassuring that Morley used values generated from her sample, although her distribution of birthweight ratio for the < 31 week sample was still skewed to the left. The Merseyside study referred to Scottish standards, presumably because they were considered the most appropriate available. If significant proportions of the oldest (and most numerous) infants were excluded by the birthweight criteria, some bias will exist because the excluded infants will be the most mature with the highest birthweight ratios. In the samples, high birthweight ratio would be associated with greater prematurity, making SGA outcomes appear better than they should.

Morley et al. [33] found no association between birthweight ratio and neurodevelopment outcome at 18 months. Hutton et al. [34] excluded 15 children with clinically diagnosed motor, learning or sensory disability. Among the remaining infants, birthweight ratio was positively associated with IQ after adjusting for social class as measured by maternal education, housing satus and number of social security benefits received.

In summary, there is little valid information concerning the effect of IUGR in very preterm infants. The first study discussed suggests possible increases in hyperactivity and disability such as cerebral palsy, which is similar to findings in term born infants. Cohort studies have difficulty in attaining sufficient power for definitive answers regarding the association with rare outcomes. Whether or not chromosomal or congenital anomaly or infectious aetiologies are excluded, cohort studies show an excess of minor neurological impairments and suggest an excess of major neurological handicap among infants born SGA. Several case–control studies have investigated the latter, especially for cerebral palsy.

Case–control studies

Neurodevelopmental Disability

Taylor and Howie [39] considered 287 singleton children with neurodevelopmental disability but without a recognised syndrome born in Dundee 1974–5. They compared them with non-disabled controls born immediately before and after each index case. Disabled children were born more prematurely (16 per cent < 38 weeks compared with 7.4 per cent), to shorter, lighter mothers with a tendency to higher parity. Even adjusting for these determinants of birthweight the disabled group were smaller for gestation than controls (mean Z scores –0.42 vs. –0.21, $P = 0.0025$). Severe hypertension, unclassified antepartum haemorrhage and preterm labour were precursors in half the SGA disabled children but only a fifth of AGA disabled children or of SGA non-disabled children. Twelve disabled children had cerebral palsy; the other disabilities were not described.

Cerebral palsy

Six case–control studies of congenitally acquired cerebral palsy born 1967–90 consider measures of IUGR. Samples vary in geographical location, control group (total or selected populations), criteria for IUGR and type of cerebral palsy considered (all [40, 41], spastic type [42], dyskinetic type [43], preterm < 37 weeks [44] and very preterm < 32 weeks [45]). All but one study excluded multiple pregnancies but no other recognised causes of growth restriction were excluded. All studies were compatible with a strong association between cerebral palsy and IUGR in infants born after 33 weeks of gestation. The risk of cerebral palsy increased with decreasing PEBW [42, 41] and those at highest risk were those with evidence of most long-standing restriction [46]. The study of dyskinetic cerebral palsy found an association between birthweight more than 2 s

Table 19.2 Odds ratios for cerebral palsy in very preterm infants by IUGR from case–control studies

Study	GA* (weeks)	IUGR definition	OR	95% CI
Topp et al. [44]	28–30	< –2s#**	0.22	0.06–0.86
	31–33	< –2 s	0.83	0.35–2.0
Murphy et al. [45]	< 32	< –2 s	0.5	0.2–1.5
	< 32	AN US+***	1.0	0.9–1.1
Uvebrant et al. [40]	28–33	< –2 s	3.0	(0.8–11.2)
	28–33	< –1SD	1.3	(0.6–2.7)
Blair and Stanley [42]	< 34	3rd percentile	1.98	(0.3–9.8)
	< 34	< 10th percentile	1.48	(0.5–4.3)

*   GA, gestational age at delivery
**   Birthweight more than 2 s below mean birthweight for gestation
*** Antenatal ultrasonic diagnosis IUGR.

below the mean and dystonic but not choreoathetoid cerebral palsy. The results for more premature infants were variable, as shown in Table 19.2.

The problem of there being no satisfactory (normal) control group with which to compare very preterm SGA births remains and the variability shown above is likely to be a function of methodological differences.

Specific Causes of IUGR

Famine

Famine-induced growth restriction, independent of social class such as that seen in the Dutch Hunger winter [47], was associated with severe growth restriction, particularly with third trimester exposure. Perinatal mortality increased and the incidence of neural tube defects increased for those exposed periconceptually but there was no increase in intellectual impairment in 18-year-old survivors, nor of cerebral palsy (Ezra Susser, 1998, personal communication), though the numbers of cerebral palsy outcomes were small.

Congenital Anomalies and Infections

Many cohort studies exclude aneuploidy, congenital anomaly and congenital infection from their IUGR samples. Central nervous system congenital anomaly and both major and minor non-central nervous system congenital anomaly [48–50], maternal rubella [51], CMV infection [52] and methyl mercury exposure [53] are known antecedents of cerebral palsy that are associated with growth restriction. The role of the growth restriction in cerebral palsy aetiology is not known. Any correlation between degree of restriction and severity of outcome could be explained either because degree of growth restriction measures the severity of the common underlying disease or because there is a causal association between the growth restriction and the cerebral damage.

Multiple Pregnancy

Multiple pregnancy is another cause of IUGR strongly associated with cerebral palsy with several postulated causal mechanisms [54], few of which include growth restriction in the causal path.

No significant differences in paediatric outcome were found between heavier and lighter monozygotic co-twins [55]. Twin pairs with larger birthweight differences scored slightly lower than those with small differences. Where birthweight differences were > 15 per cent the smaller twin scored slightly higher than the heavier twin, whereas the reverse was true for pairs with smaller birthweight differences. While birthweight difference can be the result of unequal placental sharing, differences, particularly if large, may be the result of twin–twin transfusion in which the twin with higher birthweight is the plethoric recipient with characteristically poor outcome.

In uncomplicated multiple pregnancy the degree of growth restriction tends to increase with increasing duration of gestation and this partially explains our unpublished observation that risk of cerebral palsy in twins increases with increasing PEBW, because immaturity is a stronger predictor of cerebral palsy than poor growth. Among very premature births, PEBW tends to be higher for twins with cerebral palsy than for equally premature normal twin survivors, whereas the expected relationship holds with moderately premature twins for whom risk of cerebral palsy is associated with lower PEBW. At term there is no association between PEBW and risk of cerebral palsy in twins. Growth restriction may therefore be of little importance in the aetiology of suboptimal paediatric outcomes of multiple pregnancy.

Smoking

Maternal smoking decreases gestational duration very little but more than doubles the risk of SGA birth and accounts for one-fifth to one-third of SGA births, depending on smoking prevalence [56]. It was not significantly associated with major paediatric disability in the Finnish cohort study [57], which did not report whether the slight increase in disability observed among children of smokers was seen primarily in children born SGA. Associations between smoking and softer paediatric outcomes are likely to be confounded by socioeconomic circumstance. In a study of term infants without major congenital anomaly, SGA associated with smoking (and with *first* birth) decreased neurobehavioural scores less than other causes of SGA [58].

Alcohol

A Swedish study [59] found a 12-fold increase in birthweight more than 2 *s* below mean birthweight among newborn infants of alcoholic mothers. There was an increased incidence of cerebral palsy (four of 48 (8 per cent) children born to alcoholic mothers) and a very high incidence of intellectural impairment, which correlated with deficits in birthweight for gestation.

Pre-eclampsia

Pre-eclampsia and other indicators of fetal deprivation of supply are the most common precursors of growth restriction in developed countries. Spinillo et al. [7] compared neurological development at 2 years in a cohort of 78 singleton births to pre-eclamptic mothers with a control group individually matched for gestation of delivery and birthweight, thus controlling for degree of growth restriction as well as maturity and effectively comparing the outcomes of pre-eclampsia with other causes of growth restriction. Pre-eclamptic mothers smoked less, had more years of formal education, more disseminated intravascular coagulation and were more likely to be delivered by CS. Three children with intraparenchymal haemorrhage born to pre-eclamptic mothers died, and a further three had neurological abnormalities (one with severe cerebral palsy) at 2 years, compared with one perinatal death and no abnormalities at 2 years among the newborns equally mature and equally growth restricted from other causes. Thus pre-eclampsia was associated with more paediatric disability, but these differences did not reach statistical significance. The mean gestational duration of these samples was almost 37 weeks, which is likely to account for the difference between this study and the numerous studies of preterm or low birthweight infants reporting apparently protective effects of pre-eclampsia, possible explanations for which have already been discussed. Uvebrant and Hagberg [40] grouped infants exposed to pre-eclampsia, antepartum haemorrhage (APH), placental infarction and multiple pregnancy and labelled them fetal deprivation of supply (FDS). In their case–control study many more cases than controls were

SGA, but the proportion of FDS among SGA subjects was the same for both cases and controls, suggesting that FDS aetiologies of SGA were not more strongly associated with cerebral palsy than other causes of SGA.

The origin of these discrepant results may be the dates of the cohorts (1983–8 and 1975–82 respectively) if the later cohort had more survivors of severe pregnancy-induced hypertension. Yamaguchi [8] reports that infants born to mothers with onset of pre-eclampsia before 28 weeks' gestation have a higher incidence of neurological handicap than infants born to mothers with later onset of pre-eclampsia. Another explanation may lie with differences in study design. Cohort studies have high quality exposure data, enabling a narrow focus on pre-eclampsia, but are usually too small to consider rare outcomes, while retrospective case–control studies have sufficient numbers of the rare outcome, but the exposure data quality is often poor, necessitating grouping of somewhat similar exposures.

To determine the impact of pre-eclampsia, it must be remembered that, since preterm delivery is usually a direct result of the pre-eclampsia, often through iatrogenic intervention, control for gestation of delivery is inappropriate. The relative risk of cerebral palsy with pre-eclampsia in Western Australia adjusted for multiple pregnancy but not for gestational duration is greater than unity at 1.4 [3].

Does the Risk of Impairment Vary Intrinsically with Cause or Is It Mediated only Through Severity and Timing of Growth Restriction?

In Swedish cases of cerebral palsy following intrauterine infection or chromosomal or genetic anomaly the proportion who were SGA or had evidence of fetal deprivation of supply was the same as in cerebral palsy cases without such causes [40]. Kramer et al. [60] found no convincing evidence that neonatal outcome among infants with a given degree of growth restriction was a function of the cause of the growth restriction, but subjects with chromosomal anomalies, major malformations, congenital infections or multiple birth were excluded. No significant variations in risk of spastic cerebral palsy in SGA infants by putative cause of SGA were found in Western Australia [42], but numbers for each cause were very small. In this same study no cases but several controls with congenital anomaly were below third centile birthweight for gestation. Perhaps the malformed fetus with cerebral damage who is also SGA is less likely to survive? The importance of cause of IUGR, independent of degree of restriction, to outcome seems almost self-evident, but little evidence is available.

Intermediate Factors on Causal Paths of IUGR to Poor Paediatric Outcome

There are several possible mechanisms whereby restricted growth may be associated with poor paediatric outcomes.

1. Specific causes (C) of restricted growth such as central nervous system malformations may directly cause poor paediatric outcome (PPO) and the growth restriction is then incidental.

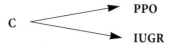

2. For cerebral palsy (**CP**), the central motor defects responsible may conceivably decrease growth rate, for example, by decreasing fetal movement.

$$\text{Central motor defects (CP)} \longrightarrow \text{IUGR}$$

3. A direct (intrinsic) consequence of growth restriction (**X**) may be responsible for cerebral damage.

$$C \longrightarrow IUGR \longrightarrow X \longrightarrow PPO$$

4. Growth restriction may increase vulnerability to another (extrinsic) factor (**Y**) that is the immediate cause of poor outcome.

$$C \longrightarrow IUGR \left.\begin{array}{l} Y \\ \text{and} \\ IUGR \end{array}\right\} \longrightarrow PPO$$

Mechanisms three and four are differentiated because extrinsic factors should be more avoidable that intrinsic factors but they are closely allied. Y, for example, could be hypoglycaemia occurring without further outside influence, but the degree of hypoglycaemia is dependent on the energy demands placed on the fetus, which could have an extrinsic source, the most likely being intrapartum stress. The idea that the undernourished fetus with low glycogen reserves is less able to withstand the hypoxic stress of labour is plausible and the role of intrapartum stress in SGA outcomes has been investigated in several studies. Dijxhoorn et al. [61] found that indicators of antepartum stress were better predictors of neonatal neurological morbidity than those of intrapartum stress and concluded that intrapartum stress did not substantially increase the risk of neurological morbidity associated with SGA. Blair and Stanley [42] came to the same conclusion estimating that, while 22 per cent of spastic cases could be attributed to being below to 10th percentile birthweight, only 2 per cent could be attributed to the combination of SGA and intrapartum hypoxia. Uvebrant and Hagberg [40] concluded that SGA infants were at lower risk of cerebral palsy as a result of intrapartum hypoxia than were AGA infants. In contrast, Berg [19] and Kyllerman [43] found that only SGA infants who exhibited signs of perinatal stress were at increased risk of childhood neurological morbidity or dystonic cerebral palsy. However, the clinical criteria from which intrapartum stress was inferred were low Apgar scores [43], requirement for resuscitation, cord knots or placenta previa [19], which may well be either the cause or the result of chronic stress and are not specific to intrapartum stress [62].

Other possible intermediate factors include meconium aspiration, hypothermia, hypoglycaemia [8, 63], polycythenia, hypocalcaemia, cerebral lesions [64, 65], damage massive pulmonary haemorrhage and even iatrogenic very preterm birth.

Conclusions

Growth restriction is defined conceptually and epidemiologically satisfactory criteria are difficult to devise. It is almost always inferred from deficits of size for gestational age, but size independent criteria are becoming more widely used.

Using primarily measures of size deficit, growth restriction has been associated with an increase in the risk of both major and minor neurological sequelae in term and moderately preterm infants. Differences in social class are likely to explain the increased risks of some aspects of poor school performance but not behavioural disturbances related to attention deficit disorder and hyperactivity. The relative risk of cerebral palsy and severe intellectual handicap increases with increasing birthweight deficit but, since these outcomes are rare, the majority of SGA infants are not affected.

Designing valid studies of effect of IUGR in infants born very preterm is difficult because there is no ideal comparison group, the effects of IUGR are overshadowed by those of prematurity and the severity of the disease underlying the growth restriction is likely to be correlated with the degree of prematurity.

It is intuitively appealing to differentiate between different aetiologies of restricted growth when studying its sequelae and this may be appropriate, particularly for malformations of the central nervous system and infections directly affecting the brain. However, observed differences in outcome between aetiologies may be mediated by differences in timing of onset and severity of restriction, timing of delivery and social class distribution.

References

1. Blair E. The undesirable consequences of controlling for birth weight in perinatal epidemiological studies. J Epidemiol Commun Health 1996;50:559–563.
2. Commey JOO, Fitzhardinge PM. Handicap in the preterm small-for-gestational age infant. J Pediatr 1979;94:779–86.
3. Blair E. Cerebral palsy in very low birthweight infants, pre-eclampsia and magnesium sulphate. Pediatrics 1996;97:780–1.
4. Allen MC. Developmental outcome and follow up of the small for gestational age infant. Semin Perinatol 1984;8:123–56.
5. Lindsay C, Thomas A, Catalano P. The effect of smoking tobacco on neonatal body composition. Am J Obstet Gynecol 1997;177:1124–8.
6. Lapillonne A, Peretti N, Ho P, Claris O, Salle B. Aetiology, morphology and body composition of infants born small for gestational age. Acta Paediatr 1997;Suppl 423:172–6.
7. Spinillo A, Stonati M, Ometto A, Fazzi E Lanzi G, Guaschino S. Infant neurodevelopmental outcome in pregnancies complicated by gestational hypertension and intra-uterine growth retardation. J Perinat Med 1993;35:45–54.
8. Yamaguchi K, Mishina J, Mitsuishi C, Nakabayashi M, Nishida H. Neonatal hypoglycaemia in infants with intrauterine growth retardation due to pregnancy-induced hypertension. Acta Paediatr Japon 1997;39(Suppl 1):S48–50.
9. Fitzhardinge PM, Steven EM. The Small-for-Date Infant I. Later Growth Patterns. Pediatrics 1972;49:671–81.
10. Neligan G, Kolvin I, Scott D, Garside R. Born too soon or born too small. London: Heinemann 1976.
11. Parkinson C, Wallis S, Harvey D. School achievement and behaviour of children who were small-for-dates at birth. Dev Med Child Neurol 1981;23:41–50.
12. Low JA, Galbraith RS, Muir D, Killen H. Pater B, Karchmar J. Intrauterine growth retardation: A study of long-term mobidity. Am J Obstet Gynecol 1982;142:670–7.
13. Rubin R, Rosenblatt C, Balow B. Psychological and educational sequelae of prematurity. Pediatrics 1973;52:352–63.
14. Dowding VM, Barry C. Cerebral palsy: social class differences in prevalence in relation to birth-weight and severity of disability. J Epidemiol Commun Health 1990;44:191–5.
15. Hawdon JM, Hey E, Kolvin I, Fundudis T. Born too small – is outcome still affected? Dev Med Child Neurol 1990;32:943–53.
16. Kjellmer I, Liedholm M, Sultan B, Wennergren M, Götborg CW, Thordstein M. Long-term effects of intrauterine growth retardation. Acta Paediatr 1997;86(Suppl 422):83–4.

17. Rantakallio P. A 14-year follow-up of children with normal and abnormal birth weight for their gestational age. Acta Paediatr 1985;74:62–9.
18. Ellenberg JH, Nelson KB. Birth weight and gestational age in children with cerebral palsy or seizure disorders. Am J Dis Child 1979;133:1044–8.
19. Berg AT. Childhood neurological morbidity and its association with gestational age, intrauterine growth retardation and perinatal stress. Paediatr Perinat Epidemiol 1988;2:229–39.
20. Berg AT. Indices of fetal growth-retardation, perinatal hypoxia-related factors and childhood neurological morbidity. Early Hum Dev 1989;19:271–83.
21. Valcamonico A, Danti L, Frusca T, Soregaroli M, Zucca S, Abrami F, et al. Absent end-diastolic velocity in umbilical artery: risk of neonatal morbidity and brain damage. Am J Obstet Gynecol 1994;170:796–801.
22. Chan FY, Pun TC, Lam P, Lam C, Lee CP, Lam YH. Fetal cerebral Doppler studies as a predictor of perinatal outcome and subsequent neurologic handicap. Obstet Gynecol 1996;87:981–8.
23. Marsál K, Ley D. Intrauterine blood flow and postnatal neurological development in growth-retarded fetuses. Biol Neonate 1992;62:258–64.
24. GRIT. When do obstetricians recommend delivery for a high-risk preterm growth-retarded fetus? Eur J Obstet Gynecol Reprod Biol 1996;67:121–6.
25. Kingdom J, Rodeck C, Kaufmann P. Umbilical artery Doppler – more harm than good? Br J Obstet Gynaecol 1997;104:393–6.
26. Soothill PW, Ajayi RA, Campbell S, Ross EM, Nicolaides KH. Fetal oxygenation at cordocentesis, maternal smoking and childhood neuro-development. Eur J Obstet Gynecol Reprod Biol 1995;59:21–4.
27. Soothill PW, Nicolaides KH, Campbell S. Prenatal asphyxia, hyperlacticaemia, hypoglacaemia, and erythroblastosis in growth retarded fetuses. BMJ 1987;294:1051–3.
28. Fancourt R, Campbell S, Harvey D, Norman AP. Follow-up study of small-for-dates babies. BMJ 1976;1:1435–7.
29. Spinillo A, Capuzzo E, Egbe TO, Fazzi E, Colonna L, Nicola S. Pregnancies complicated by idiopathic intrauterine growth retardation: Severity of growth failure, neonatal morbidity and two-year infant neurodevelopmental outcome. J Reprod Med 1995;40:209–15.
30. Henderson-Smart DJ. Postnatal consequences of chronic intrauterine compromise. Reprod Fertil Dev 1995;7:559–65.
31. Robertson C, Etches P, Kyle J. Eight-year school performance and growth of preterm, small for gestational age infants: A comparative study with subjects matched for birth weight or for gestational age. J Pediatr 1990;116:19–26.
32. Wocadlo C, Rieger I. Developmental outcome at 12 months corrected age for infants born less than 30 weeks gestation: influence of reduced intrauterine and postnatal growth. Early Hum Dev 1994;39:127–37.
33. Morley R, Brooke O, Cole T, Powell R, Lucas A. Birthweight ratio and outcome in preterm infants. Arch Dis Child 1990;65:30–4.
34. Hutton JL, Pharoah POD, Cooke RWI, Stevenson RC. Differential effects of preterm birth and small gestational age on cognitive and motor development. Arch Dis Child 1997;76:F75–81.
35. Dickson D, Forbes J. Birthweight crown-heel length and head circumference standards for 24 to 42 weeks gestation. Glasgow: Social Paediatric and Obstetric Research Unit, University of Glasgow, 1986.
36. Beeby PJ, Bhutap T, Taylor LK. New South Wales population-based birthweight percentile charts. J Paediatr Child Health 1996;32:512–18.
37. Ulrich M. Fetal growth in a population of Danish newborns, part I. Acta Paediatr Scand 1982;Suppl 292:5–17.
38. Blair E, Stanley F. Intra-uterine growth charts. Canberra; Australian Government Publishing Service, 1985.
39. Taylor DJ, Howie PW. Fetal growth achievement and neurodevelopmental disability. Br J Obstet Gynaecol 1989;96:789–94.
40. Uvebrant P, Hagberg G. Intrauterine growth in children with cerebral palsy. Acta Paediatr 1992;81:407–12.
41. Palmer L, Petterson B, Blair E, Burton P. Family patterns of gestational age at delivery and growth in utero in moderate and severe cerebral palsy. Dev Med Child Neurol 1994;36: 1108–19.
42. Blair E, Stanley FJ. Intrauterine growth and spastic cerebral palsy I. Association with birth weight for gestational age. Am J Obstet Gynecol 1990;162:229–37.
43. Kyllerman M. Dyskinetic cerebral palsy II. Pathogenetic risk factors and intra-uterine growth. Acta Paediatr Scand 1982;71:551–8.

44. Topp M, Langhoff-Roos J, Uldall P, Kristensen J. Intrauterine growth and gestational age in preterm infants with cerebral palsy. Early Hum Dev 1996;44:27–36.

45. Murphy DJ, Sellers S, MacKenzie IZ, Yudkin PL, Johnson M. Case–control study of antenatal and intrapartum risk factors for cerebral palsy in very preterm singleton babies. Lancet 1995;346:1449–54.

46. Blair E, Stanley FJ. Intrauterine growth and spastic cerebral palsy II. The association with morphology at birth. Early Hum Dev 1992;28:91–103.

47. Susser M. Timing in prenatal nutrition: A reprise of the Dutch Famine Study. Nutr Rev 1994;52:84–94.

48. Nelson KB, Ellenburg JH. Antecedents of seizure disorders in early childhood. Am J Dis Child 1986;140:1053–61.

49. Blair E, Stanley FJ. When can cerebral palsy be prevented? The generation of causal hypotheses by multivariate analysis of a case-control study. Paediatr Perinat Epidemiol 1993;7:272–301.

50. Coorssen EA, Msall ME, Duffy LC. Multiple minor malformations as a marker for prenatal etiology for cerebral palsy. Dev Med Child Neurol 1991;33:730–6.

51. Stanley F, Sim M, Wilson GS. The decline in congenital rubella syndrome in Western Australia: an impact of the school girl vaccination program? Aus J Public Health 1986;76(1):35–7.

52. Hagberg B, Hagberg G, Olow I, von Wendt L. The changing panorama of cerebral palsy in Sweden. VII. Prevalence and origin in the birth year period 1987–90. Octa Paediatr 1996;85:954–60.

53. Amin-Zaki L, Majeed MA, Elhassani SB, Clarkson TW, Greenwood MR, Doherty RA. Prenatal methylmercury poisoning. Clinical observations over five years. Am J Dis Child 1979;133:172–7.

54. Petterson B, Blair E, Watson L, Stanley F. Adverse outcome after multiple pregnancy. Bailliere's Clin Obstet Gynecol 1998;12:1–17.

55. Fujikura T, Froehlich LA. Mental and motor development in monozygotic co-twins with dissimilar birth weights. Pediatrics 1974;53:884–9.

56. Kramer MS. Determinants of low-birth weight: Methodological assessment and meta-analysis. Bull World Health Organ 1987;65:663–737.

57. Rantakallio P, Koiranen M. Neurological handicaps among children whose mothers smoked during pregnancy. Prev Med 1987;16:597–606.

58. Ounsted M, Moar VA, Scott A. Neurological development of small for gestational age babies during the first year of life. Early Hum Dev 1988;16:163–72.

59. Olegård R, Sabel K-g, Aronsson M, Sandin B, Johnsson PR, Carlsson C, et al. Effects on the child of alcohol abuse during pregnancy: Retrospective and prospective studies. Acta Paediatr Scand 1979;Suppl 274:112–21.

60. Kramer MS, Olivier M, McLean FH, Willis DM, Usher RH. Impact of intrauterine growth retardation and body proporionality on fetal and neonatal outcome. Pediatrics 1990;86:707–13.

61. Dijxhoorn MJ, Visser GHA, Touwen BCL, Huisjes HJ. Apgar score, meconium and acidaemia at birth in small-for-gestational age infants born at term, and their relation to neonatal neurological morbidity. Br J Obstet Gynaecol 1987;94:873–9.

62. Blair E, A research definition for "birth asphyxia"? Dev Med Child Neurol 1993;35:449–55.

63. Lucas A, Morley R, Cole T. Adverse neurodevelopment outcome of moderate neonatal hypoglycaemia. BMJ 1988;297:1304–8.

64. Gaffney G, Squier M, Johnson A, Flavell V, Sellers S. Clinical associations of prenatal ischaemic white matter injury. Arch Dis Child 1994;70:F101–6.

65. Burke C, Tannenberg A, Payton D. Ischaemic cerebral injury, intrauterine growth retardation and placental infarction. Dev Med Child Neurol 1997;39:726–30.

20 Long Term Implications for Adult Health

Rebecca M. Reynolds and Keith M. Godfrey

Introduction

Recent research suggests that a number of the major diseases of later life, including coronary heart disease, hypertension and non-insulin-dependent diabetes, originate through restriction of intrauterine growth and development. These diseases may be consequences of "programming", whereby a stimulus or insult at a critical, sensitive period of early life has permanent effects on body size and proportions, and on a range of physiological processes. Evidence that coronary heart disease, hypertension and diabetes are programmed came from longitudinal studies of men and women in which size at birth was related to the occurrence of the disease in middle age. People who were small or disproportionate (thin or short) at birth had high rates of coronary heart disease, raised blood pressure and cholesterol levels, and abnormal glucose–insulin metabolism. Constraint of intrauterine growth and development seems to be widespread in the population, affecting many babies whose birthweights are within the normal range. Although the influences that impair fetal development and programme adult cardiovascular disease remain to be defined, there are strong pointers to the importance of the maternoplacental capacity to satisfy the fetal nutrient requirement. Maternal nutrition can exert important effects on both the fetal nutrient demand and the maternoplacental supply capacity and may have hitherto unrecognised effects on both intrauterine development and health in later adult life.

The Concept of Programming During Early Development

During prenatal growth and development, tissues of the body grow during periods of rapid cell division. Stimuli applied at these "critical periods" of early life may alter expression of the fetal genome, leading to permanent effects on a range of physiological processes. This phenomenon is termed fetal "programming" [1]. Growth depends on nutrients and oxygen, and the fetus's main adaptation to lack of these is to slow its rate of cell division, especially in those tissues that are undergoing critical periods at the time. Even brief periods of undernutrition may permanently reduce the number of cells in particular organs and hence programme the body. Other lasting memories of fetal undernutrition include changes in the distribution of cell types, hormonal feedback, metabolic activity and organ structure [2,3].

Experimental studies in animals have shown that fetal undernutrition can programme permanent changes in blood pressure, cholesterol metabolism, insulin secretion and a range of other metabolic, endocrine and immune parameters important in human disease. For example, lifelong elevation of blood pressure in the offspring has resulted from both maternal uterine artery ligation in guinea pigs [4] and feeding pregnant rats a low protein diet during pregnancy [5].

In humans, only recently has it become apparent that some of the body's memories of early undernutrition become translated into pathology and thereby determine disease in later life. The "fetal origins" hypothesis proposes that adaptations made by the fetus in response to undernutrition lead to permanent changes in physiology and metabolism, which in turn predispose to cardiovascular, metabolic and endocrine diseases in adult life. Rickets serves as an unquestionable example of the fact that the structure of the human body can be programmed by undernutrition.

Fetal Growth and Adult Cardiovascular Disease

Coronary Heart Disease

For some time it had been argued that events in childhood might influence the pathogenesis of adult coronary heart disease [6]. The suggestion that the *intrauterine* environment may exert important long term effects on coronary heart disease susceptibility offered, however, a new point of departure for research. This hypothesis originated from studies of death rates among babies born in Britain during the early 1900s [7]. The usual certified cause of death in newborn babies at that time was low birthweight. Neonatal death rates differed considerably between one part of the country and another, being highest in some of the northern industrial towns and the poorer rural areas in the north and west. This geographical pattern in death rates was shown to resemble closely today's large variations in death rates from coronary heart disease, variations that form one aspect of the continuing north–south divide in health in Britain [7]. One possible conclusion suggested by this observation was that low rates of growth before birth are linked to the development of coronary heart disease in adult life.

The early epidemiological studies that pointed to the likely importance of programming in coronary heart disease were based on the strategy of following up men and women in middle and late life whose body measurements at birth had been recorded. The groups of birth records utilised in the initial studies in the UK came from Hertfordshire, Preston and Sheffield, and were identified as a result of the Medical Research Council's systematic search of archives and records offices. The Hertfordshire records were maintained by health visitors and included measurements of growth in infancy and details of infant feeding as well as birthweight for all babies born in the county from 1911 onwards. In Preston and Sheffield detailed obstetric records documented body proportions at birth [8,9].

A follow-up study of men and women born in Hertfordshire showed for the first time that those who had had low birthweights had increased death rates from

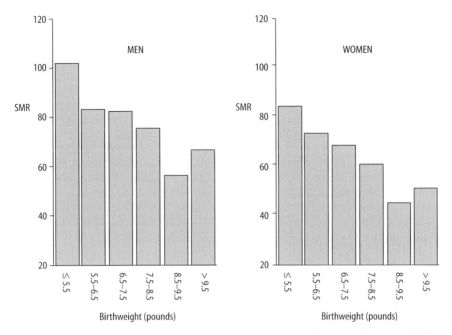

Fig. 20.1 Coronary heart disease death rates, expressed as standardised mortality ratios (SMR), in 15,726 men and women born in Hertfordshire, UK.

coronary heart disease in adult life [10]. Thus, among 15,726 men and women born during 1911–30, death rates from coronary heart disease fell progressively with increasing birthweight in both men and women (Fig. 20.1). A small rise at the highest birthweights could relate to the macrosomic infants of women with gestational diabetes. Another study, of 1,586 men born in Sheffield during 1907–25, showed that it was particularly people who were small at birth as a result of growth restriction, rather than those born prematurely, who were at increased risk of the disease [9]. The association between low birthweight and coronary heart disease has now been confirmed in studies of 80,000 nurses in the USA [11], of men in South Wales [12] and of men and women in Mysore, South India [13].

The trends in coronary heart disease with birthweight have been found to be paralleled by similar trends in two of its major risk factors – raised blood pressure and non-insulin-dependent diabetes [14,15].

Raised Blood Pressure and Hypertension

A systematic review of 34 studies examining the relation between birthweight and blood pressure in different populations around the world found strong support for an association between low birthweight and higher blood pressure in prepubertal children and adults [16]. The relationship was less consistently found in adolescence, perhaps because the tracking of blood pressure is perturbed by the adolescent growth spurt. Similarly to coronary heart disease, raised blood pressure is found in people who were SGA rather than those born prematurely.

Follow-up studies of men and women who had more detailed neonatal anthropo-metric measurements have shown that those who were disproportionate (thin or short) at birth also tend to have raised blood pressure and a greater risk of hypertension in adult life [17].

One response to the demonstration of associations between low birthweight and adult cardiovascular risk factors has been to argue that people who were exposed to an adverse environment in utero and failed to grow continue to be exposed to an adverse environment in childhood and adult life, and it is this later adverse environment that produces the effects attributed to programming in utero. There is, however, little evidence to support this argument. Rather, associations between birthweight and raised adult blood pressure, for example, are found in each social group, and are independent of influences such as smoking, alcohol intake and obesity in adult life [18].

Metabolic and Endocrine Disease

Non-insulin-dependent Diabetes and Insulin Resistance

Associations between low birthweight and altered glucose metabolism have been demonstrated in nine studies of adult men and women in Europe, the USA and Australia [19]. The prevalence of non-insulin-dependent diabetes and impaired glucose tolerance falls progressively between those who were small and those who were large at birth. The trends are strong, as illustrated by a study of 370 men aged 65 years born in Hertfordshire, shown in Table 20.1. The prevalence of non-insulin-dependent diabetes and impaired glucose tolerance fell from 40 per cent among those who weighed 5.5 pounds (2.54 kg) or less at birth to 14 per cent among those who weighed 9.5 pounds (4.31 kg) or more [14].

As for raised blood pressure, the associations between birthweight and later glucose tolerance are independent of adult lifestyle influences [18]. Adult obesity does, however, add to the intrauterine effects, such that the highest prevalence of non-insulin-dependent diabetes and impaired glucose tolerance is seen in people who were small at birth but obese as adults [14,20].

There is some evidence that a reduced number of pancreatic ß cells, and hence a reduced capacity to make insulin, may result in people who had had low

Table 20.1 Prevalence of non-insulin dependent diabetes (NIDDM) and impaired glucose tolerance in 370 men aged 59–70 years

Birthweight in pounds (kg)	Number of men	% with NIDDM or impaired glucose tolerance	Odd ratio* (95% CI)
< 5.5 (2.54)	20	40	6.6 (1.5–28)
5.5–6.5 (2.95)	47	34	4.8 (1.3–17)
6.5–7.5 (3.41)	104	31	4.6 (1.4–16)
7.5–8.5 (3.86)	117	22	2.6 (0.8–8.9)
8.5–9.5 (4.31)	54	13	1.4 (0.3–5.6)
> 9.5 (4.31)	28	14	1.0
All	370	25	

* Adjusted for current BMI.

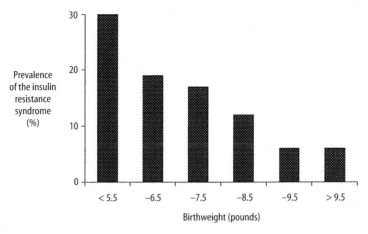

Fig. 20.2 Prevalence (%) of the insulin resistance syndrome in 407 Hertfordshire men aged 59–70 years.

birthweight being less able to withstand the stress of adult obesity. However, there is stronger evidence of insulin resistance in adults who experienced growth restriction in utero [21,22]. Further studies of Hertfordshire men showed that low birthweight was associated with the combination of impaired glucose tolerance, raised blood pressure and disturbed lipoprotein metabolism coinciding in the same patient, the so-called "insulin resistance syndrome" [22]. Fig. 20.2 shows that the prevalence of the insulin resistance syndrome fell from 30 per cent among those who weighed 5.5 pounds or less at birth to 6 per cent among those who weighed 9.5 pounds or more. Biochemically, the syndrome is characterised by raised serum insulin concentrations and it leads to coronary heart disease. Studies in Preston showed that it is particularly thinness at birth, measured by a low PI (birthweight/length^3), that is associated with a raised serum insulin concentration and its associated disorders in later life [22]. This observation has recently been confirmed in Sweden [20]. Insulin tolerance tests in a group of 103 men and women aged 47–56 years born in Preston provided more direct evidence that thinness at birth is associated with insulin resistance in adult life (Table 20.2) [21]; those who had a low PI at birth had a slower fall in blood glucose after an insulin challenge.

Table 20.2 Mean insulin resistance in 103 men and women aged 47–56 years

PI at birth (oz/in^3 × 1000)	No. of subjects	Insulin resistance* (min)
≤ 12.00	26	20.6
12.01–13.25	37	17.3
13.26–14.75	23	17.9
> 14.75	17	16.6
P for trend		*0.01*

* Half-life of blood glucose during an insulin tolerance test.

Cholesterol Metabolism and Blood Coagulation

Studies in Sheffield showed that neonates within the normal range of birthweight but with altered body proportions at birth, particularly a small AC and short body in relation to head size, have persisting disturbances of cholesterol metabolism and blood coagulation [23,24]. Disproportion in body length relative to head size is thought to result from cranial redistribution of oxygenated blood away from the trunk to sustain the brain using an adaptive response present in mammals [25]. This affects the growth of the liver, two of whose functions, regulation of cholesterol and of blood clotting, seem to be permanently perturbed [23,24]. Disturbance of cholesterol metabolism and blood clotting are both important features of coronary heart disease.

The Sheffield records included AC at birth and it was particularly reduction in this birth measurement that predicted raised serum low density lipoprotein cholesterol and plasma fibrinogen concentrations in adult life [23]. The differences in LDL concentrations across the range of AC were large: statistically equivalent to a 30 per cent difference in mortality caused by coronary heart disease. The findings for plasma fibrinogen concentrations, a measure of blood coagulability, were of similar magnitude [24].

Following on from these epidemiological observations, recent animal studies support the hypothesis that impaired fetal liver growth may be associated with reprogramming of hepatic metabolism. If pregnant guinea pigs are fed a restricted diet, their offspring have altered body proportions, with reduction in body size in relation to head size; as adults, the offspring exhibit profound elevation of serum cholesterol concentrations if fed a high cholesterol diet [26]. Experiments on rats have shown that undernutrition in utero can permanently alter the balance of the liver enzymes, phosphoenol-pyruvate carboxykinase and glucokinase, which are involved in the synthesis and breakdown of glucose respectively [27]. Feeding pregnant rats an isocaloric low protein diet changes the balance of enzyme activity in the offspring in favour of synthesis; the same diet during postnatal life has no effect on hepatic glucose metabolism [27]. It is thought that the long term effects of the low protein diet during gestation reflect enhancement of cell replication in the area around the portal vein at the expense of the cells around the hepatic vein.

Polycystic Ovary Syndrome

Although the clinical presentations and endocrinology of women with polycystic ovary syndrome are heterogeneous, two common profiles are of women with normal body weight and high serum LH concentrations, compared with women of excess body weight, androgenisation and high concentrations of plasma LH and testosterone [28]. The pathophysiology is not understood but there is evidence from both animal and human experiments suggesting that the syndrome may originate during intrauterine development.

Experimental studies in rats have shown that the pattern of gonadotrophin release by the hypothalamus is programmed by the concentration of androgens during early development [29,30]. Female rats exposed to high androgen concentrations have persisting changes in reproductive physiology, including anovulatory sterility and polycystic ovaries [31,32]. A recent study of 235 women aged 40–42 years born in Sheffield suggested that the two common forms of poly-cystic ovary syndrome may have different origins in intrauterine life [33]. Thin women with polycystic ovaries were more likely to have been born post-term and one possibility is that this could have resulted in altered hypothalamic control of LH release. Obese, hirsute women with polycystic ovaries and increased ovarian secretion of androgens tended to be of higher birthweight and to have mothers with a high BMI in pregnancy. Although more studies are needed, this does provide further evidence that patterns of hormone release and tissue sensitivity established in utero have an important influence on the development of adult disease.

Mechanisms Linking Fetal Programming with Adult Disease

Skeletal Muscle Metabolism

While the mechanisms linking restriction of fetal growth with impaired glucose tolerance and diabetes in adult life are not fully understood, there is some evidence that changes in skeletal muscle metabolism may be important. In addition to their tendency to be insulin resistant, people who were thin at birth also tend to have metabolic changes in adult life suggestive of a bias towards fuel conservation, and it has been proposed that these could indicate persistence of a fetal glucose-conserving adaptation [19].

In fetal life, insulin has a key role in stimulating cell division via the glucose–insulin–IGF-I axis [34] and insulin resistance in specific tissues, such as skeletal muscle, might conserve glucose by reducing growth. In the short term such an adaptation would result in diminished muscle mass and thinness at birth; as skeletal muscle is a major peripheral site of action of insulin in adult life, persistence of such insulin resistance could, however, result in a range of metabolic abnormalities. Magnetic resonance spectroscopy using ^{31}P has shown that adults who were thin at birth have reduced rates of glycolysis and glycolytic adenosine triphosphate (ATP) production in skeletal muscle [35]; other studies using stable isotopes and indirect calorimetry suggest they have an increased rate of fat oxidation [36,37].

Adrenocortical and Sympathoadrenal Hormonal Activity

Recent animal studies and preliminary evidence in humans suggests that impaired fetal nutrient supply may also lead to permanent alterations in fetal neuroendocrine development, resulting in long term changes in the setpoint of adrenocortical and sympathoadrenal hormonal activity. Any such changes may cause persisting alterations in both stress responses and metabolism as gluco-corticoids and sympathoadrenal hormones have potent biological effects adversely affecting carbohydrate metabolism and raising blood pressure. Exposure of pregnant rats to a variety of stressors, including low protein diets, alcohol, or non-abortive infections, increases hypothalamic–pituitary–adrenal axis (HPAA) activity and leads to an exaggerated cortisol response to stress in the offspring in adult life [38,39]. It is thought that these effects are mediated by excessive fetal glucocorticoid exposure, resulting in persisting alterations in HPAA activity. In rats these effects can be mimicked by prenatal treatment with dexamethasone, which leads to permanently increased activity of the HPAA and increased concentrations of circulating glucocorticoids. This is probably because of lifelong alterations in the numbers of glucocorticoid receptors in the hippo-campus, an important site of negative feedback control. In adult life the rats are hypertensive and glucose intolerant [40,41].

It is currently unknown whether the link between maternal exposure to low protein diets or other stressors and programming of the HPAA is mediated by fetal or maternal glucocorticoids. Evidence that maternal glucocorticoids may be important derives from animal experiments showing that the effect of maternal protein restriction on blood pressure in the offspring is abolished by maternal adrenalectomy or the administration of metyrapone during gestation [42]. Preliminary evidence suggests that maternal protein restriction during pregnancy may increase fetal exposure to maternal cortisol by reducing the levels of the enzyme 11β-hydroxysteroid dehydrogenase, which normally forms a placental barrier to maternal glucocorticoids [43].

Increased fetal glucocorticoid exposure leads not only to long term changes in glucocorticoid-inducible enzymes, but also to alterations in sympathoadrenal

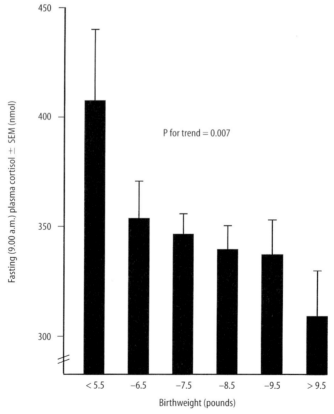

Fig. 20.3 Fasting plasma cortisol according to birthweight in 370 Hertfordshire men.

function. The latter has been demonstrated in rat experiments in which maternal glucocorticoid administration altered the differentiation of autonomic neurones and the development of adrenergic receptors and their coupling to cell transduction mechanisms [44,45].

Despite this body of animal evidence, there are as yet few studies in human populations. Evidence for programming of adrenocortical activity comes from observations that low birthweight fetuses not only have increased cortisol concentrations in umbilical cord blood, but also tend to have raised cortisol excretion in childhood [46]. That such effects may persist into adult life is suggested by a study of 60-year-old men showing that birthweight is inversely related to adult fasting plasma cortisol concentrations [47] (Fig. 20.3). Evidence for programming of sympathoadrenal function comes from the observation that resting pulse rate, an indicator of increased sympathetic nervous system activity, is raised in subjects with low birthweight [48].

Effects at Different Stages of Development

The varying critical periods during which organs and systems mature indicate that an adverse intrauterine environment at different developmental stages is likely to have specific short and long term effects. A critical period for gonadal development exists, for example, very early in gestation [49], as compared with a critical period for renal development later in gestation between 26 and 34 weeks of pregnancy [50].

Babies who are symmetrically small, short or thin are thought to have been exposed to fetal undernutrition at different stages in gestation, and follow-up studies indicate that they are predisposed to different disorders in adult life [18]. Proportionately small babies are at increased risk of raised adult blood pressure, but do not appear to develop coronary heart disease. By downregulating growth in response to undernutrition *early* in development the fetus may reduce its demand for nutrients, so making it less likely to subsequently experience relative undernutrition in late gestation [51]. The abnormalities of adult cholesterol metabolism and clotting factor synthesis in individuals who had a small AC and were disproportionately short at birth [23,24] may reflect effects on liver development resulting from cranial redistribution of blood *later in gestation* [25]. Thin babies at increased risk of the insulin resistance syndrome in adult life are thought to have reduced subcutaneous fat and skeletal muscle in consequence of fetal undernutrition in the *weeks prior to delivery* [51].

As might be expected, the predominant phenotype of fetal growth restriction and the mix of babies with different types vary greatly in different populations both around the world and within the United Kingdom. For example, data collected in the WHO study of lactational amenorrhoea have shown that babies born in China tend to be proportionately small, with symmetrical reduction of their skeletal proportions and a high PI, whereas thin babies predominate in India [51]. The long term consequences of these patterns of fetal growth restriction may contribute to geographical variations in the prevalence of coronary heart disease.

One important aspect of timing is that effects manifested late in pregnancy may commonly originate much earlier in gestation. Studies of the Dutch Hunger

Winter famine of 1944–5 [52] led to the dogma that thinness at birth, for example, results from influences operating in the last trimester of pregnancy. Animal and human studies both indicate that fetal undernutrition late in pregnancy is, however, more commonly a consequence of an inadequate materno-placental supply capacity set up much earlier in gestation [53,54]. Thus, while the short and long term effects of an acute severe famine are of great scientific importance, we must be aware that they could result in erroneous conclusions about timing in the non-famine situation.

Influences Underlying Fetal Programming

Determinants of Fetal Growth

As small size at birth and disproportion in head size, length and weight are thought to be surrogate markers for the influences that programme the human fetus, consideration of the principal determinants of fetal growth is important. The relative contributions of the intrauterine environment and the fetal genotype towards differences in fetal growth have been the subject of many studies. Although the fetal genome undoubtedly determines growth *potential* in utero, the weight of evidence from animal cross-breeding experiments [55], from studies of half-siblings related either through the mother or the father [56] and from embryo transfer studies [57] strongly suggests that the fetal genome plays a subordinate role in determining the growth that is actually achieved [58,59]. For example, in embryo transfer studies it is the recipient mother rather than the donor mother that more strongly influences the growth of the fetus; a fetus trans-ferred to a larger uterus will achieve a larger birth size [57]. Thus it seems that the dominant determinant of fetal growth is the nutritional and hormonal milieu in which the fetus develops, and in particular the nutrient and oxygen supply [60].

Maternal height and cigarette smoking are well documented as both being strongly related to size at birth; follow-up studies have, however, found that they are not related to levels of cardiovascular risk factors in the offspring [61,62]. In contrast, initial studies suggest that maternal nutrition may have important long term effects on cardiovascular risk [63].

Maternal Influences and Fetal Programming – Maternal Nutrition

Suggestions that normal variations in maternal nutrition may exert important effects on the fetus contrast with the view that regulatory mechanisms in the maternal and placental systems act to ensure that fetal growth and development are largely independent of the mother's dietary intakes. This view partly arose from studies of the Dutch Hunger Winter famine showing that extreme dietary restriction in pregnancy may exert only relatively small effects on size at birth [52], and partly from the relatively disappointing results of human interventional studies of maternal nutrition during pregnancy [64]. Recent advances indicate, however, that we have hitherto had far too simplistic an approach to assessing the true impact of maternal nutrition.

In broad terms, the size achieved by a fetus may be thought of as reflecting the combination of its aspirations for growth and the maternoplacental capacity to

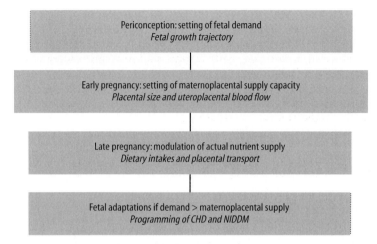

Fig. 20.4 The effects of maternal nutrition on fetal development and programming (CHD = coronary heart disease; NIDDM = non-insulin-dependent diabetes mellitus).

meet those aspirations. It is currently thought that the programming of adult cardiovascular disease may in part be a consequence of fetal adaptations invoked as a result of failure of the maternoplacental supply line to satisfy the fetal nutrient requirement (Fig. 20.4). Maternal nutrition can exert important effects on both the fetal nutrient demand and the maternoplacental supply capacity, and in reality we are only in the earliest stages of understanding its effects on both intrauterine development and health in later adult life. Specific issues that have not been adequately addressed in previous interventional studies include effects on the trajectory of fetal growth, cumulative intergenerational effects, paradoxical effects on placental growth, effects on fetal proportions and specific tissues, and the importance of the balance of macronutrients in the mother's diet and of her body composition.

The Fetal Growth Trajectory

The developing embryo consists of two groups of cells: the ICM, which develops into the fetus, and the outer trophectoderm, which becomes the placenta (see Ch. 2). Animal experiments indicate that the distribution of cells between the two masses is influenced by periconceptual alterations in maternal nutrition and hormonal status [65,66]. Alterations in cell allocation change the trajectory of fetal growth. Resetting of the growth trajectory to a lower rate may be an important fetal adaptation in early gestation because it reduces the subsequent demand for nutrients. Conversely, a fast growth trajectory increases nutrient demand and paradoxically renders the fetus more vulnerable to a poor nutrient supply in late gestation [67]. Thus, in ewes, maternal undernutrition during the last trimester has a greater adverse effect on the development of fetuses that are growing most rapidly. These fetuses make a series of adaptations in order to survive that include fetal wasting and placental oxidation of fetal amino acids to maintain lactate output to the fetus [67].

The trajectory of fetal growth is thought to increase with improvements in periconceptual nutrition and is faster in male fetuses [68]. One possibility is that the greater vulnerability of such fetuses on a fast growth trajectory could contribute to the rise in coronary heart disease with westernisation and the higher death rates in men.

Intergenerational Effects on Fetal Growth

Experimental studies in animals have shown that nutrition can have cumulative effects on reproductive performance over several generations. In one study, feeding rats a protein-deficient diet over 12 generations resulted in progressively greater fetal growth restriction over the generations; following refeeding with a normal diet it then took three generations to normalise growth and development [69].

Strong evidence for major intergenerational effects in humans has come from studies showing that a woman's birthweight influences the birthweight of her offspring [70,71]. We have, moreover, found that, whereas low birthweight mothers tend to have thin infants with a low PI, the father's birthweight is unrelated to PI at birth [54] (Table 20.3). The effect of *maternal* but not *paternal* birthweight may reflect impaired placentation in women who themselves had poor fetal growth, perhaps as a result of alterations in the uterine vasculature determined during fetal life.

Paradoxical Effects on Placental Growth

The nutrient and hormonal milieu of the fetus is strongly influenced by the placenta. Experiments in sheep in Adelaide, Australia have shown that maternal nutrition in early pregnancy can profoundly influence the growth of the placenta, and thereby alter fetal development; the effects produced crucially depend, however, on the nutritional status of the ewe in the periconceptual period [53]. In ewes that were poorly nourished around the time of conception, high nutrient intakes in early pregnancy enhanced placental growth; in ewes well nourished

Table 20.3 Mean PI (birthweight/length^3) in term pregnancies in Southampton, UK

		No. of subjects	Ponderal index at birth (kg/m^3)
Mother's own birthweight (g)	≤ 2500	28	26.2
	2500–3000	110	26.8
	3000–3500	180	27.0
	3500–4000	132	27.4
	> 4000	42	28.3
	P for trend		*< 0.0001*
Father's birthweight (g)	≤ 2500	27	27.3
	2500–3000	62	26.9
	3000–3500	138	27.2
	3500–4000	149	27.0
	> 4000	59	27.3
	P for trend		*0.9*

around conception, high intakes in early pregnancy suppressed placental growth [53]. Although this suppression appears paradoxical, in sheep farming it is common practice for ewes to be put on rich pasture prior to mating and then on poor pasture for a period in early pregnancy [72].

As part of a study designed to evaluate whether the normal variations in maternal diet found in Western communities could influence fetal growth and development, we have found evidence of a similar suppressive effect of high dietary intakes in early pregnancy on placental growth. Thus, among 538 women who delivered at term, those with high dietary intakes in early pregnancy, especially of carbohydrate, had smaller placentas, particularly if combined with low intakes of diary protein in late pregnancy [73]. These effects were independent of the mother's body size, social class and smoking, and resulted in alterations in the ratio of placental weight to birthweight (placental ratio).

Effects on placental growth may be of long term importance; a follow-up study of men born earlier this century in Sheffield [74] found a U-shaped relation between the placental ratio and later coronary heart disease. While babies with a disproportionately small placenta may suffer as a consequence of an impaired placental supply capacity, those with a disproportionately large placenta may experience fetal catabolism and wasting to supply amino acids for placental consumption [75,76]. Consequent fetal adaptations may underlie the increased adult coronary heart disease death rates in those with both low and high placental ratios.

Effects on Fetal Proportions and Specific Tissues

Studies in animals have shown that dietary manipulations during early development can have tissue-specific effects, resulting in alterations in an animal's proportions. For example, in pigs fed differing diets in the 1st year of life, those fed a protein-deficient diet had disproportionately large head, ears and genitalia compared with those fed an energy-deficient diet [2].

In humans, few studies have examined the possibility of maternal nutrition during pregnancy having tissue-specific effects on the fetus, leading to greater alterations in neonatal proportions than in birthweight. We have recently found that women with low dairy protein intakes in late pregnancy tended to have babies that were thinner at birth [54]; maternal dairy protein intakes were not, however, related to birthweight [73]. Furthermore, initial follow-up studies have shown that, while indices of maternal nutrition in pregnancy are related to the offspring's subsequent blood pressure, these effects are not mediated through alterations in birthweight [77].

The Importance of Dietary Balance and Maternal Body Composition

Experimental studies in pregnant rats have shown that maternal diets with a low ratio of protein to carbohydrate and fat alter fetal and placental growth and result in lifelong elevation of blood pressure in the offspring [5]. Follow-up studies of 40-year-old men and women whose mothers had taken part in a study of nutrition in pregnancy found that at either extreme of the balance of maternal animal protein to carbohydrate intake the offspring had both alterations in placental weight at birth and raised blood pressure in adult life [63].

Support for the thesis that alterations in fetal and placental development may result from a *low* ratio of animal protein to carbohydrate comes our observational studies of maternal nutrition in Southampton [73]. Support for the thesis that a *high* ratio of animal protein to carbohydrate may have adverse effects comes from a reanalysis of human studies providing dietary supplements to pregnant women [78]. This review of 16 trials of protein supplementation showed that supplements with a high percentage of calories derived from protein were consistently associated with lower birthweight.

Further evidence for the role of nutrition in programming comes from follow-up studies indicating that extremes of maternal body composition in pregnancy are associated with adverse long term outcomes in the offspring. Among Jamaican children, those whose mothers were *thin* in early pregnancy, having low SFT, had raised blood pressure at age 10 years [77], and in South India the prevalence of coronary heart disease was highest in men and women whose mothers had low weight in pregnancy [13].

At the other extreme of maternal body fatness, support for major effects of maternal *obesity* has come from follow-up of a cohort of men in Finland born earlier this century [79]; as in previous studies, those who had been thin at birth, with a low PI, had markedly increased coronary heart disease death rates 60 or so years later in adult life. Measurements of the mother's height and weight on admission to the labour ward also allowed derivation of the mother's BMI prior to delivery; further analyses showed the highest coronary heart disease death rates were in thin babies whose mothers had a high BMI. Modelling the data to derive contour lines of similar coronary heart disease death rates indicated that increasing BMI had little effect in tall women, but strong effects in short women [79]. One possibility is that increasing body fatness on a background of short stature caused by multigenerational undernutrition increases the fetal demand in circumstances that cannot be matched by maternal supply capacity.

The Future

The weight of evidence indicating that fetal growth restriction has long term implications for adult health is now such that we need to progress beyond epidemiological associations to greater understanding of the cellular and molecular processes that underlie them. Such an approach may allow us to use the information outlined here to reduce the prevalence of major diseases. We need to know what factors limit the delivery of nutrients and oxygen to the human fetus, how the fetus adapts to a limited supply, how these adaptations programme the structure and physiology of the body, and by what molecular mechanisms nutrients and hormones alter gene expression.

It is becoming clear that size at birth is no more than an indirect proxy measure for the actual influences that drive fetal programming. Recent observations suggest that maternal nutrition may be one influence that has important long term effects on the offspring and challenge the view that the fetus is little affected by changes in maternal nutrition, except in circumstances of famine. While we are only in the earliest stages of understanding the mechanisms that might mediate the effects of maternal nutrition on human fetal development, initial studies point to the importance of the glucose–insulin–IGF-I axis [80,81].

Birthweight is an inadequate summary measure of fetal growth, and we need to adopt a considerably more sophisticated view of maternal nutrition and fetal development. This needs to take account not only of periconceptual effects on later fetal demand and early pregnancy effects on the maternoplacental supply capacity, but also of intergenerational effects and the long term sequelae of fetal adaptations to undernutrition. Further research requires a strategy of interdependent clinical, animal and epidemiological investigations.

References

1. Lucas A. Programming by early nutrition in man. In: Bock GR, Whelan J, editors. The childhood environment and adult disease. Chichester: John Wiley, 1991;38–55.
2. McCance RA, Widdowson EM. The determinants of growth and form. Proc Royal Soc Lond 1974;185:1–17.
3. Widdowson EM, McCance RA. A review: new thought on growth. Pediatr Res 1975;9:154–6.
4. Jansson T, Persson E. Placental transfer of glucose and amino acids in intrauterine growth retardation: studies with substrate analogues in the awake guinea pig. Pediatr Res 1990;28:203–8.
5. Langley SC, Jackson AA. Increased systolic blood pressure in adult rats induced by fetal exposure to maternal low protein diets. Clin Sci 1994;86, 217–22.
6. Rose G. Familial patterns in ischaemic heart disease. Br J Prev Soc Med 1964;18:75–80.
7. Barker DJP, Osmond C. Infant mortality, childhood nutrition, and ischaemic heart disease in England and Wales. Lancet 1986; i:1077–81.
8. Barker DJP, Bull AR, Osmond C, Simmonds SJ. Fetal and placental size and risk of hypertension in adult life. BMJ 1990;301:259–62.
9. Barker DJP, Osmond C, Simmonds SJ, Wield GA. The relation of small head circumference and thinness at birth to death from cardiovascular disease in adult life. BMJ 1993;306:422–6.
10. Osmond C, Barker DJP, Winter PD, Fall CHD, Simmonds SJ. Early growth and death from cardiovascular disease in women. BMJ 1993;307:1519–24.
11. Rich-Edwards JW, Stampfer MJ, Manson JAE, Rosner B, Hankinson SE, Colditz GA, et al. Birth weight and the risk of cardiovascular disease in a cohort of women followed up since 1976. BMJ 1997;315:396–400.
12. Frankel S, Elwood P, Sweetnam P, Yarnell J, Davey Smith G. Birthweight, body mass index in middle age, and incident coronary heart disease. Lancet 1996;348:1478–80.
13. Stein CE, Fall CHD, Kumaran K, Osmond C, Cox V, Barker DJP. Fetal growth and coronary heart disease in South India. Lancet 1996;348:1269–73.
14. Hales CN, Barker DJP, Clark PMS, Cox LJ, Fall C, Osmond C, et al. Fetal and infant growth and impaired glucose tolerance at age 64. BMJ 1991;303:1019–22.
15. Barker DJP, Osmond C, Golding J, Kuh D, Wadsworth MEJ. Growth in utero, blood pressure in childhood and adult life, and mortality from cardiovascular disease. BMJ 1989;298:564–7.
16. Law CM, Shiell AW. Is blood pressure inversely related to birthweight? The strength of evidence from a systematic review of the literature. J Hypertens 1996;14:935–41.
17. Barker DJP, Godfrey KM, Osmond C, Bull A. The relation of fetal length, ponderal index and head circumference to blood pressure and the risk of hypertension in adult life. Paediatr Perinat Epidemiol 1992:6, 35–44.
18. Barker DJP. Fetal origins of coronary heart disease. BMJ 1995;311:171–4.
19. Phillips DIW. Insulin resistance as a programmed response to fetal undernutrition. Diabetologia 1996;39:1119–22.
20. Lithell HO, McKeigue PM, Berglund L, Mohsen R, Lithell U-B, Leon DA. Relation of size at birth to non-insulin dependent diabetes and insulin concentrations in men aged 50–60 years. BMJ 1996;312:406–10.
21. Phillips DIW, Barker DJP, Hales CN, Hirst S, Osmond C. Thinness at birth and insulin resistance in adult life. Diabetologia 1994;37:150–4.
22. Barker DJP, Hales CN, Fall CHD, Osmond C, Phipps K, Clark PMS. Type 2 (non-insulin-dependent) diabetes mellitus, hypertension and hyperlipidaemia (syndrome X): relation to reduced fetal growth. Diabetologia 1993;36:62–7.
23. Barker DJP, Martyn CN, Osmond C, Hales CN, Fall CHD. Growth *in utero* and serum cholesterol concentrations in adult life. BMJ 1993;307:1524–7.

24. Martyn CN, Meade TW, Stirling Y, Barker DJP. Plasma concentrations of fibrinogen and factor VII in adult life and their relation to intra-uterine growth. Br J Haematol 1995;89:142–6.

25. Rudolph AM. The fetal circulation and its response to stress. J Dev Physiol 1984;6: 11–19.

26. Kind K, Clifton P, Katsman A, Simonetta G, Robinson JS, Owens JA. Prenatal programming of glucose and cholesterol homeostasis in the guinea pig. Presented at the 36th Conference of The Australian Society for Medical Research, Adelaide, 1997; S8–2.

27. Desai M, Crowther N, Ozanne SE, Lucas A, Hales CN. Adult glucose and lipid metabolism may be programmed during fetal life. Biochem Soc Trans 1995;23:331–5.

28. Conway GS, Honour JW, Jacobs HS. Heterogeneity of the polycystic ovary syndrome: clinical, endocrine and ultrasound features in 556 patients. Clin Endocrinol 1989;30:459–70.

29. Pfeiffer CA. Sexual differences of the hypophyses and their determination by the gonads. Am J Anat 1936;58:195–225.

30. Barraclough CA, Gorski RA. Evidence that the hypothalamus is responsible for androgen-induced sterility in the female rat. Endocrinology 1961;68:68–79.

31. Barraclough CA. Production of anovulatory, sterile rats by single injections of testosterone propionate. Endocrinology 1961;68:62–7.

32. Vom Saal FS, Bronson FH. Sexual characteristics of adult female mice are correlated with their blood testosterone levels during prenatal development. Science 1980;208:597–9.

33. Cresswell JL, Barker DJP, Osmond C, Egger P, Phillips DIW, Fraser RB. Fetal growth, length of gestation, and polycystic ovaries in adult life. Lancet 1997;350:1131–5.

34. Gluckman PD, Cutfield W, Harding JE, Milner D, Jensen E, Woodhall S, et al. Metabolic consequences of intrauterine growth retardation. Acta Paediatr Suppl 1996;417:3–6.

35. Taylor DJ, Thompson CH, Kemp GJ, Barnes PRJ, Sanderson A, Radda GK, et al. A relationship between impaired fetal growth and reduced muscle glycolysis revealed by ^{31}P magnetic resonance spectroscopy. Diabetologia 1995;38:1205–12.

36. Wootton SA, Murphy JL, Wilson F, Phillips D. Energy expenditure and substrate metabolism after carbohydrate ingestion in relation to fetal growth in women born in Preston. Proc Nutr Soc 1994;53:174A (abst).

37. Phillips DIW, Caddy S, Ilic V. Intramuscular triglyceride and muscle insulin sensitivity: evidence for a causative relationship. Metabolism 1996;45:947–50.

38. Barbazanges A, Piazza PV, Le Moal M, Maccari S. Maternal glucocorticoid secretion mediates long-term effects of prenatal stress. J Neurosci 1996;16:3943–9.

39. Meaney MJ, Viau V, Bhatnagar S. (1991) Cellular mechanisms underlying the development and expression of individual differences in the hypothalamic-pituitary-adrenal stress response. J Steroid Biochem Mol Biol 1991;39:265–74.

40. Levitt NS, Lindsay RS, Holmes GE, Seckl JR. Dexamethasone in the last week of pregnancy attenuates hippocampal glucocorticoid receptor gene expression and elevates blood pressure in the adult offspring of rats. Neuroendocrinology 1996;64:412–18.

41. Lindsay RS, Lindsay RM, Waddell B, Seckl JR. Programming of glucose tolerance in the rat; role of placental β-hydroxysteroid dehydrogenase. Diabetologia 1996;39:1299–305.

42. Langley-Evans SC. Intrauterine programming of hypertension by glucocorticoids. Life Sci 1997;60:1213–21.

43. Phillips GJ, Langley-Evans SC, Benediktsson R, Seckl JR, Edwards CRW, Jackson AA. The role of dietary protein restriction during pregnancy on the activity of placental 11 β-hydroxysteroid dehydrogenase. Proc Nutr Soc 1994;53:170A.

44. Lau C, Seidler FJ, Cameron AM. Nutritional influences on adrenal chromaffin cell development: comparison with central neurones. Pediatr Res 1988;24:583–7.

45. Seidler FJ, Bell JM, Slotkin TA. Undernutrition and overnutrition in the neonatal rat: effects on noradrenergic pathways in brain regions. Pediatr Res 1980;27:191–7.

46. Clark PM, Hindmarsh PC, Shiell AW, Law CM, Honour JW, Barker DJP. Size at birth and adreno-cortical function in childhood. Clin Endocrinol 1996;45:721–6.

47. Phillips DIW, Barker DJP, Fall CHD, Seckl JR, Whorwood CB, Wood PJ, et al. Elevated plasma cortisol concentrations: a link between low birthweight and the insulin resistance syndrome? J Clin Endocrinol Metab 1998;83:757–60.

48. Phillips DIW, Barker DJP. Association between low birthweight and high resting pulse in adult life: is the sympathetic nervous system involved in programming the insulin resistance syndrome. Diabet Med 1997;14:673–7.

49. Beral V, Colwell L. Randomised trial of high doses of stilboestrol and ethisterone therapy in pregnancy: long-term follow-up of the children. J Epidemiol Community Health 1981;35:155–60.

50. Konje JC, Bell SC, Morton JJ, De Chazal R, Taylor DJ. Human fetal kidney morphometry during gestation and the relationship between weight, kidney morphometry and plasma active renin concentration at birth. Clin Sci 1996;91:169–75.

51. Barker DJP. Mothers, babies and disease in later life. London: BMJ, 1994.

52. Stein Z, Susser M, Saenger G, Marolla F. Famine and human development: the Dutch Hunger Winter of 1944–1945. New York: Oxford University Press, 1975;119–48.

53. Robinson JS, Owens JA, de Barro T, Lok F, Chidzanja S. (1994) Maternal nutrition and fetal growth. In: Ward RHT, Smith SK, Donnai D, editors. Early fetal growth and development. London: Royal College of Obstetricians and Gynaecologists, 1994;317–34.

54. Godfrey KM, Barker DJP, Robinson S, Osmond C. Mother's birthweight and diet in pregnancy in relation to the baby's thinness at birth. Br J Obstet Gynaecol 1997;104:663–7.

55. Walton A, Hammond J. The maternal effects on growth and conformation in Shire horse – Shetland pony crosses. Proc Royal Soc Lond B 1938;125:311–35.

56. Morton NE. The inheritance of human birthweight. Ann Hum Genet 1955;20:123–34.

57. Brooks AA, Johnson MR, Steer PJ, Pawson ME, Abdalla HI. Birth weight: nature or nurture? Early Hum Dev 1995;42:29–35.

58. Carr-Hill R, Campbell DM, Hall MH, Meredith A. Is birthweight determined genetically? BMJ 1987;295:687–9.

59. Snow MHL. Effects of genome on fetal size at birth. In: Sharp F, Fraser RB, Milner RDG, editors. Fetal growth, proceedings of the 20th study group, RCOG. London: Royal College of Obstetricians and Gynaecologists, 1989;1–11.

60. Ounsted M, Ounsted C. Maternal regulation of intrauterine growth. Nature 1966;212:687–9.

61. Law CM, Barker DJP, Bull AR, Osmond C. Maternal and fetal influences on blood pressure. Arch Dis Child 1991;66:1291–5.

62. Whincup PH, Cook DG, Papacosta O. Do maternal and intrauterine factors influence blood pressure in childhood? Arch Dis Child 1992;67:1423–9.

63. Campbell DM, Hall MH, Barker DJP, Cross J, Shiell AW, Godfrey KM. Diet in pregnancy and the offspring's blood pressure 40 years later. Br J Obstet Gynaecol 1996;103:273–80.

64. Kramer MS. Effects of energy and protein intakes on pregnancy outcome: an overview of the research evidence from controlled clinical trials. Am J Clin Nutr 1993;58:627–35.

65. Kleeman DO, Walker SK, Seamark RF. Enhanced fetal growth in sheep administered progesterone during the first three days of pregnancy. J Reprod Fertil 1994;102:411–17.

66. Walker SK, Hartwich KM, Seamark, RF. The production of unusually large offspring following embryo manipulation: concepts and challenges. Theriogenology 1996;45:111–20.

67. Harding JE, Liu L, Evans P, Oliver M, Gluckman P. Intrauterine feeding of the growth-retarded fetus: can we help? Early Hum Dev 1992;29:193–7.

68. Leese HJ. The energy metabolism of the pre-implantation embryo. In: Heyner S, Wiley L, editors. Early embryo development and paracrine relationships. New York: Alan R Liss, 1990;67–78.

69. Stewart RJC, Sheppard HG, Preece RF, Waterlow JC. The effect of rehabilitation at different stages of development of rats marginally malnourished for ten to twelve generations. Br J Nutr 1980;43:403–11.

70. Klebanoff MA, Meirik O, Berendes HW. Second generation consequences of small-for-dates birth. Pediatrics 1989;84:343–7.

71. Emanuel I, Filakti H, Alberman E, Evans SJW. Intergenerational studies of human birthweight from the 1958 birth cohort. 1. Evidence for a multigenerational effect. Br J Obstet Gynaecol 1992;99:67–74.

72. Slen SB. Wool production and body growth in sheep. In: Cuthbertson D, editor. Nutrition of animals of agricultural importance. Part 2. Assessment of and factors affecting the requirements of farm livestock. Oxford: Pergamon, 1969;827–48.

73. Godfrey K, Robinson S, Barker DJP, Osmond C, Cox V. Maternal nutrition in early and late pregnancy in relation to placental and fetal growth. BMJ 1996;312:410–14.

74. Martyn CN, Barker DJP, Osmond C. Mothers' pelvic size, fetal growth and death from stroke in men. Lancet 1996;348:1264–8.

75. Barker DJP, Gluckman PD, Godfrey KM, Harding J, Owens JA, Robinson JS. Fetal nutrition and adult disease. Lancet 1993;341:938–41.

76. Robinson JS, Chidzanja S, Kind K, Lok F, Owens P, Owens JA. Placental control of fetal growth. Reprod Fertil Dev 1995;7:333–44.

77. Godfrey KM, Forrester T, Barker DJP, Jackson AA, Landman JP, St E Hall J, et al. Maternal nutritional status in pregnancy and blood pressure in childhood. Br J Obstet Gynaecol 1994;101:398–403.

78. Rush D. Effects of changes in maternal energy and protein intake during pregnancy, with special reference to fetal growth. In Sharp F, Fraser RB, Milner RDG, editors. Fetal growth. London: Royal College of Obstetricians and Gynaecologists, 1989;203–29.

79. Forsen T, Eriksson JG, Tuomilehto J, Teramo K, Osmond C, Barker DJP. Mother's weight in pregnancy and coronary heart disease in a cohort of Finnish men: follow up study. BMJ 1997;315:837–40.

80. Godfrey KM, Hales CN, Osmond C, Barker DJP, Taylor KP. Relation of cord plasma concentrations of proinsulin, 32–33 split proinsulin, insulin and C-peptide to placental weight, body size and body proportions at birth. Early Hum Dev 1996;46:129–40.

81. Godfrey KM, Hales CN, Osmond C, Barker DJP, Robinson S. Nutrition in pregnancy and the concentrations of proinsulin, 32–33 split proinsulin, insulin and C-peptide in cord plasma. Diabet Med 1996;13:868–73.

Section 3
Future Advances

21 Molecular Regulation of Placental Development

James C. Cross

Introduction

Dysfunction of the placenta is generally accepted as a potential underlying cause of IUGR. Primary pathologies of the normal placenta, such as infection or infarction, can certainly restrict its ability to deliver nutrients to the fetus. In addition, though, deficiencies in the development of the placenta could also occur to restrict its function. This idea is supported by the findings of cellular and structural changes in the placenta that are associated with IUGR [1–3], many of which are suggestive of a relatively immature organ. Similar placentation changes have also been described in pre-eclampsia (PE), a fact that suggests the pathogenesis of the two syndromes may be related [4]. Because these changes may reflect a failure in development that occurred *weeks or even months before an effect on fetal growth was manifest*, an opportunity for early diagnosis and therapy thus exists. A challenge for the future will be to understand the molecular basis of these developmental changes. The last few years have seen an explosion of new information concerning the regulation of placental development resulting from a combination of cell biological studies in humans and molecular genetic studies in mice. This chapter will highlight work that is beginning to describe molecular mechanisms essential for normal placental development, which may help to explain the placental origins of IUGR.

Stages of Placental Development in Mice and Men

There are significant differences in gross anatomical structure and certain endocrine functions among placentas from different eutherian mammals [5]. These differences are curious from an evolutionary standpoint and must certainly be kept in mind when extrapolating data from one species to another. They have almost certainly discouraged scientists from applying insights gained in experimental animals to humans. Overcoming this problem is increasingly important, though, owing to the advent of "gene knockout" technology in mice. We are in the midst of a revolution in understanding the function of individual genes in mouse placental development. This should be a sufficient incentive to embrace the mouse as model to understand human placentation. Despite some differences in gross anatomy, especially on the maternal side of the placenta (see

Table 21.1 Comparison of human and mouse placental development

	Human	Mouse
chronology of development		
length of gestation	9 months	19 days
implantation (postfertilisation)	7 days	4.5 days
vascularisation of placenta	3 weeks	9 days
placental structure		
fetomaternal interface	haemochorial	haemochorial
vascular exchange structure	villous	labyrinthine
trophoblast cell types		
stem cells	villous cytotrophoblast	chorion
invasive cells	extravillous cytotrophoblast	giant cells
transport surface	syncytiotrophoblast	syncytiotrophoblast
	(monolayer)	(bilayer)

Fig. 21.1, [6]), it is readily apparent that at the cellular level there are considerable similarities in the structure and development of the placenta in different species (Table 21.1). As a consequence it is likely that the underlying molecular mechanisms governing placental development should be evolutionarily conserved. As described below, through studies of protein and gene expression patterns we are now getting glimpses that this hypothesis may be correct.

In all eutherian mammals, the placenta is formed largely from two cell lineages that have distinct embryological origins: trophoblast and mesoderm. The epithelial component of the placenta is derived from the trophoblast lineage, which first forms as the trophectoderm at the blastocyst stage. The ICM of the blastocyst gives rise to the three germ layers of the embryo proper as well as to the mesodermal cells that later make up the stromal and vascular components of the placenta (see Ch. 7). Trophoblast cell derivatives interacting with the underlying stroma develop into the fetal vascular exchange unit of the placenta – which is so variable amongst mammals. For example, in humans the surface of the placenta elaborates into a villous tree, which "floats" in a large blood-filled space, whereas in rodents a labyrinth is formed consisting of a series of small maternal blood channels.

In humans, the blastocyst implants into the uterus 7–8 days after conception in a process mediated by the trophectoderm. Soon after implantation, the trophectoderm layer gives rise to distinct differentiated cell types: a multinucleated, postmitotic syncytiotrophoblast, which covers the conceptus, and an underlying villous cytotrophoblast layer, which continues to proliferate. As development proceeds and the placenta grows, the chorionic villi are formed. Individual villi are covered by syncytiotrophoblast, and have an underlying cytotrophoblast layer with a stromal cell core within which the placental vessels form. Most of the chorionic villi remain free of the uterine wall (floating villi) and function solely in nutrient transport. Cytotrophoblast cells are a progenitor cell population that differentiates into syncytiotrophoblast as villi grow and mature. In addition, at the tips of a small proportion of villi that attach to the decidua (anchoring villi), cytotrophoblasts can also differentiate into specialised cells that migrate out of the villus, forming columns of cytotrophoblasts that contact endometrium. From the tips of these columns emerge extravillous cytotrophoblast cells that invade into the decidua and myometrium (extravillous cytotrophoblasts). Cytotrophoblast cells invade into maternal arterioles and arteries through both endovascular and perivascular migrations [7]. Endovascular cytotrophoblast cells replace the muscular walls of the arteries producing the "physiological" changes associated with the development of low resistance blood flow to the implantation site.

In rodents, as in humans, there are several distinctive trophoblast cell subtypes and structures in the mature placenta (Fig. 21.1): an outermost layer of trophoblast giant cells, an intermediate layer called the spongiotrophoblast and the innermost labyrinthine layer [8]. The labyrinthine layer is analogous in function to the floating chorionic villi. It begins to form by about day nine of mouse gestation, following the attachment of the allantois (mesoderm) to the trophoblast-derived chorion. The bulk of the labyrinthine tissue consists of two layers of trophoblast syncytia, which separate the maternal blood space from the fetal stroma/blood vessels. Mononuclear trophoblast cells also exist in the labyrinth although their function is unknown. In early gestation, the trophoblast stem population probably exists in the structure called the chorion. The trophoblast giant cells are an unusual population at the periphery of the rodent placenta. These can differentiate from precursor cells in the spongiotrophoblast layer. They are polyploid cells that form as a result of endoreduplication, in contrast to the cell fusion that occurs to produce the syncytiotrophoblast. Trophoblast giant cells in rodents are probably analogous to the extravillous cytotrophoblast cells of the human placenta: both cell types are inherently invasive, postmitotic and interact with maternal blood vessels [8].

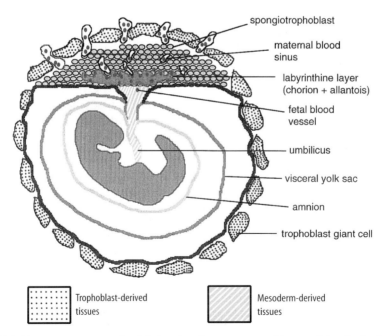

Fig. 21.1 Mouse conceptus at day 9.5 showing the structure and layers of the chorioallantoic placenta (reproduced from [6] with permission from Cross 1998, and NYAS).

Potential Origins of IUGR During Placental Development

Although several studies have shown a strong association between certain histological changes in the placenta in IUGR and PE, several authors have highlighted the variable nature of pathological lesions seen in IUGR and PE (e.g. [2,3]). It is possible that overall placental insufficiency may result even though only part of the placenta is affected. Therefore, some of this variability may be caused by failure to examine *several* representative samples of the placenta (stereological analysis – see Ch. 7). However, it also likely that placental insufficiency may arise by independent mechanisms that produce different structural changes. Given this, it has been suggested that the diseases should perhaps be subclassified according to pathological mechanism and the level at which the delivery of oxygen and nutrients to the fetus is compromised, as described by others [1,2], as follows: (a) *preplacental*: encompasses maternal effects that reduce nutrient delivery; (b) *uteroplacental*: includes defects in cytotrophoblast invasion and its remodelling of maternal spiral arteries; (c) *postplacental*: includes changes that affect the uptake of oxygen and nutrients and their delivery to the fetus. Clearly, the pathological mechanisms accounting for each type are very different, though the latter two forms may be readily explained in terms of altered placental development.

Considerable attention has been focused on studying uteroplacental insufficiency due to impaired cytotrophoblast invasion, particularly associated with PE. In particular, remodelling of the myometrial segments of the uterine arteries is inadequate in PE [9–11] (see Ch. 6). This is thought to result in higher than normal resistance to blood flow and is correlated with the development of abnormal uterine artery velocity waveforms as detected by Doppler ultrasound [12,13]. It is thought that the remodelling of decidual uterine arterial segments may be normal, in contrast to the failure of extravillous trophoblast cells to invade myometrial segments. Thus the cytotrophoblast defect in PE may be expressed later in development. Evidence of excess extravillous trophoblast proliferation is common in the PE placental bed and this, combined with evidence of arrested invasion, suggests that the placenta may be relatively immature and blocked in its normal developmental programme [4]. Consistent with this, extravillous cytotrophoblast cells in PE fail to express α1 integrin, a marker characteristic of the invasive population [14].

Though less widely documented, many of the histopathological features of PE are also observed in IUGR. Remodelling of the uterine spiral arteries may be limited to the decidual segments [15]. Atherotic lesions, which are commonly associated with PE, may also be found in IUGR [16,17]. Defects in cytotrophoblast invasion [10,18] and changes in CAM expression on extravillous cytotrophoblast cells [19] have also been reported in association with IUGR. These similarities suggest that IUGR and PE reflect different possible outcomes of a common abnormality rather than distinct syndromes [4]. Due to inadequate extravillous cytotrophoblast invasion and remodelling of spiral arteries, the fetoplacental unit is likely to become deprived later in gestation because of inadequate oxygen and nutrient delivery. This typically would result in fetal growth restriction and, in the absence of other factors, would result simply in IUGR. In contrast, PE might result in women who have complicating hypertensive or metabolic alterations – factors that would affect maternal pathophysiological responses to the altered pregnancy.

Compared with the volume of literature devoted to impaired cytotrophoblast invasion as causes of IUGR and PE, lesions in the villous placenta that would produce postplacental insufficiency are less widely documented. None the less, the IUGR placenta shows reduced villous surface area [20–22] and evidence of fetoplacental vessel pathology [23]; using three-dimensional modes of analysis, several studies have also documented a significant reduction in villous vessel branching, particularly in severe IUGR [24–26]. The presence of these last lesions provides a reasonable explanation for dramatic changes in fetoplacental blood flow detected by Doppler ultrasound of umbilical arteries in severe IUGR.

Molecular Control of Placental Development

Recently, tremendous progress has been made in identifying molecular mechanisms that control placental development. This subject has been reviewed extensively elsewhere [8,27,28] and angiogenic growth factors are reviewed in Ch. 8. The focus here is on those mechanisms related to the processes affected in the IUGR placenta, namely trophoblast differentiation and invasion and development of the fetoplacental circulation.

Factors Controlling Trophoblast Differentiation

Several transcription factors have been implicated in the regulation of trophoblast growth and differentiation in mice [28]. These include the zinc-finger transcription factors Err2 [29] and mSna [30], as well as the helix–loop–helix transcription factors Hand1 (previously called Hxt) and Mash2. In Err2 knockout mice, the conceptuses lack trophoblast cells of the chorion, thus implicating this factor in the control of trophoblast proliferation. The factors mSna, Mash2 and Hand1 are all implicated in regulating the differentiation of the invasive trophoblast giant cells in mice. The Mash2 and mSna genes are expressed in trophoblast giant cell precursors of the spongiotrophoblast, but this expression is dramatically downregulated upon giant cell differentiation. Overexpression of either factor in Rcho-1 trophoblast cells prevents giant cell differentiation [30,31]. Mash2 mutant conceptuses die at mid gestation, show a loss of giant cell precursors in the spongiotrophoblast layer and have more giant cells than normal [32]. Recent experiments [33] indicate that Mash2 functions cell-autonomously either to sustain spongiotrophoblast cell proliferation and/or survival or to block giant cell differentiation. The Hand1 gene is expressed in non-proliferating trophoblast in the outer regions of the ectoplacental cone and in trophoblast giant cells [31]. Its overexpression in Rcho-1 trophoblast cells induces growth arrest and giant cell transformation [31]. Mutation of the Hand1 gene in mice indicates that it is essential for trophoblast giant cell differentiation [34]. In addition to these positive-acting helix–loop–helix regulators, the negative helix–loop–helix factors Id-1 and Id-2 are also expressed in proliferative trophoblast [35,36] and probably regulate trophoblast development. Differentiation of Rcho-1 cells is accompanied by downregulation of Id-1 and Id-2 [31], and sustained expression of Id-1 reduces Rcho-1 differentiation [31], which is consistent with its activity in other cell types. Together these data indicate that a network of helix–loop–helix factors and mSna may interact to regulate the differentiation of trophoblast cells to the giant cell phenotype. As the giant cells are similar to the invasive, extravillous cytotrophoblast cells of the human placenta, altered activity of these factors could, in theory, play a role in the impaired cytotrophoblast invasion observed in IUGR and PE. Of these factors, homologues for Mash2 [37] and Id2 [38] have been shown to be expressed in the human placenta.

Factors Controlling Trophoblast Invasiveness

The invasion of cytotrophoblast cells is highly regulated and may be influenced by growth factors and cytokines produced either by cytotrophoblast cells themselves, having an autocrine action, or by fetal stromal and maternal decidual cells [8]. Isolated cytotrophoblast cells differentiate in vitro into cells that invade into ECM substrates, usually rich in laminin [39]. The gestational age of the placental tissue is an important determinant, because the invasive behaviour peaks in cells made from first trimester placentas compared with later stages [40]. Similarly, villous explants from first trimester placentas will develop structures that resemble anchoring villi, owing to the migration and invasion of cytotrophoblast cells from the villous tips [41]. The ability of cytotrophoblast cells to invade depends on the appropriate expression of both surface CAMs (e.g. integrins) as well as proteases that degrade the extracellular matrix (e.g. plasminogen activator and MMPs) [8]. Different integrins are expressed at specific points within the cytotrophoblast column, demarcating the stages of differentiation. Briefly, the $\alpha6$ integrin (a laminin receptor) is expressed by villous cytotrophoblast cells and is downregulated as migration occurs. Cytotrophoblast cells that migrate through the column express the $\alpha5$ integrin (a fibronectin receptor) whereas the $\alpha1$ integrin (a collagen and laminin receptor) becomes upregulated as the cells invade the decidua [39,42]. Immunoneutralisation of the $\alpha1$ integrin blocks invasion in vitro [43]. Similarly, MMP-9 (gelatinase B) is required for cytotrophoblast invasion in vitro [44]. The fact that isolated cytotrophoblast cells can differentiate into invasive cells in relatively simple in vitro conditions indicates that an intrinsic programme drives this process. Autocrine-acting cytokines may play a role. The placenta is a major source of activin during pregnancy [45–49]. The presence of activin receptors on cytotrophoblast cells suggests that activin may have autocrine or paracrine effects [50]. In vitro, activin appears to promote cytotrophoblast outgrowth from villous explants and progression towards invasion [51]. Local production of the activin antagonist, follistatin, may be one way of controlling invasion [51].

Factors Controlling Extraembryonic Mesoderm Differentiation

Mesodermal cells form during the process of gastrulation, which begins around day 6.5 and nine of mouse and human gestation, respectively. Mesoderm contributes both to the embryo proper as well as to the placenta and extraembryonic membranes. Therefore gene mutations that block gastrulation, or subsequent mesoderm migration, prevent normal placental development. However, it has become clear that different, exclusively acting genes also affect embryonic and extraembryonic mesodermal development. For example, in the *eed* [52] and *nodal* [53] mouse mutants, embryonic mesoderm formation is inhibited whereas extraembryonic mesoderm can form, and indeed appears to form excessively. Likewise, whereas *FGFR1* mutant cells are poorly able to migrate out of the primitive streak and contribute to anterior embryonic structures, they can contribute to extraembryonic mesoderm populations [54]. These genes are therefore examples of ones that control embryonic but not extraembryonic mesoderm development. However, no specific factors have been implicated in extraembryonic mesoderm specification.

Trophoblast–Mesoderm Interactions in Placental Development

Even after the trophoblast cell lineage has been segregated at the blastocyst stage in early development, it continues to interact with the ICM and its derivatives throughout development. Cell–cell interactions play major roles in trophoblast cell growth and differentiation. For example, only trophoblast cells overlying the ICM in the blastocyst continue to proliferate after implantation in the mouse [8]. Later in development, the proliferating trophoblast cell population is in contact with mesodermal cells – an interaction critical for subsequent development. Mouse embryos that lack either α4 integrin [55] or VCAM-1 [56] die at mid gestation owing to a failure in chorioallantoic fusion, demonstrating roles for these CAMs in this interaction. However, a fraction of *VCAM-1* mutants are able to undergo chorioallantoic fusion, but they still die at mid gestation showing defective formation of the labyrinthine layer [56]. This observation indicates that interactions other than cell adhesion are required between the trophoblast and mesodermal cell derivatives in order to direct trophoblast proliferation and morphogenesis of the labyrinthine layer.

There are several candidate growth factors produced by mesodermal derivatives of the placenta that could regulate trophoblast growth and differentiation. In mice, mutation of the genes encoding the growth factor scatter factor/hepatocyte growth factor (SF/HGF) and its receptor c-Met are associated with poorly developed spongiotrophoblast and labyrinth [57–59]. SF/HGF produced by the allantois probably maintains trophoblast growth [57] and in its absence trophoblast cells may undergo premature differentiation. SF/HGF and c-Met are expressed by mesenchyme and trophoblast, respectively, in the human placenta and recent data describes reduced expression in early onset IUGR [60]. Wnt2 is another signalling molecule thought to be expressed by the allantois. *Wnt2* mouse mutants show abnormal labyrinthine placental structure [61]. VEGF is produced within the placenta, and at least one of its receptors, flt-1, is expressed on trophoblast cells of mice [62] and humans [63,64]. VEGF can stimulate human trophoblast DNA replication [65] and therefore could have roles outside of its effect on vascular development (see below and Ch. 8). TGF-β is highly expressed in the placenta and can suppress cytotrophoblast invasion [51,66–68] and endocrine differentiation [69].

Vascular Development in the Fetal Placenta

The origin of the placental vessels now appears to be relatively clear, in rodents at least. Mesodermal cells within the allantois can undergo the process of vasculogenesis, in which blood vessels and blood cells form de novo. Although this occurs in a cell compartment that is separate from the yolk sac where fetal blood cell formation begins, it seems likely that similar molecular mechanisms control both. VEGF and its receptors flt-1 and flk-1 are critical for blood vessel formation throughout the conceptus [70–72], and all are all expressed in the placenta of mice [62] and humans [63,64], supporting the idea that they may play a role in fetoplacental blood vessel formation. Other factors appear to control the outgrowth, branching and survival of established blood vessels during embryonic development, as suggested by mutations of genes encoding angiopoietin-1 and its receptor Tie-2 [73–75]. The expression or activity of this system in the placenta has not been well documented though Dunk and Ahmed present some preliminary data in Ch. 8. While there may be conservation of mechanisms controlling blood vessel formation in the embryo and placenta, there are some suggestions that development of the placental vasculature may depend on some unique genes as well. Mutations in the *Arnt* [76] and *Vhl* [77] genes result in embryonic mortality due to placental defects. Interestingly, while blood vessel formation in the placenta is compromised in both these mutants, it appears to be normal in the yolk sac and embryo proper.

Modulation of Placental Development by Maternal Factors

Cytotrophoblast differentiation can potentially be modulated by environmental factors including growth factors produced by the mother and tissue oxygen levels. Embryos homozygous for a mutation in the EGF receptor show different phenotypes that are influenced by strain-specific modifier genes. Early lethality occurs soon after implantation when only trophoblast cells normally express the receptor [78], and mid-gestation lethality is associated with a small spongiotrophoblast layer [78,79]. Several members of the EGF family could potentially interact with the trophoblast EGF receptor. At the time of implantation, heparin binding EGF (HB-EGF) [80] and amphiregulin [81] are expressed by the maternal endometrium surrounding the conceptus. A role for leukaemia inhibitory factor (LIF) in trophoblast development was implied since mutation of a LIF receptor results in abnormal spongiotrophoblast morphogenesis [82]. The fact that LIF-deficient fetuses do not show this phenotype [83] suggests that maternally derived LIF affects placental development.

Tissue oxygen levels may have a significant effect on placental development. Early in the first trimester of human pregnancy, blood flow velocity in the intervillous space is normally quite low [84,85]. Direct measurements have shown that the oxygen levels in the placenta are much lower than in the endometrium until 12–13 weeks [86]. This suggests that before 12 weeks the normal environment for trophoblast development is low in oxygen. Similarly in the mouse, after implantation and the decidual reaction, there are few maternal blood vessels adjacent to the implantation site [5]. The finding that intervillous blood flow before 12 weeks is associated with poor pregnancy outcome suggests either that blood flow may physically prevent proper attachment and formation of anchoring villi [84,85], or that elevated oxygen may have a direct deleterious effect on early trophoblast development. In support of the latter hypothesis, culture of first trimester villous explants in 2.5 per cent oxygen, compared with 20 per cent oxygen, results in better maintenance of syncytiotrophoblast cell viability [87] and isolated cytotrophoblast cells continue to proliferate only in low oxygen [88]. At low oxygen levels in culture, first trimester cytotrophoblast cell invasion is blocked [88,89]. These latter data suggest the possibility that preplacental changes in oxygen delivery early in gestation could perturb cytotrophoblast invasion in such a way as to affect the ability of the placenta to deliver nutrients and oxygen later in gestation, even if the preplacental changes are corrected.

Finding the Molecular Targets in the IUGR Placenta

For those cases where abnormal placental development or function compromises fetal growth, we have a reasonable description of the cellular changes present in the placentas, though we have little concrete proof of its molecular pathological basis. The extent to which we can reduce IUGR to simple molecular models is limited by the degree to which the disease has a simple pathology. As described above, advances in molecular and cellular biology have greatly improved our understanding of how normal placental development is controlled. Therefore, we should be well poised to make reasonable and testable hypotheses. These hypotheses can be tested using two different lines of investigation.

Clues from Knockout Mice

In theory, if the molecular basis of IUGR or PE is a single gene mutation, then "knockout" mice should be reasonable models. An example may be *IGF-II* mutant mice. Fetal growth is certainly compromised in IGF-II-deficient fetuses, but it is unclear if IGF-II affects placental development per se or, rather, is required directly as a growth factor in the fetus. There is recent evidence that placental stores of glycogen are reduced in IGF-II-deficient conceptuses [90], suggesting that the placenta may be a direct target of the growth factor. With respect to placental development per se, at present many of the genes implicated in placental development have been identified by analysing the effects of severe (e.g. null) mutations, which by and large result in severe placental insufficiency and embryonic mortality. Such phenotypes are obviously more extreme that what is observed in IUGR. However, it is reasonable that more subtle mutations that reduce but do not ablate gene function may have effects that more closely resemble what is observed in IUGR and PE. Therefore, more work must be done to examine the effects of these type of mutations in the mouse model system.

Clues from the Study of Confined Placental Mosaicism and the Mouse Imprinting Map

Several authors have found that the incidence of IUGR is higher in pregnancies where there are findings of trisomy and/or confined placental mosaicism (CPM), particularly involving chromosomes 2, 7, 9, 15, 16 and 22 [91–93] – see Ch. 2. Trisomy and CPM are frequently observed together. Trisomies are thought to develop primarily through meiotic defects that may affect either the maternal or paternal gamete. The resulting trisomic fertilised egg can development as such; alternatively, the third chromosome may be lost during embryonic mitoses, resulting in a return to disomy. Depending on the lost chromosome's parent of origin it may result in a "normal" biparental disomy or uniparental disomy

(UPD). Development of UPD cells may be abnormal if the affected chromosome carries genes that are subject to genomic imprinting [92]. Genes are said to be imprinted when they are expressed from only one chromosome that is dictated by the parent of origin. For example, *Mash2* is an imprinted gene in mice that is expressed from the maternally but not the paternally derived chromosome [94]. In understanding the molecular pathogenesis of IUGR that is associated with trisomies and CPM, one needs to consider two different scenarios. In the first, trisomy may increase gene expression owing to the presence of an additional functional allele. Alternatively, CPM resulting in a UPD may result in lost of gene expression if the lost chromosome carried imprinted genes that represented the expressed alleles.

Table 21.2 shows the chromosomal map position of a few genes implicated in placental development and/or fetal growth. Cases of CPM are potentially very informative for understanding IUGR because they suggest that genes involved in its development are located on the affected chromosomes. For example, CPM involving chromosome 7 is frequently associated with IUGR [92], and several genes located on human chromosome 7 have been implicated in placental development in mice (*EGFR*, *WNT2*, *HGF* and *c-MET*). In addition, three other genes on chromosome 7 can be reasonably be implicated in regulating fetal growth, two of which encode IGF-binding proteins (*IGFBP-1*, *IGFBP-3*) and another encoding a putative signalling protein (*GRB10*). The Grb10 protein is thought to be downstream of the insulin, IGF-I and EGF receptors to downregulate signal transduction [95]. The *Grb10* gene is an especially interesting case because it is an imprinted gene, expressed only from the maternally derived allele [96]. The region of chromosome 7 where *GRB10* maps is syntenic with a proximal region of mouse chromosome 11. Robertsonian translocations in mice, resulting in duplication of maternal or paternal proximal chromosome 11, result in IUGR and fetal growth promotion respectively [97,98].

Table 21.2 Chromosome map positions of genes with defined roles in placental development or that are directly implicated in fetal growth

Gene	Protein function	Proposed function	Chromosome map position	
			Mouse	Human
ITGA4	integrin α4	placental development	2	2q31–q32
EGFR	EGF receptor	rophoblast function	11	7p12
IGFBP1	IGF-binding protein	fetoplacental growth	11	7p13p12
IGFBP3	IGF-binding protein	fetoplacental growth	11	7p13p12
GRB10	signalling adaptor	fetal growth	11	7q11.2–12
HGF	cytokine	placental development	5	7q21.1
c-MET	HGF receptor	placental development	6	7q31
WNT2	cytokine	placental development	6	7q31
RXRA	retinoid receptor	placental development	2	9q34
FLT1	VEGF receptor	fetal angiogenesis	5	13q12
LIF	cytokine	placental development	11	22q12

Conclusions

This is an exciting era in IUGR research. Breakthroughs in the understanding of placental development and in the specific cellular processes that are affected in the IUGR placenta make it reasonable to think that a molecular approach to tackling the disease is within our grasp. To complete the task, progress will depend combining our best efforts in descriptive studies of the IUGR placenta with experimental approaches in model organisms such as the genetically engineered mouse.

References

1. Ghidini A. (1996) Idiopathic fetal growth restriction: a pathophysiologic approach. Obstet Gynecol Surv 1996;51:376–82.
2. Kingdom JCP, Kaufmann P (1997) Oxygen and placental villous development: origins of fetal hypoxia. Placenta 18:613–21.
3. Salafia CM. Placental pathology of fetal growth restriction. Clin Obstet Gynecol 1997;40:740–9.
4. Cross JC. Trophoblast function in normal and preeclamptic pregnancy. Fet Matern Med Rev 1996;8:57–66.
5. Wooding FBP, Flint APF. Placentation. In: GE Lamming, editor. Marshall's physiology of reproduction, 4th edn. New York: Chapman & Hall, 1994;233–460.
6. Cross JC. Formation of the placenta and extraembryonic membranes. Ann N Y Acad Sci 1998;857:23–32.
7. Pijnenborg R, Dixon G, Robertson WB, Brosens I. Trophoblastic invasion of human decidua from 8 to 18 weeks of pregnancy. Placenta 1980;1:3–19.
8. Cross JC, Werb Z, Fisher SJ. Implantation and the placenta: key pieces of the development puzzle. Science 1994;266:1508–18
9. Gerretsen G, Huisjes HJ, Elema JD. Morphological changes of the spiral arteries in the placental bed in relation to pre-eclampsia and fetal growth retardation. Br J Obstet Gynaecol 1981;88: 876–81.
10. Khong TY, De Wolf F, Robertson WB, Brosens I. Inadequate maternal vascular response to placentation in pregnancies complicated by pre-eclampsia and by small-for-gestational age infants. Br J Obstet Gynaecol 1986;93:1049–59.
11. Brosens IA, Robertson WB, Dixon HG. The role of the spiral arteries in the pathogenesis of preeclampsia. Obstet Gynecol Ann 1972;1:177–91.
12. Lin S, Shimizu I, Suehara N, Nakayama M, Aono T. Uterine artery Doppler velocimetry in relation to trophoblast migration into the myometrium of the placental bed. Obstet Gynecol 1995;85: 760–5.
13. Iwata M, Mmatsuzaki N, Shimizu I, Mitsuda N, Nakayama M, Suehara N. Prenatal detection of ischemic changes in the placenta of the growth-retarded fetus by Doppler flow velocimetry of the maternal uterine artery. Obstet Gynecol 1993;82:494–9.
14. Zhou Y, Damsky CH, Chiu K, Roberts JM, Fisher SJ. Preeclampsia is associated with abnormal expression of adhesion molecules by invasive cytotrophoblasts. J Clin Invest 1993;9:950–60.
15. De Wolf F, Brosens I, Renaer M. Fetal growth retardation and the maternal arterial supply of the human placenta in the absence of sustained hypertension. Br J Obstet Gynaecol 1980;87:678–85.
16. Brosens I, Dixon HG, Robertson WB. Fetal growth retardation and the arteries of the placental bed. Br J Obstet Gynaecol 1977;84:656–63.
17. Althabe O, Labarrere C, Telenta M. Maternal vascular lesions in placentae of small-for-gestational infants. Placenta 1985;6:265–76.
18. Khong TY, Liddell HS, Robertson WB. Defective haemochorial placentation as a cause of miscarriage: a preliminary study. Br J Obstet Gynaecol 1987;94:649–55..
19. Zygmunt M, Boving B, Wienhard J, et al. Expression of cell adhesion molecules in the extravillous trophoblast is altered in IUGR. Am J Reprod Immunol 1997;38:295–301.
20. Teasdale F. Morphometric evaluation. Contrib Gynecol Obstet 1982;9:17–28.
21. Teasdale F. Idiopathic intrauterine growth retardation: histomorphometry of the human placenta. Placenta 1984;5:83–92.

22. Teasdale F. Histomorphometry of the human placenta in maternal preeclampsia. Am J Obstet Gynecol 1985;152:25–31.
23. Salafia CM, Pezzullo JC, Minior VK, Divon MY. Placental pathology of absent and reversed end-diastolic flow in growth-restricted fetuses. Obstet Gynecol 1997;90:830–6.
24. Jackson MR, Walsh AJ, Morrow RJ, Mullen JB, Lye SJ, Ritchie JW. (1995) Reduced placental villous tree elaboration in small-for-gestational-age pregnancies: relationship with umbilical artery Doppler waveforms. Am J Obstet Gynecol 1995;172:518–25.
25. Krebs C, Macara LM, Leiser R, Bowman AW, Greer IA, Kingdom JCP. Intrauterine growth restriction with absent end-diastolic flow velocity in the umbilical artery is associated with maldevelopment of the placental terminal villous tree. Am J Obstet Gynecol 1996;175:1534–42.
26. Hitschold TP. Doppler flow velocity waveforms of the umbilical arteries correlate with intravillous blood volume. Am J Obstet Gynecol 1998;179:540–3.
27. Rinkenberger J, Cross JC, Werb Z. Molecular genetics of implantation in the mouse. Dev Genet 1997;21:6–20.
28. Scott IC, Cross JC (1998) Transcription factors regulating the differentiation of the trophoblast cell lineage. In: D Carson, editor. Embryo implantation: molecular, cellular and clinical aspects. New York: Springer Verlag, 1999.
29. Luo J, Sladek R, Bader J-A, Matthyssen A, Rossant J, Giguere V. Placental abnormalities in mouse embryos lacking the orphan nuclear receptor ERR-β. Nature 1997;388:778–82.
30. Nakayama H, Scott IC, Cross JC. The transition to endoreduplication in trophoblast giant cells is regulated by the mSNA zinc-finger transcription factor. Dev Biol 1998;199:150–63.
31. Cross JC, Flannery ML, Blanar MA, et al. Hxt encodes a basic helix–loop–helix transcription factor that regulates trophoblast cell development. Development 1995;121:2513–23
32. Guillemot F, Nagy A, Auerbach A, Rossant J, Joyner AL. Essential role of Mash-2 in extra-embryonic development. Nature 1994;371:333–6.
33. Tanaka M, Gertsenstein M, Rossant J, Nagy A. *Mash2* acts cell autonomously in mouse spongiotrophoblast development. Dev Biol 1997;190:55–65.
34. Riley P, Anson-Cartwright L, Cross JC. The Hand1 bHLH transcription factor is essential for placentation and cardiac morphogenesis. Nat Genet 1998;18:271–5.
35. Jen Y, Manova K, Benezra R. Each member of the Id gene family exhibits a unique expression pattern in mouse gastrulation and neurogenesis. Dev Dyn 1997;208:92–106.
36. Evans SM, O'Brien TX. Expression of the helix–loop–helix factor Id during mouse embryonic development. Dev Biol 1993;159:485–99.
37. Alders M, Hodges M, Hadjantonakis AK, et al. The human Achaete-Scute homologue 2 (ASCL2,HASH2) maps to chromosome 11p15.5, close to IGF2 and is expressed in extravillus trophoblasts. Hum Mol Genet 1997;6:859–67.
38. Janatpour MJ, Israel MA, Fisher SJ. The transcriptional negative regulator Id-2 can control MMP-9 expression. Mol Biol Cell Suppl 1995;6:304a, abstr 1768.
39. Fisher SJ, Damsky CH. Human cytotrophoblast invasion. Semin Cell Biol 1993;4:183–8.
40. Fisher SJ, Cui T-Y, Zhang L, et al. Adhesive and degradative properties of human placental cytotrophoblast cells in vitro. J Cell Biol 1989;109:891–902.
41. Genbacev O, White TEK, Gavin CE, Miller RK. Human trophoblast cultures: models for implantation and peri-implantation toxicology. Reprod Toxicol 1993;7:75–94.
42. Damsky CH, Fitzgerald ML, Fisher SJ. Distribution patterns of extracellular matrix components and adhesion receptors are intricately modulated during first trimester cytotrophoblast differentiation along the invasive pathway in vivo. J Clin Invest 1992;89:210–2.
43. Damsky CH, Librach C, Lim KH, et al. Integrin switching regulates normal trophoblast invasion. Development 1994;120:3657–66.
44. Librach CL, Werb Z, Fitzgerald ML, et al. 92-kD type IV collagenase mediates invasion of human cytotrophoblasts. J Cell Biol 1991;113:437–49.
45. Petraglia F, Woodruff TK, Botticelli G, et al. Gonadotropin-releasing hormone, inhibin, and activin human placenta: evidence for a common cellular localization. J Clin Endocrinol Metab 1992;74:1184–8.
46. Petraglia F, Anceschi MM, Calza L, et al. Inhibin and activin in human fetal membranes: evidence for a local effect on prostaglandin release. J Clin Endocrinol Metab 1993;77:542–8.
47. Rabinovich J, Goldsmith PC, Librach CL, Jaffe RB. Localization and regulation of the activin-A dimer in human placental cells. J Clin Endocrinol Metab 1992;75:571–576
48. Petraglia F, Sawchenko P, Lim AT, Rivier J, Vale W. Localization, secretion, and action of inhibin in human placenta. Science 1987;237:187–9.
49. Petraglia F, Garuti GC, Calza L, et al. Inhibin subunits in human placenta: localization and messenger ribonucleic acid levels during pregnancy. Am J Obstet Gynecol 1991;165:750–8.

50. Peng C, Huang T-HJ, Jeung E-B, Donaldson CJ, Vale WW, Leung PCK, et al. Expression of the type II activin receptor gene in the human placenta. Endocrinology 1993;133:3046–9.
51. Caniggia I, Lye SJ, Cross JC. Activin is a local regulator of cytotrophoblast cell differentiation. Endocrinology 1997;138:3976–86.
52. Faust C, Schumacher A, Holdener B, Magnuson T. The eed mutation disrupts anterior mesoderm production in mice. Development 1995;121:273–85.
53. Zhou X, Sasaki H, Lowe L, Hogan BL, Kuehn MR. Nodal is a novel TGF-beta-like gene expressed in the mouse node during gastrulation. Nature 1993;361:543–7.
54. Ciruna B, Schwartz L, Harpal K, Yamaguchi T, Rossant J. Chimeric analysis of fibroblast growth factor receptor-1 (Fgfr1) function: a role for FGFR1 in morphogenetic movement through the primitive streak. Development 1997;124:2829–41.
55. Yang JT, Rayburn H, Hynes RO. Cell adhesion events mediated by alpha-4 integrins are essential in placental and cardiac development. Development 1995;121:549–60.
56. Gurtner GC, Davis V, Li H, McCoy MJ, Sharpe A, Cybulsky MI. Targeted disruption of the murine VCAM1 gene: essential role of VCAM-1 in chorioallantoic fusion and placentation. Genes Dev 1995;9:1–14.
57. Uehara Y, Minowa O, Mori C, et al. Placental defect and embryonic lethality in mice lacking hepatocyte growth factor/scatter factor. Nature 1995;373:702–5.
58. Saito S, Bladt F, Goedecke S, et al. Hepatocyte growth factor promotes the growth of cytotrophoblasts by the paracrine mechanism. J Biochem 1995;117:671–6.
59. Bladt F, Riethmacher D, Isenmann S, Aguzzi A, Birchmeier C. Essential role for the c-*met* receptor in the migration of myogenic precursor cells into the limb bud. Nature 1995;376:768–71.
60. Somerset DA, Li XF, Afford S, Strain AJ, Ahmed A, Sangha RK, Whittle MJ, Kilby MD. Ontogeny of hepatocyte growth factor (HGF) and its receptor (c-met) in human placenta: reduced HGF expression in intrauterine growth restriction. Am J Pathol 1998;153:1139–47.
61. Monkley SJ, Delaney SJ, Pennisi DJ, Christiansen JH, Wainwright BJ. Targeted disruption of the Wnt2 gene results in placentation defects. Development 1996;122:3343–53.
62. Dumont DJ, Fong GH, Puri MC, Gradwohl G, Alitalo K, Breitman ML. Vascularization of the mouse embryo: a study of flk-1, tek, tie, and vascular endothelial growth factor expression during development. Dev Dyn 1995;203:80–92.
63. Barleon B, Hauser S, Schollmann C, et al. Differential expression of the two VEGF receptors flt and KDR in placenta and vascular endothelial cells. J Cell Biochem 1994;54:56–66.
64. Ahmed A, Li XF, Dunk C, Whittle MJ, Rushton DI, Rollason T. Colocalisation of vascular endothelial growth factor and its flt-1 receptor in human placenta. Growth Factors 1995;12:235–43.
65. Charnock-Jones DS, Sharkey AM, Boocock CA, et al. Vascular endothelial growth factor receptor localization and activation in human trophoblast and choriocarcinoma cells. Biol Reprod 1994;51:524–30.
66. Graham CH, Lala PK. Mechanism of control of trophoblast invasion in situ. J Cell Physiol 1991;148:228–34.
67. Lala PK, Lysiak JJ. Role of locally produced growth factors in human placental growth and invasion with special reference to transforming growth factors. In: Hunt JS, editor. Immunobiology of reproduction. New York: Springer-Verlag, 1994;57–81.
68. Caniggia I, Taylor CV, Ritchie JW, Lye SJ, Letarte M. Endoglin regulates trophoblast differentiation along the invasive pathway. Endocrinology 1997;138:4977–88.
69. Morrish DW, Bhardwaj D, Paras MT. Transforming growth factor β1 inhibits placental differentiation and human chorionic gonadotropin and human placental lactogen secretion. Endocrinology 1991;129:22–6.
70. Shalaby F, Rossant J, Yamaguchi TP, et al. Failure of blood-island formation and vasculogenesis in Flk-1-deficient mice. Nature 1995;376:62–.
71. Fong G-H, Rossant J, Gertsenstein M, Breitman ML. Role of the Flt-1 receptor tyrosine kinase in regulating the assembly of vascular endothelium. Nature 1995;376:66–70.
72. Carmeliet P, Ferreiira V, Breier G, et al. Abnormal blood vessel development and lethality in embryos lacking a single VEGF allele. Nature 1996;380:435–9.
73. Partanen J, Puri MC, Schwartz L, Fischer KD, Bernstein A, Rossant J. Cell autonomous functions of the receptor tyrosine kinase TIE in a late phase of angiogenic capillary growth and endothelial cell survival during murine development. Development 1996;122:3013–21.
74. Suri C, Jones PF, Patan S, et al. Requisite role of angiopoietin-1, a ligand for the TIE2 receptor, during embryonic angiogenesis [see comments]. Cell 1996;87:1171–80.
75. Patan S. TIE1 and TIE2 receptor tyrosine kinases inversely regulate embryonic angiogenesis by the mechanism of intussusceptive microvascular growth. Microvasc Res 1998;56:1–21.

76. Kozak KR, Abbott B, Hankinson O. ARNT-deficient mice and placental differentiation. Dev Biol 1997;191:297–305.

77. Gnarra JR, Ward JM, Ported FD, et al. Defective placental vasculogenesis causes embryonic lethality in VHL- deficient mice. Proc Natl Acad Sci USA 1997;94:9102–7.

78. Threadgill DW, Dlugosz AA, Hansen LA, et al. Targeted disruption of mouse EGF receptor: effect of genetic background on mutant phenotype. Science 1995;269:230–4.

79. Sibilia M, Wagner EF. Strain-dependent epithelial defects in mice lacking the EGF receptor. Science 1995;269:234–8.

80. Das SK, Wang X-N, Paria BC, et al. Heparin-binding EGF-like growth factor gene is induced in the mouse uterus temporally by the blastocyst solely at the site of its apposition: a possible ligand for interaction with blastocyst EGF-receptor in implantation. Development 1994;120:1071–83.

81. Das SK, Chakraborty I, Paria BC, Wang X-N, Plowman G, Dey SK. Amphiregulin is an implantation-specific and progesterone-regulated gene in the mouse uterus. Mol Endocrinol 1995;9:691–705.

82. Ware CB, Horowitz MC, Renshaw BR, et al. Targeted disruption of the low-affinity leukemia inhibitory factor receptor gene causes placental, skeletal, neural and metabolic defects and results in perinatal death. Development 1995;121:1283–.

83. Stewart CL, Kaspar P, Brunet LJ, et al. Blastocyst implantation depends on maternal expression of leukaemia inhibitory factor. Nature 1992;359:76–9.

84. Jauniaux E, Zaidi J, Jurkovic D, Campbell S, Hustin J. Comparison of colour Doppler features and pathological findings in complicated early pregnancy. Hum Reprod 1994;9:2432–37.

85. Jauniaux E, Jurkovic D, Campbell S, Hustin J. Doppler ultrasonographic features of the developing placental circulation: correlation with anatomic findings. Am J Obstet Gynecol 1992;166:585–7.

86. Rodesch F, Simon P, Donner C, Jauniaux E. Oxygen measurements in endometrial and tropho-blastic tissues during early pregnancy. Obstet Gynecol 1992;80:283–5.

87. Watson AL, Palmer ME, Burton GJ. Problems associated with oxygen tension in the maintenance of first trimester placental tissue in organ culture. Placenta 1995;16:A.75

88. Genbacev O, Zhou Y, Ludlow JW, Fisher SJ. Regulation of human placental development by oxygen tension. Science 1997;277:1669–72.

89. Genbacev O, Joslin R, Damsky CH, Polliotti BM, Fisher SJ. Hypoxia alters early gestation human cytotrophoblast differentation/invasion in vitro and models the placental defects that occur in preeclampsia. J Clin Invest 1996;97:540–50.

90. Lopez MF, Dikkes P, Zurakowski D, Villa-Komaroff L. Insulin-like growth factor II affects the appearance and glycogen content of glycogen cells in the murine placenta. Endocrinology 1996;137:2100–8.

91. Wolstenholme J, Rooney DE, Davison EV. Confined placental mosaicism, IUGR, and adverse pregnancy outcome: a controlled retrospective U.K. collaborative survey. Prenat Diagn 1994;14:345–61.

92. Kalousek DK, Vekemans M. Confined placental mosaicism. J Med Genet 1996;33:529–33.

93. Wolstenholme J. Confined placental mosaicism for trisomies 2, 3, 7, 8, 9,16, and 22: their incidence, likely origins, and mechanisms for cell lineage compartmentalization. Prenat Diagn 1996;16:511–24.

94. Guillemot F, Caspary T, Tilghman SM, et al. Genomic imprinting of Mash2, a mouse gene required for trophoblast development. Nat Genet 1995;9:235–42.

95. He W, Rose DW, Olefsky JM, Gustafson TA. Grb10 interacts differentially with the insulin receptor, insulin-like growth factor I receptor, and epidermal growth factor receptor via the Grb10 Src homology 2 (SH2) domain and a second novel domain located between the pleckstrin homology and SH2 domains. J Biol Chem 1998;273:6860–7.

96. Miyoshi N, Kuroiwa Y, Kohda T, et al. Identification of the Meg1/Grb10 imprinted gene on mouse proximal chromosome 11, a candidate for the Silver-Russell syndrome gene. Proc Natl Acad Sci USA 1998;95:1102–7.

97. Cattanach BM, Beechey CV, Rasberry C, Jones J, Papworth D. Time of initiation and site of action of the mouse chromosome 11 imprinting effects. Genet Res 1996;68:35–44.

98. Beechey CV, Cattanach BM. Genetic imprinting map. Mouse Genome 1996;94:96–9.

22 Towards Evidence-based Management

James G. Thornton and Janet Hornbuckle

Introduction

Although evidence-based medicine (EBM) describes a type of practice with which no-one can seriously disagree [1], it has also become a buzzword that irritates some doctors who see it eroding their clinical freedom. I hope to describe some of the key features of EBM as applied to fetal growth restriction and to demonstrate that the latter view is mistaken. The problem in clinical practice is mainly to do with information, and EBM is mainly concerned with dealing with information in a sensible way [2]. Sackett [1] defined EBM as converting information needs into answerable questions, tracking down the best evidence to answer them, critically appraising the evidence for its validity (closeness to truth) and its usefulness (clinical applicability), applying the results in clinical practice and evaluating our performance.

No one is likely to take issue with this as an ideal, but in practice there are difficulties. Evidence-based management requires a lot from many people. Researchers must perform properly designed experiments to evaluate both the tests used to diagnose disease and the interventions used to treat it. Patients must participate in such experiments. Opinion leaders and textbook writers must assess the evidence from such experiments systematically. Finally, clinicians must practise in accord with such systematic evidence, while also taking into account individual patient factors and personal values.

We are a long way from this in the management of IUGR. Few of the tests we use have been evaluated properly. Most have been evaluated for the prediction of surrogate endpoints rather than for the outcomes that parents care about, namely death and handicap. Many studies have been susceptible to treatment paradox and tests are often interpreted badly. Although there have been trials of such interventions as rest, nutritional and vitamin supplementation, oxygen therapy, abdominal decompression, aspirin and NO, many have been small and inconclusive and the commonest intervention, timed delivery, has not been subjected to evaluation by a randomised trial at all. This last omission is particularly serious since such a widely used intervention has great potential for doing harm.

The lack of clear evidence makes it difficult for clinicians to take an individual patient's values properly into account. For example, it is plausible that in some circumstances early delivery might reduce mortality but increase the chance of survival with handicap. A good clinician would inform parents of this and help them decide whether they wished to maximise total survival or intact survival. Such conversations frequently take place in the area of prenatal diagnosis, but for growth restriction the data to inform them are not available at present.

In this chapter I will discuss the evidence required for managing IUGR, and end with a brief description of the ways in which such evidence might be applied to individual patients.

The Evidence

The information needs for doctors dealing with IUGR are twofold: for well-characterised tests that predict outcome reliably, and for well-evaluated interventions that reduce adverse outcomes.

Tests and their Interpretation

Much of clinical medicine is concerned with prediction. When we have made a prediction, we can apply an effective treatment if there is one. When we first meet a patient we are rarely if ever certain what the outcome will be, and a test is any item of information that can help us. It includes items from the history, and observations from the clinical examination, as well as such things as laboratory blood tests and X-ray examinations. Unfortunately tests are rarely perfect; some people with a positive result will not have the disease, and conversely some with a negative result will have it. This is why interpretation may be difficult.

Some of the tests that we use in managing IUGR are extremely well evaluated. For example, testing the karyotype of the fetus is a reliable predictor of poor outcome. If it shows triploidy or trisomy 13 the fetus will not survive into childhood. If it shows trisomy 21 there will inevitably be moderate or severe mental handicap. However, even here no test is perfect. There may be confined placental mosaicism or even a mislabelled sample. More often the tests used to predict outcome are much less accurate than this. Before we can measure the quality of a test like this we need to decide what outcome we wish the test to predict.

Gold Standards

Ideally we would like some outcome measure with which everyone can agree, a gold standard. Examples would include perinatal death and cerebral palsy. Although it might take some time to find out eventually such diagnoses are unambiguous, and we can say for certain whether the test in question predicted the outcome correctly or not. In practice, gold standards are rare and tests have to be evaluated for their prediction of less important endpoints such as low birthweight corrected for gestational age or low Apgar scores. If our test is validated only against such endpoints we must always remember that these are not really the outcomes we are interested in and that we do not know for certain the relationship between these outcomes and the gold standards.

Treatment Paradox

In a scientifically ideal world we would perform tests on a large number of people and wait to see how many, who turned out to be gold standard positive, had been predicted correctly (the true positive rate, or sensitivity). Similarly, we would measure how many, who turned out gold standard negative, had also been predicted correctly (the true negative rate, or specificity). The problem is that even with a new test, humans are rarely able to stop intervening in response to the result. If the intervention affects the gold standard outcome it will alter the measured test performance. The paradox is that test performance will be falsely improved if the abnormal results led to harmful treatment but worsened if the abnormal results led to effective intervention and a good outcome. This is why it is relatively easy to develop tests for Down's syndrome for which the gold standard diagnosis is unaffected by treatment, but difficult to develop one for perinatal death or brain damage, where treatment may have good and bad effects. The solution is as far as possible to evaluate tests in studies where the results are collected but concealed from the patient and clinician.

Concealing results is relatively easy for new tests not yet in common use and for those such as the biochemical placental function tests, which have been, perhaps prematurely, dropped from clinical use. There are difficulties for current tests, although the variation in policies between centres is such that usually there is a unit somewhere not using the test of interest. There are also difficulties concealing the result when it appears at the bedside (e.g. Doppler machines) rather than via the laboratory (biochemical tests) and this concealment may directly cause bad outcomes [3]. One possibility might be to adapt Doppler machines for research by, for example, occluding the lower part of the waveform (the diastolic part) on the operator's screen. Such machines might actually improve the measurement by excluding operator bias in the same way as random zero sphygmomanometers. It has been done for pulse oximetry in labour [4] and it is vital for the development of valid tests that researchers are aware of treatment paradox and take steps to avoid it when evaluating new tests.

Fortunately there have been a number of studies that have evaluated Doppler umbilical artery flow velocity waveforms for the prediction of perinatal death, using absent or reversed umbilical artery end-diastolic flow (ARED) as the abnormal result, and concealing the results from clinicians [5]. The results are summarised in Table 22.1. It is clear that the sensitivity and specificity of ARED for this endpoint are high, thus allowing doctors to usefully revise an individual patient's risk of having a dead baby. Unfortunately we cannot combine studies in a similar way to estimate the sensitivity and specificity of reduced EDF because different cut-off levels have been reported, and because in this group death is a much less frequent event reducing the precision of any estimate.

Similar evaluation of the biophysical profile score (BPS) is more difficult since fewer trials have concealed the test results and combining different series is almost impossible because of differing techniques and cut-off points. The large

Table 22.1 Studies of Doppler umbilical artery flow velocity waveforms

Gold standard	Positive baby dies	Negative baby lives	Total
test result			
positive (ARED)	20	72	92
negative (EDF present)	10	2,876	2,886
total	30	2,948	2,978

The sensitivity is thus 20/30 (66.6%) and the specificity 2,876/2,948 (98%).

data sets of Manning [6,7] are the best available and illustrate some of the problems. In his first series, in which results were concealed, a BPS of less than or equal to six had a sensitivity for perinatal death among normally formed fetuses of 5/7 (71 per cent) and specificity of 167/209 (80 per cent) [6]. The small number of deaths limits the precision of the estimate of sensitivity. In the later and larger series the sensitivity was 8/24 (33 per cent) and specificity 11,969/12,620 (95 per cent) for the same cut-off score [7]. However, in this series results were revealed and may have been affected by treatment paradox. It is tempting to speculate that the lower sensitivity (which may have occurred by chance) resulted from correct management preventing deaths that were otherwise destined to occur.

Interpreting Tests

By counting vertically in Table 22.1 we can see what proportion of the babies who died (gold standard positive) were detected by the test. This is the sensitivity or true positive rate (TPR). For umbilical artery Doppler this is 20/30 (66.6 per cent). We can also see how many of the babies that lived were correctly predicted by the test (the true negative rate (TNR), or specificity): 2,876/2,948 (98 per cent). These test characteristics do not vary with the prevalence of the disease and are thus a stable measure of test performance. They describe to the scientist how well the test works, but they are not much use to the doctor who knows the test result (positive or negative) and wants to know how likely it is that a particular patient has the disease or, in our example, that a particular baby will die.

To estimate this, we read Table 22.1 horizontally rather than vertically. First let us look at all the women with a positive result: 20/92 babies actually died, so the predictive value of a positive result is 22 per cent. Note that the predictive value positive is *not* the same as the sensitivity (TPR), which we have already noted was 66.6 per cent. Of those who had a negative test 2,876/2,886 eventually survived. The predictive value of a negative result is thus 99.7 per cent. Again this is *not* the same as the specificity (TNR). However, these average predictive values drawn from the combined results of a number of Doppler studies, some performed on high risk patients and some performed on low risk patients, are very misleading because the predictive value of a test varies with the prevalence of the disease.

The prevalence of perinatal death in these series is 30/2,978, that is, approximately 1 per cent. If we had applied the test to a patient whose prior risk of perinatal death was also 1 per cent we could read off the positive predictive value directly as 20/92 (22 per cent). However we usually know that our patient has a much higher or lower risk than this, even before we do any test. Table 22.2 shows how the positive predictive value varies with disease prevalence.

It is clear that the chance of the baby dying is much greater if a very high risk patient has a positive result than if a low risk patient who is simply being screened for disease has a positive result. Again, remember predictive value varies with prevalence.

Bayes' Theorem and Likelihood Ratios

Calculating the predictive value of a test result from the two by two table, as we did above, is possible only if the patient in front of you comes from a population

Table 22.2 Effect of prevalence on predictive value*

Gold standard	Positive – baby dies	Negative – baby lives	Total
a Prevalence 5000/10,000 = 50% i.e. very high risk			
test result			
+ve (ARED)	true +ve. 3,000	false +ve 100	3,100
–ve (EDF present)	false neg. 2,000	true neg. 4,900	6,900
total	5,000	5,000	10,000
+ve predictive value	3,000/3,100 = 97%		
b Prevalence 500/10,000 = 5% i.e. moderately high risk			
test result			
+ve (ARED)	true +ve 300	false +ve 190	490
–ve (EDF present)	false –ve 200	true –ve 9,310	9,510
total	500	9,500	10,000
+ve predictive value	300/490 = 61%		
c Prevalence 10/10,000 = 0.1% i.e. very low risk			
test result			
+ve (ARED)	true +ve 6	false +ve 199	205
–ve (EDF present)	false –ve 4	true –ve 9,791	9,795
total	10	9,990	1,000
+ve predictive value	6/205 = 2.9%		

* The sensitivity (60%) and specificity (98%) do not change.

with the same disease prevalence as that of the patients on whom the test was originally developed. This is often not the case. Tests are frequently developed on high risk patients in teaching hospitals, and then applied to patients in a low risk practice. Occasionally the reverse may happen, if we apply a test to someone we already know to be at particularly high risk.

Doctors need a way of calculating the predictive value of a test from the information that they are likely to have available, namely the prevalence of the disease and the test characteristics. It can be done! In this next section I make two changes to the two by two tables. First, I consider a hypothetical test with 90 per cent sensitivity (true positive rate) and 80 per cent specificity (true negative rate). Secondly I change all rates to odds. A risk of 1 in 4 is the same as odds of 1:3; a risk of 90 per cent is the same as odds of 90:10 or 9:1. Both these changes make the mathematics easier (Table 22.3a).

Let us now redraw our two by two table to show the crucial information (Table 22.3b). The top row gives us the information we need but don't have: the predictive value positive. The odds of having the disease with a positive test are 18:16 or 9:8, or slightly better than evens. The disease prevalence gives us the odds before the test result (i.e. 20:80 or 1:4). We call these the *prior odds*. What we need from the test is a single measure, the diagnostic value that changed the prior odds of 1:4 to *posterior odds* of 9:8. The answer is the ratio between the true positive

Table 22.3 Bayes' theorem: the likelihood ratio as the relationship between prior odds and posterior odds (two by two table for an imaginary test with a sensitivity (TPR) of 90% and a specificity (TNR) of 80% applied to a population with 20% risk of disease)

Gold standard	Positive baby dies	Negative baby lives	Total
a			
test +ve	18	16	34
test −ve	2	64	66
total	20	80	100
	TPR 90%	FPR 20%	
b			
test +ve	9	8	
test −ve			
prior odds	1	4	
LR +ve	9	2	

Calculation:
9:8 = posterior odds; 1:4 = prior odds; 9:2 = likelihood ratio.
Prior odds × likelihood ratio = posterior odds.
$1/4 \times 9/2 = 9/8$

rates (90 per cent) and the false positive rate (20 per cent). This is called the *likelihood ratio of a positive result* (LR +ve) because it is the ratio between the likelihood of having a positive result if the disease is present against the likelihood of having a positive result if the disease is absent. The LR +ve for this test is thus 9:2. The relationship between these three figures is:

$$\text{prior odds} \times \text{likelihood ratio} = \text{posterior odds}$$
$$1:4 \times 9:2 \qquad = 9:8$$

This is Bayes' theorem. It comes in a number of different versions but this one, the odds–likelihood ratio form, is the most useful for doctors. A dichotomous test will have two likelihood ratios, one for a positive result and one for a negative result. If the doctor knows the LR for the test result and the prior odds, calculation of the individual patient's risk is easy.

Varying the Cut-off Values

Up till now we have used the Doppler result as if it were either positive or negative. In practice there are a range of results. The worst is reversed EDF, followed by absent EDF, reduced EDF and best of all normal EDF. Unfortunately, few researchers have reported mortality for all these various cut-off points so we cannot plot the likelihood ratios for different cut-off values for the prediction of death. However, some workers have reported results for different cut-offs for the surrogate endpoint of fetal hypoxaemia [8]. The likelihood ratio for severely reduced EDF (A/B ratio > 4.5) is 25:1. We can use this easily in practice. Imagine a healthy woman undergoing a screening Doppler test in whom the EDF is reduced. Her prior odds of hypoxaemia might be estimated at, say, 1:1,000. The posterior odds become 1:1,000 × 25 = 25:1,000 or 1 in 40 (i.e. even with an abnormal result the baby is still probably *not* hypoxaemic). Conversely, imagine a woman with high blood pressure and vaginal bleeding whose baby has the same A/B ratio. If we estimate her prior odds of hypoxaemia as evens (1:1) the posterior odds become $1:1 \times 25 = 25:1$. The baby is almost certainly hypoxaemic and her obstetrician may advise immediate delivery.

Test Evaluation Summary

If tests are to be used properly to practise evidence-based medicine they must be evaluated for the prediction of the outcomes that really matter to parents, namely the gold standard of death or handicap. They must be evaluated in studies that avoid treatment paradox so that accurate and stable test characteristics, the sensitivity specificity and likelihood ratio, can be calculated. Doctors who interpret these tests need to know the likelihood ratios for each level of result and must interpret them in the light of the patient's prior risk using Bayes' theorem. In future there will probably be many more tests for possible causes of growth restriction. Whether these are new Doppler tests, biochemical tests or even genetic tests for, say, uniparental disomy (UPD) [9,10], mutations in leptin or other genes [11,12], or for mitochondrial disease, they should be evaluated and interpreted this way.

Effective Treatment

Some treatments, such as salpingectomy for ruptured tubal pregnancy, or in vitro fertilisation for bilateral tubal blockage, treat such well-defined diseases, and are so much better than any alternative, that no one doubts their effectiveness. Few treatments are so clear cut. Often disease definitions are hazy, the prognosis is variable, whatever is done, and treatment is only partially effective. Frequently research studies appear to conflict, and clinical practice varies even between experts. Fetal growth restriction is much more like this. How is the doctor who wishes to practise evidence-based medicine to choose? We need to first decide what is the best type of evidence and then to identify that evidence.

Clinical Trials

Why Have Clinical Trials?

We measure treatment effectiveness by comparing a group of patients given the treatment (the intervention or treatment group), with another group not given it (the control group). If an effective treatment is already known then the control group will usually be given the established treatment and the experimental group the new treatment. If the two groups are otherwise similar, and the treatment group has better outcomes, we conclude that the treatment was effective. Difficulties arise if the two groups were not really comparable, or the play of chance misled us.

Incomparable groups usually result from a poorly designed experiment, in which the results for one or other group are susceptible to bias. Bias results if there is a systematic error in our measurements. This is different from random variation in that it will not be affected by increasing the sample size. Of course we can never be certain that there is no systematic error, but in a treatment comparison there will be no problem so long as any bias affects treatment and control groups equally, since it will cancel itself out. The result is subject to bias only if some systematic error affects the measurements of one group and not the other. Unfortunately bias can enter in many ways and is often extremely difficult to eradicate.

Historical comparisons will be subject to bias if other aspects of treatment are improving, so that patients treated today usually do better than those in the past. Comparisons between patients treated by different doctors or in different hospitals are often biased, since any doctor evaluating a treatment is usually an expert, and will certainly be an enthusiast. On the one hand, one might expect the investigator's patients to do better than those treated by other doctors, or by the doctor concerned before he or she developed special expertise in this treatment method. On the other hand, the more difficult cases may be referred to the expert, so biasing results *against* this doctor's treatment. Yet again, the investigator, as an expert, may be able to make the diagnosis in milder cases, possessing particularly good diagnostic skills for the condition, thus biasing results *in favour* of this treatment.

Even if the same doctor administers the treatment, a non-randomised comparison of cases treated one way with those treated another may be misleading. For example, many people have compared the outcome of breech babies delivered vaginally with those delivered by CS and usually concluded that those delivered by CS are more likely to survive. The conclusion can be justified only if both groups were comparable to start with. This is unlikely. Babies delivered after a rapid labour, at night, or who were thought to be unlikely to survive anyway because they were premature or abnormal are all or more likely to be delivered vaginally, thus biasing the results against vaginal delivery.

Matching

If we know what factors are related to outcome, we can match cases and controls for these factors to make the two groups similar. For example growth-restricted pregnancies could be matched by gestational age and Doppler waveform. However, we can never match exactly. There will always be some difference in gestational age between cases in the treatment and control groups. More importantly we can rarely match for, or even know about, all the possible factors that might affect outcome. A subtle factor can still bias results if it was unequally distributed between groups. You cannot match for unknown risk factors.

The best way to ensure that two groups of patients are matched for unknown, as well as known, risk factors is to select them at random. This means using the toss of a coin, random number tables, or other forms of computer-generated random numbers to select which patients get the new treatment and which are given placebo or control therapy.

Randomised Controlled Trials

Not all apparently randomised trials are of equal quality. The results may still be biased if the design was poor. Sometimes patients are allocated to treatment or placebo groups alternately, by day of the week, or last digit of hospital number. At first sight this may seem satisfactory but since the doctors know the group allocation when they enter the trial there is scope for entry bias.

Sources of Bias

Postrandomisation Exclusions

Bias can also occur if patients are more likely to be excluded from the trial in one group than the other. For example we might wish to compare two policies for timing delivery in growth restriction. Women are allocated at random, half to immediate delivery, and half to delivery, say, two weeks later (see Fig. 22.1). Some women allocated to the delay group will develop a serious new problem such as bleeding or hypertension during the two weeks, necessitating delivery early anyway. If we remove them from analysis we introduce bias in favour of delay, because we have removed women with problems from that group. Similar exclusions may occur in the immediate delivery group. Perhaps the neonatal intensive care unit is found to be full when we come to deliver. If the baby and mother are both well the obstetrician may decide to delay delivery, but if a problem has arisen with either the baby or mother she will probably go ahead with delivery anyway and arrange either for extra staff to be brought in or for some babies to be transferred elsewhere. If we excluded those babies allocated to immediate delivery who for one reason or another had their delivery delayed we would again be biasing our results against immediate delivery.

In the jargon there is risk of bias if there are any "postrandomisation exclusions", and we avoid the problem by analysing the trial by "intention to treat". So long as we compare the two groups as chance allocated them, we can be sure that no bias has crept in. It may seem strange to include the results for some women who got delivered early in the "delay" group and some women got delivered late in the early delivery group, but there is no other way to avoid bias. Of course, we must ensure that compliance is high if we really want to find out whether a drug or procedure can work.

Biased Assessment of Outcome

Even if the two groups of patients in a trial are exactly comparable, bias may be introduced if the investigators recording the outcomes know which form of care has been received. The solution is not to tell them. If the doctors do not know which group the patient is in, they are said to be blinded, and their assessment of outcome cannot be influenced. This is a particular problem with "soft" outcomes whose measurement is not totally objective.

The Placebo Effect

If patients believe that the treatment they received works, this may be a self-fulfilling prophecy. This is the placebo effect. Trials of many treatments for premenstrual tension, for example, have shown high cure rates among patients given inactive medicine. Usually the active treatment has been no better, and investigators have concluded that the treatment was ineffective. If no placebo had been used, the treatment might have been wrongly given the credit for the improvement. Patients are also said to be "blinded" when they do not know which treatment they are receiving. A trial is said to be "double blind" when neither the patient nor the investigator knows which treatment is being given. Blinding is often not necessary. If the endpoint is unambiguous, like death or CS, blinding at the stage of outcome assessment is unnecessary, although it may still be necessary during the treatment period. If blinding is not possible, but the outcome of interest is susceptible to observer bias, it may be possible to eliminate it by having independent observers make the assessment.

Co-interventions

If a trial is not blinded, either the investigators or the patients may behave differently towards the treatment and control groups. This may make the results difficult to interpret. A good example is oxygen therapy for growth restriction. The trials [13] suggest a non-significant beneficial effect. However, all the participants were aware whether they were receiving oxygen, so that those in the treatment group probably spent more time in bed tied to their oxygen cylinder, and also smoked less for fear of explosions. Pragmatists who wish only to help the baby may not be too concerned if the beneficial effect of oxygen therapy was mediated via increased rest or decreased smoking. However, those investigators who want to understand whether oxygen itself really works directly will wish to perform trials where control patients breathe air via matched cylinders. Such trials are planned (Johanson and Lindow, personal communication).

Statistical Problems with Trials

These occur because of random variation: the play of chance. Random variation differs from bias in that increasing the sample size will reduce it. There are two ways that the play of chance can mislead:

1. We may think there is a difference, when all we saw was chance variation. This is called a *type 1* or *alpha error*.
2. We may fail to realise that there is a real difference. This is called a *type 2* or *beta error*.

A number of statistical tests have been used to avoid making them.

Tests to Avoid Type 1 Error

The results of an experiment usually take the form of a series of observations on a treatment and control group. These may be continuous measures, such as birthweights, or dichotomous variables, such as death rates. We will concentrate on dichotomous outcomes. If the mortality rates are identical between treatment and control groups we won't be misled into a false belief that the treatment was effective. The difficulty arises when there is a difference and we want to know whether it occurred by chance or was caused by the treatment. Most statistical tests tell us how likely it was to occur by chance. This is the familiar P value. By convention we call $P < 0.05$ statistically significant. This means that there was a less than 5 per cent chance that the difference we observed, or one more extreme, would occur by chance if the treatments were equally effective. Although hallowed by tradition, this method of presenting results simply tells us that we have not made a type 1 error. If $P > 0.05$ we do not know whether there really is no important difference, or whether our trial was too small. Nor does the P value tell us the likely size of any difference. A very small and clinically unimportant difference may be statistically highly significant if a large study has been performed.

Type 2 Error

Here we are concerned with a false negative trial result and the probability that a trial has failed to show a real effect. The probability of a negative result depends on the particular size of treatment effect we wish to detect; there is a range of values corresponding to the range of possible treatment effects. It is cumbersome to look at all the probabilities of making a type 2 error. However, it is possible to look for the probability of failing to detect a particular size of effect. One important effect size is the effect that would be clinically meaningful so that, if it were confirmed, doctors would change over treatment. Clearly the ability of a particular trial to exclude a large effect is greater than its ability to exclude a small effect. We call this the *power* of the trial. Power is the opposite of type 2 error; that is, for a type 2 error beta, power is 1-beta.

Odds Ratios and their Confidence Intervals

A good way to look at treatment effects is to consider the risks or odds of the bad outcome with the treatment relative to the control therapy. In this way the effect of the treatment is given in the form of a relative risk (RR) or more commonly an odds ratio (OR). An OR of 1, like a likelihood ratio of 1, indicates that the treatment does not alter the odds of adverse outcome. An OR below 1 indicates that the odds of adverse outcome are reduced by treatment and an OR above 1 that treatment increases these odds. An OR of 0.5 indicates a halving of the odds, and an OR of 2 a doubling. The 95 per cent confidence interval (CI) can be calculated for an OR. An OR of 0.5 with a 95 per cent CI of 0.25–1 indicates that we have found a halving in the odds of the outcome, and we can be 95 per cent confident that the true effect of treatment lies between an OR of 0.25 and 1. This corresponds to a P value of 0.05 since the CI just includes 1.

To put it another way, the 95 per cent CI indicates the size of treatment effect that has been excluded with a probability of 0.05. We can be fairly confident that the true effect is no larger or smaller than this.

Multiple Tests of Significance

A major problem with many trials is that it is unclear that only one hypothesis was tested. Sometimes investigators perform multiple tests of significance on a range of endpoints. This reduces the power of the study because it makes it more likely that an apparently significant result could have occurred by chance. For example, it is virtually certain that if 20 tests of significance were performed on independent outcome measures in a trial of an ineffective treatment that one of them would apparently have a P value below 0.05. To avoid this investigators should clearly specify the hypothesis they wish to test, and to define the sample size, the endpoints and the statistical tests to be used in the primary analysis, before any data are collected. In the jargon the analysis should be "hypothesis driven" rather than "data driven". Of course, secondary analyses can be made on the data obtained in the trial but it should be made clear when this is the case. Depending on the extent to which such secondary analyses are supported by other evidence, they should usually be regarded as hypothesis generating rather than hypothesis testing.

Meta-analysis

Type 2 errors are minimised by large trials. Unfortunately these are difficult and expensive to perform so they do not exist for many interventions. One solution is to combine the results of such trials as have been performed. The statistics need not concern us, but the results can be conveniently presented as ORs for each trial separately, and the typical OR and CI for all the trials combined plotted beneath them. The danger with such analyses is that trials with weak methodology may be included and give a misleading result. Unfortunately many of the trials reported in obstetrics have contained one or more of the fundamental methodological flaws listed above [14–17]. Another risk is that trials that showed negative results may be less likely to be published. It is therefore important that authors of meta-analyses both record the quality of the trials they include and search for unpublished trials. This is not easy but the Cochrane Collaboration is working to help reviewers generate reviews that follow these principles. In obstetrics this is coordinated by the Cochrane Pregnancy and Childbirth Group, which can be contacted at the address given in the appendix to this chapter.

Trials of Therapy for Fetal Growth Restriction

Bed rest has never been evaluated in a randomised trial and low dose aspirin as treatment for established disease is ineffective [18]. Maternal hyperoxygenation is promising, but published trials have been small and not placebo controlled [13]. This leaves timed delivery, which obstetricians tend to use in one of two ways. Some restrict it to fetuses already in imminent danger of dying, and delay delivery until there are established CTG changes, reversed umbilical artery Doppler waveforms, fetal venous pulsation, or signs of cerebral decompensation. Even though no trials have been performed, timed delivery used like this probably prevents some perinatal death.

Other obstetricians argue that, since growth restriction is a risk factor for cerebral palsy [19] and possibly low IQ [20,21], and infants with antepartum acidosis or with certain abnormalities of Doppler waveform or fetal heart rate tend to have impaired developmental outcomes [20–25], it is plausible that even earlier delivery will improve long term neurodevelopment. However, supporting evidence is weak and the rate of cerebral palsy in association with premature delivery has increased in some countries [19,26–28]. Nor is there an animal model for cerebral palsy or developmental delay. Nevertheless the idea is attractive and widely believed to be plausible. The GRIT study detailed below is designed to measure the effect of varying timed delivery this way.

The GRIT Study

The trial uses obstetrician uncertainty as the main entry criterion. Eligible patients are between 24 and 36 completed weeks and the fetus is failing to thrive, but, after taking all factors into account, the obstetrician is uncertain whether or not it is better to deliver immediately. With parental consent the clinical details, including gestational age and the results of the latest ultrasound and umbilical artery flow velocity waveforms, are recorded and the patient is randomised to either "deliver" or "delay". "Delivery" is usually within 24 hours of randomisation at a convenient time for the staff and patient, although it may be deferred to complete a steroid course. "Delay" means waiting until delivery can safely be delayed no longer (i.e. until there is a significant worsening of Doppler or biophysical parameters, or FHR decelerations), or the passage of time is such that the balance of risks tilts in favour of delivery.

Randomisation like this is ethical. It would be unethical to randomise if the responsible doctor had a clear preference for one or other treatment. Some would even argue that if doctors have no clear preference and can help other patients in future, it is unethical not to participate. This use of uncertainty in trial design is widespread and has other advantages. It maximises possible recruitment, so that patients with a wide range of gestational ages and degrees of fetal jeopardy will be entered. The results will be more generalisable than if more narrow entry criteria had been used. It has the disadvantage that there is little meaning in giving the trial results as a single recommendation. Some subgroups are likely to benefit from delivery and some from delay. The participants must be stratified into narrower subgroups before analysis.

The primary outcome measures are survival to hospital discharge, and the Griffiths developmental quotient measured at 2 years [29]. At the time of writing, 397 participants have been recruited over 4 years (target 600). The gestational

Table 22.4 Gestational age and UA Doppler results for 470 babies randomised to GRIT (Aug '99)

| Umbilical artery doppler | Gestation (completed weeks) | | | | | | | | | | | | |
	24	25	26	27	28	29	30	31	32	33	34	35	36
reversed EDF	1		4	2	3	3	4	6				1	
absent EDF	2	1	7	10	25	25	25	25	20	13	3	3	
severely reduced		1	2		2	4	3	21	24	22	31	25	10
Mod. reduced/normal			1	4	8	9	9	16	20	16	29	24	6

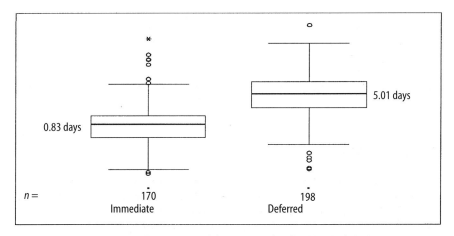

Fig. 22.1 Randomisation to delivery interval in the GRIT study [30].

age and umbilical artery Doppler results immediately prior to randomisation are shown in Table 22.4, and the randomisation to delivery intervals is shown graphically in Fig. 22.1. The median difference between the two groups was 4 days.

Results

Although interim results have been presented to the GRIT collaborators at twice yearly meetings, they are not presented here to avoid prejudicing publication of the final report and to prevent overinterpretation. At collaborators' meetings the results are presented after stratification into subgroups and interpreted in the light of participants' prior beliefs using Bayesian statistical methods. These involve formally measuring the prior beliefs of the doctors involved before the trial results are available [30], and then estimating how much the actual results alter these beliefs [31–33]. Open analysis of interim results is not only permitted but also encouraged. Although some experts have been concerned that open analysis may reduce recruitment, this has not been observed so far. Even if interim results make doctors certain how to manage particular clinical scenarios they will usually simultaneously make them less sure how to manage other scenarios, such as the same results 2 weeks later or earlier. The trial will recruit until April 2001 so that outcomes at 2 years of age will be available in 2003. If successful this will help obstetricians place one of the most central aspects of the management of growth restriction on an evidence base.

Applying the Evidence to Individual Patients

Finally let me return to individual patients. They are all different. Does EBM really suggest that everyone should be treated the same? Nothing could be further from the truth. Practitioners of EBM are just as keen as anyone else to ensure that patients are treated in ways that accord with their own value systems. EBM does not impede this; rather it makes it possible by providing the factual evidence about the likely outcomes after various treatments on which patients can decide, taking into account their personal values. For example, it is impossible for patients to weigh up correctly the relative risks of perinatal death and survival with or without handicap after various treatments for growth restriction without first knowing what these risks are. Only properly evaluated tests, interpreted properly taking into account prior risks, and treatments evaluated by randomised controlled trials, can ever provide this evidence. When the risks of various treatment options are defined various tools are available, notably decision analysis to help with decision making [34]. However, the evidence must come first.

Appendix: Useful Addresses for Reviewers

For the Cochrane Pregnancy and Childbirth Group contact:

Mrs Sonja Henderson, Administrator/Professor James P Neilson, Coordinating Editor, Liverpool Women's Hospital NHS Trust, Crown Street, Liverpool L8 7SS, UK tel +44 151 702 4066; fax +44 151 702 4024; email sonjah@liverpool.ac.uk

There are also national Cochrane centres all round the world. The UK one is:

UK Cochrane Centre, Summertown Pavilion, Middle Way, Oxford OX2 7LG
tel +44 1865 516300; fax +44 1865 516311; email general@cochrane.co.uk

There are also many Cochrane centre websites, for example:

http://hiru.mcmaster.ca/cochrane/centres/UK/default.htm

References

1. Sackett DL, Rosenberg WM, Gray JA, Haynes RB, Richardson WS. Evidence based medicine: what it is and what it isn't. BMJ 1996;312(7023):71–2.
2. Cooke IE, Sackett DL. Evidence based obstetrics and gynaecology. In: Cooke IE, Sackett DL, editors. Evidence-based obstetrics and gynaecology. Bailliere's Clin Obstet Gynaecol 1996;10:535–49.
3. Cox DN, Wittman BK, Hess M, Ross AG, Lind J, Lindahl S. The psychological impact of diagnostic ultrasound. Obstet Gynecol 1987;70:673–6.
4. Johnson N. Development and potential of fetal pulse oximetry. Contemp Rev Obstet Gynaecol 1992;3:193–200.
5. Thornton JG, Lilford RJ. Do we need randomised trials of antenatal tests of fetal wellbeing? Br J Obstet Gynaecol 1993;100:197–200.
6. Manning FA, Platt LD, Sipos L. Antepartum fetal evaluation: development of a fetal biophysical profile. Am J Obstet Gynecol 1980;136:787–95.
7. Manning FA, Morrison I, Lange IR, Harman CR, Chamberlain PF. Fetal assessment based on fetal biophysical profile scoring: experience in 12,620 referred high-risk pregnancies 1. Perinatal mortality by frequency and etiology. Am J Obstet Gynecol 1985;151:343–50.
8. Tyrell S, Obaid AH, Lilford RJ. Umbilical artery Doppler velocimetry as a predictor of fetal hypoxia and acidosis at birth. Obstet Gynecol 1989;74:332–7.
9. Spence JE, Perciaccante RG, Greig GM, Willard HF, Ledbetter DH, Hejtmancik JF, et al. Uniparental disomy as a mechanism for human disease. Am J Hum Genet 1988;42:217–26.
10. Hall JG. Genomic imprinting: review and relevance to human diseases. Am J Hum Genet 1990;46:857–73.
11. Koistinen HA, Koivisto VA, Andersson S, Karonen SL, Kontula K, Oksanen L, et al. Leptin concentration in cord blood correlates with intrauterine growth. J Clin Endocrinol Metab 1997;82:3328–30.
12. Liebel RL. And finally genes for human obesity. Nat Genet 1997;16:218–20.
13. Johanson R, Lindow SW, van der Elst C, Jaquire Z, van der Westhuizen S, Tucker A. A prospective randomised comparison of the effect of continuous O_2 therapy and bedrest on fetuses with absent end-diastolic flow on umbilical artery Doppler waveform analysis. Br J Obstet Gynaecol 1995;102(8):662–5.
14. Grimes DA. Randomisation controlled trials: "it ain't necessarily so". Obstet Gynecol 1991;78:703–4.
15. Schulz KF, Chalmers I, Grimes DA, et al. Assessing the quality of randomization from reports of controlled trials published in obstetrics and gynecology journals. JAMA 1994;272:125–8.
16. McDonough PG. "Leaky randomization": standard practice-but is it correct? Fertil Steril 1995;64:216–17.
17. Grimes DA, Schulz KF. Methodology citations and the quality of RCTs in obstetrics and gynecology. Am J Obstet Gynecol 1996;174:1312–15.
18. CLASP Collaborative Group. CLASP: a randomised trial of low-dose aspirin for the prevention and treatment of pre-eclampsia among 9364 pregnant women. Lancet 1994;343: 619–29.
19. Nelson KB, Ellenberg JH. Antecedents of cerebral palsy. Multivariate analysis of risk. New Engl J Med 1986;315:81–6.
20. Naeye RL, Peters EC. Antenatal hypoxia and low IQ values. Am J Dis Child 1987;141:50–4.
21. Sung I-K, Vohr B, Oh W. Growth and neurodevelopmental outcome of very low birth weight infants with intrauterine growth retardation: comparison with control subjects matched by birth weight and gestational age. J Paediatr 1993;123:618–24.

22. Todd AL, Trudinger BJ, Cole MJ, Cooney GH. Adverse fetal welfare and outcome at 2 years. J Matern Fetal Invest1991;1(2):101.
23. Soothill PW, Ajayi RA, Campbell E, Ross EM, Candy JDCA, Snijders RM, et al. Relationship between fetal acidemia at cordocentesis and subsequent neurodevelopment. Ultrasound Obstet Gynaecol 1992;2(2):80–3.
24. Gaudier FL, Goldenberg RL, Nelson KG, Peralta-Carcelen M, Johnson SE DuBard MB, et al. Acid base status and subsequent neurosensory impairment in surviving 500 to 1000 gm infants Am J Obstet Gynecol 1994;170:48–53.
25. Goldstein RF, Thompson RJ, Oehler JM, Brazy JE. Influence of acidosis, hypoxemia, and hypotension on neurodevelopmental outcome in very low birth weight infants. Pediatrics 1995;95: 238–43.
26. Hagberg B, Hagberg G, Olow I, Von Wendt L. The changing panorama of cerebral palsy in Sweden. Acta Paediatr Scand 1989;78:283–90.
27. Stanley FJ, Watson L. The cerebral palsies in western Australia: trends, 1968–1981. Am J Obstet Gynecol 1988;158:89–93.
28. Pharoah POD, Cooke T, Cooke RWI, Rosenbloom L. Birthweight specific trends in cerebral plasy. Arch Dis Child 1990;65:602–6.
29. Griffiths R. The abilities of young children. A comprehensive system of mental measurement for the first eight years of life. High Wycombe, Bucks: The Test Agency, 1970.
30. GRIT Study Group. When do obstetricians recommend delivery for a high-risk preterm growth-retarded fetus? Eur J Obstet Gynaecol Reprod Biol 1996;67:121–6.
31. Thornton JG, Lilford RJ. Preterm breech babies, and randomised trials of rare conditions [commentary]. Br J Obstet Gynaecol 1996;103:611–13.
32. Lilford RJ, Braunholz D. The statistical basis of public policy: a paradigm shift is overdue. BMJ 1996;313:603–7.
33. Freedman L. Bayesian statistical methods. BMJ 1996;313:569–70.
34. Thornton JG, Lilford RJ, Johnson N. Decision analysis in medicine. BMJ 1992;304:1099–103.

23 The Internet and Medicine

Mark Walker, Graeme Smith and Rory Windrim

Medical Informatics and the Modern Physician

Part of the art of medicine into the next millennium will be the management of information. At present, it is estimated that the experienced clinician uses about 2 million pieces of information to manage his or her patients [1,2]. However, the doubling time of biomedical information is currently about 19 years, which is equivalent to a fourfold increase during the average practice lifetime [2]. The body of literature on HIV alone doubles every 22 months [3]. In order to practise up to date medicine, physicians must be able to access, synthesise and implement new information into their clinical practice. Aiding practitioners in this goal is the accessibility of information provided through the medium of the Internet. In this chapter we will review the evolution of the Internet and its impact on health care from the perspective of both physicians and patients. Useful medical websites will also be reviewed and summarised.

The Internet

The Internet has fuelled the information revolution to an unprecedented level. It has impacted on the way we communicate, do business and spend our recreational time. In the health care field, there has been a paradigm shift for physicians from the traditional role of the gatekeeper of information to partner in information. The Internet has a wealth of resources for both providers and consumers. For physicians, previously pain-staking literature searches can be conducted through many of the publically available search engines. For health care consumers, there are infinite numbers of websites that will provide them with information on their particular ailment. Patients will often arrive at their appointment armed with the latest search from the Internet and ask their physician, "what do you think about the use of heparin for intrauterine growth restriction?", for example.

History of the Internet

The Internet began as a small scale network set up between four universities in California and Utah. It was funded by the Advanced Research Projects Agency

(ARPA) of the Department of Defense in the United States [4]. The military wanted to devise a way for US authorities to maintain communication in the event of a nuclear attack. At the time, network communications were linked serially, where each link depended on the link before it. An ingenious new approach was devised where the network was more like a fishnet, where information could flow through one of many paths. If one section of the network was disabled then information could travel along an alternate route. This network, called ARPANET, became operational in 1969. Soon other academic institutions joined their networks to ARPANET and the growing system began to be known as the Internet. The Internet received a large boost from the National Science Foundation in 1986 with the creation of NSFNET, which supported the development of regional academic computer networks. This agency then funded a private corporation, Advanced Network and Services Inc. (ANS), to create ANSNET, a high speed national network that interconnected the regional networks in all parts of the United States [5]. Thus the framework of the Internet was created. Private industry has since taken over most of the regional and long distance Internet connections. The Internet has flourished and is growing at an exponential rate.

Internet Milestones

Some milestones in the history of the Internet are shown in Table 23.1.

Anatomy of the Internet

The Internet, put simply, is a global network of computers. Information is stored on remote computers running special software, which are called *servers*. Servers host all the information that is in web pages. When we go to our favourite location on the Internet we are actually connecting to a remote server that is sending the graphics and text of that web page.

When we access the web, we do so through an *Internet service provider (ISP)*. Examples of ISPs are America Online (AOL), Compuserve, Netcom and Worldcom. When connected to our provider, we can then seek out information that is stored on servers thoughout the globe. For home users, Internet access is

Table 23.1 Milestones

Date	Event
1969	ARPANET developed
1971	ARPANET grows to 31 hosts
1972	First email program
1982	The term "Internet" first used
1984	1,000 Internet hosts
1990	100,000 Internet hosts
1992	World Wide Web developed
1996	150 countries connected to Internet
1996	40 million users
1998	100 million users

usually through a dial-up account with a modem. At professional institutions, Internet access is through a *local area network (LAN)*.

There are many ways to communicate information on the Internet. The two most popular are electronic mail (email), and the World Wide Web (WWW). The WWW was originally developed by physicists at CERN (Centre European pour la Recherche Nucleaire) to allow for research collaboration between the many scientists who were involved in the centre. The basic protocols and standards that they developed formed the basis of what we now know as the Web.

The software that we use to interface with the Internet or "surf the net" is called a *browser*. The two most popular browsers at the time of writing are Netscape Navigator and Microsoft Explorer. These programs provide a graphical interface with the Internet. Browsers function by converting hypertext mark-up language (HTML), which is the computer language used to write web pages, into text. Each subsequent generation of browser has more sophisticated features. For instance, Netscape Navigator 5.0 will provide multimedia capabilities and database functionality, as does Explorer 5.0 (which is now available).

All computers on the Internet have a name. This name is called the *uniform resource locator* or *URL*. Some examples of URLs are Microsoft.com. and Netscape.com. URLs are like an address: when you type them into the browser they take you to that location. Useful URLs related to obstetrics are listed in Table 23.2.

Table 23.2 Obstetrics and gynaecological societies websites

Society	URL
Royal College of Obstetricians and Gynecologists	www.rcog.org.uk/
American College of Obstetricians and Gynecologists	www.acog.com/
Society of Obstetricians and Gynecologists of Canada	www.sogc.medical.org/
Royal Australian and New Zealand College of Obstetricians and Gynecologists	www.racog.edu.au/
International Society of Perinatal Obstetricians	www.bgsm.edu/ISPO/
Dutch Society for Obstetrics and Gynecology	http://ourworld.compuserve.com/homepages/NVOG/
Society for Maternal Fetal Medicine	www.acog.org/spo/index.html

Websites

The number of sites on the Internet and the WWW is growing at a staggering rate on a daily basis. Anyone with basic computer knowledge and Internet access can essentially set up their own website. As such, there are justified concerns regarding the quantity and varying quality of medical information that physicians and their patients can access. While physicians should be able to critically evaluate what they are reading, this is not usually the case for patients. Significant misinformation, or non-evidence-based medicine, exists and is readily retrievable. This could lead to harm. However, the Internet has the potential to be an invaluable tool for communication, collaboration and patient information. Physicians need to be proactive in discussions with patients about which sites are good sources of information and also sites of which they should be wary.

To this extent, there are several excellent sites that have attempted to provide a critical evaluation of other sites and to provide an up to date view of the literature. Some of these will now be discussed.

Health On the Net (HON) (http://www.hon.ch/)

The Health On the Net Foundation is based in Geneva University Hospital, Switzerland. It is currently funded by both the public sector and private individuals. This is an international initiative that has sprung from a meeting in 1995 on the use of the Internet and World Wide Web for telematics in health care.

The Foundation is dedicated to realising the benefits of the Internet and related technologies in the fields of medicine and healthcare. The purpose of the Foundation is to advance the development and application of new information technologies, notably in the fields of health and medicine.

In conjunction with the Molecular Imaging and Bioinformatics Laboratory at Geneva University Hospital, a robot has been developed to search the Internet for specific medical listings using keywords. The robot, MARVIN (Multi-Agent Retrieval Vagabond on Information Networks), has a medical dictionary of 12,000 keywords that are weighted by relevance and specificity in medicine. Using these keywords, MARVIN searches the WWW selecting documents relevant to the medical field.

Within the HON page, there are five different search engines (*MedHunt, 2DHunt, BioHunt, HON index* and *ExPASy index*) that use the databases created by MARVIN. The most relevant to clinical medicine is MedHunt. When you use MedHunt to search a topic, it seeks pages in its database that correspond to the request. For each page, a score is calculated that takes into account the location of the topic as it appears in the page (e.g. Title, URL, text, etc.). These locations are weighted. For instance, a topic or keyword that appears in the title of the page will have a higher score than if the term is present only in the body of the text. The higher the score, the more likely it is that the page corresponds to the keyword or topic. Graphical appearance for the score is also given depending on whether the entire page, a paragraph, or a line pertains to the topic. However, the scores do not represent a critical evaluation of the page, but only the relation between the search question and the page.

The HON has set a code of conduct (*HONcode*) in an attempt to unify the quality of medical information on the WWW. This was done in response to the varying quality of medical information presently available. By complying with the HONcode principles and displaying the HONcode logo on their website, web owners commit themselves to this high standard of practice. The principles include such things as: advice only from medically trained professionals, maintenance of confidentiality, use of specific references and links, provision of evidence-based medicine, and clear outlining of where support for the website (e.g. industrial funding, private funding or grant support) has been obtained.

Online Mendelian Inheritance in Man (OMIM)
(http://www3.ncbi.nlm.nih.gov/Omim/)

This site is an excellent database of human genes and genetic disorders. It is authored and maintained by the National Center for Biotechnology Information

(NCBI) at Johns Hopkins University. The database contains information in the forms of text, pictures and references including an extensive catalogue of MEDLINE articles and gene sequence information. This database is primarily intended for use by physicians as true to life graphic images are available to download by a link to the image archive at *Neonatology on the Web*. There are different parts of OMIM that can be searched on a particular topic as well as links to OMIM allied resources.

As an example of a search using the term "IUGR" on the OMIM database, factor V deficiency came up as one of the specific genetic aetiologies. Further expansion of this found alternative titles including all the known thrombophilias. Text, references and clinical synopses were available as well as other database links.

Centre for Evidence-based Medicine (http://cebm.jr2.ox.ac.uk/)

This is the flagship of the EBM movement (see Ch. 22). It is authored and maintained by the Oxford University group. It contains links to their resources including support materials to the EBM book by members of this group, information of the Journal of Evidence-based Medicine, critically appraised topics, and a useful collection of analytical tools for EBM.

Health Information Research Unit (HiRU)
(http://hiru.mcmaster.ca/main.htm)

The Health Information Research Unit at McMaster University in Canada conducts research in evidence-based health informatics. Its research is directed towards supporting evidence-based health care and the evaluation of various novel methods to overcome health care information problems. It is a member of the Cochrane Collaboration providing links to the Cochrane Library. Guidelines, information and other links relating to these topics are provided.

These are but a small sample of useful websites available to physicians. Of concern is the vast number of sites, potentially of dubious quality, that patients may obtain information from. Essentially, anyone with a working knowledge of computers and use of recent software can set up their own website and provide "help/information". Patients are turning more and more to the Internet for a "second opinion" [6]. Information may be obtained from "chat rooms" or support groups/associations, or from a medical organisation/institution website having pages devoted to public information regarding various diseases. Finally, individuals can access almost the entire published medical literature through any of the free Medline websites listed in Table 23.3. These sources represent an increasing level of sophistication in obtaining and processing the information; frequently, they also represent an increasing level of accuracy. "Chat rooms" are a popular source that can be particularly problematic. People send in questions to which *anyone* can respond. The responders, for the most part, are other people who have gone through the same process or had the same complication. Their responses may reflect their own (or their physicians') interpretations of what they've been told, which may not be accurate. Individuals or groups appear to use the Internet to validate their feelings and anxieties in an attempt to obtain reassurance from people having gone through similar experiences previously. We recently sent an anonymous question about the aetiology of "our baby"

Table 23.3 Key Internet sites to bookmark

Medline source	URL	Description
PubMed	www.ncbi.nlm.nih.gov/PubMed/	free from the National Library of Medicine in the United States; uses standard Boolean query structure; abstracts available
Internet Grateful Med	igm.nlm.nih.gov/	free from the National Library of Medicine in the United States; uses standard Boolean and query structure; abstracts available; also has link to Lonesome Doc, which provides access to full text documents
Aries Systems Corporation & Knowledge Finder®	www.kfinder.com	guest account available for 31 days, then you need a paid subscription; this is a "must see" – allows for searching the medline database with "fuzzy logic"; you type in a question as opposed to keywords and MESH headings; search is returned with abstracts ranked in order of relevance
Societies of interest to obstetrics and gynecology	www.museum.state.il.us/isas/obsoc.html	this site has links to many of the national societies of obstetrics and gynaecology across the world
Instructions to authors in the health sciences	www.mco.edu/lib/instr/libinsta.html	this site contains links to websites that provide instructions to authors for over 2,000 journals in the health sciences

with IUGR and received replies (which anyone can read) ranging from accurate aetiological information (placental problems, drugs, alcohol, nutrition, etc.) to speculation about specific nutritional deficiencies, use of "too many ultrasounds" and physician incompetence! Recommendations regarding therapy included bed rest (for which there is *no* good evidence; see Ch. 16), megadoses of vitamin supplementation, oxygen therapy, and holistic and naturopathic suggestions. There are sites on the Internet where patients can obtain information from a physician or health care provider. However, these responses may reflect medical practice in that physician's country (remember, this is world-wide access!), which may or may not be appropriate to your standard of treatment. An example of this is the aggressive treatment of a "shortening" cervix seen on transvaginal ultrasound. Apparently, cervical cerclage has become the most common surgical procedure in the USA for this reason, with no evidence of its usefulness. Clearly patients should be warned about the potential quality of information available. The risk of misinformation may become translated into risk of adverse outcomes, including unnecessary anxiety, inappropriate requests for termination of pregnancy, misguided refusal of testing or treatment and loss of satisfaction with the physician–patient relationship.

Access to institutional websites and free medline searching has already resulted in patients presenting to their physician's office with printouts of abstracts and articles downloaded from the Internet. This trend represents a growing challenge to busy clinicians who may find themselves counselling anxious parents with a great deal of information, potentially both accurate and inaccurate. In order for these encounters to be both non-threatening to the physician and beneficial to the patient, practitioners will be forced to maintain a current knowledge of the literature and be able to appraise critically what they are reading. More effort in medical schools and postgraduate training will have to be directed at the teaching and practice of evidence-based medicine.

It would be useful for physicians to avail themselves of Internet access to see what their patients can access. The use of descriptive hierarchies may help to delineate the potential quality of the information. These include *.edu* (educational institutions), *.net* (network organisations), *.mil* (military), *.com* (commercial organisations), *.gov* (government), *.org* (other organisations). In the *.edu* domain, a subdomain would be a university name. Providing a list of useful sites that are of good quality information may be helpful to patients and might prevent inappropriate anxiety or decision making. Our governing bodies would go a long way in public relations by providing sites for patients to access information (e.g. SOGC, ACOG, RCOG, etc.).

References

1. Pauker SG, Gorry GA, Kassirer JP, Schwartz WB. Towards the simulation of clinical cognition. Taking a present illness by computer. Am J Med 1976;60:981–96.
2. Wyatt J. Use and sources of medical knowledge [see comments]. Lancet 1991;338:1368–73.
3. Sengupta IN, Kumari L. Bibliametric analysis of AIDS literature. Scientometrics 1991;20:297–315.
4. Lynch DC. Internet system handbook. Reading, Mass: Addison-Welsey, 1993.
5. Kassirer JP. The next tranformation in the delivery of health care [editorial]. N Engl J Med 1995;332:52–4.
6. Hart A. Second opinion. Internet World 1998;42–8.

Index

(IUGR = intrauterine growth restriction; HCG = human chorionic gonadotrophin; AFP = alpha fetoprotein; SGA = small for gestational age)

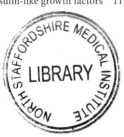